Chronic Abdominal and Visceral Pain

Chronic Abdominal and Visceral Pain

THEORY AND PRACTICE

edited by

Pankaj Jay Pasricha
University of Texas Medical Branch
Galveston, Texas, U.S.A.

William D. Willis
University of Texas Medical Branch
Galveston, Texas, U.S.A.

G. F. Gebhart
University of Pittsburgh
Pittsburgh, Pennsylvania, U.S.A.

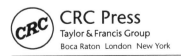

CRC Press
Taylor & Francis Group
Boca Raton London New York

CRC Press is an imprint of the
Taylor & Francis Group, an **informa** business

CRC Press
Taylor & Francis Group
6000 Broken Sound Parkway NW, Suite 300
Boca Raton, FL 33487-2742

First issued in paperback 2019

© 2010 by Taylor & Francis Group, LLC
CRC Press is an imprint of Taylor & Francis Group, an Informa business

No claim to original U.S. Government works

ISBN-13: 978-0-8493-2897-8 (hbk)
ISBN-13: 978-0-367-38996-3 (pbk)

A CIP record for this book is available from the British Library.

Library of Congress Cataloging-in-Publication Data available on application

Visit the Taylor & Francis Web site at
http://www.taylorandfrancis.com

and the CRC Press Web site at
http://www.crcpress.com

Preface

If anything ail a man, so that he does not perform his functions, if he have a pain in his bowels even,—for that is the seat of sympathy,—he forthwith sets about reforming—the world. – Henry David Thoreau (1817–1862)

There is almost no physician who has not encountered the problem of chronic visceral pain at some point in his or her career. Visceral and abdominal pain is a major clinical problem, affecting up to 25% of the general U.S. population. It may be part of a well-defined syndrome such as irritable bowel syndrome or chronic pancreatitis or be the sole or dominant clinical manifestation as in functional abdominal pain and dyspepsia. Patients with such pain present to a variety of medical specialists including gastroenterologists, cardiologists (noncardiac chest pain), gynecologists (pelvic pain syndromes) or urologists (interstitial cystitis etc.), anesthesiologists. The last two decades have seen impressive progress in the neurobiology of somatic pain and this is now beginning to be translated into clinical practice with the advent of several new classes of analgesics, particularly for neuropathic syndromes. By contrast, despite its prevalence, chronic visceral pain remains poorly understood, leading to significant difficulty in diagnosis and management. Much of modern medicine has tended to dismiss chronic visceral pain, in part because changes in function and structure of visceral organs are more subtle than those seen in somatic structures (a deformed and swollen knee for instance). Indeed, the term "functional pain" is often used (pejoratively) for these patients, generally in association with a referral to a clinical psychologist.

The editors of this book feel fortunate and privileged to be able to assemble leading experts from across the world to write the first definitive and comprehensive work on this subject and one that is truly "bench to bedside." Conceptually, this book is divided into four sections. The first deals with a global overview of visceral pain, its distinctive features and social impact. The second section, written by many of the authors who have defined the paradigms in this field, provides a detailed discussion of the neurobiological, immunological, and psychological basis of visceral pain, as provided by the study of both animal models and human subjects. The next section deals with the growing array of molecular targets for treatment of visceral pain as well as current conventional and alternative approaches used in the clinic. The final section consists of a detailed discussion of individual syndromes covering the gamut of problems encountered by the practicing physician. In most instances, two leading authorities in the field have provided a state-of-the-art summary of the pathophysiology and management of these conditions, often bringing unique insight as well as practical tips.

The reader can approach this book in many different ways. For the novice clinician or researcher, if read as written, it will be an easily understood journey of discovery from basic anatomic and physiological principles to an understanding of the complex balance of pathophysiological factors that make up a given clinical syndrome and rational approaches to treatment of the same. For the expert, individual chapters can be perused with ease for an in-depth and up-to-date review of the topic. Either way, we are confident that the experience will be rewarding and stimulating.

It is clear that visceral pain syndromes are complex, possibly more so than their somatic counterparts. The editors of this book hope that we have been able to put together a compilation of work that will provide the beginning of a rational approach to this symptom and the recognition of the real suffering it causes.

Pain is real when you get other people to believe in it. If no one believes in it but you, your pain is madness or hysteria.– Naomi Wolf (b. 1962)

Pankaj Jay Pasricha
William D. Willis
G. F. Gebhart

Contents

SECTION III: THERAPY FOR VISCERAL PAIN: SCIENTIFIC BASIS AND PRACTICE ASPECTS

Contributors

Elie D. Al-Chaer Departments of Pediatrics, Neurobiology and Developmental Sciences, Center for Pain Research, College of Medicine, University of Arkansas for Medical Sciences, Little Rock, Arkansas, U.S.A.

Q. Aziz Department of Gastrointestinal Science, University of Manchester, Hope Hospital, Salford, U.K.

Fernando Azpiroz Digestive System Research Unit, University Hospital Vall d'Hebron, Autonomous University of Barcelona, Barcelona, Spain

Jane C. Ballantyne Department of Anesthesia and Critical Care, Harvard Medical School, and Division of Pain Medicine, Massachusetts General Hospital, Boston, Massachusetts, U.S.A.

Klaus Bielefeldt Division of Gastroenterology, Hepatology and Nutrition, University of Pittsburgh Physicians, Pittsburgh, Pennsylvania, U.S.A.

Lori A. Birder Departments of Medicine and Pharmacology, University of Pittsburgh School of Medicine, Pittsburgh, Pennsylvania, U.S.A.

L. Ashley Blackshaw Department of Gastroenterology, Hepatology and General Medicine, Nerve-Gut Research Laboratory, Royal Adelaide Hospital, Discipline of Physiology, School of Molecular and Biomedical Sciences, Department of Medicine, University of Adelaide, Adelaide, South Australia, Australia

Stuart M. Brierley Department of Gastroenterology, Hepatology and General Medicine, Nerve-Gut Research Laboratory, Royal Adelaide Hospital, Discipline of Physiology, School of Molecular and Biomedical Sciences, University of Adelaide, Adelaide, South Australia, Australia

Charles D. Brooker Pain Management Research Institute, Royal North Shore Hospital, St. Leonard's, New South Wales, Australia

Luis F. Buenaver Department of Psychiatry and Behavioral Sciences, Johns Hopkins University School of Medicine, Baltimore, Maryland, U.S.A.

Michael Camilleri Clinical Enteric Neuroscience Translational and Epidemiological Research (C.E.N.T.E.R.) Program, Mayo Clinic College of Medicine, Rochester, Minnesota, U.S.A.

Fernando Cervero Anesthesia Research Unit (Faculty of Medicine), Faculty of Dentistry and McGill Center for Pain Research, McGill University, Montreal, Quebec, Canada

Harpreet K. Chadha Department of Anatomical Sciences and Neurobiology, University of Louisville School of Medicine, Louisville, Kentucky, U.S.A.

Premjit S. Chahal Department of Internal Medicine, University of Iowa Carver College of Medicine, Iowa City, Iowa, U.S.A.

Lin Chang Center for Neurovisceral Sciences and Women's Health, Division of Digestive Diseases, Department of Medicine, David Geffen School of Medicine at UCLA, and VA, Greater Los Angeles Healthcare System, Los Angeles, California, U.S.A.

Michael J. Cousins Pain Management Research Institute, Royal North Shore Hospital, St. Leonard's, New South Wales, Australia

Danita Czyzewski Departments of Psychiatry and Behavioral Sciences and Pediatrics, Texas Children's Hospital, Baylor College of Medicine, Houston, Texas, U.S.A.

Ram Dickman The Neuro-Enteric Clinical Research Group, Southern Arizona VA Health Care System, and University of Arizona Health Sciences Center, Tucson, Arizona, U.S.A.

Douglas A. Drossman UNC Center for Functional GI and Psychiatry, Division of Gastroenterology and Hepatology, University of North Carolina at Chapel Hill, Chapel Hill, North Carolina, U.S.A.

Andrew W. DuPont Department of Medicine, Division of Gastroenterology and Hepatology, University of Texas Medical Branch, Galveston, Texas, U.S.A.

Robert Edwards Department of Psychiatry and Behavioral Sciences, Johns Hopkins University School of Medicine, Baltimore, Maryland, U.S.A.

Ronnie Fass The Neuro-Enteric Clinical Research Group, Section of Gastroenterology, Department of Medicine, Southern Arizona VA Health Care System, and University of Arizona Health Sciences Center, Tucson, Arizona, U.S.A.

G. F. Gebhart Center for Pain Research, University of Pittsburgh, Pittsburgh, Pennsylvania, U.S.A.

Maria Adele Giamberardino Department of Medicine and Science of Aging, "G. d'Annunzio" University of Chieti, Chieti, Italy

Michael S. Gold Department of Biomedical Sciences, Dental School, Program in Neuroscience, and Department of Anatomy and Neurobiology, Medical School, University of Maryland, Baltimore, Maryland, U.S.A.

Douglas Gourlay The Wasser Pain Management Center, Mount Sinai Hospital, Toronto, Ontario, Canada

David S. Greenbaum College of Human Medicine, Michigan State University, Michigan, U.S.A.

Smita L. S. Halder Division of Gastroenterology, Dyspepsia Center, Mayo Clinic College of Medicine, Rochester, Minnesota, U.S.A.

Lucinda Harris Division of Gastroenterology and Hepatology, Mayo Clinic, Scottsdale, Arizona, U.S.A.

Jennifer A. Haythornthwaite Department of Psychiatry and Behavioral Sciences, Johns Hopkins University School of Medicine, Baltimore, Maryland, U.S.A.

Howard Heit Georgetown University School of Medicine, Washington, D.C., U.S.A.

Margaret Heitkemper Department of Biobehavioral Nursing, University of Washington, Seattle, Washington, U.S.A.

Peter Holzer Department of Experimental and Clinical Pharmacology, Medical University of Graz, Graz, Austria

Charles H. Hubscher Department of Anatomical Sciences and Neurobiology, University of Louisville School of Medicine, Louisville, Kentucky, U.S.A.

Ezidin G. Kaddumi Department of Anatomical Sciences and Neurobiology, University of Louisville School of Medicine, Louisville, Kentucky, U.S.A.

Stephen Kennedy Nuffield Department of Obstetrics and Gynecology, University of Oxford, John Radcliffe Hospital, Oxford, U.K.

Indumathi Kuncharapu University of Texas Medical Branch, Galveston, Texas, U.S.A.

G. Richard Locke III Division of Gastroenterology, Dyspepsia Center, Mayo Clinic College of Medicine, Rochester, Minnesota, U.S.A.

Emeran A. Mayer Center for Neurovisceral Sciences and Women's Health, David Geffen School of Medicine at UCLA, Los Angeles, California, U.S.A.

Sebastiano Mercadante Anesthesia and Intensive Care Unit, Pain Relief and Palliative Care Unit, Law Maddalena Cancer Center, Palermo, Italy

Mulugeta Million CURE/Digestive Diseases Research Center, and Center for Neurovisceral Sciences and Women's Health, Division of Digestive Diseases, Department of Medicine, University of California Los Angeles, and VA Greater Los Angeles Healthcare System, Los Angeles, California, U.S.A.

Jane Moore Nuffield Department of Obstetrics and Gynecology, University of Oxford, John Radcliffe Hospital, Oxford, U.K.

Bruce Naliboff VA Greater Los Angeles Healthcare System, Los Angeles, California, U.S.A.

T. J. Ness Department of Anesthesiology, School of Medicine, University of Alabama at Birmingham, Alabama, U.S.A.

Pankaj Jay Pasricha Department of Internal Medicine, Division of Gastroenterology and Hepatology, and Enteric Neuromuscular Disorders and Pain Center, University of Texas Medical Branch, Galveston, Texas, U.S.A.

Donald D. Price Departments of Oral Surgery and Neuroscience, University of Florida Colleges of Dentistry, Public Health, and Health Professions, and Medicine, and McKnight Brain Institute, Gainesville, Florida, U.S.A.

Satish S. C. Rao Department of Internal Medicine, University of Iowa Carver College of Medicine, Iowa City, Iowa, U.S.A.

David R. Robinson Center for Pain Research, University of Pittsburgh, Pittsburgh, Pennsylvania, U.S.A.

Michael E. Robinson Department of Clinical and Health Psychology, University of Florida Colleges of Dentistry, Public Health and Health Professions, and Medicine, and McKnight Brain Institute, Gainesville, Florida, U.S.A.

Abhishek Sharma Department of Gastrointestinal Science, University of Manchester, Hope Hospital, Salford, U.K.

Robert J. Shulman Department of Pediatrics and Children's Nutrition Research Center, Texas Children's Hospital, Baylor College of Medicine, Houston, Texas, U.S.A.

Victor S. Sierpina University of Texas Medical Branch, Galveston, Texas, U.S.A.

Yvette Taché CURE/Digestive Diseases Research Center, and Center for Neurovisceral Sciences and Women's Health, Division of Digestive Diseases, Department of Medicine, University of California Los Angeles, and VA Greater Los Angeles Healthcare System, Los Angeles, California, U.S.A.

Jan Tack Department of Internal Medicine, Division of Gastroenterology, University Hospital Gasthuisberg, University of Leuven, Herestraat, Leuven, Belgium

Richard J. Traub Department of Biomedical Sciences and Research Center for Neuroendocrine Influences on Pain, University of Maryland Dental School, Baltimore, Maryland, U.S.A.

Nimish Vakil University of Wisconsin School of Medicine and Public Health, Madison, Marquette University College of Health Sciences, Milwaukee, Wisconsin, U.S.A.

G. Nicholas Verne Department of Medicine, University of Florida Colleges of Dentistry, Public Health and Health Professions, and Medicine, and McKnight Brain Institute, Gainesville, Florida, U.S.A.

Arnold Wald Department of Medicine, Section of Gastroenterology and Hepatology, University of Wisconsin School of Medicine and Public Health, Madison, Wisconsin, U.S.A.

William D. Willis Department of Neuroscience and Cell Biology, University of Texas Medical Branch, Galveston, Texas, U.S.A.

John H. Winston Department of Internal Medicine, Division of Gastroenterology and Hepatology, and Enteric Neuromuscular Disorders and Pain Center, University of Texas Medical Branch, Galveston, Texas, U.S.A.

Naoki Yoshimura Departments of Urology and Pharmacology, University of Pittsburgh School of Medicine, Pittsburgh, Pennsylvania, U.S.A.

1 ▌ Distinctive Clinical and Biological Characteristics of Visceral Pain

T. J. Ness
Department of Anesthesiology, School of Medicine, University of Alabama at Birmingham, Alabama, U.S.A.

INTRODUCTION

In the natural sciences, there has long been a continuous conceptual battle between the "lumpers" and the "splitters"—those who wish to lump together phenomena with similarities as variations of an overriding mechanism and those who wish to split observed events into multiple independent phenomena with their own unique mechanisms. Nowhere is this lumper versus splitter dichotomy more apparent than in the field of pain research. Some would extrapolate all findings related to one type of painful stimulus to all types of painful stimuli in all sites. Others would claim that there can be no generalization of pathways or function for any pains arising from different parts of the body. Obviously, there is a middle ground where general principles may apply to many systems, but there may be mechanisms specific to individual systems. Such is the case with visceral pain.

Clinically, visceral pain is common. It keeps gastroenterologists, cardiologists, urologists, gynecologists, general surgeons, and internists of all kinds busy on a daily basis in their attempt to diagnose and treat its causes. Until recently, our knowledge related to pain arising from the internal organs of the body was extrapolated from studies related to heating and poking the surface of the body, but studies in the last two decades gave evidence that this is an overextrapolation that contains many inaccuracies. There are differences in the clinical experience of visceral pain when compared with that of cutaneous pain, and these differences have been confirmed in psychophysical studies comparing the two types of pain. There are also clear differences in the neurobiology of visceral pain systems when compared with those of superficial pain systems. This chapter will present an overview of these differences with an emphasis on human studies, and will defer an in-depth description of basic science studies to subsequent chapters. This chapter builds on previous reviews of this topic (1–6), and many primary sources may be found in those other sites. The terms "superficial" and "cutaneous" are used interchangeably, and to avoid ambiguity, the term "somatic" is avoided, since pain arising in deep, nonvisceral somatic structures such as muscles and joints share many of the characteristics of pain arising from the internal organs of the body.

CLINICAL VISCERAL PAIN

The viscera, when they are healthy, give rise to minimal conscious sensation. Fullness, gurgles, and a sensation of gas are the consequences of ingestion or sources of a need for elimination. In day-to-day activities, these sensations often increase to levels of mild discomfort, but when viscera become diseased or inflamed, the same stimuli that produce innocuous sensations can become an overwhelming source of sensations that can stop all activity and can demand complete attention. Nausea occurs commonly with visceral pains as do other autonomic responses such as sweating to the point of diaphoresis, piloerection, and dyspnea. It is clinical lore that visceral pains produce strong emotional responses to the point that they may appear out of proportion to the perceived intensity of the pain. Strong emotions are not only evoked by visceral sensations but also serve to evoke further visceral sensations such that a positive feedback effect is possible with pain producing anxiety, which produces more pain. For this reason, there is a poor correlation between the amount of definable visceral pathology and the distress/pain intensity produced by that pathology.

The observation that pathology and symptomatology may not agree is readily apparent in numerous visceral pain disorders. For example, chronic pancreatitis typically has a definable pathology, but alterations in pain are not consistently correlated with the degree of changes in radiographic or laboratory findings. Other disorders such as irritable bowel syndrome, noncardiac chest pain, and postcholecystectomy syndrome appear to have no histopathological bases and so are termed "functional." They are often associated with altered patterns/pressures associated with motility, production of gas, and ingestion of food or beverage, but measures of "altered" activity are often within physiological limits. Hence the term "visceral hypersensitivity" was coined to describe discomfort and pain in the absence of obvious visceral pathology (7).

The clinical feature of visceral pain that is considered its hallmark finding is its poor and unreliable localization. Researchers and thinkers from Lewis (8) to Procacci et al. (9) to the present (1–6) have debated concepts of "true" visceral pain versus "referred" visceral pain—the distinction between them being some element of localization. True visceral pain (or splanchnic pain) has no structural localization, but referred visceral pain has perceived localization to nonvisceral sites. Generally stated, visceral pains are deep and diffuse, with generalized localization to body regions and not to specific organs of origin. Unless experienced on multiple events so that an association is formed between certain sensations and a particular organ (as in recurrent cardiac angina), often the only organ-related localization that is possible is when physical examination manipulations serve to directly stimulate the painful organ or when particular body functions (e.g., urination) lead to the evocation of pain. Visceral pain originating from a focal pathology can be felt in several different areas at the same time or can migrate throughout a region even though the site of origin does not appear to change. Sites of pain sensation, when localized, are typically sensed in deep tissues that receive afferent inputs at the same spinal segments as visceral afferent entry. Hence, a "mapping" of referred pain sites can lead to a mapping of visceral afferent pathways. What is called referred pain in the clinical literature appears to be two separate phenomena: (i) the sensation is transferred to another site (e.g., angina can be felt in the chest, neck, and arm), and/or (ii) same-segmental sites become more sensitive to inputs applied directly to those other sites (e.g., flank muscle becomes sensitive to palpation when passing a kidney stone). The latter phenomenon is also described as secondary somatic hyperalgesia. Motor responses evoked by visceral stimuli are also segmental in nature, with a generalized increase in muscle tone to the point of spasm.

Like most other pains, in females, most clinically relevant visceral pains are affected by the menstrual cycle, with an apparent flare in pain intensity during the perimenstrual period. This appears to be true for irritable bowel syndrome (10), kidney stones (11), and interstitial cystitis (12), as well as gynecological pains (13). Arendt-Nielsen et al. (14) examined the effect of gender and the menstrual cycle on both experimental and visceral pain and found that normal healthy populations have some gender- or cycle-related effects, but that in subjects with clinical disease syndromes, these differences and effects are magnified.

CLINICAL SUPERFICIAL PAIN

Superficially applied noxious stimuli appear to produce more consistent responses than stimuli applied to visceral structures. In contrast to the viscera, the surface of our body continuously generates conscious sensations, and there is a clear localization of sensations to very small surface areas. In nonhairy skin areas, adjacent painful stimuli can be discriminated to within millimeters. Pain can be evoked from any body surface in a reliable fashion, and the intensity of the evoked stimulus is highly consistent unless actual tissue damage occurs with secondary inflammation. Likewise, superficial sensations from a specific site are always reliably localized to the same site and do not "migrate" to other body areas in the absence of nerve injury. Injury to the surface of our body inspires motion with "fight or flight" behavioral responses, highly localized flexion-withdrawal reflexes, and stimulus-linked alterations in ongoing activities. Hypersensitivity, when it occurs in superficial structures, is always associated with inflammation or nerve injury. All these noted phenomena are different from the equivalent phenomena evoked by visceral stimuli.

PSYCHOPHYSICAL STUDIES OF VISCERAL SENSATION

To determine whether uncontrolled clinical observations are indeed representative of responses evoked by visceral pain rather than a nonspecific characterization of chronic pain, psychophysical studies have been performed using controlled visceral and nonvisceral stimuli in both healthy subjects and those with clinical diagnoses of painful visceral disorders. Visceral stimuli have included chemical, electrical, thermal, and mechanical stimuli (15). Most studies have not attempted to compare responses to visceral stimuli with those evoked by cutaneous stimuli in a side-by-side comparison. An exception to this is a study by Strigo et al. (16), which directly compared sensations evoked by balloon distension of the esophagus with sensations evoked by thermal stimulation of the midchest skin. Using graded intensities of both distending and thermal stimuli, it was possible to match the intensity of evoked sensations produced at the two different sites. Consistent with clinical lore, visceral sensations were poorly localized, and equal intensities of reported sensation produced greater emotional responses when the visceral stimulus was employed (this will be discussed to a greater extent below). Normal subjects undergoing urinary bladder distension also report higher unpleasantness ratings than intensity ratings produced by identical levels of visceral stimulation (17). In the study by Strigo et al. (16), there was a tight temporal link between the thermal cutaneous stimulus and the evoked sensations. In contrast, there was a poor temporal correlation with the esophageal stimulus in that a sustained, relatively high intensity of sensation was perceived even after terminating the distending esophageal stimulus. Kwan et al. (18) observed similar findings related to the temporal correlation between visceral stimuli and sensation when they examined the sensations evoked by rectal distension in normal subjects. They were able to simultaneously to measure and control volumes and pressures of distension within a rectal balloon and had subjects report sensations evoked by this stimulus using a real-time, computer-driven visual analog scale. In general, visceral sensations outlasted the visceral stimulus. Further, after five repeated distensions, pain ratings increased markedly as did unpleasantness ratings, suggesting a sensitization phenomenon. Other psychophysical studies have also demonstrated that a sensitization process can occur with sequentially repeated stimuli. Specifically, repeated distension of the gut may lead to increasing intensities of pain/discomfort when the same organ is distended (19) and may also sensitize neighboring visceral structures (20). Hence, in these studies of normal healthy control subjects, a minimally insensate organ became hypersensitive with the presentation of recurrent abnormal afferent input.

Psychophysical studies have demonstrated evidence of hypersensitivity to visceral stimuli in virtually all clinically relevant visceral pain disorders. This includes hypersensitivity to gastric distension in patients with functional dyspepsia (21), intestinal and rectal distension in patients with irritable bowel syndrome (7,22), biliary and/or pancreatic duct distension in patients with postcholecystectomy syndrome or chronic pancreatitis (23), and bladder distension in patients with interstitial cystitis (17). In all cases, pain and/or discomfort were experienced at intensities of stimulation lower than required to produce the same quality and intensity of sensation in a healthy population. It is notable that in many cases, the hypersensitivity was limited to the particular organ system being studied. An example of this was reported by Aspiroz (24), who observed hypersensitivity to gastric distension but normal sensitivity in the duodenum and upon cutaneous testing in subjects with functional dyspepsia. Others have reported more whole-body effects. For example, Verne et al. (25) reported hypersensitivity to thermal testing in all dermatomes in subjects with irritable bowel syndrome, but the hypersensitivity was greatest in those dermatomes closest to those corresponding to rectal "viscerotomes."

Evidence of subpopulations within a single clinical diagnosis has also been presented. Testing of rectal sensitivity in irritable bowel patients using random order, graded distension found that some subjects test as reliably hypersensitive, with consistent lowering of thresholds independent of the order of stimulus intensity presentation, and others appear to be hypervigilant, with greater sensitivity associated with progressively increasing intensities of stimulation (26). A recent study examining the effects of urinary bladder sensations evoked by distension in subjects with the diagnosis of interstitial cystitis (17) observed possible subpopulations when thermal thresholds for pain evocation were examined. Both a high–thermal sensitivity group and a low-normal–thermal sensitivity group were apparent. It is notable that all psychophysical studies that have measured various psychological factors such as depression, anxiety, and hypervigilance have identified differences between the clinically diseased populations and their associated healthy controls (17,25). As a consequence, dissociating potential psychological modifiers of sensory reports from other, more neurophysiological pathologies has proved to be a difficult and at sometimes insurmountable methodological problem.

NEUROANATOMY OF VISCERAL PAIN

Basic science studies have demonstrated that from the level of gross anatomy to the microscopic determination of both peripheral and central afferent terminals, visceral sensory pathways are diffusely organized and distributed (diagrammatic summary in Fig. 1). Rather than mimicking the precise organization of cutaneous sensory afferent pathways, which travel in defined peripheral nerves and extend into a limited number of spinal segmental nerves organized in a unilateral, somatotopic fashion, visceral sensory afferent nerve fibers originate from multiple branchings of nerve fascicles organized into weblike plexuses scattered through the thoracic and abdominal cavities that extend from the prevertebral region to reach the viscera by predominantly perivascular routes. Injection of neuronal tracing agents into focal sites within viscera may easily result in the labeling of cell bodies in the dorsal root ganglia of 10 or more spinal levels in a bilaterally distributed fashion (27). The central spinal projections of visceral afferent neurons have been demonstrated by Sugiura et al. (28) to branch within the spinal cord and to spread over multiple spinal segments located both rostral and caudal to the level of entry. In these studies, individual C-fiber cutaneous afferents were demonstrated to form tight "baskets" of input to the superficial laminae of localized spinal cord segments, but individual C-fiber visceral afferents were demonstrated to terminate in superficial and deep laminae bilaterally in more than 10 spinal segments. Visceral afferents have also been noted to be neurochemically different than cutaneous afferents, with the expression of differing receptor subtypes for chemical stimuli (29).

Visceral sensory processing is uniquely different from cutaneous sensory processing in that there are peripheral sites of the visceral neuronal synaptic contact that occurs with the cell bodies of prevertebral ganglia such as the celiac ganglion, superior mesenteric ganglion, and

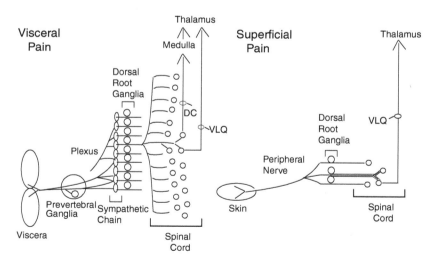

Figure 1 Diagrammatic representation of visceral and superficial pain pathways. Visceral pain pathways are much more diffuse, with multiple peripheral branchings, pathways through prevertebral ganglia, and the sympathetic chain to cell bodies residing bilaterally within multiple dorsal root ganglia. Central projections of visceral afferents also demonstrate significant branching to interact with spinal cord dorsal horn neurons in multiple laminae of multiple spinal segments. Major projections of these dorsal horn neurons to supraspinal structures then travel via dorsal column and ventrolateral quadrant pathways. Superficial pain pathways are, in contrast, much more organized, with distinct peripheral nerves, a limited number of spinal segmental sites of entry, and focal, heavy interaction with a limited number of dorsal horn neurons. Supraspinal connections of these dorsal horn neurons travel predominantly in the ventrolateral quadrant.

pelvic ganglion. This synaptic contact can lead to alterations in local visceral function that is outside of central control. The gut also carries the enteric nervous system as a self-contained "little brain" regulating the complex functions of digestion/absorption.

The location of the dorsal root ganglion neurons innervating the viscera appears to follow the original location of the structural precursors of the viscera during embryological development. Thoracic organs arose near somites corresponding to thoracic segments. Most abdominal organs arose near somites corresponding to mid-to-low thoracic and upper lumbar spinal segmental structures. Organization appears more complicated in the realm of urogenital/pelvic structures, where a dual innervation is apparent with afferents from lower thoracic–upper lumbar segments and from sacral segments. The testes and ovaries both originate relatively high in the abdomen and so carry with them a thoracic innervation. The urinary bladder arises from structures that traverse the developing umbilicus and is still connected to it by the residual urachus. It has a similar thoracolumbar innervation, with sensory inputs extending up to the T10 level. However, like all structures that physically open their orifices to sacral dermatomes (rectum, genital structures), it also has a dual spinal innervation that includes local sacral inputs (the pelvic nerve; S2–S4). An apparent "gap" in the innervation of urogenital structures is simply the absence of those nerves associated with the hindlimb bud (L3–S1). Mixed with spinal innervations are the wandering inputs and outputs of the vagus nerve and an elaborate local ganglionic circuitry. The result is that pelvic organs such as the urinary bladder, gynecological structures, and the lower gastrointestinal (GI) tract have a complex and doubly diffuse neuroanatomy. Taken together, from a macro- to microscopic level, there is an imprecise and diffuse organization of visceral primary inputs that would be sufficient to explain the imprecise and diffuse localization of visceral events by the central nervous system. However, upon entering the central nervous system, additional mechanisms are at work that lead to additional impreciseness. When quantitatively examined, spinal dorsal horn neurons with visceral inputs have multiple, convergent inputs from other viscera, from joints, from muscle, and from cutaneous structures. This presents a substrate that may explain the phenomenon of referred pain as a misinterpretation of spinal dorsal horn neuronal activity as being due to input from other more commonly activated structures, but it also means that the convergence of inputs from multiple viscera onto the same spinal neurons further contributes to the impreciseness of the localization of the source of pain, since activity in these neurons could reflect visceral, myofascial, articular, or cutaneous pathology. In contrast, neurons with exclusively cutaneous input are commonly identified in the spinal dorsal horn, in particular from nonhairy skin. As such, there is no ambiguity associated with the activation of these neurons and a higher order "interpretation" of their activity.

DIFFERENCES IN SPINAL PATHWAYS

Once transmission has occurred at a spinal level, the information must be passed to higher sites of processing. There is good evidence that visceral pain follows pathways that are different from those used for the perception of superficial pain. There now exist at least 10 clinical reports from six different neurosurgical groups in the United States, Europe, and Asia who have demonstrated that a midline myelotomy of the spinal cord (ablation of dorsal midline region) produces analgesia for visceral pain related to pelvic and lower abdominal organs (30–37) and for upper abdominal organs such as the stomach, pancreas, and hepatobiliary systems (38,39). Traditionally, it has been taught that the primary pathways for pain-related information from the dorsal horn of the spinal cord to the brain are via the ventrolateral quadrant white matter of the spinal cord. Tracts located within the ventrolateral quadrant include the classic spinothalamic and spinoreticular tracts as well as the spinomesencephalic and spinohypothalamic tracts. The ventrolateral quadrant of the spinal cord is clearly important for cutaneous pain sensation because lesions of those areas of white matter lead to pinprick analgesia in contralateral dermatomes below the level of the lesion. It is for this reason that the observation that surgical lesions of the dorsal midline of the spinal cord produce clinical analgesia was considered so contrary to dogma. Fortunately, there are good basic science data to support these clinical observations. In primates, dorsal midline lesions reduce the activity of thalamic neurons evoked by colorectal distension (40). In rats, effects of similar lesions have been demonstrated to reduce or abolish thalamic neuronal responses and/or behavioral responses to colorectal distension (30,41), duodenal distension (42), pancreatic stimulation (43), and hypersensitivity following lower extremity osteotomy (44). Whereas dorsal midline lesions affect visceral inputs to the nucleus gracilis of the medulla (45), these lesions do not affect visceral inputs to the ventrolateral medulla (41). Hence, it would appear that the dorsal midline pathway is one of at least two ascending pathways important to the perception of visceral pain. Spinal neurons with viscerosomatic convergence and axonal extensions into the dorsal columns have been demonstrated for primates (46) and rats (30).

FUNCTIONAL IMAGING OF VISCERAL SENSATION

Identification of supraspinal central nervous system sites of increased activity during visceral stimulation has been possible in humans using positron emission tomography and functional magnetic resonance imaging technologies. Recently reviewed by Derbyshire (47), such studies have revealed some consistencies, but are most notable for the multitude of sites that demonstrate increased regional blood flow. Rectal distension and urinary bladder distension both produce increased blood flow in select areas of the thalamus, hypothalamus, mesencephalon, pons, and medulla. Cortical sites of processing include the anterior and mid-cingulate cortex, the frontal and parietal cortices, and in the cerebellum (47,48). The best study of its kind comparing visceral pain sensation with cutaneous pain sensation is that of Strigo et al. (49). Similar to their psychophysical studies described above, these investigators matched the intensity of pain sensation produced by esophageal distension with that produced by heating of the skin of the mid-chest region and measured alterations in cerebral blood flow during the differing types of stimulation. Cutaneous and esophageal pain sensations were associated with a similar activation of the secondary somatosensory and parietal cortices plus the thalamus, basal ganglia, and cerebellum. Cutaneous pain evoked a higher activation of the anterior insular cortex bilaterally than did esophageal pain and also selectively activated the ventrolateral prefrontal cortex. Esophageal pain led to the activation of the inferior primary somatosensory cortex bilaterally, the primary motor cortex bilaterally, and a more anterior locus of the anterior cingulate cortex than cutaneous pain. This all suggests some shared components of sensation from the same segmental structures, but also a selective activation of some structures by superficial versus visceral pain.

EFFECTS OF STRESS ON VISCERAL PAIN

When nervous, one feels "butterflies" or "a pit" in the stomach. "Gut wrenching" emotions can also evoke profound changes in heart rate, breathing, and all other visceral functions. There is little doubt that the emotional state can alter sensations from and function of the viscera but the reverse situation also appears to be true: visceral pain evokes strong emotions, stronger than those evoked by equal intensities of superficial pain. This has been demonstrated in numerous observational studies, but was most definitively demonstrated in the study by Strigo et al. (16) (discussed above), which compared balloon distension of the esophagus with thermal stimulation of the mid-chest skin. Matched intensities of both distending and thermal stimuli were presented and the magnitude of emotional responses was then quantified using several tools designed to dissect out the affective components of clinical pain. Word selection from the McGill Pain Questionnaire suggested a stronger affective component to the sensation evoked by esophageal distension compared with that by the thermal stimulus. Greater anxiety was evoked by esophageal distension as measured by the Spielberg State-Trait Anxiety Inventory. Stressful life events have been viewed as classic "triggers" for the evocation of diffuse abdominal complaints of presumed visceral origin. As a consequence, these findings suggest that a positive feedback phenomenon can occur where visceral pain produces anxiety, which increases visceral pain, which in turn increases anxiety, in an unending cycle.

To dissect out purely physiological from psychological mechanisms of pain, we must sometimes turn to animal models. Unfortunately, there are severe limits to the interpretation of emotional experiences in animals. As a consequence, there are limited basic scientific data that can address issues related to the emotional impact of visceral stimuli. It is possible to demonstrate aversion to a stimulus by demonstrating alterations in behavior performed by an animal so that it might avoid the experience of such a stimulus but the existent literature is limited. There is a greater amount of literature related to the easier-to-interpret effects of experimental manipulations known to induce changes in pain-related behavioral, reflex, and neuronal responses.

Stress-induced analgesia (or hypoalgesia) has been a long-recognized phenomenon associated with cutaneous pain sensation. Soldiers may sustain severe wounds but feel pain only after the battle subsides. However, it would appear that stress-induced hyperalgesia is the correlate phenomenon associated with visceral pain sensation. In animal models, classic behavioral stressors such as a cold-water swim or restraint stress produce an elevation in thresholds for the evocation of responses to thermal stimuli (stress-induced analgesia), but the same animals have an increased vigor of visceromotor responses to visceral stimuli (50–52). This phenomenon appears to be associated with early-in-life events and can be modified by gonadal hormones, neurokinins, corticotrophin-releasing factor, and mast cell function. Genetic factors also play a part, since rats with high measures of anxiety on experimental testing also had increased responsiveness to visceral stimuli (53). Mechanisms that underlie this phenomenon may include central nervous system changes. The same research group has also demonstrated that alterations of the central nervous system induced by injections of corticosteroids or mineralocorticoids into the amygdala produce increased measures of anxiety and also produce augmented responses to visceral stimuli (54–56). A hypersensitivity to visceral stimulation was measured as an increased vigor of visceromotor responses and as increased responses of spinal dorsal horn neurons to colon or urinary bladder distension. Given the multiple interaction effects that have been noted between manipulations known to alter emotional state and visceral sensitivity, there can be little doubt that the two are linked at a basic neurophysiological level.

SILENT AFFERENTS IN THE VISCERA

As stated earlier, an important feature of sensation related to the viscera is that it is normally absent (or minimal), but under certain conditions, it can become intense, dominating all life events. As noted in the previous section, there can be psychological and other higher order processing modulation that occurs, but the simplest explanation to date for the conversion from silence to prominence is that the viscera have a high number of afferents that are normally "silent," with minimal or no activation produced by mechanical and/or other noxious stimuli presented to their transducer endings (57). However, in the presence of inflammation (58), ischemia [e.g., Ref. (59)], or specific chemical messengers [e.g., purines (60)], these same afferents acquire spontaneous activity and polymodal reactivity and so begin transmitting messages related to visceral events to the central nervous system. An extended discussion related to the role of particular substances producing particular alterations in subsets of particular afferents from particular organ systems is beyond the scope of this chapter. Suffice it to say that such alterations are common in visceral afferent systems and are uncommon in systems related to superficial pain sensation.

The "awakening" of previously silent afferents gives a neurophysiological substrate to explain a transition from minimal sensation to intense sensation, but given the quantitative scarcity and diffuse distribution of visceral afferents to the spinal cord, such an awakening must produce its profound neurophysiological effects either due to the direct potent actions of the neurotransmitters released or due to an amplification process of the central nervous system. Our own studies suggest the latter (61–63). In our study, most neurons excited exclusively by cutaneous stimuli appear to be subject to counter-irritation (noxious stimuli presented to distant sites produce neuronal inhibition), whereas half of the neurons excited by visceral stimuli are not subject to this "negative-feedback" effect, but rather appear to be part of a "positive-feedback" loop where nonsegmental excitatory inputs lead to neuronal activation. A formal study of this phenomenon by others may test the validity and generalization of this observation.

ARE ALL VISCERAL PAINS THE SAME?

We began this chapter by noting the conceptual differences between lumpers and splitters. We have proceeded to split off visceral pain from superficial pain, but have managed to lump together all visceral pains as though they were one entity. At present, there is insufficient information to make any additional distinctions. It would appear that the general anatomical organization of structures related to most, if not all, viscera follows a similar pattern of diffuseness at a peripheral level and utilizes similar spinal mechanisms of processing and transmission. Visceral structures with a matched pair (i.e., ovaries, kidneys), based on clinical symptomatology, appear to have some lateralization of their afferents to the central nervous system. The chemical and mechanical stimuli adequate to activate primary afferents of differing organ systems appear to vary according to organ and according to afferent pathway (64). This is logical, given the differing functions performed by these organs and their exposure to the external world (i.e., the bladder is sterile, whereas the lower GI tract is full of coliform bacteria). Ascending pathways of sensation that utilize the dorsal midline region of the spinal cord appear to vary in their distance from the midline. All in all, every organ system is unique in some ways, but systems related to the various internal organs are more like each other than they are like systems encoding for superficial pain. This is not to say that there are no similarities between visceral and superficial pain. Primary afferent cell bodies associated with visceral nociception reside within dorsal root ganglia and the initial processing of sensory information (excluding cranial nerve inputs) occurs at the level of the dorsal horn of the spinal cord. Most, if not all, doral horn neurons receiving visceral input also respond to cutaneous stimuli. Most sites of higher processing in the brain activated by noxious visceral stimuli are also activated by noxious cutaneous stimuli.

Where visceral pains differ from superficial pain is in the encoding properties of visceral primary afferent transducers and in their distribution to and within the central nervous system. The final consequence of these dissimilarities is a difference in localization and a difference in the magnitude of emotional and autonomic responses. Altogether, these differences lead to the distinctive clinical and biological characteristics of visceral pain.

REFERENCES

1. Al-Chaer ED, Traub RJ. Biological basis of visceral pain: recent developments. Pain 2002; 96:221.
2. Ness TJ, Gebhart GF. "Mechanisms of Visceral Pain" in the Neurological Basis of Pain. Pappagallo M, ed. New York: McGraw-Hill, 2004:95.
3. Ness TJ. "Visceral Pain in Cancer" in Cancer Pain: Pharmacologic Interventional and Palliative Care. In: Oscar DeLeon Cassasola, Saunders-Elsevier, 2006; 85–94.
4. Cervero F, Laird JM. Understanding the signaling and transmission of visceral nociceptive events. J Neurobiol 2004; 61:45.
5. Cervero F. Visceral pain-central sensitization. Gut 2000; 47(Suppl 4):iv56.
6. McMahon SB, Dmitrieva N, Koltzenberg M. Visceral pain. Br J Anaesth 1995; 75:132.
7. Mertz H. Visceral hypersensitivity. Aliment Pharmacol Ther 2003; 17:623.
8. Lewis T. In: Pain. London: McMillan, 1942.
9. Procacci P, Maresca M, Cersosimo RM. Visceral pain: pathophysiology and clinical aspects. Adv Exp Med Biol 1991; 298:175.
10. Heitkemper MM, Jarrett M. Patterns of gastrointestinal and somatic symptoms across the menstrual cycle. Gastroenterol 1992; 102:505.
11. Giamberardino MA et al. Modulation of pain and hyperalgesia from the urinary tract by algogenic conditions of the reproductive organs in women. Neurosci Lett 2001; 304:61.
12. Powell-Boone T et al. Menstrual cycle affects urinary bladder sensation in subjects with interstitial cystitis. J Urol 2005; 174:1832–1836.
13. Bajaj P et al. A comparison of modality-specific somatosensory changes during menstruation in dysmenorrheic and nondysmenorrheic women. Clin J Pain 2002; 18:180.
14. Arendt-Nielsen L, Bajaj P, Drewes AM. Visceral pain: gender differences in response to experimental and clinical pain. Eur J Pain 2004; 8:465.
15. Drewes AM, Gregersen H, Arendt-Nielsen L. Experimental pain in gastroenterology: a reappraisal of human studies. Scand J Gastroenterol 2003; 38:1115.
16. Strigo IA et al. Psychophysical analysis of visceral and cutaneous pain in human subjects. Pain 2002; 97:235.
17. Ness TJ et al. Psychophysical evidence of hypersensitivity in subjects with interstitial cystitis. J Urol 2005; 173:1983.
18. Kwan CL et al. The relationship between rectal pain, unpleasantness, and urge to defecate in normal subjects. Pain 2002; 97:53.
19. Ness TJ, Metcalf AM, Gebhart GF. A psychophysiological study in humans using phasic colonic distension as a noxious visceral stimulus. Pain 1990; 43:377.
20. Munakata J et al. Repetitive sigmoid stimulation induces rectal hyperalgesia in patients with irritable bowel syndrome. Gastroenterology 1997; 112:55.
21. Salet GA et al. Responses to gastric distension in functional dyspepsia. Gut 1998; 42:823.

22. Ritchie J. Pain from distension of the pelvic colon by inflating a balloon in the irritable colon syndrome. Gut 1973; 14:125.
23. Corazziari E, Shaffer EA, Hogan WJ, et al. Functional disorders of the biliary tract and pancreas. Gut 1999; 45 Suppl 2:II48.
24. Aspiroz F. Hypersensitivity in functional gastrointestinal disorders. Gut 2002; 51 Suppl I:i25.
25. Verne GN, Robinson ME, Price DD. Hypersensitivity to visceral and cutaneous pain in the irritable bowel syndrome. Pain 2001; 93:7.
26. Naliboff BD et al. Evidence for two distinct perceptual alterations in irritable bowel syndrome. Gut 1997; 41:505.
27. Ness TJ, Gebhart GF. Characterization of neurons responsive to noxious colorectal distension in the T13-L2 spinal cord of the rat. J Neurophysiol 1988; 60:1419.
28. Sugiura Y et al. Quantitative analysis of central terminal projections of visceral and somatic primary afferent fibers in the guinea pig. J Comp Neurol 1993; 332:315.
29. Zhong Y et al. Bladder and cutaneous sensory neurons of the rat express different functional P2X receptors. Neuroscience 2003; 120:667.
30. Hirshberg RM et al. Is there a pathway in the posterior funiculus that signals visceral pain? Pain 1996; 67:291.
31. Nauta HJ et al. Surgical interruption of a midline dorsal column visceral pain pathway: case report and review of the literature. J Neurosurg 1997; 86:538.
32. Nauta HJ et al. Punctate midline myelotomy for the relief of visceral cancer pain. J Neurosurg 2000; 92:125.
33. Becker R et al. The punctate midline myelotomy concept for visceral cancer pain control–case report and review of the literature. Acta Neurochir Suppl 2002; 79:77.
34. Becker R, Sure U, Bertalanffy H. Punctate midline myelotomy: a new approach in the management of visceral pain. Acta Neurochir (Wien) 1999; 141:881.
35. Filho OV et al. CT–guided percutaneous punctate midline myelotomy for the treatment of intractable visceral pain: a technical note. Stereotact Funct Neurosurg 2001; 77:177.
36. Fink RA. Neurosurgical treatment of nonmalignant intractable rectal pain: microsurgical commissural myelotomy with the carbon dioxide laser. Neurosurgery 1984; 14:64.
37. Gildenberg PL, Hirshberg RM. Limited myelotomy for the treatment of intractable cancer pain. J Neurol Neurosurg Psychiatry 1984; 47:94.
38. Kim YS, Kwon SJ. High thoracic midline dorsal column myelotomy for severe visceral pain due to advanced stomach cancer. Neurosurgery 2000; 46:85.
39. Hwang S-L et al. Punctate midline myelotomy for intractable visceral pain caused by hepatobiliary or pancreatic cancer. J Pain Symptom Manage 2004; 27:79.
40. Al-Chaer ED, Feng Y, Willis WD. A role for the dorsal column in nociceptive visceral input into the thalamus of primates. J Neurophysiol 1998; 79:3143.
41. Ness TJ. Evidence for ascending visceral nociceptive information in the dorsal midline and lateral spinal cord. Pain 2000; 87:83.
42. Feng Y et al. Epigastric antinociception by cervical dorsal column lesions in rats. Anesthesiology 1998; 89:411.
43. Houghton AK, Wang CC, Westlund KN. Do nociceptive signals from the pancreas travel in the dorsal column? Pain 2001; 89:207.
44. Houghton AK, Hewitt E, Westlund KN. Dorsal column lesion prevent mechanical hyperalgesia and allodynia in osteotomy model. Pain 1999; 82:73.
45. Al-Chaer ED et al. Pelvic visceral input into the nucleus gracilis is largely mediated by the postsynaptic dorsal column pathway. J Neurophysiol 1996; 76:2675.
46. Al-Chaer ED, Feng Y, Willis WD. Comparative study of viscerosomatic input onto postsynaptic dorsal column and spinothalamic tract neurons in the primate. J Neurophysiol 1999; 82:1876.
47. Derbyshire SWG. A systematic review of neuroimaging data during visceral stimulation. Am J Gastroenterol 2003; 98:12.
48. Athwal BS et al. Brain responses to changes in bladder volume and urge to void in healthy men. Brain 2001; 124:369.
49. (49) Strigo IA et al. Differentiation of visceral and cutaneous pain in the human brain. J Neurophysiol 2003; 89:3294.
50. Coutinho SV et al. Neonatal maternal separation alters stress–induced responses to viscerosomatic nociceptive stimuli in rat. Am J Physiol Gastrointest Liver Physiol 2002; 282:G307.
51. Gue M et al. Stress-induced visceral hypersensitivity to rectal distension in rats: role of CRF and mast cells. Neurogastroenterol Motil 1997; 9:271.
52. Bradesi S et al. Stress-induced visceral hypersensitivity in female rats is estrogen-dependent and involves tachykinin NK1 receptors. Pain 2003; 102:227.
53. Gunter WD et al. Evidence for visceral hypersensitivity in high-anxiety rats. Physiol Behav 2000; 69:379.
54. Qin C et al. Visceromotor and spinal neuronal responses to colorectal distension in rats with aldosterone onto the amygdala. J Neurophysiol 2003; 90:2.
55. Qin C et al. Corticosterone acts directly at the amygdala to alter spinal neuronal activity in response to colorectal distension. J Neurophysiol 2003; 89:1343.

56. Qin C, Greenwood–Van Meerveld B, Foreman RD. Spinal neuronal responses to urinary bladder stimulation in rats with corticosterone and aldosterone onto the amygdala. J Neurophysiol 2003; 90:2180.
57. Michaelis M, Habler HJ, Janig W. Silent afferents: a separate class of primary afferents? Clin Exp Pharmacol Physiol 1996; 23:99.
58. Habler HJ, Janig W, Koltzenberg M. Activation of unmyelinated afferent fibres by mechanical stimuli and inflammation of the urinary bladder in the cat. J Physiol 1990; 425:545.
59. Pan HL, Chen SR. Myocardial ischemia recruits mechanically insensitive cardiac sympathetic afferents in cats. J Neurophysiol 2002; 87:660.
60. Rong W, Spyer KM, Burnstock G. Activation and sensitization of low and high threshold afferent fibres mediated by P2X receptors in the mouse urinary bladder. J Physiol 2002; 541:591.
61. Ness TJ, Gebhart GF. Inflammation enhances reflex and spinal neuron responses to noxious visceral stimulation in rats. Am J Physiol Gastrointest Liver Physiol 2001; 280:G649–G657.
62. Ness TJ, Gebhart GF. Interactions between visceral and cutaneous nociception. I. Noxious cutaneous stimuli inhibit visceral nociceptive neurons and reflexes. J Neurophysiol 1991; 66:20–28.
63. Ness TJ, Gebhart GF. Interactions between visceral and cutaneous nociception in the rat. II. Noxious visceral stimuli inhibit cutaneous nociceptive neurons and reflexes. J Neurophysiol 1991; 66:29–39.
64. Blackshaw LA, Gebhart GF. The pharmacology of gastrointestinal nociceptive pathways. Curr Opin Pharmacol 2002; 2:642.

2

Epidemiology and Socioeconomic Impact of Visceral and Abdominal Pain Syndromes

Smita L. S. Halder and G. Richard Locke III
Division of Gastroenterology, Dyspepsia Center, Mayo Clinic College of Medicine, Rochester, Minnesota, U.S.A.

INTRODUCTION

Pain in the chest, abdomen, or pelvis is a common experience. For some people, this happens just now and then, but for others this is a daily occurrence. Community surveys have suggested that 25% of people have intermittent abdominal pain, 20% have chest pain, and 24% of women have pelvic pain. Only a minority of these people seek care. The population that seeks care is different from those who do not, and thus population-based studies are needed to truly understand the epidemiology of these visceral and abdominal pain syndromes. These conditions are associated with diminished quality of life, and when people do seek care, they incur significant medical expense. This review will outline the epidemiology of the main visceral and abdominal pain syndromes a clinician is likely to encounter.

ABDOMINAL PAIN

Abdominal pain can be an indication of a specific underlying disease, but in many sufferers, establishing a diagnosis is difficult, especially if the pain is longstanding, recurrent, and without specific pathophysiological abnormality. Such pain is thought to be visceral in origin, because most often it has an indistinct, crampy character and is poorly localized. The terminology used to describe abdominal pain of no specific etiology is as diverse and confusing as the theories surrounding its existence. Surgeons refer to it as nonspecific abdominal pain, older textbooks comment on nonorganic pain, and pain in children is known as recurrent abdominal pain (RAP). Whatever term clinicians, researchers, or patients themselves use to describe this condition is somewhat arbitrary. For convenience, the terms "visceral pain" and "functional abdominal pain" will be used interchangeably throughout this chapter.

Epidemiology of Abdominal Pain

The symptom of abdominal pain is common in the community, with prevalence rates between 22% and 28% (1–3). Women are more likely than men to complain of abdominal pain and bloating. It is noteworthy that only one in five of people in the community with abdominal pain had consulted a physician about their symptoms. In contrast, the majority of respondents complain of impairment in carrying out usual activities due to the pain, with the level of impairment similar between the sexes. This implies that abdominal pain impacts upon the daily lives of a vast number of people in whom no formal diagnosis is made.

The natural history of abdominal pain in the adult population is largely unknown. Abdominal symptoms have been observed to relapse and remit over the course of a year (4). The overall prevalence rate remains constant, but this is accounted for by considerable symptom turnover. The onset rate is about 10% and the disappearance rate is 35%. Prevalence rates are stable because the absolute numbers of people with onset and disappearance are matched.

Burden of Functional or Visceral Abdominal Pain on Health Care

Functional abdominal pain makes up a major component of the clinical spectrum of hospital admissions for abdominal pain. This is not a new problem. In 1966, abdominal pain for which no definite explanation could be found was the 10th most common cause of admission to hospital for any reason in men and the sixth most common cause in women (5). Of those who were admitted with undiagnosed abdominal pain, there was a higher preponderance of young females, and there was a significant excess of people with a previous admission for psychiatric reasons. The situation has not changed to the present day. Up to 67% of consecutive admissions to a teaching hospital surgical ward are for "nonspecific" abdominal pain (6). In Britain, the mean cost to the National Health Service (NHS) per patient was estimated at £807, which was mainly attributed to the in-patient stay. Extrapolating to the whole of the United Kingdom, the economic burden of nonspecific abdominal pain was postulated to be in excess of £100 million per year.

Abdominal Pain in the Elderly

Abdominal pain is also a common complaint in the elderly (7,8). Information is less widely available on the epidemiology of pain in this sector of the population. Yet clearly, abdominal pain has an impact on the lives of older people in a fashion similar to their younger counterparts. In a study of 70-year-olds, epigastric pain was the most commonly cited location and over half of the participants were affected in their ability to work or carry out daily activities due to abdominal pain (8). In a survey of 65- to 93-year-olds, one-fourth complained of frequent abdominal pain. A diagnosis of functional abdominal pain is difficult to make in the elderly as organic diseases are more common. Also, elderly people may have coexisting illnesses or be on medications that have gastrointestinal (GI) side effects. Thus the actual proportion of the elderly with functional abdominal pain is not known.

SPECIFIC VISCERAL AND ABDOMINAL PAIN SYNDROMES
Irritable Bowel Syndrome

The irritable bowel syndrome (IBS) is a chronic GI disorder characterized by RAP that is associated with defecation. The symptoms do not have a structural or biochemical explanation (9,10). Many population-based surveys around the globe have assessed the individual symptoms of IBS (11) and estimated the prevalence to be between 8% and 22% (12,13). The prevalence of IBS is higher in women and lower in the elderly (7,14,15).

Although many studies have assessed the prevalence of IBS, data regarding incidence are much more difficult to obtain. Information on symptom onset and disappearance can be obtained by repeated surveys over time (4,16). Roughly 10% of the general population will report the onset of IBS symptoms over a one-year period (4,16). Approximately one-third of people with IBS symptoms will report symptom resolution over time (4). The incidence of a clinical diagnosis of IBS has been estimated to be 196 to 260 per 100,000 person-years (17,18). This is not the true incidence of IBS but rather the rate at which the diagnosis of IBS is made in the clinic. These numbers may seem low; however, when multiplied by 30 years of disease duration and then doubled to reflect the rate of those seeking health care, the result is 12%, which matches the prevalence reported in the symptom surveys. It is noteworthy that these incidence rates are also much higher than the rates reported for colorectal cancer and inflammatory bowel disease, which are 50 and 10 per 100,000 person-years, respectively (19,20).

The cost of IBS is high in terms of health care utilization (outpatient costs, hospitalization costs, and prescription costs) and employer costs (15,21) IBS accounts for 25% to 50% of referrals to gastroenterologists, 96,000 hospital discharges, 3 million physician visits, and 2.2 million prescriptions annually (21). Although only 9% of people with IBS symptoms in the community seek care annually (15), these people miss more days from work and have more physician visits for both GI and non-GI complaints than the general population. By one estimate (15), people with IBS incur an extra $313 per person per year in charges compared with controls. If extrapolated to the U.S. population, the resulting cost of IBS is $8 billion per year.

Numerous studies have shown that the quality of life of individuals with IBS is lower than that of the general population and even lower than that of individuals with congestive heart failure (22). Many patients with IBS have multiple non-GI symptoms (e.g., fatigue and musculoskeletal pain), and while this association is unexplained, it can confound epidemiological association studies (10).

Dyspepsia

Dyspepsia is not a condition, but rather a set of symptoms of which upper abdominal pain or discomfort is the predominant complaint. In cross-sectional surveys, the prevalence of dyspepsia (3,14,23–26) has ranged from 3% to 44%. Why this large variation? The first consideration is whether the study included the symptom of heartburn in the definition of dyspepsia. Heartburn is experienced by 20% of the population weekly and 40% annually (27). There is significant overlap between upper abdominal symptoms and heartburn (23,27), and clinical studies have shown that many people with dyspepsia have reflux even in the absence of heartburn (28). If heartburn is ignored, the surveys suggest that 15% to 20% of the population experience dyspepsia over the course of a year. The second issue is whether patients who have symptoms of IBS in addition to their symptoms of dyspepsia are included. Approximately 30% of people with dyspepsia will also report IBS symptoms (3). Exclusion of people with IBS will decrease the prevalence estimate of dyspepsia down to 10% or even 3% (25).

The prevalence of dyspepsia is similar for men and women (3,23–26). Many studies have demonstrated that the prevalence actually decreases with age (14,23,25,26). In one study, Caucasians were found to have a lower prevalence of dyspepsia than non-Caucasians (25).

The previous section summarized the proportion of people who have symptoms of dyspepsia. However, these studies have not subjected these people to a diagnostic evaluation in order to determine whether or not they had functional dyspepsia. Many of these authors have, in fact, assumed that the majority of these people have functional dyspepsia. When determining the prevalence of functional dyspepsia, the investigators often exclude people who report a history of peptic ulcer disease, and approximately 8% of the population will report such a history (3,23). However, most people have not had any investigations and some people may report a history of peptic ulcer without having had any testing. Obviously, the absence of evaluation makes it very difficult to get a true estimate of the prevalence of functional dyspepsia. Still, the few studies that have evaluated people with dyspepsia in the community have not identified significant disease (24,29,30).

As compared to the number of cross-sectional studies done to estimate the prevalence of dyspepsia and functional dyspepsia, far fewer studies provide incidence data. Like IBS, these studies have surveyed a cross section of the community on two or more occasions, one to five years apart (4,16,26,31). Approximately 10% of the population will report the onset of dyspepsia over the course of one year. Talley et al. calculated the annual incidence of dyspepsia and found it to be 56 per 1000 person-years (4). This figure is hard to interpret by itself. However, this rate of 5600 per 100,000 person-years is over 500 times larger than the current annual incidence of gastric cancer (10 per 100,000 person-years) (11).

Chronic Functional Abdominal Pain Syndrome

Functional abdominal pain syndrome is defined as "pain for at least six months that is poorly related to gut function and is associated with some loss of daily activities" (32). In functional abdominal pain syndrome, there is no disordered bowel motility, and thus bowel disruption is not a prominent feature. Pain is judged functional only when an organic reason can be safely excluded and is considered to exist in the absence of structural or biochemical abnormalities.

Functional abdominal pain syndrome, in its strictest form, is relatively infrequent in the general population. In the U.S. householder study, which examined the frequency of functional GI disorders in an unselected population, functional abdominal pain syndrome was seen in 2% of the respondents (25). Despite the low prevalence, the socioeconomic impact of functional abdominal pain syndrome was immense, with sufferers missing three times as many workdays in the previous year compared to those without abdominal symptoms (25). Patients who are referred to gastroenterologists have further cost implications, because they undergo numerous diagnostic procedures and treatments and make a disproportionate number of health care visits.

Noncardiac Chest Pain/Functional Chest Pain

Chest pain is an alarm symptom that brings hundreds of thousands of people to seek health care worldwide each year (33). In the population, 28% of people report experiencing some form of chest pain in the past year (27). Due to the high prevalence and serious morbidity of coronary artery disease, the complaint of chest pain is treated as cardiac in origin until proven otherwise. Still, 10% to 20% of patients admitted to a coronary care unit are shown to have an esophageal disease (34). The challenge for health care providers has been differentiating those with acute coronary syndromes from those with other causes for chest pain.

Noncardiac chest pain (NCCP) is defined by the absence of significant stenoses in the major epicardial coronary arteries. Each year, about 450,000 people with chest pain have normal coronary angiograms (35). Despite the high number of people suffering from NCCP, little is known about the epidemiology or natural history of chest pain in the community. Moreover, little population-based data have been published to date that help characterize NCCP in the community. The prevalence of NCCP has been estimated to be 23% based on self-report only (27). The prevalence in the community is similar by gender (25,27,36) but a higher female-to-male ratio is seen in tertiary care referral centers (37). It has been observed that there is significant overlap between NCCP and frequent gastroesophageal reflux symptoms.

Anorectal Pain (Proctalgia)

Little epidemiologic data exist on functional anorectal pain. Proctalgia can be associated with organic or functional disorders; the two most common functional disorders are levator ani syndrome and proctalgia fugax. The main differences between them are the nature and duration of pain. The pain of levator ani syndrome is described as a dull ache or pressure-like discomfort that can last for hours. The estimated prevalence of levator ani syndrome lies between 7% and 11.3%, with a higher rate seen in females and those under 45 years of age (25,38).

Proctalgia fugax is characterized by sudden and severe shooting pain in the rectal area that lasts for seconds-to-minutes and then disappears completely until the next episode. This syndrome is more common than levator ani, with 14% of those questioned in a population survey reporting at least one episode and 5% reporting at least six episodes yearly (39).

RAP in Children

Abdominal pain is a prominent feature in the life of the average child, with 12-month period prevalence rates varying from 20% in a population sample (40) to 44% in a general practice cohort (41). In up to one-fifth of affected children, episodes are recurrent and interspersed by symptom-free periods, and this is termed RAP (41). In the majority of children, the abdominal pain is vague and typically situated in the periumbilical area. Physical examination is strikingly normal and laboratory investigations unremarkable. Because an organic diagnosis is made in less than 10% of cases, this has led to the long-held belief that most childhood abdominal pain is functional in origin (42).

RAP is defined by at least three discrete episodes of pain over a period of at least three months. Physical examination reveals no abnormality and laboratory investigations are unremarkable. Studies dating back to the 1950s (43) have reported that 10% of children aged 5 to 14 years suffered from RAP. Subsequent published prevalence rates have varied from 9% to nearly 25% (41,44,45). Whether there is a sex difference in the prevalence rates is disputed, but it is generally acknowledged that as children get older, incidence rates are higher in girls than in boys. In the late adolescent years, there is a sharp decline in incidence.

In many ways, the burden of illness is similar to unexplained abdominal pain in adults. Only 30% of emergency hospital visits for abdominal pain result in a definitive diagnosis (46), and in up to one-third of emergency appendectomies performed for abdominal pain, the appendix is normal (47). The financial impact of abdominal pain is overshadowed by the effects on the child. Many school days are lost through recurrent clinic visits or hospitalizations, which, in addition to the disruption of social activities, may be detrimental to the child's well-being and development.

Abdominal Pain for Life?

RAP is regarded by pediatricians to be a short-term phenomenon with no long-standing clinical consequences. However, there is comparatively little literature on the long-term outcome in children with RAP. Studies from clinical samples suggest that between 25% and 50% continue to experience symptoms into adulthood and have higher rates of psychiatric disorders (40).

Conversely, medically unexplained symptoms in adult life, including unexplained hospitalizations, are associated with experiencing abdominal pain in childhood (48,49). Overall, this evidence adds weight to the theory that RAP is a childhood form of functional disorder. For some, the natural history of abdominal pain may be life long.

CONCLUSIONS

The chapter has reviewed the epidemiology of abdominal pain and the most well-recognized functional GI disorders. These symptoms are each common in the community, with one out of four people reporting RAP. Although many of these people have not had diagnostic testing to exclude organic diseases, the current literature suggests that most of these people have functional GI disorders. The remainder of this book will cover why people have these symptoms and what can be done to help them. Improved understanding of these conditions is necessary to alleviate suffering and reduce the economic burden of these syndromes.

REFERENCES

1. Sandler RS et al. Abdominal pain, bloating, and diarrhea in the United States: prevalence and impact. Dig Dis Sci 2000; 45(6):1166.
2. Talley N, Zinsmeister AR, Melton LJ III. Irritable bowel syndrome in a community: symptom subgroups, risk factors and health care utilization. Am J Epidemiol 1995; 142:76.
3. Talley N et al. Dyspepsia and dyspepsia subgroups: a population-based study. Gastroenterology 1992; 102(4 Pt 1):1259.
4. Talley NJ et al. Onset and disappearance of gastrointestinal symptoms and functional gastrointestinal disorders. Am J Epidemiol 1992; 136(2):165.
5. Rang E, Fairbairn A, Acheson E. An enquiry into the incidence and prognosis of undiagnosed abdominal pain treated in hospital. Br J Prev Soc Med 1970; 24(1):47.
6. Sheridan W et al. Non-specific abdominal pain: the resource implications. Ann R Coll Surg Engl 1992; 74(2):181.
7. Talley N et al. Prevalence of gastrointestinal symptoms in the elderly: a population-based study. Gastroenterology 1992; 102(3):895.
8. Kay L, Jorgensen T, Schultz-Larsen K. Abdominal pain in a 70-year-old Danish population. An epidemiological study of the prevalence and importance of abdominal pain. J Clin Epidemiol 1992; 45(12):1377.
9. Thompson WG et al. Functional bowel disorders and functional abdominal pain. Gut 1999; 45 (Suppl 2):II43.
10. Talley NJ, Spiller R. Irritable bowel syndrome: a little understood organic disease? Lancet 2002; 360(9332):555.
11. Locke GR. The epidemiology of functional gastrointestinal disorders in North America. Gastroenterol Clin North Am 1996; 25(1):1.
12. Saito YA, Schoenfeld P, Locke GR III. The epidemiology of irritable bowel syndrome in North America: a systematic review. Am J Gastroenterol 2002; 97:1910.
13. Talley N et al. Epidemiology of colonic symptoms and the irritable bowel syndrome. Gastroenterology 1991; 101:927.
14. Agreus L et al. The epidemiology of abdominal symptoms: prevalence and demographic characteristics in a Swedish adult population. A report from the Abdominal Symptom Study. Scand J Gastroenterol 1994; 29(2):102.
15. Talley NJ et al. Medical costs in community subjects with irritable bowel syndrome. Gastroenterology 1995; 109(6):1736.
16. Agreus L et al. Irritable bowel syndrome and dyspepsia in the general population: overlap and lack of stability over time. Gastroenterology 1995; 109:671.
17. Rodriquez LG et al. Detection of colorectal tumor and inflammatory bowel disease during follow-up of patients with initial diagnosis of irritable bowel syndrome. Scand J Gastroenterol 2000; 35:306.
18. Locke GRI et al. The incidence of clinically diagnosed irritable bowel syndrome in the community. Gastroenterology 1999; 116:A76.
19. Greenlee RT et al. Cancer statistics. CA Cancer J Clin 2000; 50(1):7.
20. Loftus EV, Sandborn WJ. Epidemiology of inflammatory bowel disease. Gastroenterol Clin North Am 2002; 31(1):1.
21. Sandler RS et al. The burden of selected digestive diseases in the United States. Gastroenterology 2002; 122(5):1500.
22. El-Serag H, Olden K, Bjorkman D. Health-related quality of life among persons with irritable bowel syndrome: a systematic review. Aliment Pharmacol Ther 2002; 16:1171.
23. Jones R et al. Dyspepsia in England and Scotland. Gut 1990; 31(4):401.

24. Bernersen B, Johnsen R, Straume B. Towards a true prevalence of peptic ulcer: the Sorreisa gastro-intestinal disorder study. Gut 1990; 31:989.
25. Drossman DA et al. U.S. householder survey of functional gastrointestinal disorders. Prevalence, sociodemography, and health impact. Dig Dis Sci 1993; 38(9):1569.
26. Kay L, Jorgensen T. Epidemiology of upper dyspepsia in a random population. Scand J Gastroenterol 1994; 29:1.
27. Locke GR III et al. Prevalence and clinical spectrum of gastroesophageal reflux: a population-based study in Olmsted County, Minnesota. Gastroenterology 1997; 112:1448.
28. Klauser A et al. What is behind dyspepsia?. Dig Dis Sci 1993; 38(1):147.
29. Bytzer P, Hansen J, Schaffalitzky de Muckadell O. Empirical H2-blocker therapy or prompt endoscopy in management of dyspepsia. Lancet 1994; 343:811.
30. Castillo J et al. Overlap of IBS and dyspepsia: how much is explained by upper abdominal pain associated with bowel habit?. Gastroenterology 2002; 126(4 Suppl 2):A371.
31. Jones R, Lydeard S. Dyspepsia in the community. Br J Clin Pract 1992; 46:95.
32. Drossman D et al. Rome II: a multinational consensus document on functional gastrointestinal disorders. Gut 1999; 45(Suppl II):II1.
33. Goodacre S et al. The health care burden of acute chest pain. Heart 2005; 91(2):229.
34. Alban Davies J. Anginal pain of esophageal origin: Clinical presentation, prevalence, and prognosis. Am J Med 1992; 92(Suppl 5A):5S.
35. Ockene I et al. Unexplained chest pain in patients with normal coronary arteriograms: a follow-up study of functional status. N Engl J Med 1980; 303:1249.
36. Eslick GD, Jones MP, Talley NJ. Non-cardiac chest pain: prevalence, risk factors, impact and consulting—a population-based study. Aliment Pharmacol Ther 2003; 17(9):1115.
37. Cormier L et al. Chest pain with negative cardiac diagnostic studies. Relationship to psychiatric illness. J Nerv Ment Dis 1988; 176:351.
38. Whitehead WE et al. Functional disorders of the anus and rectum. Gut 1999; 45(Suppl 2):II55.
39. Thompson WG. Proctalgia fugax. Dig Dis Sci 1981; 26(12):1121.
40. Hotopf M et al. Why do children have chronic abdominal pain, and what happens to them when they grow up? Population-based cohort study. BMJ 1998; 316(7139):1196.
41. Huang R, Palmer L, Forbes D. Prevalence and pattern of childhood abdominal pain in an Australian general practice. J Paediatr Child Health 2000; 36(4):349.
42. Apley J. The Child with Abdominal Pains. Oxford: Blackwell Scientific Publications, 1975.
43. Apley J, Naish N. Recurrent abdominal pains: a field study of 1000 school children. Arch Dis Child 1958; 33:165.
44. Scharff L. Recurrent abdominal pain in children: a review of psychological factors and treatment. Clin Psychol Rev 1997; 17(2):145.
45. Boey C, Yap S, Goh K. The prevalence of recurrent abdominal pain in 11 to 16-year-old Malaysian schoolchildren. J Paediatr Child Health 2000; 36(2):114.
46. Williams N et al. Incidence of non-specific abdominal pain in children during school term: population survey based on discharge diagnoses. BMJ 1999; 318(7196):1455.
47. Heafield R et al. Outcome of emergency surgical admissions for non-specific abdominal pain. Gut 1990; 31:A1167, 1990.
48. Hotopf M et al. Childhood risk factors for adults with medically unexplained symptoms: results from a national birth cohort study. Am J Psychiatry 1999; 156(11):1796.
49. Hotopf M et al. Childhood predictors of adult medically unexplained hospitalisations. Results from a national birth cohort study. Br J Psychiatry 2000; 176:273.

3 | Overview of Pain and Sensitization

Michael S. Gold

Department of Biomedical Sciences, Dental School, Program in Neuroscience, and Department of Anatomy and Neurobiology, Medical School, University of Maryland, Baltimore, Maryland, U.S.A.

WHAT IS PAIN?

The International Association for the Study of Pain (IASP) has defined pain as an unpleasant sensory and emotional experience associated with noxious stimuli or described in such terms (1). Implicit in this definition are two important features of pain. First and foremost is that pain is a perception that occurs in a conscious brain, requiring activation of multiple cortical areas to produce an "experience." In contrast, "nociception" is the term used to describe activity in either the peripheral or the central nervous system (CNS) evoked by noxious stimuli. Importantly, nociception may or may not result in the perception of pain. The implication of this distinction is that pain not only requires consciousness, but also an intact nervous system and a nervous system that has developed sufficiently such that activity in subcortical nociceptive circuits is able to influence activity in the appropriate cortical circuits (2). Second, pain has both sensory and emotional content. This notion is supported by data from brain imaging studies as well as deficits observed in patients following specific brain injuries. Imaging data indicate that noxious stimuli result in the activation of SI and SII sensory cortices, brain areas critical for sensory discrimination (3–5). Noxious stimuli also result in the activation of brain areas critical for processing of emotion, such as the amygdala and the anterior cingulate cortex (4,6–8). The relative contribution of each of these areas can be manipulated experimentally, resulting in differences in perception (9). Furthermore, patients suffering unilateral damage to SI and SII cortex, which would eliminate sensory, but not affective components of pain, report vague unpleasantness in response to noxious stimulation of body regions contralateral to the site of brain injury (10,11). A third feature of pain, not implied in the IASP definition, is that it involves a cognitive component. In other words, pain has meaning and its meaning can impact both the sensory and the emotional experience. For example, a little abdominal discomfort following a bowl of chili in a person prone to intestinal gas may mean something very different, and will likely be perceived very differently, from the abdominal discomfort experienced by a person recently hospitalized for a bleeding ulcer.

Pain Is Unique Compared to Other Sensory Modalities

There are several other aspects of pain that distinguish it from other sensory modalities. First, unlike other sensory modalities such as taste, vision, or audition, pain is a submodality of somatosensory processing. Somatosensation involves the detection of mechanical, thermal, and chemical stimuli impinging on structures outside the CNS. At low intensities, these stimuli are not perceived as painful. At higher intensities, each of these stimuli may result in tissue damage. Such intense stimuli are referred to as noxious and are generally perceived as painful. For somatic structures such as skin and muscle distinct afferent populations are involved in encoding non-noxious and noxious stimuli (13). Low-threshold mechanoreceptors and warm and cool fibers encode non-noxious stimuli, and nociceptors encode noxious stimuli. However, because many noxious stimuli will activate both low-threshold and nociceptive afferents, the quality of pain associated with these stimuli is often influenced by activity in low-threshold afferents. Visceral structures such as the colon (14) and the esophagus (15) are innervated by both low-threshold and high-threshold afferents. However, even the

Box 1   Theories on the Perception of Pain

Three major theories have dominated views about how noxious stimulation of peripheral tissue may ultimately be perceived as pain. One is the labeled line theory. The idea here is that like other sensory modalities, such as vision and audition, there are specialized neural pathways dedicated to the perception of pain. The result would be a dedicated neural pathway, or labeled line, from the periphery to the brain, activity in which would result in the perception of pain. A second is the frequency-encoding theory. This theory is based on the observation that for other sensory modalities, the amount of neural activity encodes the intensity of a stimulus. The prediction of this theory was that there would be neurons that could encode stimulus intensity over a wide range, and at some level of activity, the perception of the stimulus would change from nonpainful to painful. The Gate Control Theory by Melzack and Wall (12) was an alternative to both of these theories, incorporating aspects of both, but formally proposing a third mechanism for the perception of pain that depended on neural circuitry. Melzack and Wall proposed that the perception of pain depended on the relative activity in a number of different neurons that were interconnected in ways that enabled these neurons to influence, either directly or indirectly, the activity of other neurons in the circuit. Data from studies designed to elucidate the complexity of the neural circuitry underlying the perception of pain, particularly that arising from visceral structures, indicates that fundamental aspects of each of these theories are correct.

low-threshold afferents appear to encode stimulus intensity into the noxious range. This difference between visceral and other somatic structures may contribute to the observation that the ability to distinguish the modality of noxious stimuli impinging on the viscera is relatively poor.

A second, unique aspect of pain is that it demands attention and, more importantly, action. From an evolutionary perspective, this makes intuitive sense, as tissue integrity, and, ultimately, survival may depend on escape from noxious stimuli. Consequently, noxious stimuli result in the activation of neural circuits that enable not only rapid escape from the stimulus, as is observed in a withdrawal reflex, but also cardiovascular changes that facilitate whole body "fight or flight" responses (16). Thus, again in contrast to other sensory modalities, the response to acute noxious stimuli can be measured with changes in a host of autonomic measures such as heart rate and blood pressure. These responses may change in the face of tissue injury or prolonged noxious stimulation where behavioral changes conducive to wound healing, such as inactivity, may come to predominate (6).

A third unique aspect of pain is that application of the same stimulus, for example, a contact probe at 48°C, does not always produce the same perception. This dynamic nature of pain appears to reflect a number of mechanisms. As mentioned above, cognitive factors are but one class of mechanisms that influence the perception of pain. The impact of cognitive factors has been eloquently demonstrated in studies employing distraction (17) and/or hypnotic suggestion (9) to alter the perception of pain. Other factors include (i) the state of the organism, which is influenced by variables such as nutritional status (18,19) and diurnal fluctuations of physiological processes (20); (ii) the age of the organism (21), and (iii) the history of the organism (22,23). The history of the organism, particularly, that associated with previous noxious stimulation may have a particularly profound impact on the perception of pain. This impact may be observed within seconds (24) as well as over the lifetime of the organism (23).

Following tissue injury or in the presence of disease, there may be changes in pain perception that are the most clinically relevant. These changes in pain signal the presence of injury and disease and serve as a primary motivation for patients to seek medical attention. Undertreated, this pain may have serious deleterious consequences, as pain has been shown to suppress immune function (25), thereby slowing recovery or worsening the progression of a disease (26). Furthermore, persistent pain may develop into a disease in its own right as it may persist following resolution of initiating causes or in the absence of any apparent underlying pathology.

PAIN TERMINOLOGY

Specific terms are used to describe the increase in pain observed in the presence of injury or disease. An increase in pain in response to normally painful stimuli is referred to as hyperalgesia (27). In contrast, the perception of pain in response to stimuli that are normally not perceived as painful is referred to as allodynia (1,27). One of the most common positive signs (28) associated with peripheral neuropathy is pain in response to light brushing of skin, a normally innocuous stimulus (29). Pain in response to such innocuous stimuli is referred to as dynamic mechanical allodynia. Hyperalgesia may reflect an increase in the excitability of tissue nociceptors, as well as neurons in the CNS involved in nociceptive processing. This increase in excitability is referred to as sensitization. In contrast, dynamic mechanical allodynia appears to be conveyed by low-threshold afferents impinging on a sensitized CNS (30). The vast majority of dorsal horn neurons receiving input from visceral structures also receive input from somatic structures (so-called convergent input), in particular, those overlying the visceral organ in question. Consequently, injury or inflammation of a visceral structure may result in hyperalgesia or allodynia in the somatic structure overlying the inflamed visceral organ. Such hyperalgesia and allodynia is called referred hyperalgesia and referred allodynia, and again reflects sensitization of neurons within the CNS (31).

Ascending Circuitry

The perception of noxious stimulation of peripheral tissue depends on the transmission of a signal from the site of stimulation to a number of distinct regions in the cerebral cortex. In most peripheral structures, the first step in the transmission of such information involves the activation of a nociceptor, or receptor activated by noxious stimuli, located in the peripheral terminal of an afferent (sensory) axon or fiber, commonly referred to as a nociceptive afferent. These afferents synapse on distinct classes of neurons within the spinal cord and trigeminal dorsal horn. Subpopulations of neurons within the dorsal horn project to discrete nuclei within the thalamus (i.e., ventral posterior lateral thalamus) as well as other structures in the brain stem [i.e., parabrachial nucleus and periaquaductal gray (PAG)]. From the thalamus, information is conveyed to cortical areas involved in sensory processing or those involved in processing emotional or affective information (32). While this ascending pathway may sound like a labeled line, it is important to keep in mind that the system is far more complicated than that. At each step of the pathway, nociceptive and non-nociceptive information appears to be processed in parallel. This is particularly true at supraspinal sites, where evidence of nociceptive-specific neurons, those that are selectively activated by noxious stimulation, is rare, and evidence of nociceptive-specific nuclei at supraspinal sites is nonexistent.

An interesting distinction between transducers in other specialized senses and transducers in nociceptive neurons is that transducers in specialized senses transduce a single form of energy, while those in nociceptive afferents transduce several forms of energy. For example, transient receptor potential channel V1 where V is for vanniloid (TRPV1) [formerly vanniloid receptor 1 (VR1)], a protein thought to be responsible for the transduction of temperatures between 42°C and 48°C is also activated by protons and capsaicin, the "hot" compound in chili peppers (36). Transient receptor potential channel M8 where M is for Melastatin (TRPM8) [also known as cold and menthol responsive channel 1 (CMR-1)], a protein thought to be responsible for the transduction of temperatures between 30°C and 20°C is also activated by

Box 2 The Implication of Free Nerve Endings

Signaling within the nervous system depends on electrical activity or changes in membrane potential. The implication of this fact is the particular form of energy that constitutes a stimulus [e.g., electromagnetic radiation, volatile chemicals, a pinprick (mechanical), or a change in temperature (thermal)] must be converted into an electrical signal. The process of converting energy of the environment into an electrical signal is referred to as transduction. The electrical signal is referred to as a generator potential. Specialized cell types such as photoreceptors (vision) and hair cells (audition) are responsible for transduction in the special senses. In the somatosensory system, specialized cells types are either responsible for transduction of low-threshold mechanical stimuli (e.g., Golgi tendon organ) or aid in the transduction of low-threshold mechanical stimuli (e.g., Pacinian corpuscle). Consequently, low-threshold mechanosensitive afferents terminate at these specialized cell types. In contrast, peripheral terminals of nociceptive afferents are not associated with any particular cell type, and are therefore said to have free nerve endings. An important implication of the observation that nociceptive afferents terminate in free nerve endings is that protein complexes necessary for stimulus transduction must be present in the afferent terminals. Indeed, nociceptive afferents have been shown to express a full array of proteins thought to underlie thermal transduction (33) and chemotransduction (34). And while specific mechanisms mediating mechanotransduction are still being actively investigated, studies of isolated sensory neurons in vitro suggest that nociceptive afferents express proteins necessary for mechanotransduction (35).

Box 3 Transduction in Visceral Afferents

While afferents innervating visceral structures appear to express many of the transducers present in afferents innervating somatic tissue, transduction of many stimuli in visceral tissue may in fact involve specialized cell types. Epithelial cells in the bladder have been shown to store adenosine triphosphate (ATP) and release this transmitter in a Ca^{2+}-dependent manner (44). More importantly, these cells have been shown to release ATP in response to a variety of stimuli, including mechanical (stretch), thermal, and chemical (44). ATP has also been shown to be released following stimulation of the colon with a variety of stimuli (45). ATP receptors are present on primary afferent neurons, including those that innervate the bladder (46) and colon (45,47). Thus, release of ATP from bladder or colon epithelial cells in response to a variety of stimuli will result in the activation of visceral afferents expressing ATP receptors. This places the ATP receptor at a critical point of convergence following activation of visceral tissue. Furthermore, because ATP receptor–mediated currents may be increased in the presence of inflammation (47–49), ATP-dependent transduction may contribute to the increase in visceral pain observed in the presence of inflammation. Consequently, blocking ATP receptors may be an effective way of blocking visceral pain. Indeed, several lines of preclinical data indicate that this is the case (44,46).

the cooling compound menthol (37,38). Channels originally thought to signal a decrease in tissue pH, acid sensing ion channel 2 (ASIC2), and ASIC3 [also known as dorsal root acid sensing ion channel (DRASIC)] (39–41) appear also to be involved in mechanotransduction (42,43).

Descending Pathways

While the neural circuitry enabling the perception of noxious stimuli in the periphery is referred to as the ascending system, there are also neural circuits originating from supraspinal sites that influence nociceptive activity in the spinal cord and in primary afferents. This system is referred to as the descending system (50,51). Initial descriptions of this system suggested that the neural circuitry was dedicated to the suppression of pain. Indeed electrical and/or chemical stimulation of the PAG, a region of gray matter that surrounds the cerebral aqueduct between the third and the fourth ventricle, results in the selective suppression of pain, leaving others sensory modalities intact (52). This form of pain suppression is referred to as stimulation-produced analgesia, and appears to be mediated via both the presynaptic inhibition of primary afferent input into the dorsal horn and the inhibition of dorsal horn projection neurons (50,51). The PAG receives input from collaterals of ascending fibers as well as from higher brain centers such as the amygdala, hippocampus, and hypothalamus (16). Output of the PAG is to the rostroventral medulla as well as other sites in the pons and medulla. Projections from these sites descend to the dorsal horn. Importantly, this circuit is a primary mechanism underlying the actions of exogenous analgesics such as morphine (50,51).

More recently, it is becoming clear that pain may also be facilitated via neural circuitry associated with descending pathways (53). Electrophysiological recording in the rostroventral medulla revealed two populations of neurons: one that stopped firing immediately before the initiation of a nociceptive reflex (so-called "off cells") and another that began firing prior to the initiation of a nociceptive reflex (so-called "on cells"). Stimulation within the PAG or the exogenous administration of opioids resulted in both the suppression of nociceptive reflexes and the off cell pause. Conversely, increased activity in on cells resulted in the facilitation of nociceptive reflexes (54). These data formed the basis for the suggestion that the perception of pain can be both increased and decreased by circuitry within the brain.

While investigators have focused on the dorsal horn as the primary site of descending modulation of nociception, there is compelling evidence suggesting that this bidirectional modulation also occurs at afferent peripheral terminals. The circuitry underlying modulation of nociception at the peripheral terminal involves sympathoadrenal and hypothalamic-pituitary-adrenal axes. Antinociception is mediated by inhibitory peptides such as β-endorphin and enkephalin, released from the pituitary and the adrenal medulla as well as immune cells (55). An increase in nociception is mediated by epinephrine released from the adrenal medulla (56,57).

Mechanisms of Sensitization—Transducers

In an effort to identify mechanisms underlying hyperalgesia and allodynia observed in the presence of injury and disease, scientists have studied mechanisms underlying both ascending and descending pathways. As described above, the first step in the ascending pathway is stimulus transduction. Single-unit recording of nociceptive afferents indicates that peripheral terminals are sensitized in the presence of injury or inflammation (13). There are at least three mechanisms that could account for the observed increase in excitability. The first is a change in tissue properties, such that stimuli are conveyed to afferent terminals more readily. Analysis of changes in tissue mechanics observed in the presence of inflammation suggests that changes in tissue properties may contribute to nociceptor sensitization (58).

A second mechanism that may account for the sensitization of nociceptor terminals is a change in the transduction process. In the case of visceral structures, such as the bladder or colon, where release of ATP appears to contribute to stimulus transduction, an increase in the release of ATP would contribute to an apparent increase in the excitability of nociceptive terminals. As indicated above, following inflammation of the colon (47) and bladder (59), an increase in evoked release of ATP has been observed. Alternatively, there may be changes in the properties of protein/protein complexes underlying stimulus transduction. Again, as mentioned above, inflammation results in an increase in the magnitude of ATP-evoked currents in sensory neurons (48,49). Thus, even if there were no changes in ATP release, an increase in the sensitivity of ATP receptors would contribute to nociceptor sensitization. Inflammation-induced changes in the properties of other transducers, such as those underlying changes in pH (60), receptors for inflammatory mediators such as bradykinin (61), and receptors for neurotrophins such as brain-derived neurotrophic factor (62–64), have also been described.

TRPV1, a transducer for noxious heat (36), protons (36) and the activation of intracellular signaling cascades (65), is one of the most thoroughly characterized transducers. Inflammation results in several changes in the expression and biophysical properties of TRPV1, which all enable this channel to play a critical role in inflammatory hyperalgesia. There is an increase in channel density that appears to reflect in increase protein translation (66). The desensitization of the channel appears to be significantly attenuated (67), enabling the channel to more readily contribute to repeated nociceptor activation. The channel itself may also be sensitized, such that temperature threshold for channel activation is significantly lowered (68). Importantly, there is evidence that the threshold for channel activation may be lowered to approximately 37°C, a threshold that would mean the channel could be activated at resting body temperatures. This observation has led to the suggestion that TRPV1 may mediate ongoing pain associated with inflammation (69). Inflammation-induced changes in TRPV1 illustrate the multiplicity of ways in which changes in transducers and/or their properties may contribute to the sensitization of nociceptive afferents.

Mechanisms of Sensitization—Ion Channels

In order for the membrane depolarization that follows stimulus transduction to impact the CNS, it must be converted into an action potential. This requires another set of specialized proteins referred to as voltage-gated ion channels. These channels are opened or closed in response to changes in membrane potential. Voltage-gated Na+ channels (VGSC) mediate the rapid depolarization of the action potential. VGSCs consist of an α- and up to two β-subunits (70). The α-subunit contains the voltage sensor and ion channel. Nine α-subunits have been identified, which differ with respect to their pharmacological sensitivity and biophysical properties. Phosphorylation of VGSC α-subunits results in changes in biophysical properties of the channel (71). β-subunits also influence the biophysical properties of VGSCs and are instrumental in targeting VGSCs to specific sites in the cell membrane (72). Thus, there are a number of ways in which changes in VGSCs may contribute to the sensitization of nociceptive afferents in the presence of tissue injury or disease. Those that have been observed include (i) changes in the expression of α-subunits (73), (ii) changes in the expression of β-subunits (74,75), (iii) changes in the relative distribution of α-subunits in the cell membrane (76), and (iv) changes in the biophysical properties of VGSCs (77). The relative density of VGSCs available for activation determines action potential threshold, and the ability of a neuron to fire repetitive action potentials. Therefore, an increase in channel density will result in a decrease in action potential threshold and an increase in the neuronal firing frequency. Because β-subunits can increase the rate of channel activation (78), an increase in β-subunit may also decrease action potential threshold as well as the magnitude of the generator potential necessary to reach action potential threshold. Some VGSC α-subunits have a lower threshold for activation than others (76,79), and thus a shift in the relative distribution of α-subunits from high threshold to low threshold would result in a decrease in action potential threshold. Finally, because the biophysical properties such as the voltage dependence of channel activation, the voltage dependence of channel availability, and rates of channel activation and inactivation may be influenced by phosphorylation state of the α-subunit (71), the appropriate changes in channel phosphorylation may also result in decreases in action potential threshold and/or the ability of the channel to sustain multiple action potentials.

Voltage-gated K^+ channels (VGPCs) are primarily responsible for membrane repolarization following the depolarization mediated by VGSCs. The density and biophysical properties of VGPCs also influence other aspects of the action potential waveform including action potential threshold and the magnitude and duration of the after hyperpolarization that occurs following an action potential. Other types of K^+ channels such as Ca^{2+}-modulated K^+ channels [big conducatance Ca^{2+} modulated K^+ channel (BK) and small conducatance Ca^{2+} activated K^+ channel (SK)], voltage-independent, or leak K^+ channels [i.e., two-pore potassium channels such as TWIK related K^+ channel 1 where TWIK stands for tandem of p domains in a weak inward rectifier K^+ channel (TREK-1) and TWIK related arachidonic acid stimulated K^+ channel (TRAAK)], and ligand-regulated K^+ channels [such as KQT related K^+ channel (KCNQ) or inward rectifying K^+ channel (Kir) channels] may also influence properties of the action potential waveform. Because some of these K^+ channels may have a low threshold for activation or even be active at the resting membrane potential, they may influence the extent to which membrane depolarization that occurs following stimulus transduction is able to drive activation of VGSCs, and therefore impact action potential initiation (80). Because these channels may influence the magnitude and/or decay of the afterhyperpolarization, they can influence interspike interval and action potential burst duration (80). Finally, because these channels may influence action potential duration (81), they may have a secondary influence on the amount of Ca^{2+} that enters the neuron via voltage-gated Ca^{2+} channels (VGCCs). The amount of Ca^{2+} entry can again influence the excitability of afferent terminals via Ca^{2+}-modulated K^+ channels (82). Ca^{2+} may also influence transmitter release, which occurs at both peripheral and central terminals of nociceptive afferents. The peripheral release of transmitter may further contribute to nociceptor sensitization via a direct action back on the afferent terminal as well as a secondary facilitation of the inflammatory process (83). In short, a wide variety of K^+ channels are able to influence the excitability of nociceptive afferents in a multiplicity of ways. Importantly, both acute (84) and persistent (85–87) changes in K^+ channels have been described in response to inflammatory mediators and/or inflammation as well as other forms of tissue injury (88).

As suggested above, VGCCs constitute a third class of ion channels that may also contribute to the sensitization of nociceptor terminals. In addition to their secondary influence on nociceptive excitability via modulation of K^+ and Cl^- channels (82,89,90) and transmitter release, there is evidence that VGCCs contribute directly to the sensitization of nociceptive afferents. The most compelling evidence has been obtained for low-threshold, or T-type VGCCs (91,92). Pharmacological evidence suggests that these channels influence action potential threshold and therefore nociceptive threshold (91). There is also evidence that when present in sufficient density, these channels may also mediate a sustained depolarization following action potential initiation that is of sufficient magnitude to induce subsequent action

Box 4 Action Potentials in the Sensory Neuron Cell Body

Researchers have long appreciated that the density of voltage-gated channels in the cell body of sensory ganglia is sufficient to support neural activity. However, because of the T-junction, action potentials may travel from afferent terminal to terminal without invading the sensory neuron cell body. Thus, it was not immediately clear why the density of channels within the cell body should be high enough to support action potential generation. However, recent evidence suggests that action potentials in the sensory neuron cell body may serve several purposes. It turns out that Ca^{2+} transients associated with neural activity invading the cell body may be critical for regulating transcriptional and translational machinery, and therefore a number of cellular processes such as nerve formation (97). Activity-evoked Ca^{2+} transients may also be sufficient to drive transmitter release within the ganglia (98), providing a mechanism for "cross talk" between sensory neurons, which is thought to amplify signals initiated in the periphery (99,100). In the presence of nerve injury, activity may even be initiated from within sensory ganglia, a change thought to contribute to ongoing pain associated with nerve injury (101).

potential generation (93). While the impact of injury on the density, distribution, or properties of low-threshold VGCCs has yet to be investigated in detail (94), there is evidence of both acute (95) and persistent changes in high-threshold VGCCs (94,96).

Mechanisms of Sensitization—Structural Changes

Structural changes in primary afferent neurons may also contribute to the manifestation of injury-induced increases in excitability. While sensitization of transducers or changes in the properties of ion channels may contribute to an increase in receptive field size, there is also evidence of a sprouting in peripheral terminals. In the presence of inflammation, increases in neuropeptides such as calcitonin gene–related peptide (CGRP) have been reported, as well as the growth-associated protein, GAP-43 (102,103). Sprouting within central terminals would also be manifest as an increase in receptive field size, and there is evidence for sprouting of central terminals in the presence of (104,105), or in response to (106,107) inflammation and nerve injury (108). Another structural change that may contribute to an increased pain associated with tissue injury or disease has been referred to as a "phenotypic switch." This term has been applied to sensory neurons that begin to express different properties such as the neuropeptide substance P that is normally only expressed in nociceptive afferents (109). Expression of such neuropeptides in low-threshold afferents would amplify nociceptive signaling in the spinal cord and may contribute to mechanical allodynia.

Mechanisms of Sensitization—Receptors

In addition to the thermo- and mechanoreceptors described above, a vast array of chemoreceptors has been identified that contribute to that activation and/or sensitization of nociceptive neurons (34). Chemoreceptors are most often described in terms of the compounds or agonists that activate them, such as glutamate receptors or substance P receptors. They are also classified according to whether they are directly coupled to ion channels (ionotropic receptors) or to second-messenger pathways (metabotropic receptors). Metabotropic receptors are further subclassified according to the second-messenger pathway(s) initiated following receptor activation. The largest family of metabotropic receptors is the guanine nucleotide–binding protein (G-protein)–coupled receptors. Additional metabotropic receptor families include those bearing intrinsic protein tyrosine kinase domains (i.e., Trk receptors), receptors that associate with cytosolic tyrosine kinases (i.e., non–tyrosine kinase receptors such as cytokine receptors and integrins), and protein serine/threonine kinases [i.e., transforming growth factor (TGF)-β receptors].

Unlike mechano- or thermotransduction, which ultimately must result in neuronal activation, chemoreceptors may be either excitatory or inhibitory. A number of factors impact whether or under what conditions a receptor will be excitatory or inhibitory. For example, in most neurons in adult animals, the ionotropic γ-aminobutyric acid (GABA) receptor (GABAA receptor) is inhibitory. The GABAA receptor is a Cl^- channel and because the concentration of intracellular Cl^- is usually low and the concentration of extracellular Cl^- is generally high, the equilibrium potential for Cl^- is usually below action potential threshold. However, following tissue injury, the intracellular concentration of Cl^- may be increased as a result of changes in the expression of Cl^- transporters (110). Consequently, activation of GABAA receptors may result in membrane depolarization sufficient for action potential generation. Similarly, because the concentration of intracellular Cl^- is always relatively high in primary afferent neurons, a decrease in action potential threshold may enable GABAA receptor activation to generate action potentials in primary afferents (83).

Different chemoreceptors preferentially couple to different second-messenger pathways (see below). Thus, a common mechanism influencing whether a receptor will be excitatory or inhibitory is the second-messenger pathway activated by a particular receptor. In primary afferent neurons, adenosine A2 receptors appear to couple to stimulatory G-proteins, resulting in the activation of adenylate cyclase, an increase in cyclic adenosine monophosphate (cAMP), the activation of protein kinase A (PKA) and ultimately nociceptor sensitization (111,112). In contrast, adenosine A1 receptors appear to couple to inhibitory G-proteins, resulting in the inhibition of adenylate cyclase, a decrease in cAMP and PKA activity and a reversal of sensitization (111). The relative balance between excitatory and inhibitory processes will depend on a number of factors, including receptor properties (i.e., binding affinity for transmitter or ligand), relative receptor density, and the history of the neuron. The balance between excitation and inhibition is further complicated in the CNS, where there is excitatory and inhibitory neural circuitry that is influenced by excitatory and inhibitory receptor activation.

Recent evidence suggests that two additional factors critically impact receptor function. The first of these is the ability of receptors or receptor subunits to form complexes. There are a number of ionotropic receptors that are assembled from a number of distinct receptor subunits. For example of GABAA receptors, which are composed of two α, two β, and a single γ subunit (most commonly). Several receptors particularly relevant for nociception may be assembled from either multiples of the same subunit (homomultimers) or multiples of different subunits (heteromultimers). For example, ionotropic ATP receptors (referred to as P2X receptors) may be formed from homomultimers of P2X2 or P2X$_3$ as well as heteromultimers of P2X2/3 (113). Importantly, the biophysical properties and/or pharmacology of heteromultimers are distinct. Therefore, the stoichiometry of subunit assembly will impact the properties of evoked currents. Recently, the issue has proven to be even more complex, as there are at least preliminary data of functional interaction between distinct ionotropic receptor subtypes. For example, there is evidence of functional interaction between ATP receptors (P2X5) and proton receptors (ASIC3), which dramatically alters proton activation of the ASIC3 receptor (114). The issue is complicated still further by evidence to suggest that G-protein–coupled receptors form functional interactions that influence receptor affinity, signaling, and trafficking (115–117).

"Receptor trafficking" is a term used to describe processes underlying receptor localization, internalization, and reinsertion in neuronal membranes. While many of the mechanisms underlying receptor trafficking have yet to be fully elucidated, it is clear that these processes play a critical role in neural plasticity and therefore are likely to contribute to both peripheral and central sensitization observed following tissue injury (118,119).

Mechanisms of Sensitization—Second-Messenger Pathways

Molecules released or activated following ligand binding to a receptor that leads to changes in cellular processes are referred to as second messengers. The sequence of cellular events associated with the release/activation of second messengers is referred to as a second-messenger pathway. Second-messenger pathways underlie the sensitization of both peripheral and central neurons. The detail to which many of these pathways have been elucidated is extraordinary, and far beyond the scope of the present chapter. Nevertheless, several general concepts have arisen from detailed analysis of second-messenger pathways that are particularly important to the understanding of pain and sensitization. These include the duration of a second-messenger–mediated change in cellular processes, the history of the neuron, cross talk between second-messenger pathways, and the influence of target of innervation.

A primary function of second-messenger–mediated signaling pathways is that they enable the amplification of cellular events in terms of the magnitude of the event, its cellular distribution, and its duration. The duration of an event is tightly regulated and depends both on the second-messenger pathway utilized and on the presence of cellular processes responsible for the termination/reversal of the event. There are second-messenger–mediated events that occur on the millisecond-to-minute time scale, other events that occur over minutes to hours and others still that may require days or longer. Classical second-messenger–signaling pathways involve the activation of PKA or protein kinase C (PKC). These two kinases appear to be critical for the initiation of inflammatory hyperalgesia (120–122) as well as changing the properties of ion channels thought to underlie inflammatory hyperalgesia (123). It has long been known that activation of PKC may involve the activation of phospholipase C (PLC), which cleaves phosphatidylinositol 4,5-bisphosphate (PIP2), resulting in the liberation of diacylglycerol (DAG) and inositol trisphosphate (IP3). Liberated IP3 causes the release of Ca^{2+} from internal stores, and DAG and Ca^{2+} may act as coactivators of PKC. More recently, it has been demonstrated that PIP2 may directly regulate the activity of specific ion channels. Consequently, PLC-mediated cleavage of PIP2 may result in the activation of some ion channels (124) or the inhibition of others (125). More recently, a number of additional, rapid second-messenger cascades have been identified that underlie sensitization of nociceptive afferents, including the nitric oxide (NO)/ guanylate cyclase (GC)/protein kinase G (PKG) pathway (126), ceramide sphingomyelinase pathway (127), and at least two myelin-associated protein kinase (MAPK) pathways, including extracellular signal-related/mitogen-activated potein kinase (ERK) (128) and p38 (66). Some of the kinase-mediated changes in nociceptor excitability are relatively short lived as the apparent result of phosphatase activity. However, in the face of limited phosphatase activity, some of the kinase-mediated changes in excitability may last many tens of minutes. While not well documented in nociceptive systems, there is evidence of changes in ion channel and/or receptor distribution following the activation of specific second-messenger pathways (129). These changes appear to involve cytoskeletal proteins and may last for minutes to hours.

Even longer-lasting changes appear to ultimately reflect changes in protein synthesis. Changes in transcription and translation have both been documented and may be driven by a number of distinct second-messenger pathways (34). Time-dependent activation of second-messenger pathways in a series of different cell types, developing over many days, appears to underlie the maintenance of pain observed, following nerve injury (130).

Cross talk between second-messenger pathways appears to be the norm and is a phenomenon that has important implications for the interpretation of experiments designed to characterize second-messenger pathways mediating the sensitization of nociceptive neurons. "Cross talk" is the term used to describe the observation that the activation of one second-messenger pathway may lead to modulation and/or activation of a second pathway. This sort of interaction may occur at a number of levels starting from the receptor and ending at the effector molecule. Interactions between PKA- and PKC-dependent pathways have been well documented and depend on the actions of a number of different second messengers including G-protein subunits, adenylate cyclase isoforms, and Ca^{2+} (131). Interestingly, a relatively novel mechanism of interaction between PKA and PKC pathways was recently identified and actually occurs upstream of activation of PKA. An increase in cAMP in a subpopulation of nociceptive neurons results in the activation of a cAMP-activated guanine exchange factor (Epac) in addition to, and/or instead of, the activation of PKA (132). Epac, in turn, appears to mediate the activation of two phospholipases, PLC and PLD, both of which are critical for the activation of an isoform of PKC. An example of an interaction that occurs at the effector level is the kinase-mediated modulation of BK channels, depending on the splice variant of the α subunit of the BK channel (slo); the ability of PKA to phosphorylate the channel may depend on whether the channel has been phosphorylated by PKC (133).

Several lines of evidence indicate that the second-messenger pathway(s) activated by an inflammatory mediator in naive tissue may not be the same second-messenger pathway activated by the inflammatory mediator in tissue previously injured, thereby highlighting the importance of "history" on the response to injury. Importantly, the response of an organism to reinjury may be exacerbated or prolonged (22,134). Evidence that this change in the response to reinjury may reflect a change in second-messenger coupling was suggested by data from a model employing two inflammatory insults (22). In naive tissue, administration of the inflammatory mediator PGE2 results in nociceptor sensitization mediated by the activation of PKA- and PKG-dependent second-messenger cascades. This sensitization appears to last for approximately 60 minutes. However, in tissue previously inflamed, PGE2 results in hyperalgesia lasting more than 24 hours that appears to be mediated by the activation of a PKC-dependent pathway (22).

The observation that activation of the NO/GC/PKG pathway may produce different results depending on whether inflammation is present provides another example of the influence of "history" on second-messenger signaling. The NO pathway is involved in the modulation of afferent activity, underlying the action of bradykinin (135,136) and PGE2 (137), where in naive tissue activation of this pathway appears to mediate nociceptor sensitization via modulation of a VGSC (137). In the presence of persistent inflammatory hyperalgesia, however, the NO pathway appears to mediate the antinociceptive effects of peripheral opioids via activation of a potassium channel (138).

The role of NO-dependent pathways in the modulation of afferent excitability also illustrates the importance of target of innervation on the mechanisms underlying injury-induced changes in nociception as different subpopulations of afferents that are either sensitized, inhibited, or unaffected by the activation of NO-dependent pathways (139). For example, intradermal activation of this pathway is pronociceptive, suggesting that intradermal afferents are sensitized, following the activation of this pathway (139). Conversely, subcutaneous activation of this pathway is antinociceptive (139), suggesting that activation of this pathway can decrease the excitability of cutaneous afferents. The suggestion that both populations of neurons may innervate the same site in some tissues comes from the observation that there are subpopulations of dural afferents that could be distinguished according to whether they were sensitized, inhibited, or unaffected by NO (140).

Second-messenger–mediated pathways leading to long-term changes in neuronal properties involve changes in protein synthesis and therefore engage translational and transcriptional machinery. A number of second-messenger pathways underlying short-term changes in neuronal properties, such as those associated with Ca^{2+} influx or MAPK activation are also involved in mediating changes in protein synthesis. Activity-mediated Ca^{2+} influx is clearly involved in initiating changes in protein synthesis (97). Much more widely studied, however, is the impact of neurotrophic factors such as nerve growth factor (NGF) and glial-derived neurotrophic factor. Molecules such as NGF were originally shown to activate specific receptors, forming a trophic factor/receptor complex, which was internalized, transported back to the cell body, and translocated into the nucleus where it was thought to regulate transcriptional activity through binding to DNA at specific sites (141). More recently, it has been shown that these signaling molecules are able to initiate a number of distinct second-messenger cascades (142) and that downstream targets such as ERK and p38 are also involved in regulating transcriptional and translational machinery (66,143).

Mechanisms of Sensitization—CNS Changes

Many of the processes underlying central sensitization are analogous to those observed in the peripheral nervous system. For example, there is evidence that central sensitization reflects an increase in synaptic strength (analogous to transduction in the periphery), which reflects changes in the biophysical properties (144), density (145–148), and/or distribution of receptors critical to enabling postsynaptic neurons in the spinal cord dorsal horn (or at higher sites) to respond to excitatory input from nociceptive afferents. Similarly, there is evidence of changes in VGSCs (149) and VGPCs (150) associated with tissue injury, which mediate increases in the excitability of dorsal horn neurons. Interestingly, upregulation of a VGSC α subunit NaV1.3 occurs in both the spinal cord and the thalamus following spinal cord injury, where it appears to be critical for mediating sensitization of these CNS neurons (151). There is also evidence of phenotypic changes in CNS neurons following injury (110,152). As indicated above, the balance between inhibitory and excitatory input to CNS neurons is a critical factor influencing output. The importance of this balance is highlighted by the observation that pain associated with some forms of injury may reflect a loss of inhibition. A loss of inhibition may reflect a decrease in inhibitory receptors (153) as well as a structural change in the form of a loss of inhibitory interneurons (154).

There is also evidence for both segmental and suprasegmental changes in circuitry that appears to contribute to central sensitization, or at least increases in nociceptive processing following injury. For example, there is evidence for a segmental interaction between lumbosacral and thoracolumbar regions of the spinal cord, which may contribute to increases in the area of referred pain observed in the presence of inflammation of the colon (see Traub Chapter 7 this volume). The observation that pain associated with injury may reflect a shift in the balance of descending input to the spinal cord is an example of a change in suprasegmental circuitry; which a number of investigators have reported following injury, with a decrease in descending inhibition and/or an increase in descending facilitation (53).

Caveats and Qualifications

While it is true that, in general terms, sensitization will involve common processes such as increases in inward currents and/or excitatory input and decreases in outward currents or inhibitory input, it is also true that the exact nature of these processes are influenced by a number of important factors. Several of these factors have been discussed above. These include (i) timing and or duration of an injury, as the underlying mechanisms mediating pain can and do change over the time course of an injury (130), (ii) history of the organism, as previous injury (22), as well as developmental experiences (23) impact the response to subsequent injury, (iii) the type of injury, as the response to nerve injury (155) may be distinct from that associated with inflammation (156), and (iv) site of injury, which may not only influence second-messenger pathways utilized, but the relative involvement of various ion channels (120).

There are at least two additional factors that also appear to influence mechanisms of sensitization. First, there is sex and/or gonadal status of the organism. While debate continues over whether there is a difference between men and women with respect to pain threshold and pain tolerance (157–159), there is little debate over the question about whether there is a sex difference in the expression of persistent, particularly inflammatory, pain. Women, in general, are more likely to suffer from inflammatory pain that is often more intense and longer lasting than that in men (159–161). While there are a number of mechanisms that may contribute to this difference, evidence from both clinical and preclinical studies suggests that gonadal hormones, in particular estrogen, may be a critical factor. Its mechanisms of action are complex, as estrogen has been shown to influence structures relevant to nociception throughout the body. Timing, with respect to estrogen cycling or the sustained application of estrogen (as in the case of hormone replacement therapy), site of action, and dependent measures of nociception all appear to be important factors when assessing the impact of estrogen on specific aspects of nociceptive processing (120).

A second factor that appears to influence the response to injury and pain, if not sensitization, is genetic background. Mutations in specific genes have recently been linked to two pain disorders: erythmalgia (162) and hemiplegic migraine (163). More subtle changes in specific genes have also been shown to influence the response to noxious stimulation and analgesics and the likelihood of developing a pain condition. These include single-nucleotide polymorphisms in genes encoding the μ-opioid receptor (164), an isoform of cytochrome P450 (165), melanocortin receptor-1 (166), and a catalytic enzyme catechol-*O*-methyl transferase (COMT) (167). Specific haplotype blocks of COMT correlate with both pain tolerance and threshold ratings and increased likelihood of developing a pain syndrome (168).

SUMMARY AND CONCLUSIONS

The inability to treat pain adequately, particularly persistent pain, continues to be a major problem in health care. The dearth of effective therapeutic interventions with minimal side effects is due to a number of factors related to the complexity of nociceptive signaling. These include the fact that pain is a submodality within the larger somatosensory system, that the response to injury is dynamic, that the type of injury impacts the response and consequently the underlying mechanisms of pain, that history of the organism impacts the response to subsequent injury, that demographic factors such as age and sex impact the response to injury, and that the site of injury impacts the response and consequently underlying mechanisms of pain. As indicated in chapters throughout the rest of this volume, all of these factors are particularly relevant to visceral pain. Despite the complexity of nociceptive processing and a therapeutic armament that has not kept pace with advances in our understanding of this complexity, there is still reason for optimism that effective therapeutic interventions are not far off. There are two main reasons for this optimism, particularly with respect to the prospects for novel treatments for visceral pain. The first is that preclinical results with novel interventions have been promising (169,170). The second is that several exciting targets have been identified that appear to function at points of convergence of discrete cellular pathways.

ACKNOWLEDGMENTS

I would like to thank Dr. Joel Greenspan for helpful comments during the preparation of this manuscript. Some of the work described in this manuscript was supported by NIH grants AR049555 and NS41384.

REFERENCES

1. Merskey H, Bogduk N. Classification of Chronic Pain, IASP Press, Seattle, 1994:240.
2. Lee SJ et al. Fetal pain: a systematic multidisciplinary review of the evidence. JAMA 2005; 294: 947–954.
3. Chen JI et al. Differentiating noxious- and innocuous-related activation of human somatosensory cortices using temporal analysis of fMRI. J Neurophysiol 2002; 88:464–474.
4. Coghill RC, McHaffie JG, Yen YF. Neural correlates of interindividual differences in the subjective experience of pain. Proc Natl Acad Sci USA 2003; 100:8538–8542.
5. Moulton EA et al. Regional intensive and temporal patterns of functional MRI activation distinguishing noxious and innocuous contact heat. J Neurophysiol 2005; 93:2183–2193.
6. Rainville P, Bushnell MC, Duncan GH. Representation of acute and persistent pain in the human CNS: potential implications for chemical intolerance. Ann N Y Acad Sci. 2001; 933:130–141.
7. Ribeiro SC et al. Interface of physical and emotional stress regulation through the endogenous opioid system and μ-opioid receptors. Prog Neuropsychopharmacol Biol Psychiatry 2005.

8. Zubieta JK et al. Regional μ opioid receptor regulation of sensory and affective dimensions of pain. Science 2001; 293:311–315.

9. Rainville P et al. Dissociation of sensory and affective dimensions of pain using hypnotic modulation. Pain 1999; 82:159–171.

10. Ploner M, Freund HJ, Schnitzler A. Pain affect without pain sensation in a patient with a postcentral lesion. Pain 1999; 81:211–214.

11. Head H, Holmes G. Sensory disturbances from cerebral lesions. Brain 1911; 34:102–154.

12. Melzack R, Wall PD. Pain Mechanisms: a new theory. Science 1965; 150:971–979.

13. Caterina MJ, Gold MS, Meyer RA. Molecular biology of nociceptors. In: Hunt S, Koltzenburg M, eds. The Neurobiology of Pain. Oxford: Oxford University Press, 2005:1–33.

14. Sengupta JN, Gebhart GF. Characterization of mechanosensitive pelvic nerve afferent fibers innervating the colon of the rat. J Neurophysiol 1994; 71:2046–2060.

15. Sengupta JN, Kauvar D, Goyal RK Characteristics of vagal esophageal tension-sensitive afferent fibers in the opossum. J Neurophysiol 1989; 61:1001–1010.

16. Bandler R, Shipley MT. Columnar organization in the midbrain periaqueductal gray: modules for emotional expression? Trends Neurosci 1994; 17:379–389.

17. Johnson MH, How does distraction work in the management of pain? Curr Pain Headache Rep 2005; 9:90–95.

18. Lieberman HR et al. Mood, performance, and pain sensitivity: changes induced by food constituents. J Psychiatr Res 1982; 17:135–145.

19. Frye CA, Cuevas CA, Kanarek RB. Diet and estrous cycle influence pain sensitivity in rats. Pharmacol Biochem Behav 1993; 45:255–260.

20. McGivern RF, Berntson GG. Mediation of diurnal fluctuations in pain sensitivity in the rat by food intake patterns: reversal by naloxone. Science 1980; 210:210–211.

21. Gibson SJ, Farrell M. A review of age differences in the neurophysiology of nociception and the perceptual experience of pain. Clin J Pain 2004; 20:227–239.

22. Aley KO et al. Chronic hypersensitivity for inflammatory nociceptor sensitization mediated by the epsilon isozyme of protein kinase C. J Neurosci 2000; 20:4680–4685.

23. Ren K et al. Characterization of basal and re-inflammation-associated long-term alteration in pain responsivity following short-lasting neonatal local inflammatory insult. Pain 2004; 110:588–596.

24. Mendell LM, Wall PD. Responses of single dorsal cord cells to peripheral cutaneous unmyelinated fibres. Nature 1965; 206:97–99.

25. Shavit Y et al. Stress, opioid peptides, the immune system, and cancer. J Immunol 1985; 135: 834s–837s.

26. Lewis JW et al. Stress and morphine affect survival of rats challenged with a mammary ascites tumor (MAT 13762B). Nat Immun Cell Growth Regul 1983; 3:43–50.

27. Merskey H et al. Pain terms: a list with definitions and notes on usage. Recommended by the IASP subcommittee on taxonomy. Pain 1979; 6:249–252.

28. Backonja MM. Defining neuropathic pain. Anesth Analg 2003; 97:785–790.

29. Backonja MM, Stacey B. Neuropathic pain symptoms relative to overall pain rating. J Pain 2004; 5:491–497.

30. Koltzenburg M, Lundberg LER, Torebjörk HE. Dynamic and static components of mechanical hyperalgesia in human hairy skin. Pain 1992; 51:207–219.

31. Mayer EA, Naliboff B, Munakata J. The evolving neurobiology of gut feelings. Prog Brain Res 2000; 122:195–206.

32. Price DD. Central neural mechanisms that interrelate sensory and affective dimensions of pain. Mol Interv 2002; 2:339,392–403.

33. Tominaga M, Caterina MJ. Thermosensation and pain. J Neurobiol 2004; 61:3–12.

34. Gold MS. Molecular basis of receptors. In: Merskey H, Loeser JD, Dubner R, eds. The paths of pain 1975–2005. Seattle: IASP Press, 2005.

35. McCarter GC, Reichling DB, Levine JD, Mechanical transduction by rat dorsal root ganglion neurons in vitro. Neurosci Lett 1999; 273:179–182.

36. Caterina MJ et al. The capsaicin receptor: a heat-activated ion channel in the pain pathway. Nature 1997; 389:816–824.

37. McKemy DD, Neuhausser WM, Julius D, Identification of a cold receptor reveals a general role for TRP channels in thermosensation. Nature 2002; 416:52–58.

38. Peier AM et al. A TRP channel that senses cold stimuli and menthol. Cell 2002; 108:705–715.

39. Chen CC et al. A sensory neuron-specific, proton-gated ion channel. Proc Natl Acad Sci USA 1998; 95:10240–10245.

40. Waldmann R et al. Molecular cloning of a non-inactivating proton-gated Na+ channel specific for sensory neurons. J Biol Chem 1997; 272:20975–20978.

41. Waldmann R et al. A proton-gated cation channel involved in acid-sensing. Nature 1997; 386: 173–177.

42. Page AJ et al. Different contributions of ASIC channels 1a, 2, and 3 in gastrointestinal mechanosensory function. Gut 2005; 54:1408–1415.

43. Kellenberger S, Schild L. Epithelial sodium channel/degenerin family of ion channels: a variety of functions for a shared structure. Physiol Rev 2002; 82:735–767.

44. Birder LA. More than just a barrier: urothelium as a drug target for urinary bladder pain. Am J Physiol Renal Physiol 2005; 289:F489–F495.
45. Wynn G et al. Purinergic mechanisms contribute to mechanosensory transduction in the rat colorectum. Gastroenterology 2003; 125:1398–1409.
46. North RA. P2X3 receptors and peripheral pain mechanisms. J Physiol 2004; 554:301–308.
47. Wynn G et al. Purinergic component of mechanosensory transduction is increased in a rat model of colitis. Am J Physiol Gastrointest Liver Physiol 2004; 287:G647–G657.
48. Dang K et al. Gastric ulcers evoke hyperexcitability and enhance P2X receptor function in rat gastric sensory neurons. J Neurophysiol 2005; 93:3112–3119.
49. Xu GY, Huang LY. Peripheral inflammation sensitizes P2X receptor-mediated responses in rat dorsal root ganglion neurons. J Neurosci 2002; 22:93–102.
50. Basbaum AI, Fields HL. Endogenous pain control systems: brainstem spinal pathways and endorphin circuitry. Annu Rev Neurosci 1984; 7:309–338.
51. Fields HL, Basbaum AI. Brainstem control of spinal pain-transmission neurons. Annu Rev Physiol 1978; 40:217–248.
52. Reynolds DV. Surgery in the rat during electrical analgesia induced by focal brain stimulation. Science 1969; 164:444–445.
53. Porreca F, Ossipov MH, Gebhart GF. Chronic pain and medullary descending facilitation. Trends Neurosci 2002; 25:319–325.
54. Fields HL, Heinricher MM, Mason P. Neurotransmitters in nociceptive modulatory circuits. Annu Rev Neurosci 1991; 14:219–245.
55. Stein C, Schäfer M, Hassan AH. Peripheral opioid receptors. Ann Med 1995; 27:219–221.
56. Khasar SG, et al. Estrogen regulates adrenal medullary function producing sexual dimorphism in nociceptive threshold and beta-adrenergic receptor-mediated hyperalgesia in the rat. Eur J Neurosci 2005; 21:3379–3386.
57. Khasar SG, Green PG, Levine JD. Repeated sound stress enhances inflammatory pain in the rat. Pain 2005; 116:79–86.
58. Cooper B. Contribution of edema to the sensitization of high-threshold mechanoreceptors of the goat palatal mucosa. J Neurophysiol 1993; 70:512–521.
59. Birder LA et al. Feline interstitial cystitis results in mechanical hypersensitivity and altered ATP release from bladder urothelium. Am J Physiol Renal Physiol 2003; 285:F423–F429.
60. Yiangou Y et al. Increased acid-sensing ion channel ASIC-3 in inflamed human intestine. Eur J Gastroenterol Hepatol 2001; 13:891–896.
61. Dray A, Perkins M. Bradykinin and inflammatory pain. Trends Neurosci 1993; 16:99–104.
62. Cho HJ et al. Expression of mRNA for brain-derived neurotrophic factor in the dorsal root ganglion following peripheral inflammation. Brain Res 1997; 749:358–362.
63. Fukuoka T et al. Brain-derived neurotrophic factor increases in the uninjured dorsal root ganglion neurons in selective spinal nerve ligation model. J Neurosci 2001; 21:4891–900.
64. Michael GJ et al. Nerve growth factor treatment increases brain-derived neurotrophic factor selectively in TrkA-expressing dorsal root ganglion cells and in their central terminations within the spinal cord. J Neurosci 1997; 17:8476–8490.
65. Prescott ED, Julius D. A modular PIP2 binding site as a determinant of capsaicin receptor sensitivity. Science 2003; 300:1284–1288.
66. Ji RR et al. p38 MAPK activation by NGF in primary sensory neurons after inflammation increases TRPV1 levels and maintains heat hyperalgesia. Neuron 2002; 36:57–68.
67. Shu X, Mendell LM. Acute sensitization by NGF of the response of small-diameter sensory neurons to capsaicin. J Neurophysiol 2001; 86:2931–2938.
68. Tominaga M et al. The cloned capsaicin receptor integrates multiple pain-producing stimuli. Neuron 1998; 21:531–543; [see comments].
69. Reeh PW, Petho G. Nociceptor excitation by thermal sensitization—a hypothesis. Prog Brain Res 2000; 129:39–50.
70. Catterall WA. Molecular mechanisms of gating and drug block of sodium channels. Novartis Found Symp 2002; 241:206–218; discussion 218–232.
71. Fitzgerald EM et al. Cyclic AMP-dependent phosphorylation of the tetrodotoxin-resistant voltage-dependent sodium channel SNS. J Physiol (Lond) 1999; 516:433–446.
72. Isom LL. I. Cellular and molecular biology of sodium channel beta-subunits: therapeutic implications for pain? I. Cellular and molecular biology of sodium channel beta-subunits: therapeutic implications for pain?. Am J Physiol Gastrointest Liver Physiol 2000; 278:G349–G353.
73. Lai J et al. Voltage-gated sodium channels and hyperalgesia. Annu Rev Pharmacol Toxicol 2004; 44:371–397.
74. Takahashi N et al. Expression of auxiliary beta subunits of sodium channels in primary afferent neurons and the effect of nerve injury. Neuroscience 2003; 121:441–450.
75. Shah BS et al. Beta3, a novel auxiliary subunit for the voltage-gated sodium channel, is expressed preferentially in sensory neurons and is upregulated in the chronic constriction injury model of neuropathic pain. Eur J Neurosci 2000; 12:3985–3990.
76. Flake NM et al. Absence of an association between axotomy-induced changes in sodium currents and excitability in DRG neurons from the adult rat. Pain 2004; 109:471–480.

77. Cummins TR, Waxman SG. Downregulation of tetrodotoxin-resistant sodium currents and upregulation of a rapidly repriming tetrodotoxin-sensitive sodium current in small spinal sensory neurons after nerve injury. J Neurosci 1997; 17:3503–3514.
78. Patton DE et al. The adult rat brain beta 1 subunit modifies activation and inactivation gating of multiple sodium channel alpha subunits. J Biol Chem 1994; 269:17649–17655.
79. Gold MS. Sodium channels and pain therapy. Cur Op Anaesthesiol 2000; 13:565–572.
80. Rudy B. Diversity and ubiquity of K channels. Neuroscience 1988; 25:729–749.
81. Zhang XF, Gopalakrishnan M, Shieh CC. Modulation of action potential firing by iberiotoxin and NS1619 in rat dorsal root ganglion neurons. Neuroscience 2003; 122:1003–1011.
82. Cordoba-Rodriguez R et al. Calcium regulation of a slow post-spike hyperpolarization in vagal afferent neurons. Proc Natl Acad Sci USA 1999; 96:7650–7657.
83. Willis WD Jr., Dorsal root potentials and dorsal root reflexes: a double-edged sword. Exp Brain Res 1999; 124:395–421.
84. Nicol GD, Vasko MR, Evans AR. Prostaglandins suppress an outward potassium current in embryonic rat sensory neurons. J Neurophysiol 1997; 77:167–176.
85. Dang K, Bielefeldt K, Gebhart GF. Gastric ulcers reduce A-type potassium currents in rat gastric sensory ganglion neurons. Am J Physiol Gastrointest Liver Physiol 2004; 286:G573–G579.
86. Stewart T, Beyak MJ, Vanner S. Ileitis modulates potassium and sodium currents in guinea pig dorsal root ganglia sensory neurons. J Physiol 2003; 552:797–807.
87. Yoshimura N, de Groat WC. Increased excitability of afferent neurons innervating rat urinary bladder after chronic bladder inflammation. J Neurosci 1999; 19:4644–4653.
88. Everill B, Kocsis JD. Nerve injury reduces total potassium conductance of two of three identified currents in adult cutaneous afferent dorsal root ganglion neurons. Soc Neurosci Abs 1997; 23:1745.
89. Gold MS, Shuster MJ, Levine JD. Role of a slow Ca2+-dependent slow afterhyperpolarization in prostaglandin E2-induced sensitization of cultured rat sensory neurons. Neurosci Lett 1996; 205:161–164.
90. Lancaster E et al. Calcium and calcium-activated currents in vagotomized rat primary vagal afferent neurons. J Physiol 2002; 540:543–556.
91. Altier C, Zamponi GW. Targeting Ca2+ channels to treat pain: T-type versus N-type. Trends Pharmacol Sci, 2004; 25:465–470.
92. Bourinet E et al. Silencing of the Cav3.2 T-type calcium channel gene in sensory neurons demonstrates its major role in nociception. Embo J 2005; 24:315–324.
93. White G, Lovinger DM, Weight FF. Transient low-threshold Ca2+ current triggers burst firing through an afterdepolarizing potential in an adult mammalian neuron. Proc Nat Acad Sci 1989; 86:6802–6806.
94. Hogan QH et al. Painful neuropathy decreases membrane calcium current in mammalian primary afferent neurons. Pain 2000; 86:43–53.
95. Borgland SL et al. Prostaglandin E(2) inhibits calcium current in two sub-populations of acutely isolated mouse trigeminal sensory neurons. J Physiol 2002; 539:433–444.
96. Baccei ML, Kocsis JD. Voltage-gated calcium currents in axotomized adult rat cutaneous afferent neurons. J Neurophysiol 2000; 83:2227–2238.
97. Fields RD, Lee PR, Cohen JE. Temporal integration of intracellular Ca2+ signaling networks in regulating gene expression by action potentials. Cell Calcium 2005; 37:433–442.
98. Matsuka Y et al. Concurrent release of ATP and substance P within guinea pig trigeminal ganglia in vivo. Brain Res 2001; 915:248–255.
99. Amir R, Devor, M. Chemically mediated cross-excitation in rat dorsal root ganglia. J Neurosci 1996; 16:4733–4741.
100. Amir R, Devor M. Functional cross-excitation between afferent A- and C-neurons in dorsal root ganglia. Neuroscience 2000; 95:189–195.
101. Devor M. Unexplained peculiarities of the dorsal root ganglion. Pain 1999; 6(suppl):S27–S35.
102. Byers MR. Dynamic plasticity of dental sensory nerve structure and cytochemistry. Arch Oral Biol 1994; 39(suppl):13S–21S.
103. Reinert A, Kaske A, Mense S. Inflammation-induced increase in the density of neuropeptide-immunoreactive nerve endings in rat skeletal muscle. Exp Brain Res 1998; 121:174–180.
104. Ma QP, Tian L. Cholera toxin B subunit labeling in lamina II of spinal cord dorsal horn following chronic inflammation in rats. Neurosci Lett 2002; 327:161–164.
105. Yoshimura M et al. Functional reorganization of the spinal pain pathways in developmental and pathological conditions. Novartis Found Symp 2004; 261:116–124; discussion 124–131, 149–154.
106. Ling QD et al. The pattern and distribution of calcitonin gene-related peptide (CGRP) terminals in the rat dorsal following neonatal peripheral inflammation. Neuroreport 2003; 14:1919–1921.
107. Ruda MA et al. Altered nociceptive neuronal circuits after neonatal peripheral inflammation. Science 2000; 289:628–631.
108. Belyantseva IA, Lewin GR. Stability and plasticity of primary afferent projections following nerve regeneration and central degeneration. Eur J Neurosci 1999; 11:457–468.
109. Woolf CJ. Phenotypic modification of primary sensory neurons: the role of nerve growth factor in the production of persistent pain. Philos Trans R Soc Lond B Biol Sci 1996; 351:441–448.

110. Coull JA et al. Trans-synaptic shift in anion gradient in spinal lamina I neurons as a mechanism of neuropathic pain. Nature 2003; 424:938–942.

111. Taiwo YO, Levine JD. Direct cutaneous hyperalgesia induced by adenosine. Neuroscience 1990; 38:752–762.

112. Gold MS et al. Hyperalgesic agents increase a tetrodotoxin-resistant Na+ current in nociceptors. Proc Natl Acad Sci USA 1996; 93:1108–1112.

113. North RA. Molecular physiology of P2X receptors. Physiol Rev 2002; 82:1013–1067.

114. Spelta V et al. Extracellular ATP enhances ASIC3—like current in ischemia sensing neurons through an electrically quiet ion channel. Soc Neurosci Abs Program 859.4, 2004.

115. Wang HL et al. Heterodimerization of opioid receptor-like 1 and μ-opioid receptors impairs the potency of micro receptor agonist. J Neurochem 2005; 92:1285–1294.

116. Law PY et al. Heterodimerization of μ- and delta-opioid receptors occurs at the cell surface only and requires receptor-G protein interactions. J Biol Chem 2005; 280:11152–11164.

117. Pfeiffer M et al. Heterodimerization of substance P and μ-opioid receptors regulates receptor trafficking and resensitization. J Biol Chem 2003; 278:51630–51637.

118. Wang H, Woolf CJ. Pain TRPs. Neuron 2005; 46:9–12.

119. Tao YX et al. Impaired NMDA receptor-mediated postsynaptic function and blunted NMDA receptor-dependent persistent pain in mice lacking postsynaptic density-93 protein. J Neurosci 2003; 23:6703–6712.

120. Gold MS, Flake NM. Inflammation-mediated hyperexcitability of sensory neurons. Neurosignals 2005; 14:147–157.

121. Khasar SG et al. A novel nociceptor signaling pathway revealed in protein kinase C epsilon mutant mice. Neuron 1999; 24:253–260.

122. Taiwo YO et al. Mediation of primary afferent peripheral hyperalgesia by the cAMP second messenger system. Neuroscience 1989; 32:577–80.

123. Gold MS, Levine JD, Correa AM. Modulation of TTX-R INa by PKC and PKA and their role in PGE2-induced sensitization of rat sensory neurons In vitro [In Process Citation]. J Neurosci 1998; 18:10345–10355.

124. Chuang HH et al. Bradykinin and nerve growth factor release the capsaicin receptor from PtdIns(4,5)P2-mediated inhibition. Nature 2001; 411:957–962.

125. Huang CL, Feng S, Hilgemann DW. Direct activation of inward rectifier potassium channels by PIP2 and its stabilization by Gbetagamma. Nature 1998; 391:803–806.

126. Ferreira SH. The role of interleukins and nitric oxide in the mediation of inflammatory pain and its control by peripheral analgesics. Drugs 1993; 46(suppl 1):1–9.

127. Zhang YH, Vasko MR, Nicol GD. Ceramide, a putative second messenger for nerve growth factor, modulates the TTX-resistant Na(+) current and delayed rectifier K(+) current in rat sensory neurons. J Physiol 2002; 544:385–402.

128. Zhuang ZY et al. Phosphatidylinositol 3-kinase activates ERK in primary sensory neurons and mediates inflammatory heat hyperalgesia through TRPV1 sensitization. J Neurosci 2004; 24:8300–8309.

129. Misonou H et al. Regulation of ion channel localization and phosphorylation by neuronal activity. Nat Neurosci 2004; 7:711–718.

130. Zhuang ZY et al. ERK is sequentially activated in neurons, microglia, and astrocytes by spinal nerve ligation and contributes to mechanical allodynia in this neuropathic pain model. Pain 2005; 114: 149–159.

131. Selbie LA, Hill SJ. G protein-coupled-receptor cross-talk: the fine-tuning of multiple receptor-signalling pathways. Trends Pharmacol Sci 1998; 19:87–93.

132. Hucho TB, Dina OA, Levine JD. Epac mediates a cAMP-to-PKC signaling in inflammatory pain: an isolectin B4(+) neuron-specific mechanism. J Neurosci 2005; 25:6119–6126.

133. Zhou XB et al. A molecular switch for specific stimulation of the BKCa channel by cGMP and cAMP kinase. J Biol Chem 2001; 276:43239–43245.

134. Villarreal CF et al. The role of Na(V)1.8 sodium channel in the maintenance of chronic inflammatory hypernociception. Neurosci Lett 2005; 386:72–77.

135. Holthusen H. Involvement of the NO/cyclic GMP pathway in bradykinin-evoked pain from veins in humans. Pain 1997; 69:87–92.

136. Nakamura A, Fujita M, Shiomi, H. Involvement of endogenous nitric oxide in the mechanism of bradykinin-induced peripheral hyperalgesia. Br J Pharmacol 1996; 117:407–412.

137. Aley KO, McCarter G, Levine JD. Nitric oxide signaling in pain and nociceptor sensitization in the rat. J Neurosci 1998; 18:7008–7014.

138. Sachs D, Cunha FQ, Ferreira SH. Peripheral analgesic blockade of hypernociception: activation of arginine/NO/cGMP/protein kinase G/ATP-sensitive K+ channel pathway. Proc Natl Acad Sci USA 2004; 101:3680–3685.

139. Vivancos GG, Parada CA, Ferreira SH. Opposite nociceptive effects of the arginine/NO/cGMP pathway stimulation in dermal and subcutaneous tissues. Br J Pharmacol 2003; 138:1351–1357.

140. Levy D, Strassman AM. Modulation of dural nociceptor mechanosensitivity by the nitric oxide-cyclic GMP signaling cascade. J Neurophysiol 2004; 92:766–772.

141. Levi-Montalcini R et al. Nerve growth factor: from neurotrophin to neurokine. Trends Neurosci 1996; 19:514–520.

142. Bonnington JK, McNaughton PA. Signalling pathways involved in the sensitisation of mouse nociceptive neurones by nerve growth factor. J Physiol 2003; 551:433–446.
143. Obata K et al. Differential activation of extracellular signal-regulated protein kinase in primary afferent neurons regulates brain-derived neurotrophic factor expression after peripheral inflammation and nerve injury. J Neurosci 2003; 23:4117–4126.
144. Guo H, Huang LY. Alteration in the voltage dependence of NMDA receptor channels in rat dorsal horn neurones following peripheral inflammation. J Physiol 2001; 537:115–123.
145. Dolan S et al. Up-regulation of metabotropic glutamate receptor subtypes 3 and 5 in spinal cord in a clinical model of persistent inflammation and hyperalgesia. Pain 2003; 106:501–512.
146. Guan Y et al. Inflammation-induced upregulation of AMPA receptor subunit expression in brain stem pain modulatory circuitry. Pain 2003; 104:401–413.
147. Guo W et al. Activation of spinal kainate receptors after inflammation: behavioral hyperalgesia and subunit gene expression. Eur J Pharmacol 2002; 452:309–318.
148. Ohtori S et al. Up-regulation of substance P and NMDA receptor mRNA in dorsal horn and preganglionic sympathetic neurons during adjuvant-induced noxious stimulation in rats. Ann Anat 2002; 184:71–76.
149. Hains BC et al. Altered sodium channel expression in second-order spinal sensory neurons contributes to pain after peripheral nerve injury. J Neurosci 2004; 24:4832–4829.
150. Hu HJ, Glauner KS, Gereau RWt. ERK integrates PKA and PKC signaling in superficial dorsal horn neurons. I. Modulation of A-type K+ currents. J Neurophysiol 2003; 90:1671–1679.
151. Hains BC, Saab CY, Waxman SG. Changes in electrophysiological properties and sodium channel Nav1.3 expression in thalamic neurons after spinal cord injury. Brain 2005.
152. Iadarola MJ et al. Enhancement of dynorphin gene expression in spinal cord following experimental inflammation: stimulus specificity, behavioral parameters and opioid receptor binding. Pain 1988; 35:313–326.
153. Kohno T et al. Peripheral axonal injury results in reduced μ opioid receptor pre- and post-synaptic action in the spinal cord. Pain 2005; 117:77–87.
154. Scholz J et al. Blocking caspase activity prevents transsynaptic neuronal apoptosis and the loss of inhibition in lamina II of the dorsal horn after peripheral nerve injury. J Neurosci 2005; 25:7317–7323.
155. Noguchi K et al. Axotomy induces preprotachykinin gene expression in a subpopulation of dorsal root ganglion neurons. J Neurosci Res 1994; 37:596–603.
156. Cho HJ et al. Expression of mRNAs for preprotachykinin and nerve growth factor receptors in the dorsal root-ganglion following peripheral inflammation. Brain Res 1996; 716:197–201.
157. Craft RM, Mogil JS, Aloisi AM. Sex differences in pain and analgesia: the role of gonadal hormones. Eur J Pain 2004; 8:397–411.
158. Fillingim RB, Ness TJ. Sex-related hormonal influences on pain and analgesic responses. Neurosci Biobehav Rev 2000; 24:485–501.
159. Berkley KJ. Sex differences in pain. Behav Brain Sci 1997; 20:371–380.
160. LeResche L. Epidemiology of temporomandibular disorders: implications for the investigation of etiologic factors. Crit Rev Oral Biol Med 1997; 8:291–305.
161. Unruh AM. Gender variations in clinical pain experience. Pain 1996; 65:123–67.
162. Yang Y et al. Mutations in SCN9A, encoding a sodium channel alpha subunit, in patients with primary erythermalgia. J Med Genet 2004; 41:171–174.
163. Ophoff RA et al. Familial hemiplegic migraine and episodic ataxia type-2 are caused by mutations in the Ca2+ channel gene CACNL1A4. Cell 1996; 87:543–552.
164. Fillingim RB et al. The A118G single nucleotide polymorphism of the μ-opioid receptor gene (OPRM1) is associated with pressure pain sensitivity in humans. J Pain 2005; 6:159–167.
165. Stamer UM et al. Impact of CYP2D6 genotype on postoperative tramadol analgesia. Pain 2003; 105:231–238.
166. Mogil JS et al. The melanocortin-1 receptor gene mediates female-specific mechanisms of analgesia in mice and humans. Proc Natl Acad Sci USA 2003; 100:4867–4872.
167. Zubieta JK et al. COMT val158met genotype affects μ-opioid neurotransmitter responses to a pain stressor. Science 2003; 299:1240–1243.
168. Diatchenko L et al. Genetic basis for individual variations in pain perception and the development of a chronic pain condition. Hum Mol Genet 2005; 14:135–143.
169. Yoshimura N et al. Gene therapy of bladder pain with herpes simplex virus (HSV) vectors expressing preproenkephalin (PPE). Urology 2001; 57:116.
170. Honore P et al. TNP-ATP, a potent P2X3 receptor antagonist, blocks acetic acid-induced abdominal constriction in mice: comparison with reference analgesics. Pain 2002; 96:99–105.

4 | Neuroanatomy of Visceral Pain: Pathways and Processes

Elie D. Al-Chaer
*Departments of Pediatrics, Neurobiology and Developmental Sciences, Center for Pain Research,
College of Medicine, University of Arkansas for Medical Sciences, Little Rock, Arkansas, U.S.A.*

William D. Willis
*Department of Neuroscience and Cell Biology, University of Texas Medical Branch,
Galveston, Texas, U.S.A.*

PERIPHERAL PATHWAYS
The Enteric Nervous System

The gastrointestinal (GI) tract and accessory organs (e.g., liver and biliary tree) have a rich sensory innervation (1). Sensory afferents from the digestive tract project to the central nervous system (CNS) in the vagus and spinal sensory nerves. However, some enteric reflexes (e.g., mucosal stroking) are retained after connections to the CNS are severed indicating that the neural network of the enteric nervous system (ENS) contains the elements necessary for assimilation of information and coordinated motor output (2). These intrinsic sensory neurons in the enteric neural networks do not project to the CNS and therefore are not believed to contribute to gut sensations per se. This chapter will focus on extrinsic primary afferents because these tend to be more involved in visceral sensory processing and relay to the CNS.

Projections to the Central Nervous System

Unlike somatic (i.e., nonvisceral) tissue, the viscera are innervated by two sets of primary afferent fibers that project to distinct regions of the CNS. Innervation of the GI tract from the esophagus through the transverse colon is provided by vagal afferent fibers originating in the nodose ganglia and projecting centrally to the nucleus of the solitary tract. The remaining lower bowel is innervated by pelvic nerve afferent fibers, originating in the sacral (human; lumbosacral in rat) dorsal root ganglia, and projecting centrally to the sacral spinal cord. The entire GI tract is also innervated by afferent fibers in the splanchnic nerves projecting to the T5-L2 segments of the spinal cord. For example, colonic afferent fibers project in both the pelvic and the splanchnic nerves (3,4). Because these afferents run in mixed-nerve bundles that contain the autonomic outflow from the CNS, they are often referred to as parasympathetic and sympathetic afferents. This terminology is a misnomer because "parasympathetic" and "sympathetic" are terms reserved exclusively for autonomic motor function. The correct terminology refers to them as "vagal, pelvic, or splanchnic nerves" because these terms accurately describe the route the three kinds of afferents follow to the brainstem and spinal cord. Aside from the visceral afferents in vagal, splanchnic, and pelvic nerves, somatic afferents that innervate the striated musculature of the pelvic floor project to the sacral spinal cord via the pudendal nerve.

In contrast to somatic afferent fibers, visceral afferents have no end organs or morphological specialization. Endings of vagal and spinal sensory neurons terminate within the muscle, mucosal epithelia, and ganglia of the ENS (5). Spinal afferents terminate also in the serosa and mesenteric attachments and form a dense network around mesenteric blood vessels and their intramural tributaries.

Vagal afferent endings in the mucosa are in close association with the lamina propria adjacent to the mucosal epithelium where they monitor the chemical nature of luminal contents, either following their passage across the epithelium or via input from epithelial enteroendocrine cells. Nutrients cross the epithelium to reach the afferent nerve terminals in the lamina propria. In addition, luminal nutrients release messenger molecules [e.g., cholecystokinin and 5-hydroxytryptamine (HT)] from mucosal enteroendocrine cells. These molecules activate afferent terminals that lie in close proximity in the lamina propria (6).

Spinal afferents are subdivided into splanchnic and pelvic afferents. They follow the path of sympathetic and parasympathetic efferents that project to the gut wall. Axons of spinal afferents are almost exclusively thinly myelinated A-delta and unmyelinated C fibers; they exhibit chemosensitivity, thermosensitivity, and/or mechanosensitivity. There are two physiological classes of nociceptive viscerosensory receptors: (i) low-threshold afferents that respond initially to physiological distension but continue to encode levels of distension that cause pain; and, (ii) high-threshold afferents that respond to noxious distension (7). Experimental data suggest that the viscera also contain spinal nociceptive afferent fibers that are normally considered "silent" but maybe sensitized by inflammation. Silent nociceptors do not respond at all in the normal intestine but become responsive to distension when the intestine is injured or inflamed (8). This receptor behavior illustrates how mechanosensitivity is not fixed either in terms of the threshold for sensory activation or the relationship between stimulus and response. Injury and inflammation decrease the threshold and increase the magnitude of the response for a given stimulus—a phenomenon known as peripheral sensitization (9).

The distribution of these fibers also varies among organs. High-threshold receptors exclusively innervate organs from which pain is the only conscious sensation (i.e., ureter, kidney, lungs, heart), but are relatively few in organs that provide innocuous and noxious sensations (e.g., colon, stomach, and bladder) , innervated mostly by low-threshold receptors.

Spinal afferents have multiple receptive fields extending over a relatively wide area. Those in the serosa and mesenteric attachments respond to distortion of the viscera during distension and contraction. Other endings detect changes in the submucosal chemical milieu following injury, ischemia, or infection and may play a role in generating hypersensitivity. Intramural spinal afferent fibers have collateral branches that innervate blood vessels and enteric ganglia. These contain and release neurotransmitters during local axon reflexes that influence GI blood flow, motility and secretory reflexes (10). Spinal afferents en route to the spinal cord also branch into collaterals that innervate prevertebral sympathetic ganglia neurons. The same sensory information is thereby transmitted to information processing circuits in the spinal cord, ENS, and prevertebral ganglia. The main transmitters are glutamate, calcitonin gene-related peptide and substance P, and both peptides are implicated in the induction of neurogenic inflammation.

Sensory transduction in visceral afferents depends upon the modulation of ion channels and/or receptors on the sensory nerve terminal (6). Mechanosensitivity may arise indirectly following the release of chemical mediators such as adenosine triphosphate, which, in turn, act on purinergic receptors present on afferent nerve terminals. Alternatively, there may be direct activation via mechanosensitive ion channels in these afferent nerve terminals. Mechanical deformation of the nerve ending opens or closes ion channels, depolarizing the terminal to threshold and causing action potential firing.

CENTRAL PATHWAYS

Upon entering the dorsal horn, visceral afferents terminate in spinal cord laminae I, II, V, and X (11). Visceral afferents constitute less than 10% of afferent inflow into the spinal cord. This is a relatively small percentage when one considers the large surface area of some organs. Both anatomical and electrophysiological studies have demonstrated viscerosomatic convergence in both the dorsal horn and supraspinal centers (11–15). There is also evidence of viscerovisceral convergence onto these second-order neurons. Examples include the convergence of pelvic visceral inputs such as colon/rectum, bladder, uterine cervix, and vagina (3,11). Along with the low density of visceral nociceptors and the functional divergence of visceral input within the CNS, viscerovisceral convergence in the spinal cord may explain poorly localized visceral pain.

Visceral information carried by the pelvic nerve converges onto spinal neurons in the lumbosacral segments of the cord and that carried by the splanchnic nerves onto thoracolumbar segments (16). Centrally, ascending pathways involved in the transmission of visceral nociceptive information include the spinothalamic tract (STT) , spinohypothalamic tract, spinosolitary tract, spinoreticular tract, spinoparabrachial tract, and other tracts located in the anterolateral quadrant (ALQ) . In addition, a number of recent studies have pointed to a role

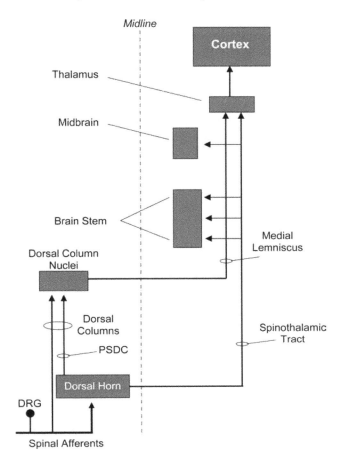

Figure 1 Schematic illustration of ascending spinal pathways and related centers involved in visceral nociceptive processing. *Abbreviations*: DRG, dorsal root ganglia; PSDC, postsynaptic dorsal column.

of the dorsal column in viscerosensory processing, opening the door for a new role of the dorsal column in visceral pain (17,18). For a schematic illustration of these pathways, see Figure 1.

Pathways in the Anterolateral Quadrant

Pathways ascending in the ALQ of the spinal cord, such as the STT, are known to be important in transmitting signals evoked by noxious cutaneous stimuli and have been proposed to carry nociceptive information of visceral origin (19). The role of the ALQ in cutaneous nociception is supported by a large amount of experimental and clinical evidence; however, the data pertinent to the role of the ALQ in processing noxious visceral information is not conclusive.

Transection of the ventral quadrant of the spinal cord in the dog raised the threshold for cutaneous nociception (20); this observation was used as an experimental basis for the introduction of cordotomy as a treatment of pain in humans (21). Several investigators have found that ventrolateral cordotomy produced somatic analgesia on the side contralateral to the lesion in monkeys (22–24). It is interesting, however, that reactions to painful stimuli applied to one side of the body in cats are not prevented by hemisecting the contralateral cord (25,26). Even a bilateral lesion often fails to prevent reactions to noxious stimuli in cats (27). The discrepancies between the observations reported in the cat and those reported in the dog may be due to a more prominent STT in the latter (28).

Spinothalamic Tract

The STT in humans is regarded as the pathway that mediates the sensations of pain, cold, and warmth, and it also contributes to touch (29–31). This idea is based largely on the results of anterolateral cordotomies performed in the 20th century to relieve pain (19,21) or deficits due to damage to the spinal cord by disease or trauma (32–34). Results of experimental studies of primates in which changes in behavioral responses to noxious stimuli before and after spinal lesions were measured, proved to be consistent with the clinical evidence (22,25,35).

The cells of origin of the STT have been mapped in monkeys, cats, and rats (31). It may be safe to assume that the pattern in monkeys is closest to that in human organization. In monkeys, a large fraction of STT cells is located in the lumbar and sacral enlargements, and these cells are concentrated in the marginal zone and neck of the dorsal horn in laminae I and IV to VI (36,37). However, some spinothalamic cells are located in other laminae, including lamina X, which is around the central canal, and in the ventral horn. Comparison of the populations of STT cells projecting to the lateral thalamus, including the ventral posterior lateral (VPL) nucleus, and those projecting to the medial thalamus, including the central lateral nucleus, show clear differences between the two (36). Laterally projecting spinothalamic neurons are more likely to be situated in laminae I and V, whereas medially projecting cells are more likely to be situated in the deep dorsal horn and in the ventral horn. Most of the cells project to the contralateral thalamus, although a small fraction projects ipsilaterally. A large group of STT cells is also located in segments C1 and C2 (37), in lamina VIII bilaterally, and in laminae I to VII contralaterally to the thalamic target.

The projections of the STT have been traced to the thalamus in humans, as well as in monkeys, cats, rats, and other experimental animals (31). The axons of spinothalamic neurons often decussate through the ventral white commissure at a very short distance from the cell body (36). They initially enter the ventral funiculus and then shift into the lateral funiculus as they ascend. Axons from STT cells of lamina I ascend more dorsally in the lateral funiculus than do the axons of STT cells in deeper layers of the dorsal horn (38).

Most STT cells studied have cutaneous receptive fields and respond to noxious and often also to innocuous mechanical stimulation of the skin (39–41). They can also be activated by stimulation of visceral afferent fibers. Many STT cells in the cat and monkey are excited by stimulation of cardiopulmonary visceral afferents (42,43) and of the greater splanchnic nerve (44,45). STT neurons can also be excited by distension of the gall bladder (46), the kidney (47), the ureter (48), or the urinary bladder (49). Milne et al. (49) recorded from STT cells in the upper lumbar and sacral segments of the monkey spinal cord in response to urinary bladder distension and noxious testicular stimulation. Thoracic and cervical STT neurons in the monkey were also excited by stimulation of A-delta and C-fiber cardiopulmonary sympathetic afferents that pass through the stellate ganglion (50–52). On the other hand, lumbosacral STT neurons are inhibited by noxious stimulation of visceral and somatic afferent fibers that enter thoracic segments (53,54). These observations are consistent with the idea that modulation of spinal nociceptive transmission might involve neuronal connections in high cervical segments (55).

In the rat, colorectal distension excited unidentified tract cells in the lumbosacral cord (56). Many of these units were antidromically activated by stimulation of the ventral quadrant of the cervical spinal cord; they also responded to tail movements and cutaneous stimuli on the scrotum and the perineal area. On the other hand, deep STT cells activated by innocuous stimuli or proprioceptive input were also inhibited by urinary bladder distension (49,57). Recently, Palecek et al. (58) reported that ureter distention evoked Fos expression in STT neurons located in laminae I, III to VII, and X of the rat spinal cord.

Clinically, unilateral anterolateral cordotomy is most effective for the treatment of unilateral pain, especially when somatic structures are involved. By contrast, bilateral anterolateral cordotomy has been proposed and performed for the relief of diffuse intractable visceral pain (19,30,59); however, pain relief is often accompanied by complications (30), including extremity paresis, bowel, bladder, and sexual dysfunction, respiratory difficulty and occasionally dysesthesias due to the development of a central pain state. In addition, recurrence of pain is often reported within a few months after an initially successful operation (19,30). These observations leave the door open for other spinal pathways to be involved in viscerosensory processing.

Pathways in the Dorsal Funiculus

The dorsal funiculus, also referred to as the dorsal column in animals or the posterior column in man, contains collateral branches of primary afferent fibers that ascend from the dorsal root entry level all the way to the medulla (31). In addition, it contains the ascending axons of tract cells of the dorsal horn (60–65). These tract cells form the postsynaptic dorsal column pathway, which along with primary afferent axons, travels in the dorsal column and synapses in the dorsal column nuclei. The dorsal funiculus is subdivided into two components, one known as the fasciculus gracilis, containing the ascending afferents from levels caudal to the midthoracic region, and the other fasciculus cuneatus, containing the ascending afferents that originate from midthoracic to upper cervical levels. The gracilis and cuneatus fasciculi terminate at the level of the lower medulla in the nucleus gracilis and the nucleus cuneatus, respectively, collectively known as the dorsal column nuclei.

Classical teaching holds that the dorsal column subserves graphesthesia, two-point discrimination, and kinesthesia. This concept was adopted at the turn of the 20th century (33,66–68) and was based on the pathologic alterations observed in certain disease states associated with dorsal column lesions and on the skimpy knowledge of spinal tracts available at that time. On the other hand, the evidence for the importance of the dorsal column pathway in the transmission of visceral nociceptive information is compelling. It rests on the great effectiveness of limited midline myelotomy in reducing intractable pelvic cancer pain in humans (69–74) and on a number of groundbreaking experimental observations (12–15,17,18).

In an early report on visceral nociceptive fibers in the dorsal column, awake human subjects experienced unbearable, excruciating pain when the dorsal column or medial aspect of the nucleus gracilis was probed mechanically (75). The pain was referred to the sacral region and perineum. Subsequent studies observed that the sensation of visceral distension was retained following extensive anterolateral cordotomy (76) and that the sensation of duodenal distension was unaffected by a differential spinal block that abolished the sensation of cutaneous pinprick (77) suggesting that these sensations were mediated by a posterior column pathway.

More direct clinical evidence comes from successful neurosurgical procedures aimed at treating intractable visceral pain. These procedures have often accidentally severed dorsal column axons in and around the midline. Commissural myelotomy was introduced as a technique to produce bilateral analgesia by interrupting the decussating axons of the spinothalamic and spinoreticular tracts by means of a longitudinal midline incision extending over several segments (59). The rostrocaudal extent of commissural myelotomy was later reduced to a localized lesion made stereotaxically by inserting a metal electrode into the midline at the C1 level with the patient awake (69–72). The clinical result was an unexpectedly widespread distribution of pain relief, similar to that found with open commissural myelotomy, despite the small extent of the lesion and its location well rostral to the decussation of most of the STT. Similar successes were reported later using limited midline myelotomy to treat pelvic visceral cancer pain (73). This result compelled a major revision in thinking regarding pain pathways in the spinal cord (30). Hirshberg et al. reported eight clinical cases where pelvic visceral cancer pain was successfully treated using a limited posterior midline myelotomy (74). The lesion was placed in the midline at the T10 level of the spinal cord and extended a few millimeters rostrocaudally. Following surgery, the pelvic pain was found to be markedly reduced or eliminated without any demonstrable postoperative neurological deficit. The extent of the lesion in one of the patients was examined histologically postmortem and was found to interrupt axons of the posterior columns at and adjacent to the midline and anteriorly to the level of the posterior gray commissure. More recent studies have lent further support for the concept that neurosurgical interruption of a midline posterior column pathway provides significant pain relief without causing adverse neurological sequelae in cancer patients with visceral pain refractory to other therapies (78–80).

Early experimental evidence that described the dorsal column as the pathway of splanchnic afferents was obtained in rabbits, cats, and dogs (81) and led to the conclusion that the sense of visceral distension may be dependent on the integrity of this afferent projection system. Responses to splanchnic nerve stimulation were recorded "in logical time relationships," in the ipsilateral fasciculus gracilis of the spinal cord, the ipsilateral nucleus gracilis, the region of decussation of the medial lemniscus, the medial lemniscus at various levels in the medulla, pons and caudal thalamus, and in the VPL nucleus of the thalamus, suggesting a continuous pathway for splanchnic input that "parallels that for proprioception from the limbs and trunk" (82). Nociceptive activity, including responses to uterine and vaginal distension, has also been demonstrated in neurons of the dorsal column nuclei (65,83–86). These nociceptive responses could be triggered by unmyelinated primary afferent fibers that have been shown to ascend in the dorsal column directly to the dorsal column nuclei (87–89). Alternatively, they could be mediated through the postsynaptic dorsal column pathway (90–93). More recent studies in primates and rodents have shown that a lesion of the dorsal column can dramatically reduce the responses of neurons in the ventral posterolateral nucleus of the thalamus (12,14,94,95) and in the dorsal column nuclei (13,15,85) to mechanical distension of normal and acutely inflamed colons. They have identified the dorsal column as being more important in visceral nociceptive transmission than the spinothalamic and spinoreticular tracts. In rats and monkeys, colorectal distension stimulates the firing of viscerosensitive VPL thalamic neurons. After a dorsal column lesion at T10 level, the responses are reduced despite ongoing stimulation. A similar lesion of the STT at T10 does not achieve the same effect (12,14). The dorsal column also has a role in signaling epigastric nociception (94,96).

The correspondence between these functional studies in experimental animals and the findings from human neurosurgical studies are consistent with accumulating evidence that strongly supports the concept that the dorsal column projection system is critical for visceral pain sensation.

Postsynaptic Dorsal Column Pathway

The postsynaptic dorsal column pathway arises from cells distributed medial to laterally in lamina III in the dorsal horn, as well as from a few cells just lateral to lamina X (63,91,97–99). The trajectories of postsynaptic dorsal column fibers are somatotopically organized in the dorsal column (74,100,101).

Although the postsynaptic dorsal column pathway in rats may not have a role in cutaneous pain (13,15,102), the postsynaptic dorsal column cells in rats and monkeys were shown to respond to both mechanical and chemical irritation of viscera (13,15). They receive inputs from the colon, the ureter, the pancreas and epigastric structures (96). Presumably, the visceral information is relayed together with cutaneous epicritic information in the medial lemniscus to the thalamus (103).

REPRESENTATION OF VISCERAL SENSATION IN THE BRAIN

In contrast to most other sensory modalities, the neuroanatomical substrates in the brain for pain sensation in general and visceral pain, in particular, have only recently begun to be elucidated. Major advances in this field have come through functional anatomical and physiological studies in nonhuman primates and rats, which have identified substrates that underlie findings from functional imaging and microelectrode studies in humans.

Thalamic Representation of Visceral Sensation

The thalamus plays a major role as a site of convergence of somatic and visceral inputs. Visceral inputs into the thalamus were examined using electrical stimulation of visceral nerves (82,104–106), or natural stimulation of visceral organs (107–110). In monkeys, medial thalamus receives viscerosomatic input via thoracic STT neurons (111), whereas neurons in lateral thalamus are activated by input through the STT and the dorsal column (14). Lateral thalamic neurons can also be excited by colorectal distension or urinary bladder distension and by convergent input elicited by noxious stimulation of somatic receptive fields in proximal lower body regions (107). In fact, the majority of lateral thalamic somatosensory neurons in squirrel monkeys receive somatovisceral and viscerovisceral inputs from naturally stimulated visceral organs (112). In the rat, neurons in and near the thalamic ventrobasal complex respond to stimulation of different visceral organs, including the uterus, the cervix, the vagina, and the colon (12,14,113). Colorectal distension or colon inflammation excites neurons in the ventral posterolateral nucleus of thalamus (12,14,112,113) and in the medial thalamus at the level of the nucleus submedius (114).

On the other hand, the sensation of angina can be evoked by microstimulation in the region of the thalamic principal sensory nucleus (the ventrocaudal nucleus) in humans (115)—a nucleus that corresponds to the ventral posterior nucleus in the cat and the monkey (116,117). Microstimulation in the area ventral and posterior to the ventrocaudal thalamus in the human brain evoked visceral pain sensations and triggered in some cases pain "memories" (118). Electrical stimulation of the thalamic ventrobasal complex in animals inhibits viscerosensory processing in normal rats but facilitates visceral hypersensitivity in rats with neonatal colon pain (119). These observations coupled with an extensive repertoire of experimental data suggest that the thalamus, particularly the posterolateral nucleus, is involved in the processing of visceral information, including both noxious and innocuous visceral inputs.

Viscero-Cortical Pain Processing

The application of functional magnetic resonance imaging and positron-emission tomography has identified a network of brain areas that process visceral sensation from the esophagus (120), stomach (121), and the anorectum (122). Results of these studies suggest that visceral sensation is primarily represented in the secondary somatosensory cortex. Unlike somatic sensation, which has a strong homuncular representation in the primary somatosensory cortex, visceral representations in the primary somatosensory cortex are vague and diffuse (120). This might account for visceral sensation being poorly localized in comparison with somatic sensation. Nevertheless, visceral sensation is represented in paralimbic and limbic structures (e.g., anterior insular cortex, amygdala, and anterior and posterior cingulate cortex), and prefrontal and orbitofrontal cortices (123,124), areas that purportedly process the affective and cognitive components of visceral sensation. Neuroimaging data suggests that differences also exist in the cortical representation of various visceral organs and in the upper versus lower GI tract. For example, the primary sensory motor cortex shows more prominent upper gut representation and the prefrontal and orbitofrontal cortices show greater lower gut representation (125).

Differential cortical activation is also seen when comparing sensation from the visceral and somatic regions of the GI tract, for example, sensations from the esophagus versus the anterior chest wall (126) or the rectum versus the anal canal (122). Brain processing for esophageal and anterior chest wall sensations occurred in a common brain network consisting of secondary somatosensory and parietal cortices, thalamus, basal ganglia, and cerebellum (126). However, differential processing of sensory information from these two areas occurred within the insular, primary sensory, motor, and anterior cingulate and prefrontal cortices. This is consistent with knowledge that similarities exist for visceral and somatic pain experience and might also explain the individual's ability to distinguish between the two modalities and generate differential emotional, autonomic, and motor responses when each modality is individually stimulated.

Gender differences in cortical representation of visceral sensation also occurred among healthy volunteers. Activation in the sensory motor and parieto-occipital areas is common in both males and females following rectal distension; however, greater activation in the anterior cingulate/prefrontal cortices was found in women (127). These gender differences in the processing of sensory input substantiate reports that perceptual responses are exaggerated in female patients with chronic abdominal pain.

REFERENCES

1. Grundy D, Scratcherd T. Sensory afferents from the gastrointestinal tract. In: Wood JD, ed. Handbook of Physiology: The Gastrointestinal System, Motility, and Circulation. Vol. 1. Bethesda, Maryland: American Physiological Society, 1989:593–620.
2. Wood JD. Physiology of the enteric nervous system. In: Johnson LR, Alpers DH, Christensen J, et al., eds. Physiology of the Gastrointestinal Tract. 3rd ed. Vol. 1. New York: Raven Press, 1994:423–482.
3. Berkley KJ, Hubscher CH, Wall PD. Neuronal responses to stimulation of the cervix, uterus, colon, and skin in the rat spinal cord. J Neurophysiol 1993; 69:545–556.
4. Traub RJ, Hutchcroft K, Gebhart GF. The peptide content of colonic afferents decreases following colonic inflammation. Peptides 1999; 20:267–273.
5. Berthoud HR, Kressel M, Raybould HE, et al. Vagal sensors in the rat duodenal mucosa: distribution and structure as revealed by in vivo DiI-tracing. Anat Embryol (Berl) 1995; 191:203–212.
6. Kirkup AJ, Brunsden AM, Grundy D. Receptors and transmission in the brain-gut axis: potential for novel therapies I. Receptors on visceral afferents. Am J Physiol 2001; 280:G787–G794.
7. Sengupta JN, Gebhart GF. Characterization of mechanosensitive pelvic nerve afferent fibers innervating the colon of the rat. J Neurophysiol 1994; 71:2046–2060.

8. McMahon SB, Koltzenberg M. Silent afferents and visceral pain. In: Fields HL, Liebeskind JC, eds. Pharmacological Approaches to the Treatment of Chronic Pain: New Concepts and Critical Issues. Progress in Pain Research and Management. Vol. 1. Seattle, Washington, D.C.: IASP Press, 1994:11–30.
9. Cervero F, Laird JM. Role of ion channels in mechanisms controlling gastrointestinal pain pathways. Curr Opin Pharmacol 2003; 3:608–612.
10. Maggi CA, Meli A. The sensory-efferent function of capsaicin-sensitive sensory neurons. Gen Pharmacol 1988; 19:1–43.
11. Sugiura Y, Terui N, Hosoya Y, et al. Quantitative analysis of central terminal projections of visceral and somatic unmyelinated (C) primary afferent fibers in the guinea pig. J Comp Neurol 1993; 332:315–325.
12. Al Chaer ED, Lawand NB, Westlund KN, et al. Visceral nociceptive input into the ventral posterolateral nucleus of the thalamus: a new function for the dorsal column pathway. J Neurophysiol 1996; 76:2661–2674.
13. Al Chaer ED, Lawand NB, Westlund KN, et al. Pelvic visceral input into the nucleus gracilis is largely mediated by the postsynaptic dorsal column pathway. J Neurophysiol 1996; 76:2675–2690.
14. Al Chaer ED, Feng Y, Willis WD. A role for the dorsal column in nociceptive visceral input into the thalamus of primates. J Neurophysiol 1998; 79:3143–3150.
15. Al Chaer ED, Feng Y, Willis WD. Comparative study of viscerosomatic input onto postsynaptic dorsal column and spinothalamic tract neurons in the primate. J Neurophysiol 1999; 82:1876–1882.
16. Traub RJ. Evidence for thoracolumbar spinal cord processing of inflammatory, but not acute colonic pain. Neuroreport 2000; 11:2113–2116.
17. Al-Chaer ED, Feng Y, Willis WD. Visceral pain: a disturbance in the sensorimotor continuum. Pain Forum 1998; 7(3):117–125.
18. Willis WD, Al-Chaer ED, Quast MJ, et al. A visceral pain pathway in the dorsal column of the spinal cord. The Neurobiology of Pain. The National Academy of Science. Proc Natl Acad Sci USA 1999; 96(14):7675–7679.
19. White JC, Sweet WH. Pain and the Neurosurgeon. Springfield: Charles C Thomas, 1969.
20. Cadwalader WB, Sweet JE. Experimental work on the function of the anterolateral column of the spinal cord. JAMA 1912; 56:1490–1493.
21. Spiller WG, Martin E. The treatment of persistent pain of organic origin in the lower part of the body by division of the anterolateral column of the spinal cord. JAMA 1912; 58:1489–1490.
22. Vierck CJ, Luck MM. Loss and recovery of reactivity to noxious stimuli in monkeys with primary spinothalamic cordotomies, followed by secondary and tertiary lesions of other cord sectors. Brain 1979; 102:233–248.
23. Poirier LJ, Bertrand C. Experimental and anatomical investigation of the lateral spino-thalamic and spino-tectal tracts. J Comp Neurol 1955; 102:745–757.
24. Yoss RE. Studies of the spinal cord. Part 3. Pathways for deep pain within the spinal cord and brain. Neurology 1953; 3:163–175.
25. Kennard MA. The course of ascending fibres in the spinal cord essential to the recognition of painful stimuli. J Comp Neurol 1954; 100:511–524.
26. Ranson SW, von Hess CL. The conduction within the spinal cord of the afferent impulses producing pain and the vasomotor reflexes. Am J Physiol 1915; 38:128–152.
27. Casey KL, Morrow TJ. Supraspinal nocifensive responses of cats: spinal cord pathways, monoamines and modulation. J Comp Neurol 1988; 270:591–605.
28. Hagg S, Ha H. Cervicothalamic tract in the dog. J Comp Neurol 1970; 139:357–374.
29. Willis WD. The Pain System. Basel: Karger, 1985.
30. Gybels JM, Sweet WH, eds. Neurosurgical Treatment of Persistent Pain. Basel: Karger, 1989.
31. Willis WD, Coggeshall RE. Sensory Mechanisms of the Spinal Cord. 3rd ed. New York: Plenum Press, 2004.
32. Gowers WR. A case of unilateral gunshot injury to the spinal cord. Trans Clin Lond 1878; 11:24–32.
33. Head H, Thompson T. The grouping of afferent impulses within the spinal cord. Brain 1906; 29:537–741.
34. Noordenbos W, Wall PD. Diverse sensory functions with an almost totally divided spinal cord. A case of spinal cord transection with preservation of part of one anterolateral quadrant. Pain 1976; 2:185–195.
35. Vierck CJ, Greenspan JD, Ritz LA. Long-term changes in purposive and reflexive responses to nociceptive stimulation following anterolateral chordotomy. J Neurosci 1990; 10:2077–2095.
36. Willis WD, Kenshalo DR, Leonard RB. The cells of origin of the primate spinothalamic tract. J Comp Neurol 1979; 188:543–574.
37. Apkarian AV, Hodge CJ. Primate spinothalamic pathways: I. A quantitative study of the cells of origin of the spinothalamic pathway. J Comp Neurol 1989; 288:447–473.
38. Apkarian AV, Hodge CJ. Primate spinothalamic pathways: II. The cells of origin of the dorsolateral and ventral spinothalamic pathways. J Comp Neurol 1989; 288:474–492.
39. Trevino DL, Maunz RA, Bryan RN, et al. Location of cells of origin of the spinothalamic tract in the lumbar enlargement of cat. Exp Neurol 1972; 34:64–77.
40. Willis WD, Trevino DL, Coulter JD, et al. Responses of primate spinothalamic tract neurons to natural stimulation of the hindlimb. J Neurophysiol 1974; 37:358–372.

41. Giesler GJJ, Menétrey D, Guilbaud G, et al. Lumbar cord neurons at the origin of the spinothalamic tract in the rat. Brain Res 1976; 118:320–324.
42. Ammons WS, Girardot MN, Foreman RD. T_2-T_5 spinothalamic neurons projection to medial thalamus with viscerosomatic input. J Neurophysiol 1985; 54:73–89.
43. Ammons WS. Cardiopulmonary sympathetic afferent excitation of lower thoracic spinoreticular and spinothalamic neurons. J Neurophysiol 1990; 64:1907–1916.
44. Hancock MB, Foreman RD, Willis WD. Convergence of visceral and cutaneous input onto spinothalamic tract cells in the thoracic spinal cord of the cat. Exp Neurol 1975; 47:240–248.
45. Foreman RD, Hancock MB, Willis WD. Responses of spinothalamic tract cells in the thoracic spinal cord of the monkey to cutaneous and visceral inputs. Pain 1981; 11:149–162.
46. Ammons WS, Blair RW, Foreman RD. Responses of primate T1-T5 spinothalamic neurons to gallbladder distension. Am J Physiol 1984; 247:R995–R1002.
47. Ammons WS. Characteristics of spinoreticular and spinothalamic neurons with renal inputs. J Neurophysiol 1987; 58:480–495.
48. Ammons WS. Primate spinothalamic cell responses to ureteral occlusion. Brain Res 1989; 496: 124–130.
49. Milne RJ, Foreman RD, Giesler GJJ, et al. Convergence of cutaneous and pelvic visceral nociceptive inputs onto primate spinothalamic neurons. Pain 1981; 11:163–183.
50. Blair RW, Weber RN, Foreman RD. Characteristics of primate spinothalamic tract neurons receiving viscerosomatic convergent inputs in T_3-T_5 segments. J Neurophysiol 1981; 46:797–811.
51. Chandler MJ, Zhang J, Foreman RD. Vagal, sympathetic and somatic sensory inputs to upper cervical (C_1-C_3) spinothalamic tract neurons in monkeys. J Neurophysiol 1996; 76:2555–2567.
52. Hobbs SF, Chandler MJ, Bolser DC, et al. Segmental organization of visceral and somatic input onto C_3-T_6 spinothalamic tract cells of the monkey. J Neurophysiol 1992; 68:1575–1588.
53. Foreman RD, Hobbs SF, Oh U-T, et al. Differential modulation of thoracic and lumbar spinothalamic tract cell activity during stimulation of cardiopulmonary sympathetic afferent fibers in the primate. A new concept for visceral pain. In: Dubner R, Gebhart GF, Bond MR, eds. Proceedings of the 5th World Congress on Pain. New York: Elsevier, 1988:227–231.
54. Hobbs SF, Oh U-T, Chandler MJ, et al. Evidence that C_1 and C_2 propriospinal neurons mediate the inhibitory effects of viscerosomatic spinal afferent input on primate spinothalamic tract neurons. J Neurophysiol 1992; 67:852–860.
55. Chandler MJ, Zhang J, Qin C, et al. Spinal inhibitory effects of cardiopulmonary afferent inputs in monkeys: neuronal processing in high cervical segments. J Neurophysiol 2002; 87(3):1290–1302.
56. Ness TJ, Gebhart GF. Characterization of neuronal responses to noxious visceral and somatic stimuli in the medial lumbosacral spinal cord of the rat. J Neurophysiol 1987; 57:1867–1892.
57. Milne RJ, Foreman, RD, Willis WD. Responses of primate spinothalamic neurons located in the sacral intermediolateral gray (Stilling's nucleus) to proprioceptive input from the tail. Brain Res 1982; 234:227–236.
58. Palecek J, Paleckova V, Willis WD. Fos expression in spinothalamic and postsynaptic dorsal column neurons following noxious visceral and cutaneous stimuli. Pain 2003; 104:249–257.
59. Armour D. On the surgery of the spinal cord and its membranes. Lancet 1927; 2:691–697.
60. Uddenburg N. Studies on modality segregation and second-order neurons in the dorsal funiculus. Experientia 1966; 15:441–442.
61. Uddenberg N. Functional organization of long, second-order afferents in the dorsal funiculus. Exp Brain Res 1968; 4:377–382.
62. Petit D. Postsynaptic fibres in the dorsal columns and their relay in the nucleus gracilis. Brain Res 1972; 48:380–384.
63. Rustioni A. Nonprimary afferents to the nucleus gracilis from the lumbar cord of the cat. Brain Res 1973; 51:81–95.
64. Angaut-Petit D. The dorsal column system: I. Existence of long ascending postsynaptic fibres in the cat's fasciculus gracilis. Exp Brain Res 1975; 22:457–470.
65. Angaut-Petit D. The dorsal column system: II. Functional properties and bulbar relay of the postsynaptic fibres of the cat's fasciculus gracilis. Exp Brain Res 1975; 22:471–493.
66. Brown-Sequard E. Lectures on the physiology and pathology of the central nervous system and on the treatment of organic nervous affections. Lancet 1868; 2:593–823.
67. Stanley E. A case of disease of the posterior columns of the spinal cord. Med-chir Trans 1840; 23:80–84.
68. Davidoff RA. The dorsal columns. Neurology 1989; 39:1377–1385.
69. Hitchcock ER. Stereotactic cervical myelotomy. J Neurol Neurosurg Psychiatr 1970; 33:224–230.
70. Hitchcock ER. Stereotactic myelotomy. Proc Roy Soc Med 1974; 67:771–772.
71. Schwarcz JR. Stereotactic extralemniscal myelotomy. J Neurol Neurosurg Psychiatr 1976; 39:53–57.
72. Schwarcz JR. Spinal cord stereotactic techniques, trigeminal nucleotomy, and extralemniscal myelotomy. Appl Neurophysiol 1978; 41:99–112.
73. Gildenberg PL, Hirshberg RM. Limited myelotomy for the treatment of intractable cancer pain. J Neurol Neurosurg Psychiatr 1984; 47:94–96.
74. Hirshberg RM, Al-Chaer ED, Lawand NB, et al. Is there a pathway in the posterior funiculus that signals visceral pain. Pain 1996; 67:291–305.

75. Foerster O, Gagel O. Die Vorderseitenstrangdurchschneidung beim menschen. Eine klinisch-patho-physiologisch-anatomische studie. Z Gesampte Neurol Psychiatr 1932; 138:1–92.
76. White JC. Sensory innervation of the viscera: studies on visceral afferent neurones in man based on neurosurgical procedures for the relief of intractable pain. Res Publ Ass Nerv Ment Dis 1943; 23:373–390.
77. Sarnoff SJ, Arrowood JG, Chapman WP. Differential spinal block. IV. The investigation of intestinal dyskinesia, colonic atony, and visceral afferent fibers. Surg Gynec Obstet 1948; 86:571–581.
78. Nauta HJ, Hewitt E, Westlund KN, et al. Surgical interruption of a midline dorsal column visceral pain pathway. Case report and review of the literature. J Neurosurg 1997; 86(3):538–542.
79. Nauta HJ, Soukup VM, Fabian RH, et al. Punctate midline myelotomy for the relief of visceral cancer pain. J Neurosurg 2000; 92(suppl 2):125–130.
80. Kim YS, Kwon SJ. High thoracic midline dorsal column myelotomy for severe visceral pain due to advanced stomach cancer. Neurosurgery 2000; 46(1):85–92.
81. Amassian VE. Fiber groups and spinal pathways of cortically represented visceral afferents. J Neurophysiol 1951; 14:445–460.
82. Aidar O, Geohegan WA, Ungewitter LH. Splanchnic afferent pathways in the central nervous system. J Neurophysiol 1952; 15:131–138.
83. Ferrington DG, Downie JW, Willis WD. Primate nucleus gracilis neurons: responses to innocuous and noxious stimuli. J Neurophysiol 1988; 59:886–907.
84. Cliffer KD, Hasegawa T, Willis WD. Responses of neurons in the gracile nucleus of cats to innocuous and noxious stimuli: basic characterization and antidromic activation from the thalamus. J Neurophysiol 1992; 68:818–832.
85. Berkley KJ, Hubscher CH. Are there separate central nervous system pathways for touch and pain? Nat Med 1995; 1:766–773.
86. Berkley KJ, Hubscher CH. Visceral and somatic sensory tracks through the neuraxis and their relation to pain: lessons from the rat female reproductive system. In: Gebhart GF, ed. Visceral Pain. Seattle: IASP Press, 1995:195–216.
87. Conti F, De Biasi S, Giuffrida R, et al. Substance P-containing projections in the dorsal columns of rats and cats. Neuroscience 1990; 34:607–621.
88. Patterson JT, Head PA, McNeill DL, et al. Ascending unmyelinated primary afferent fibers in the dorsal funiculus. J Comp Neurol 1989; 290:384–390.
89. Patterson JT, Coggeshall RE, Lee WT, et al. Long ascending unmyelinated primary afferent axons in the rat dorsal column: immunohistochemical localizations. Neurosci Lett 1990; 108:6–10.
90. Uddenberg N. Functional organization of long, second-order afferents in the dorsal funiculus. Exp Brain Res 1968; 4:377–382.
91. Bennett GJ, Seltzer Z, Lu GW, et al. The cells of origin of the dorsal column postsynaptic projection in the lumbosacral enlargements of cats and monkeys. Somatosensory Res 1983; 1:131–149.
92. Bennett GJ, Nishikawa N, Lu GW, et al. The morphology of dorsal column postsynaptic (DCPS) spino-medullary neurons in the cat. J Comp Neurol 1984; 224:568–578.
93. Noble R, Riddell JS. Cutaneous excitatory and inhibitory input to neurones of the postsynaptic dorsal column system in the cat. J Physiol 1988; 396:497–513.
94. Feng Y, Cui M, Al-Chaer ED, et al. Epigastric antinociception by cervical dorsal column lesions in rats. Anesthesiology 1998; 89(2):411–420.
95. Ness TJ. Evidence for ascending visceral nociceptive information in the dorsal midline and lateral spinal cord. Pain 2000; 87(1):83–88.
96. Willis WD, Al-Chaer ED, Quast MJ, et al. A visceral pain pathway in the dorsal column of the spinal cord. Proc Natl Acad Sci USA 1999; 96(14):7675–7679.
97. Rustioni A. Non-primary afferents to the cuneate nucleus in the brachial dorsal funiculus of the cat. Brain Res 1974; 75:247–259.
98. Rustioni A, Hayes NL, O'Neill S. Dorsal column nuclei and ascending spinal afferents in macaques. Brain 1979; 102:95–125.
99. Giesler GJ, Nahin RL, Madsen AM. Postsynaptic dorsal column pathway of the rat. I. Anatomical studies. J Neurophysiol 1984; 51:260–275.
100. Cliffer KD, Giesler GJ Jr. Postsynaptic dorsal column pathway of the rat. III. Distribution of ascending afferent fibers. J Neurosci 1989; 9:3146–3168.
101. Wang CC, Willis WD, Westlund KN. Ascending projections from the area around the spinal cord central canal: a phaseolus vulgaris leukoagglutinin study in rats. J Comp Neurol 1999; 415(3):341–367.
102. Giesler GJ Jr, Cliffer KD. Postsynaptic dorsal column pathway of the rat. II. Evidence against an important role in nociception. Brain Res 1985; 326(2):347–356.
103. Willis WD, Westlund KN. Neuroanatomy of the pain system and of the pathways that modulate pain. J Clin Physiol 1997; 14(1):2–31.
104. McLeod JG. The representation of the splanchnic afferent pathways in the thalamus of the cat. J Physiol 1958; 94:439–452.
105. Patton HD, Amassian VE. Thalamic relay of splanchnic afferent fibers. Am J Physiol 1951; 167:815–816.

106. Dell P, Olson R. Projections thalamiques, corticales et cerebelleuses des afferences viscerales vagales. Soc Biol 1951; 145:1084–1088.

107. Chandler MJ, Hobbs SF, Qing-Gong F, et al. Responses of neurons in ventroposterolateral nucleus of primate thalamus to urinary bladder distension. Brain Res 1992; 571:26–34.

108. Davis KD, Dostrovsky JO. Properties of feline thalamic neurons activated by stimulation of the middle meningeal artery and sagittal sinus. Brain Res 1988; 454:89–100.

109. Rogers RC, Novin D, Butcher LL. Hepatic sodium and osmoreceptors activate neurons in the ventrobasal thalamus. Brain Res 1979; 168:398–403.

110. Emmers R. Separate relays of tactile, pressure, thermal, and gustatory modalities in the cat thalamus. Proc Soc Exp Biol Med 1966; 121:527–531.

111. Ammons WS, Girardot MN, Foreman RD. T_2-T_5 spinothalamic neurons projecting to medial thalamus with viscerosomatic input. J Neurophysiol 1985; 54(1):73–89.

112. Brüggemann J, Shi T, Apkarian AV. Squirrel monkey lateral thalamus: II. Viscero-somatic convergent representation of urinary bladder, colon, and esophagus. J Neurosci 1994; 14:6796–6814.

113. Berkley KJ, Guilbaud G, Benoist J, et al. Responses of neurons in and near the thalamic ventrobasal complex of the rat to stimulation of uterus, cervix, vagina, colon, and skin. J Neurophysiol 1993; 69:557–568.

114. Kawakita K, Sumiya E, Murase K, et al. Response characteristics of nucleus submedius neurons to colorectal distension in the rat. Neurosci Res 1997; 28(1):59–66.

115. Lenz FA, Gracely RH, Hope EJ, et al. The sensation of angina can be evoked by stimulation of the human thalamus. Pain 1994; 59:119–125.

116. Hirai T, Jones EG. A new parcellation of the human thalamus on the basis of histochemical staining. Brain Res Rev 1989; 14:1–34.

117. Jones EG. The Thalamus. New York: Plenum, 1985.

118. Davis KD, Tasker RR, Kiss ZHT, et al. Visceral pain evoked by thalamic microstimulation in humans. Neuroreport 1995; 6:369–374.

119. Saab CY, Park YC, Al-Chaer ED. Thalamic modulation of visceral nociceptive processing in adult rats with neonatal colon irritation. Brain Res 2004; 1008(2):186–192.

120. Aziz Q, Andersson JL, Valind S, et al. Identification of human brain loci processing esophageal sensation using positron emission tomography. Gastroenterology 1997; 113:50–59.

121. Ladabaum U, Minoshima S, Hasler WL, et al. Gastric distention correlates with activation of multiple cortical and subcortical regions. Gastroenterology 2001; 120:369–376.

122. Hobday DI, Aziz Q, Thacker N, et al. A study of the cortical processing of ano-rectal sensation using functional MRI. Brain 2001; 124:361–368.

123. Silverman DH, Munakata JA, Ennes H, et al. Regional cerebral activity in normal and pathological perception of visceral pain. Gastroenterology 1997; 112:64–72.

124. Mertz H, Morgan V, Tanner G, et al. Regional cerebral activation in irritable bowel syndrome and control subjects with painful and nonpainful rectal distention. Gastroenterology 2000; 118:842–848.

125. Derbyshire SW. A systematic review of neuroimaging data during visceral stimulation. Am J Gastroenterol 2003; 98:12–20.

126. Strigo IA, Duncan GH, Boivin M, et al. Differentiation of visceral and cutaneous pain in the human brain. J Neurophysiol 2003; 89:3294–3303.

127. Kern MK, Jaradeh S, Arndorfer RC, et al. Gender differences in cortical representation of rectal distension in healthy humans. Am J Physiol 2001; 281:G1512–G1523.

5 | The Neurobiology of Visceral Nociceptors

Stuart M. Brierley
Department of Gastroenterology, Hepatology and General Medicine, Nerve-Gut Research Laboratory, Royal Adelaide Hospital, Discipline of Physiology, School of Molecular & Biomedical Sciences, University of Adelaide, Adelaide, South Australia, Australia

L. Ashley Blackshaw
Department of Gastroenterology, Hepatology and General Medicine, Nerve-Gut Research Laboratory, Royal Adelaide Hospital, Discipline of Physiology, School of Molecular and Biomedical Sciences, Department of Medicine, University of Adelaide, Adelaide, South Australia, Australia

INTRODUCTION

As detailed in other chapters, several syndromes may be attributed to overactivity of visceral nociceptors. Even if they have other etiologies, their symptoms may be alleviated by targeting visceral nociceptors. Irritable bowel syndrome (IBS) is a good example of a condition with unknown or multiple etiology, and is the most common disorder diagnosed by gastroenterologists [1]. Many IBS symptoms originate from the colon and rectum, which must therefore be conveyed by the visceral nociceptors innervating these organs. Afferent endings innervating the colon and rectum will be the area of focus of this chapter, although much of our understanding of the colorectal sensory innervation can be applied to other viscera. This chapter deals firstly with anatomical and functional specialization of visceral afferents, with comparisons between nociceptive and non-nociceptive populations in different pathways. Second, it discusses examples of modulation of visceral afferents via specific ionotropic and metabotropic receptors, and thirdly it includes recent evidence for the identity of mechanotransduction mechanisms.

IRRITABLE BOWEL SYNDROME

IBS is defined by the Rome II criteria as a functional bowel disorder in which there is the presence of continuous or recurrent abdominal pain or discomfort that is relieved with defecation or associated with a change in bowel habit [2]. IBS is a common disease afflicting approximately 10% of the population [1,3–6]. IBS patients report reduced quality of life [5,7], with several extraintestinal symptoms [5]. Estimates of the total cost of IBS per annum in the United States is $25 billion through direct costs of health-care use and indirect costs of absenteeism from work [1].

IBS can be subclassified into three groups based on altered bowel habit: constipation predominant, diarrhea-predominant, and alternating [5,8–11]. Another subclass has now been added, postinfectious IBS [12]. However, despite this heterogeneous population of patients, enhanced colonic mechanosensation is a hallmark of all subtypes of IBS and as such increased perception of mechanical distension of the distal colon/rectum has become the best-characterized clinical manifestation of IBS [1,13,14]. The extent of this enhanced colonic sensation is considerable, as a colorectal distending volume of approximately 60 mL evokes pain in less than 10% of normal subjects compared with greater than 50% of IBS patients. Therefore there is leftward shift in the psychophysical function of IBS patients suggesting the presence of hyperalgesia in IBS [13]. There is a general agreement that this visceral hypersensitivity and hyperalgesia correlates well with the overall severity of the disease [1,15], which is significant as pain is the symptom that affects quality of life the most [7].

There are various mechanisms, which are thought to be involved in the visceral hypersensitivity experienced by IBS patients; however, there is no clear consensus, which may reflect the heterogeneity of the disease. The hypothesized mechanisms include sensitization of the extrinsic sensory afferent endings within the gut wall, hyperexcitability of dorsal horn neurons, and modulation of the brain responses to information signalled by the gut. Recent evidence from behavioral and functional imaging studies of patients with IBS suggests that changes occur at the level of the primary afferent neuron and/or spinal cord but not in higher cortical centers (16,17), thereby supporting the notion that peripheral mechanosensation plays an important role in the etiology of this disease. In particular, there is circumstantial evidence suggesting that hypersensitivity of lumbar splanchnic afferents induces hyperalgesia in IBS patients (16,18). Consistent with the role of peripheral mechanisms, subsets of IBS patients have increased numbers of inflammatory cells in the colonic mucosa (19), while activated mast cells have been found in close proximity to colonic nerves, which correlate with abdominal pain in IBS patients (15), suggesting that activation or sensitization of extrinsic sensory endings within the gut wall may play a key role in IBS. Recent hypotheses support this notion by suggesting a low-grade inflammatory response at the level of the gut wall could be involved (12,15).

By contrast, postinfectious IBS patients appear to have a clearer etiology as they describe an acute onset of symptoms (as classified by Rome II criteria) after a gastroenteritis episode but previously have entirely normal bowel habit (12,20). For patients who had experienced gastroenteritis, the relative risk of developing IBS within the following year was approximately 11 times greater (12). These patients typically have diarrhea-predominant IBS and account for 6% to 17% of the IBS population (11). A role for stress in the pathophysiology of IBS has also been suggested, with psychological and environmental stressors associated with onset and symptom exacerbation, possibly via central mechanisms or via activation of sensitized immune cells within the gut wall (5,6,20–26).

SENSORY INNERVATION OF THE GASTROINTESTINAL TRACT

The sensory, or afferent, innervation of the gastrointestinal tract mediates sensations from the gut and initiates reflex control of digestive function. The afferent fibers innervating the gastrointestinal tract follow two main anatomical branches, the vagal pathway and the spinal pathway. Vagal afferents have axons which project directly into the brainstem to the nucleus tractus solitarius whereas their cell bodies are located in the nodose ganglia. Vagal afferents are important in the sensory innervation of the upper gastrointestinal tract, in particular the esophagus and stomach (27,28). However, the vagal innervation decreases down the length of the gastrointestinal tract and is sparse in the distal colon (27,29). As such, vagal fibers are asso-ciated with sensation in the upper gut such as fullness, bloating, and nausea, and induce vomiting. In contrast, pain evoked from the upper gut is probably mediated via spinal nerves.

Spinal afferent endings are distributed throughout the gut and have their cell bodies located within the dorsal root ganglia (DRG). The central projections of these afferent neurons enter the spinal cord and make synaptic contacts in the dorsal horn. Activation of spinal afferents may be associated with vague sensations of fullness, bloating, discomfort, and pain from the stomach and small bowel. However, in the rectum and distal colon, spinal afferents also give rise to more specific, graded perceptions of fullness, urgency, and discomfort, in addition to pain evoked by more intense stimulation.

Sensory information from the distal colon/rectum travels to the central nervous system (CNS) through spinal afferents via two distinct spinal anatomical pathways: the lumbar splanchnic nerves (LSNs), which terminate in the thoracolumbar spinal cord, and the paired pelvic nerves, which terminate in the lumbosacral spinal cord (Fig. 1). The thoracolumbar afferents, which have receptive fields in the colonic wall, travel via the lumbar colonic nerves via by way of the insertions into the colonic wall and into the mesenteric attachment of the colon, where they juxtapose with blood vessels supplying the colon. These afferent fibers then pass through the inferior mesenteric ganglion into the intermesenteric nerves containing the LSNs (30–35). The lumbosacral afferents travel though an entirely separate anatomical pathway via the paired pelvic nerves, which pass through the major pelvic ganglion to the lumbosacral spinal cord (34–37). Afferents in each pathway can also travel through the hypogastric nerve and innervate the colon traveling in different directions via the major pelvic ganglia and inferior mesenteric ganglia (38).

In the rat, the afferent innervation of the descending colon and rectum originates in the thoracolumbar DRG, at the anatomical levels of T_{13}-L_2, and the lumbosacral DRG, at the anatomical levels of L_6-S_2 (39). The splanchnic innervation of the colon in rat comprises

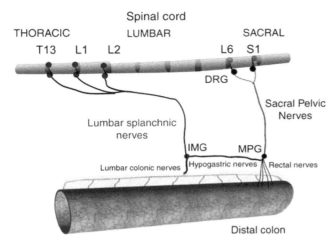

Figure 1 (*See color insert*) Extrinsic spinal innervation of the colon. The sensory information from the distal colon/rectum travels to the central nervous system through spinal afferents via two distinct anatomical pathways: the lumbar splanchnic nerves, which terminate in the thoracolumbar spinal cord, and the paired pelvic nerves, which terminate in the lumbosacral spinal cord. The thoracolumbar afferents, with receptive fields in the colonic wall, travel via the lumbar colonic nerves via the insertions into the colonic wall and into the mesenteric attachment of the colon, where they juxtapose with blood vessels supplying the colon. These afferent fibers then pass through the IMG and pass into the intermesenteric nerves containing the LSN. The lumbosacral afferents travel though an entirely separate anatomical pathway via the rectal nerves, which pass through the MPG and into the paired pelvic nerves to the lumbosacral spinal cord. Afferents in each pathway can also travel through the hypogastric nerve and innervate the colon traveling in different directions via the MPG and IMG. *Abbreviations*: IMG, inferior mesenteric ganglion; LSN, lumbar splanchinic nerves; MPG, major pelvic ganglion; DRG, dorsal root ganglia.

approximately 1500 afferent fibers and 1250 efferent fibers (34), compared with the pelvic innervation of the colon comprising approximately 1600 afferent fibers and 3200 efferent fibers (40). Other reports indicate that significantly more colonic afferents are present in the T_{13}-L_2 ganglia than in the L_6-S_2 ganglia (41).

Previous studies in rat have reported a range in size of retrogradely labeled colonic primary afferents between 12 and 30 μm in diameter (42), with the mean cell diameters of thoracolumbar and lumbosacral cells being approximately equal (28 μm). These cells are therefore classified as small- to medium-sized, indicating that the majority of retrogradely labeled colonic neurons are Aδ or C fiber afferents (see below). In the mouse, a similar afferent distribution to the rat is observed in thoracolumbar DRG, although the distribution is slightly wider at the anatomical levels of T_8-L_1; lumbosacral afferents similarly originate from DRG at the anatomical levels of L_6-S_1 (43). There are no studies to date, which have compared the relative proportion of afferent and efferent fibers from either the thoracolumbar or lumbosacral innervation of the mouse colon/rectum. However, a comparison of the two pathways reveals a greater preponderance of retrogradely labeled afferent cells within the thoracolumbar DRG (43). The majority (92%) of retrogradely labeled cells in mouse thoracolumbar and lumbosacral DRG have diameters of 11 to 30 μm, suggesting that these cells can also be classified as small- to medium-sized, and therefore give rise to function as Aδ or C fiber afferents.

Anatomical Identification of Visceral Afferent Endings

Unlike the cutaneous afferent innervation, where A fibers innervate specific anatomical structures like Merkel cells, Ruffini endings, Hair Lanceolates, and Pacinian or Meissner corpuscles, the dogma associated with the vast majority of visceral sensory endings has been for many years that the peripheral arborizations of small myelinated and unmyelinated afferent fibers terminate as free nerve endings without any clear anatomic specialization. Despite this, it is clear from numerous studies utilizing neuronal tracing techniques that these peripheral terminals of vagal and spinal afferents can be localized within the different layers gastrointestinal tract, giving an indication to their physiological characteristics and functional roles. Three types of specialized endings have been identified in the gut wall, intraganglionic laminar endings (IGLEs), intramuscular arrays (IMAs), and mucosal endings (Fig. 2).

Intraganglionic Laminar Endings

Vagal IGLEs are special terminal structures that are located within the myenteric plexus throughout the gastrointestinal tract of a variety of species including rats, mice, and guinea pigs. IGLEs, traced from nodose ganglia are distributed throughout the entire gastrointestinal

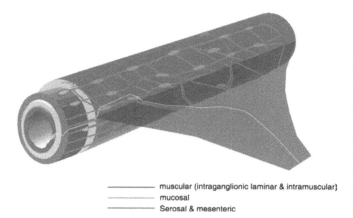

——————— muscular (intraganglionic laminar & intramuscular)
——————— mucosal
——————— Serosal & mesenteric

Figure 2 (*See color insert*) Several different classes of mechanoreceptor within the gastrointestinal tract. Mucosal afferents have been extensively documented throughout the upper gastrointestinal tract in addition to the distal colon and perianal mucosa. Mucosal fibers are silent at rest; respond to fine stroking of the luminal surface with rapidly adapting responses, and are unresponsive to distension. Intramuscular arrays (IMAs) have been documented anatomically and are special terminal structures that have a parent axon that branches several times before terminating within the circular and longitudinal muscle layers. IMAs have been suggested to be in-series tension receptors that serve as stretch or length detectors that possibly respond to both passive stretch and active contraction of the muscle. Intraganglionic laminar endings (IGLEs) have been documented anatomically and are typically characterized as single axons entering a myenteric ganglion that have ramifying endings on the surfaces of the ganglia that are flattened, highly arborizing "leaf-like" processes. IGLEs have been recently shown to be the specialized transduction sites of mechanosensitive tension-sensitive vagal afferent neurons and tension-sensitive rectal mechanoreceptors (rIGLES). Mesenteric and serosal afferents have endings that are located close to or on blood vessels or at branching points of capillaries supplying the serosa. They are classified by their response to probing or distortion of the colon but not to low-intensity circular stretch or fine mucosal stroking. However, these afferents can be activated briefly by intense stretch or distortion of the mesenteric attachment and high intensity colonic distension.

tract, with greatest densities in the stomach, in particular the corpus (6.3 IGLEs/mm^2), the antrum (3.8 IGLEs/mm^2), and the forestomach (2.8 IGLEs/mm^2). The density of IGLEs in other regions of the gastrointestinal tract is highest in the proximal duodenum (3.3 IGLEs/mm^2) with very few IGLEs in the distal colon (0.2 IGLEs/mm^2) (44–47). IGLEs are typically characterized as single axons entering a myenteric ganglion that have ramifying endings on the surfaces of the ganglia that are flattened, highly arborizing "leaf-like" processes (44–46, 48–52). In many cases, a single axon gives rise to several IGLEs of various sizes in different ganglia (48,49). These endings have been hypothesized to detect mechanical shearing forces between the orthogonal muscle layers (51,53). It has recently been demonstrated, using a combination of rapid anterograde tracing and in vitro electrophysiology, that IGLEs are specialized transduction sites of mechanosensitive vagal afferent neurons in the guinea pig esophagus (48–50). These studies show that morphologically identified IGLEs in the esophagus correspond with the receptive fields or "hot spots" of distension-sensitive afferents (48–50).

Spinal IGLEs, with special terminal structures that are located within the myenteric plexus in the guinea pig rectum, have been classified as rectal IGLEs (rIGLEs). These rIGLEs specifically innervate the rectum but not the distal colon, probably via the pelvic nerves from the sacral DRG (54,55). These rIGLEs share characteristics of vagal IGLEs in the upper gastrointestinal tract in that they display branched, flattened, lamellar endings with multiple clusters. However, rIGLEs are approximately 10-fold smaller ($\sim$630 μm^2) than vagal IGLEs innervating the guinea pig esophagus (6900 μm^2) and stomach (6100 μm^2) with fewer leaflets and less-extensive branching patterns (48,49,54,56,57). Using a combination of anterograde tracing and electrophysiological techniques, it has been demonstrated that rIGLEs are functionally similar to vagal IGLEs in the upper gut as are mechanotransduction sites, which are sensitive to both distension and muscle contraction (48,49,54–56). These morphologically identified rIGLEs in the rectum correspond with the receptive fields or "hot spots" of low threshold, slowly adapting, distension-sensitive mechanoreceptors (54–56).

Intramuscular Arrays

Vagal IMAs are special terminal structures with a parent axon that branches several times before terminating within the circular muscle layers. The size of the arrays can vary from several hundred microns to several millimeters in length (58). In the muscle layers, the individual terminals run for several millimeters, creating a distinct pattern of parallel elements that are commonly associated with interstitial cells of Cajal (29,45,46,49,58). In contrast to IGLEs, IMAs have a distinctly different distribution, and are concentrated in the forestomach, lower esophageal sphincter, and pyloric sphincter. The highest concentration of IMAs is in the forestomach (17.3 IMAs/mm^2), with fewer in the corpus (2.9 IMAs/mm^2) and antrum (0.6 IMAs/mm^2) (47). IMAs have been suggested to be in-series tension receptors that serve as stretch or length detectors, which possibly respond to both passive stretch and active contraction of the muscle (45,47,51). In the guinea pig esophagus, using a combination of rapid anterograde tracing and in vitro electrophysiology, there was no evidence to support the suggestion that IMs function as length receptors (49). Similarly, spinal IMAs have been located within the guinea pig colon; however, as yet they do not have a known functional correlate (54).

Mucosal Endings
The evidence for mucosal afferents arises mainly from electrophysiological studies (see below). Anterograde tracing from the nodose ganglia revealed vagal endings within the mucosa of the upper gastrointestinal tract. These fibers pass through the muscle layers and submucosa and have multiple branching axons within the lamina propria of both villi and crypts, and have been located mainly within rat duodenum and jejunum (51,59). Tracing from the thoracic DRG of the cat revealed spinal afferent endings in the esophagogastric junction (60), some of which were located in the squamous epithelium.

Functional Classification of Afferent Subtypes
Much of the terminology used in the classification of visceral afferents has been translated from that used in the study of cutaneous sensation. These physiological classifications are based on afferent conduction velocities, which in turn, relate to axon diameter and the degree of myelination and their responsiveness to mechanical and thermal stimuli (61). Cutaneous afferents can be subdivided into three classes based on conduction velocity alone: Aβ fibers, Aδ fibers, and C-fibers. Each of these classes has subclasses of afferents based on mechanosensory responses. Large diameter myelinated Aβ fibers can be subclassified into rapidly adapting mechanoreceptors, which respond exclusively to movement of the skin but not to static indentation and slowly, adapting mechanoreceptors, which respond to both (61). Aδ fibers have thin axons and a thin myelination and can be subclassified into either be low-threshold down hair (D-hair) mechanoreceptors, which have relatively large receptive fields, nociceptive neurons high-threshold (AM) mechanoreceptors (61,62). Small-diameter unmyelinated C-fibers can be subclassified into one of two classes. C-mechanonociceptors, have high mechanical thresholds and respond to mechanical but not thermal stimuli. Polymodal C-fibers that respond to mechanical and thermal stimuli are termed C-mechanoheat receptors. These C-fibers are designed to transmit exclusively noxious information in response to noxious stimuli (61,62). Thus cutaneous afferents have highly specific functions and as such different classes of sensory neurons carry information for distinct sensory modalities. By contrast, studies of visceral afferents throughout the gastrointestinal tract have demonstrated that conduction velocities are limited to either small diameter unmyelinated C-fibers or thinly myelinated Aδ fibers (35,36,63–68). However, visceral afferent fibers differ considerably in their basic physiological properties as they can signal normal functional events in addition to signaling pain in noxious environments (36). Moreover, studies of colonic afferents have shown little correlation between conduction velocities and functional properties either in the lumbar or in the sacral colonic afferents (67,69). In contrast to cutaneous afferents, visceral afferents lack a standardized nomenclature of afferent subclasses. As such, visceral afferents have been classified based on the layer of gut containing their receptive field, on the type of mechanical stimuli that they are responsive to, or their general response properties. However, the location of the receptive fields of the endings of their receptive field is crucial in determining their mechanical sensitivity and responsiveness to varying mechanical stimuli.

Combinations of in vivo and in vitro electrophysiological techniques have led to the identification and classification of three distinct patterns of afferent endings distributed within the wall of the gastrointestinal tract. Recent in vitro preparations have allowed manipulation of isolated afferent receptive fields resulting in a more controlled application of mechanical and chemical stimuli. Vagal and spinal afferents can be loosely divided into four classes: distension/tension sensitive, mucosal, serosal/mesenteric, and silent nociceptors.

Distension/tension Sensitive Afferents

Afferents within the wall of the gastrointestinal tract that respond broadly to distension or stretch of a region of gut have been extensively characterized. However, to add complexity, these afferents have been described by a variety of names including distension-sensitive, tension-sensitive, stretch-sensitive, muscular afferents, tonic, phasic, and low-threshold, high-threshold and wide dynamic range fibers to name but a few. Recent reviews indicate differences in the signals generated by these receptors in the vagal and spinal pathway (28,51,63,70). For example in the upper gastrointestinal tract, tension receptors have low resting activity and have low thresholds of activation. These afferents are responsive to both distension and contraction of the gut with a slowly adapting, linear relationship to wall tension and reach maximal responses within the physiological range of distension (28,51,63,70). By contrast, spinal afferents have higher thresholds of activation and encode within both physiological and noxious intensities of stimulation (28,51,63,70). Because of different response profiles, it has been suggested that vagal afferents are involved in physiological regulation, such as triggering reflexes controlling gastrointestinal function and satiety and fullness, whereas spinal afferents are responsible for mediating pain in addition to other sensations. Vagal tension-sensitive afferents respond in a graded manner to circular tension with slowly adapting responses (48,49,71,72) and are insensitive to fine mucosal stimulation (71). The receptive fields of these stretch-sensitive afferents in the esophagus and stomach correspond with morphologically identified IGLEs demonstrating that IGLEs are the specialized transduction sites of tension-sensitive vagal afferent neurons (48–50).

Distension of the colorectum has been the primary stimulus used to study LSN and pelvic nerve afferents in a multitude of species. As such, afferents that respond to colonic or rectal stretch, applied either directly in vitro or indirectly using balloon distension in vivo, have been identified and characterized (36,66,67,69,73–79). Distension-sensitive colonic afferents recorded from the LSN of the cat generally display spontaneous activity and have been classified into four categories with response patterns to distension ranging between tonic and phasic (67). Two percent are Type I units, which displayed rapidly adapting responses, 10% were Type II units that displayed slowly adapting responses, while 31% were Type III units displaying transient responses that adapted to steady state. The remaining 48% were Type IV units responding with steady state discharges. Eighty-five percent of Type I to III units had activation thresholds below 25 mmHg, while 45% of Type IV units had activation thresholds above 25 mmHg (67). These afferents also respond to contraction of the colon, while 43% of units could be activated by a discrete probing stimulus with mechanoreceptive sites identified near to or on the arteries of the colonic wall. Overall, these results indicate heterogeneous populations of distension-sensitive afferents from the LSN, and that distension may not be the primary adequate stimulus for all LSN afferents.

In contrast to LSN afferents in the cat, pelvic nerve distension-sensitive colonic afferents generally display little or no spontaneous activity and have low thresholds to intraluminal pressure (36,37,64). Moreover, pelvic nerve afferents can be classified into units with either rapidly adapting phasic (47%) or tonic (53%) responses, with most phasic afferents classed as Aδ-fibers while most tonic afferents were classed as C-fibers. Afferents with tonic responses respond linearly to increasing intraluminal pressure throughout innocuous and noxious intensities of distension. These slowly adapting responses correspond best with Type III or IV units in the LSN, while rapidly adapting fibers correspond best with Type II LSN fibers. There also appears to be a greater mechanosensitivity of distension-sensitive pelvic nerve afferents relative to LSN afferents in the cat.

Recordings from the pelvic nerve in rat colon show similar findings to those seen in the pelvic nerves of cats. Distension-sensitive pelvic nerve afferents can be classified into dynamic responses, which displayed slow adaptation (45%) or tonic nonadapting (55%) responses (64). These phasic afferents were only transiently excited during filling or emptying of the colon, whereas tonic afferents were discharged throughout the distension stimulus. These afferents could be subclassified as low threshold, responding to 10 mmHg or less (77%), or high threshold, responding to greater than 28 mmHg (23%).

More recently, various in vitro preparations have been developed to allow greater accessibility of receptive fields utilizing a combination of stretch, stoking, and probing stimuli to classify all afferent subtypes, not just distension or stretch-sensitive afferents. In rat, distal colon muscular afferents have been identified, which respond with an excitation that adapts during the stimulus (76,77). In addition to responding to circular stretch, these afferents also responded to focal compression of their receptive field via blunt probing but not to fine mucosal stroking (76,77). However, these afferents only account for 5% to 19% of the LSN innervation and are optimally activated by maintained circular stretch. Similarly, in the guinea pig distal colon, there are few stretch-sensitive mechanoreceptors; however, in the rectum there is a high density of stretch-sensitive mechanoreceptors that display low thresholds and slowly adapting response to maintained distention (54,55). The receptive fields of these low-threshold, slowly adapting, stretch-sensitive mechanoreceptors correspond with morphologically identified IGLEs in the rectum termed rIGLEs (54–56). These specialized rectal mechanoreceptors also bear many similarities to vagal IGLE mechanoreceptors in the upper gut described above (54,55).

In a recent study, muscular afferents in the mouse LSN and pelvic nerves, were activated by low-intensity circular stretch and focal compression of their receptive fields. These afferents closely resemble muscular afferents described in the LSN of the rat colon in vitro (74,76,77) and the distension-sensitive, low-threshold afferents described in vivo in the LSN of the cat (67) and in the pelvic nerves of the cat (67,73,79) and rat (69,75). The proportion of muscular LSN afferents (10%) found in the mouse study is similar to previous reports of muscular afferents in the LSN of rat using an in vitro technique (76,77). Stretch-sensitive pelvic nerve afferents constituted over 50% of the total mechanosensitive pelvic nerve-afferent population in this study (muscular and muscular/mucosal afferents combined). This is a similar proportion to the distension-sensitive afferents responding to mechanical stimulation of the colon and anal canal described in both rat (64) and cat (36) (Fig. 3).

Although stretch-sensitive afferents were recorded from both pathways in the mouse study, they differed in five critical aspects. First, stretch-sensitive pelvic nerve afferents (including muscular/mucosal afferents), greatly outnumber stretch-sensitive LSN afferents (~50% vs. 10% respectively). Second, pelvic nerve afferent receptive fields, in particular those of muscular/mucosal afferents, are located in the rectum. Third, LSN muscular afferents are less likely to respond to focal compression of their receptive field at lower stimulus intensities (<1 g), suggesting they have higher thresholds. Fourth, pelvic nerve muscular and muscular/mucosal afferents have greater responses to both probing and stretch. Finally, pelvic nerve muscular and muscular/mucosal afferents display a more maintained response to stretch compared with LSN muscular afferents.

Overall, these findings would indicate that the pelvic nerves are better equipped to respond to stretch, particularly of the distal colon and rectal wall. These pelvic nerve afferents

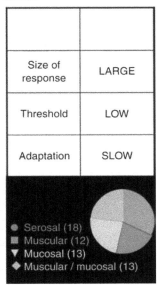

Figure 3 Key characteristics of the mechanical responsiveness of splanchnic and pelvic afferents in mouse colon determined in vitro (80), and distribution of the different subtypes according to frequency of occurrence. Note that serosal and mesenteric afferents comprise the majority of afferents in the splanchnic innervation, whereas endings within the colonic wall comprise the largest proportion of pelvic afferents.

are also activated at lower stimulation intensities and respond more robustly to tonic stretch than those found in the LSN. The sustained response of pelvic nerve afferents during maintained stretch suggests that they are more likely to signal tonic changes in the caliber or wall tension of the distal colon and rectum, such as during the presence of stool or gas. In contrast, LSN muscular afferents, with their higher stimulus response threshold and their more completely adapting responses, would be better tuned to signal the onset of higher-intensity mechanical events, such as muscular contraction or passage of material, which are of a more acute nature. Due to the different receptive field distributions of LSN and pelvic nerve afferents, signaling of muscular contraction or passage of material in the more oral region of the distal colon is likely to be signaled via LSN muscular afferents, whilst the presence of stool or gas in the rectum and most aboral regions of the distal colon is likely to be transmitted via the pelvic nerve muscular and muscular/mucosal afferents.

Data in the literature therefore indicate that muscular afferents, as a whole, are responsive to small changes in intraluminal pressure, respond to colonic stretch or distension with a linear relationship to wall tension, and are likely to encode these stimuli well into the noxious range. However, major differences exist between the LSN and pelvic nerve innervation.

Mucosal Afferents

Mucosal afferents in the vagal pathway have been extensively documented throughout the upper gastrointestinal tract. These afferents are silent at rather than respond to fine stroking of the luminal surface with rapidly adapting responses, and are unresponsive to distension. Moreover, they are polymodal as they are also chemosensitive to a range of chemical and osmotic stimuli including serotonin, bradykinin, purines, prostaglandins and cholecystokinin (28). Recent in vitro studies have highlighted the relative importance of these afferents in terms of their exact location, proportions, and modality (71,72). The major role of vagal mucosal receptors is thought to be in the generation of sensations such as satiety, nausea, and vomiting, with a minor role in direct generation of reflex responses (28).

Mucosal afferents in the lower gastrointestinal tract have not been studied as extensively as those in the upper gut; however, spinal mucosal afferents have been characterized functionally in the colon, anal canal, and perianal mucosa. In the distal colon, mucosal afferents were first identified using an in vitro preparation and recording from the LSN. These colonic mucosal afferents have similar properties to vagal mucosal afferents, responding to fine tactile stimulation of the mucosa with a 10 mg von Frey hair and did not respond to circumferential stretch of the colon. Mucosal afferents account for 24% of the colonic afferents recorded from the rat LSN and are also polymodal as they are responsive to a variety of chemical stimuli, including 5-hydroxytryptamine (5-HT), NaCl, HCl, bile, and capsaicin (74,76).

In mouse colon, both pelvic nerve and LSN pathways have been shown to contain mucosal afferents (80). These afferents are consistent with previous reports of mucosal afferents throughout the gastrointestinal tract, suggesting that these afferents may respond to particulate material within the colonic lumen. In the mouse, afferents sensitive to mucosal stroking account for nearly 50% of the pelvic nerve afferent population (including both mucosal and muscular/mucosal afferents—see below) but only 4% of the LSN innervation (mucosal afferents) (80). These afferents exhibited different distributions, with pelvic nerve mucosal and muscular/mucosal afferents localized in the rectum and most aboral regions of the distal colon while the few LSN mucosal afferents were found more orally in the distal colon. Although the responsiveness of individual afferents to mucosal stroking is similar between the two pathways, these results suggest that fine mechanical stimulation of the colonic mucosa is signaled predominantly via the pelvic nerve pathway to the lumbosacral spinal cord. In particular, this signal occurs when mechanical stimulation of the colonic mucosa occurs in the distal colon/ rectum. The high proportion of pelvic nerve mucosal afferents recorded in this study may in fact correspond to the large proportion of distension-insensitive pelvic nerve afferents reported previously in vivo (36,64), which could not be ascribed any function.

Afferents with similar properties to mucosal afferents have been identified from the pelvic nerves in vivo, with receptive fields in the anal canal of the cat (36,78) and perianal mucosa of the rat (69). In the anal canal of the cat, these afferents responded to proximodistal shearing stimuli within the lumen, had discrete receptive fields, and were usually not activated by distension. The afferents also had significantly faster conduction velocities than colonic afferents (36). Similarly, afferents documented in the perianal mucosa of the rat responded with a burst of firing to stoking of the mucosa or by rotation or movement of the experimental balloon within the colon. These afferents also had discrete receptive fields with the majority unresponsive to colorectal distension (69). Unlike the distension sensitive afferents (which were C-fibers), the majority of these perianal mucosal afferents were classified as Aδ fibers (64). As mucosal afferents are sensitive to mechanical deformation of the mucosa, they may respond to particulate material within the lumen, which can refine the quality of perceived stimuli and alter reflexes controlling motility (81,82).

Muscular/Mucosal Afferents

Muscular/mucosal afferents, a class of afferent that responds to both circumferential stretch and low-intensity mucosal stroking (10 mg), comprise 23% of the pelvic nerve afferent innervation of the mouse colon (80) and display similar properties to the vagal tension/mucosal afferents recorded from the ferret esophagus (71). Muscular/mucosal afferents are found only in the pelvic nerves, not in the LSN, and are clustered in the lower distal colon and rectum. In response to fine mucosal stroking, these afferents display similar graded responses to mucosal receptors. However, a proportion of them display greater responses to circumferential stretch than muscular afferents. Thus these afferents are able to detect both low-threshold events in the lumen plus distension of the rectum. In order to achieve this, it is likely that the muscular/mucosal afferent has two receptive fields. Overall, these data suggest that pelvic muscular/mucosal and mucosal afferents contribute equally in the signaling of fine mucosal stimulation to the CNS at similar intensities. Although muscular/mucosal and muscular afferents are activated by similar loads of circumferential stretch and contribute equally in the signaling of colonic stretch across their receptive fields, muscular/mucosal afferents signal a more intense signal to the spinal cord.

Serosal/Mesenteric Afferents

Spinal afferent fibers with endings within the serosa and mesenteric attachment of the colon have been reported in the cat, rat, and mouse (65,67,74,76,77,80). These afferents have endings that are located close to or on blood vessels or branching points of capillaries supplying the serosa and can have between one and seven punctate receptive fields (36,65,67,69,73,74,76,83). Recordings from the LSN show that punctate mechanical stimulation or stretch of the mesentery elicits afferent firing (65,67). These afferents are also capable of responding to distension with a rapidly adapting response, particularly at noxious intensities of distension (67), and are polymodal as the majority respond to chemical stimuli including 5-HT, NaCl, HCl, bile, bradykinin, and capsaicin (73,76,77). Recent in vitro studies in rat colon have demonstrated that serosal/mesenteric afferents account for between 50% and 80% of the afferents recorded from the LSN (76,77). These afferents are classified by their response to probing or distortion of the colon, but not to circular stretch or fine mucosal stroking and have small (2–4 mm^2) punctate receptive fields (74,76,77). Serosal afferents also display a greater sensitivity to mechanical stimulation on the serosal surface compared with the mucosal surface (76). It is possible that these afferents could relate to the high threshold (or phasic) mechanoreceptors that have been described previously as they have low resting activity and respond only to noxious intensities of distension. As such, they are likely to be considered mechanonociceptors.

Although serosal and mesenteric afferents were originally thought to be a single population; in a recent in vitro study in mouse, mesenteric afferents were abundant, but clearly restricted to the LSN and never encountered in recordings of pelvic nerve afferents, indicating the two populations are distinct in their organization. It is perhaps surprising that such a large population of mesenteric afferents exists for the signaling of relatively rare events such as twisting and torsion of the mesentery; therefore it is possible that these afferents have an as yet unidentified physiological role. Whatever their role, they are quite specific to the colon, as opposed to the rectum. Overall, serosal afferents were the most abundant population, accounting for approximately one-third of all fibers found in both LSN and pelvic nerve pathways. Although each pathway contributes equally in terms of numbers of serosal afferents, they differ in several features. First, pelvic nerve serosal afferents are generally clustered more distally, particularly in the rectum. Second, pelvic nerve serosal afferents responded across a wider stimulus range than LSN afferents and finally, pelvic nerve serosal afferents displayed a more intense and maintained response to focal compression than LSN afferents. Consequently, these pathways send very different signals to the spinal cord. In particular, pelvic nerve serosal afferents in more aboral regions of the distal colon and rectum would respond at lower stimulation intensities and generate a more intense and sustained afferent barrage in response to acute mechanical events. It is possible that serosal afferents in each pathway may signal transient, sharp pain at the onset of contraction or distension due to rapid transit of contents or experimental balloon inflation, during which acute intense mechanical stimulation might be achieved.

Silent Nociceptors

Silent nociceptors have been mainly studied in somatic tissues, where some have been characterized as chemonociceptors, and as a consequence have been implicated in the transmission of noxious stimuli (61,63). Large populations of afferents in the viscera that are silent at rest and are insensitive to innocuous and noxious colorectal distension (35,36,63,67) have been suggested to be "silent nociceptors." The term "silent nociceptor" was coined to describe these silent afferents, which subsequently generate spontaneous activity and mechanosensitivity during and after inflammation or chemical application (28,35,63). For example, recordings from the rat pelvic nerves reveal colonic afferents that are unresponsive to colorectal distension up to 100 mmHg. However, after 30 minutes treatment with acetic acid, these afferents developed spontaneous activity and started to respond to distension as low as 10 mmHg (35). It has been suggested that many of the afferents described previously as silent nociceptors, due to their insensitivity to distension, may in fact be another class of afferent for which colonic distension is not an adequate stimulus, and these afferents are then sensitized by inflammation or chemical application (63,76). Indeed colonic mucosal afferents described in the rat and mouse share many features with afferents that have been called silent nociceptors. These mucosal afferents (described above) are normally insensitive to distension, show no resting activity, respond to chemical stimuli, and may develop spontaneous firing after exposure to chemical stimuli during a study (76). This same study, which used a variety of mechanical stimuli (circular stretch, fine mucosal stroking, and probing) to identify subclasses of colonic afferents, showed that 6% of the afferents recorded initially had no mechanoreceptive fields, were not spontaneously active, and could not be classed as muscular, serosal, or mucosal afferents. However, these afferents were recruited during application of chemicals (NaCl, HCl, bile, and capsaicin) during the investigation of another mechanically sensitive unit, and retesting mechanical responsiveness revealed that these afferents became responsive to mechanical probing (76). More recently, another class of chemically recruited afferent has been documented in mouse colon. These afferents were mechanically insensitive and were recruited by the addition of αβ-methylene adenosine 5'-triphosphate (αβ-meATP), bradykinin, or capsaicin, but remained mechanically insensitive (84,85). These mechanically insensitive chemically recruited afferents represent a reasonably large population (approximately a quarter) and are restricted almost exclusively to the LSN. Importantly, these afferents appear to be distinct from the previously described "silent nociceptors" in skin and "chemospecific afferents" in colon because they remained insensitive to mechanical stimuli after they had been recruited by chemical stimuli and provide evidence for a novel class of truly chemospecific colonic afferents that are primarily confined to the LSN pathway. The existence of mechanically insensitive afferents in healthy animals that are responsive to chemical stimulation suggests the presence of a highly tuned early warning system to alert the CNS about injury to the colon without the complication of having to signal mechanical events simultaneously. This would result in an unambiguous signal about the chemical environment, which may be interpreted in a specific way and give rise to specific sensory and motor outcomes. Clearly, further investigation is required in the classification and existence of visceral silent nociceptors.

Chemical Modulation of Visceral Afferents

A multitude of receptors and ion channels have been shown to be involved in altering afferent firing within the gastrointestinal tract. These targets are numerous and can be classified into either having excitatory or inhibitory effects on afferent discharge and have been the subject of a multitude of recent reviews (28,70,86–93). Excitatory targets include the purinoceptor $P2X_3$, the bradykinin B2 receptor, and the transient receptor potential vanilloid receptor 1 (TRPV1) (formerly known as VR1), along with a number of serotonergic, glutamatergic, eicosanoid, and protease-activated receptors. Inhibitory targets include gabaergic, galanin, and somatostatin receptors (SSTR1–5). Many of these have been implicated in the transmission of pain in a number of systems (67,73,94–106), and may also alter mechanosensitivity either directly or indirectly (106–112). Some, including P2X$_3$, B2 and TRPV1 receptors, have been shown to be increased in patients with gastrointestinal disease (113–116). Not all of these are covered here, but a few examples are provided of mechanisms that have stimulated interest in recent years.

P2X$_3$ Receptors

P2X$_3$ is a member of the P2X purinoceptor family of ATP-gated ion channels (98,99). Studies in rat, monkey, and mouse DRG have localized the expression of P2X$_3$ receptors to small diameter primary afferent neurons (C-fibers) in DRG, usually those that bind the lectin Isolectin-B4 (43,117–125); functionally, P2X$_3$-mediated currents have been detected in these same neurons (98,99,122,126–130). As such, P2X$_3$ receptors have been strongly implicated in nociception and pain (94–99), although it should be noted that the majority of these studies have been performed in DRG that are devoid of colonic innervation (39,43). These data suggest that P2X$_3$ receptors may play a role in the processing of nociceptive information through either homomeric P2X$_3$ channels or P2X$_{2/3}$ heteromultimeric channels expressed either separately or together on individual neurons (98,99,124,127,131).

Activation of P2X$_3$ receptors by ATP or the more selective agonist α,β-meATP evokes excitation of gastrointestinal afferents in the jejunum, gastroesophageal region, and colon (50,72,123,132). The proportion of afferents that respond to these agonists varies between different species and different regions of the gastrointestinal tract. In rat jejunum, α,β-meATP activates 100% of mesenteric afferents (132) whereas 89% of vagal tension receptors were activated in the guinea pig esophagus (50). By contrast, in the mouse esophagus, only 30% of mucosal and 43% of tension receptors respond to α,β-meATP (72), while no afferents in the ferret esophagus responded (133). Lower down the gastrointestinal tract, 65% of distension sensitive pelvic colonic afferents in the rat respond to ATP or α,β-meATP (123); in mouse colon, 40% of LSN serosal afferents responded to α,β-meATP compared with only 7% of pelvic nerve serosal afferents. A recent in vitro study in mouse showed that 40% of LSN afferents responded to α,β-meATP, which was reflected in the number of retrogradely labeled colonic thoracolumbar DRG neurons exhibiting P2X$_3$-like immunoreactivity (LI) (134). Significantly fewer (7%) pelvic nerve afferents responded to α,β-meATP and only 19% of lumbosacral DRG neurons exhibited P2X$_3$ immunoreactivity. Endogenous sources of ATP that may activate afferents are several, including enteric and sympathetic neurons, endothelial and inflammatory cells, and cell damage.

Bradykinin Receptors

Bradykinin is one of the best-established chemical nociceptive stimuli and most physiologically relevant to tissue injury and pain. The direct effects of bradykinin are mediated via two G protein-coupled receptors: B$_1$, which is highly inducible in states of inflammation or injury (135) and B$_2$, which is constitutively expressed (135,136). Evidence suggests a role for B$_2$ receptors in acute inflammatory events, such as edema and inflammatory pain, whereas B$_1$ receptors appear to be involved in chronic inflammatory responses, including certain forms of persistent hyperalgesia (137). This suggests B$_2$ is a good target in normal conditions while B$_1$ may be a good target of interest in studies of altered afferent function in visceral inflammation. Bradykinin has been shown to be an important mediator of pain and irritation in skin, muscle, joints, vasculature, and all visceral organs (67,73,100–106). Bradykinin excites 55% of skin C-fibers in rat (104), 71% of joint afferents in cat (102), and 100% of cardiac afferents in cat (138). Almost 100% of guinea pig airway vagal afferents responded to bradykinin, with the exception of fast-conducting fibers with cell bodies in the nodose ganglion, which were unresponsive (139). In the gastrointestinal tract, bradykinin powerfully activates all mesenteric spinal afferents tested via B$_2$ receptors in an in vitro rat jejunum preparation (106,140). Some of these effects are also mediated via bradykinin-induced release of prostaglandins (106,140). In the cat colon, bradykinin evokes a response in 67% of LSN afferents recorded in vivo (73), while a study of nine pelvic distension-sensitive colonic afferents in rats in vivo showed that 77% of them responded to bradykinin (69). In mouse colon, bradykinin evoked responses in 66% of serosal afferents (84), an effect that was mediated via B_2 receptors, and responses to probing were potentiated after bradykinin. In this study, another group of bradykinin-responsive LSN afferents were mechanically insensitive. Fewer (11%) mouse pelvic nerve serosal afferents responded to bradykinin, and no mechanically insensitive pelvic nerve afferents were recruited by bradykinin. This suggests differences in the way each pathway signals bradykinin activation and reveals a chemospecific population of afferents. Interestingly, B_1 but not B_2 receptor protein is significantly increased in the intestines of both active ulcerative colitis and Crohn's disease patients compared with controls (116), but the relationship of this to symptoms is not known.

Recently it has been demonstrated that bradykinin activation of afferent fibers may have numerous downstream effects, including the production of 12-lipoxygenase metabolites of arachidonic acid that activate vanilloid (TRPV) receptors (104) and which are involved directly in mechanical, thermal, and pH sensitivity (95,109). A similar mechanism is responsible for bradykinin activation of the mechano- and thermosensitive channel TRPA1 (141).

Transient Receptor Potential Vanilloid Receptor 1

TRPV1 belongs to the transient receptor potential (TRP) channel family and is activated by heat, protons, and vanilloid ligands such as capsaicin (94–96,142–149). Studies have localized the expression of TRPV1 receptors on small diameter primary afferent neurons (C-fibers) in DRG, usually with $P2X_3$, while functionally TRPV1-mediated currents have been detected in these same neurons. As such, TRPV1 receptors have been strongly implicated in nociception and pain (94–99), including thermal nociception and inflammatory hyperalgesia and allodynia (97), and neuropathic pain (150). Although as is the case with $P2X_3$ receptors, it should be noted that the majority of these studies have been performed in levels of DRG, which are devoid of colonic innervation (39,43). A recent report demonstrated differences in TRPV1 expression between cutaneous and visceral afferents. This study showed, using immunohistochemistry, that 69% of rat DRG neurons innervating the urinary bladder expressed TRPV1, in contrast to only 32% of DRG neurons innervating the skin (151).

The response to TRPV1 activation is generally regarded as involving two phases: an initial excitation leading to transmitter release, followed by desensitization and damage after prolonged or repeated exposure (94,96,144,152,153). In the gastrointestinal tract, capsaicin evokes a powerful excitation of discharge in all classes of vagal and spinal afferents; however, the relative proportion varies between location and species (71,74,109,154–156). Early reports in the cat found that the majority of vagal and spinal afferents were activated by capsaicin (157). Similarly, in the mouse, 80% of isolated retrogradely labeled colonic lumbosacral DRG cells responded to capsaicin (158). By contrast, in the rat, in isolated retrogradely labeled cells capsaicin evoked responses in 42% of nodose ganglion cells (154), and 46% of colonic lumbosacral DRG cells (155). Capsaicin activated 29% of rat colonic LSN afferents, including 17% of mucosal afferents, 40% of serosal afferents, and no muscular afferents. In the mouse colon, 61% of splanchnic afferents responded to capsaicin (3 µM) and 82% of thoracolumbar colonic DRG neurons showed TRPV1-LI. Significantly fewer (47%) pelvic nerve afferents responded to capsaicin and 50% of lumbosacral colonic neurons showed TRPV1-LI. In the rat stomach, capsaicin activated 32% of spinal afferents (74). One notable finding is the ability of capsaicin to cause mechanical desensitization in vitro in gastroesophageal (156), jejunal (109), and LSN colonic preparations (85). However, in the gastroesophageal preparation, mechanical desensitization was also observed in capsaicin unresponsive afferents in addition to capsaicin-responsive afferents. The desensitization and subsequent degeneration of primary afferents by capsaicin is thought to follow from uncontrolled cation influx into afferent endings, resulting in depolarization block and subsequent osmotic damage (153). Expression of TRPV1 is increased in colonic nerve fibers of patients with inflammatory bowel disease (114), and in patients with rectal hypersensitivity (159) while administration of TRPV1 antagonists can attenuate disease severity in dextran sulphate sodium-induced colitis in mice (160). The involvement of TRPV1 in pain in the clinic may be implicated from the low levels of pH often encountered in the stomach and esophagus, particularly where ulceration and inflammation are present. Furthermore, the temperature threshold of TRPV1 to heat is considerably reduced after exposure of colonic sensory neurons to 5-HT (158), which may indicate the channels are active at normal body temperature in situations of increased 5-HT concentration in the gut—see below.

Serotonin (5-hydroxytryptamine)
The majority of 5-hydroxytryptamine (5-HT) in the body is found in the gastrointestinal tract, primarily contained within enterochromaffin cells and is released by meals, toxins, and chemotherapeutic agents (161,162). 5-HT is implicated in postinfectious IBS patients by increased numbers of enterochromaffin cells (163), increased mast cell populations (15,164), increased postprandial 5-HT release (162,165), and a decrease in symptoms using serotonergic antagonists (1,166). Metabolism of 5-HT may also be disrupted in both IBS and IBD (167). 5-HT release is well known to activate vagal afferent endings in the upper gastrointestinal tract (168–170). 5-HT also activates cutaneous nociceptive primary afferents contributing to a role in inflammatory pain (171). More recently it was shown that rat colonic LSN afferents also respond to 5-HT (77). Fifty-six percent of LSN afferents responded to 5-HT via both 5-HT_3 and non–5-HT_3 receptors, which correlates with the percentage of thoracolumbar DRG cell bodies retrogradely labeled from the colon that display 5-HT_3 receptors (77). In the rat 5-HT_1, 5-HT_2 and 5-HT_3 receptor subtypes have been demonstrated to modulate responses to noxious colorectal distension (172), and serotonergic activation of visceral sensory neurons may increase their sensitivity to other sensory modalities (158).

Glutamate
Glutamate is a major transmitter in the CNS and can act via the activation of four separate receptor types. (i) ionotropic N-methyl-d-aspartate (NMDA) receptors, (ii) α-amino-3-hydroxy-5-methyl-4-isoxazolepropionic acid (AMPA) receptors, (iii) kainate receptors, and (iv) metabotropic glutamate (mGlu) receptors. Peripheral ionotropic GluR (iGluR) receptors have been suggested to be involved in visceral pain transmission, via activation by endogenous glutamate. This follows from the observation that NMDA receptor antagonists reduce responses to mechanical stimuli in splanchnic and pelvic afferents in rat colon and they decrease the visceromotor response to colorectal distension (173). NMDA receptor antagonists also reduced the response of vagal afferent fibers innervating the rat stomach (174). Similarly, AMPA/kainate receptor antagonists also reduced the response of vagal afferent fibers innervating the rat stomach (174). Actions of glutamate are also mediated via mGlu receptors, some of which are inhibitory G-protein-coupled receptors. Glutamate can inhibit vagal afferent mechanosensitivity, when administered in the presence of kynurenate to block iGluR. This inhibition can be mimicked by selective group II and III mGluR agonists (175). Conversely, group III mGluR antagonists can increase mechanosensitivity to intense stimuli (175). Therefore there appears to be a delicate balancing act in the way in which endogenous or exogenous glutamate can act via mGluR and iGluR to regulate primary afferent mechanosensitivity (175). Whether or not this interplay occurs on spinal afferents as it does in vagal afferents is yet to be determined.

γ-Amino Butyric Acid
γ-Amino butyric acid (GABA) has a major inhibitory role in the CNS, which mediates its effect via three classes of receptors, the ionotropic GABA_A, GABA_C receptors, and the G-protein-coupled GABA_B receptors. GABA_B receptor agonists inhibit vagal afferent mechanosensitivity in the upper gastrointestinal tract and GABA_B receptors are expressed on gastric vagal afferent neurons. This peripheral action is associated with a reduction in triggering of transient lower esophageal relaxations (TLESRs) (87,176–179), which are the major cause of acid reflux. This has led to interest in these receptors as therapeutic targets for gastroesophageal reflux disease by reducing TLESRs and therefore reflux episodes. More recently, inhibitory actions of GABA_B receptors have been demonstrated on pelvic afferents from rat colon (180), suggesting they may have a peripheral antinociceptive action. Endogenous activation of peripheral GABA_B receptors on afferent endings is probably minimal, whereas endogenous GABA release is much more important in the CNS. Thus peripheral GABA_B receptors may provide a naïve but convenient target for reducing afferent excitability.

Galanin
Galanin is found throughout the CNS and enteric nervous systems. Three G protein–coupled receptors (GalR1-3) mediate the effects of galanin. Galanin causes inhibition of mechanosensitivity in 80% of mouse and 58% of ferret gastroesophageal afferents, respectively, whereas 12% displayed potentiated responses (181). The inhibitory effects are likely to be mediated via

GalR1 and/or 3 receptors and the potentiating effects via GalR2 receptors (181) based on their known coupling mechanisms.

Proteinase-activated Receptors

Proteinase-activated receptor (PARs) are a peculiar family of G-protein-coupled receptors, consisting of four receptors PAR1-4 (182). These receptors are activated by binding of a tethered ligand, following its cleavage by serine proteases such as mast cell tryptase, thrombin, and trypsin. As such they are likely to be important when mast cells degranulate following inflammation (183,184). This is highlighted by recent studies suggesting an important role for PAR1 in the pathogenesis of experimental colitis (86,183,184). Notably, PAR-2 agonists have been shown to evoke discharge of rat jejunal mesenteric afferents (185), whilst PAR-2 can sensitize TRPV1 to induce hyperalgesia (186).

Voltage-gated Na+ Channels

Voltage-gated Na+ channels (NaV) can be classified into two broad classes on the basis of their sensitivity to the NaV blocker tetrodotoxin (TTX): TTX-sensitive and TTX-resistant (TTX-R). The TTX-R channels are of particular interest because colitis induces increased neuronal excitability in mouse thoracolumbar DRG neurons via a $Na v1.8\,Na^+$ current (187). The role of these channels in visceral pain is described in detail elsewhere in Chapters 6.

Somatostatin

SSTR1–5 have been detected throughout the rat gastrointestinal tract (188), and clinical studies show that a somatostatin analog decreases colorectal pain in patients with IBS (189). This correlates with a reduction in the mechanical sensitivity of high threshold intestinal afferents by somatostatin analogs (190). The results of this study suggested the SST2 receptor may be the most important in modulation of visceral afferent sensitivity.

Mechanotransduction Mechanisms in Visceral Afferents

Mechanotransduction is fundamental to the perception of distension, contraction, mucosal contact, and a number of other visceral stimuli. Understanding the molecular basis of mechanotransduction may therefore hold the key to designing effective therapies for visceral pain. The number of candidate molecules as mechanotransducers is increasing with the discovery of novel molecules and improved understanding of established molecules. The major candidates are two families of ion channels: the degenerin/epithelial sodium channel (DEG/ENaC) family, and the TRP family. The DEG/ENaCs in mammals comprise mainly of the acid sensing ion channels (ASICs) and ENaCs (191,192). Candidate TRP channels in mechanotransduction are TRPV1, V4, C1, and A1 (109,193–195). ASICs were first implicated in mechanotransduction by their close relation to invertebrate channels, without which there are deficits in touch perception (196). It is clear from knockout, patch clamp and expression studies that ASIC1, 2, and 3 coexist in the same sensory neurons, and that they form heteromultimeric channels (192,197). A role for ASICs in mammalian mechanotransduction was indicated by studies of cutaneous mechanoreceptors in mutant mice lacking individual ASIC family members. These are rapidly adapting (RA) and slowly adapting (SA) mechanoreceptors; D-hair receptors; A-fiber mechanonociceptors (AM), and high threshold C-fibers. Disruption of ASIC2 (also known as BNC1) reduced responses of RA and SA mechanoreceptors (198). Disruption of ASIC3 (also known as DRASIC) reduced the responsiveness of AM nociceptors, whereas RA mechanoreceptors in contrast showed increased mechanosensitivity (199). The ASIC1 gene (also known as ASIC) gives rise to two proteins (ASIC1a and 1b) through alternative splicing. Disruption of ASIC1a had no effect on any cutaneous mechanoreceptors (200). Recordings of different classes of colonic LSN afferents and vagal gastroesophageal afferents revealed that disruption of ASIC1a increased the mechanical sensitivity of all afferents in both locations (200). Disruption of ASIC2 had varied effects (201): increased mechanosensitivity in gastroesophageal mucosal endings, decreases in gastroesophageal tension receptors, increases in colonic serosal endings, and no change in colonic mesenteric endings. In $ASIC3^{-/-}$ mice, all splanchnic endings had markedly reduced mechanosensitivity (Table 1) (201). Thus it would appear that ASIC3 makes a critical positive contribution to mechanosensitivity in visceral afferents. The presence of ASIC1a appears to provide an inhibitory contribution to the ion

Table 1 Summary of Effects of ASIC Disruption on Mechanosensory Responses in Each Afferent Subtype and Effects on Digestive Function in Conscious Animals

	Gastroesophageal		Gastric Emptying	Colonic		Fecal Pellet Output
	Mucosal	Tension		Serosal	Mesenteric	
ASIC1a	↑	↑	↓	↑	↑	↔
ASIC2	↑	↓↓	↔	↑↑	↔	↓
ASIC3	↔	↓↓	↔	↓↓	↓↓	↔

Source: From Ref. 20.

channel complex, while the role of ASIC2 differs widely across subclasses of afferents. These findings contrast sharply with the effects of ASIC1, 2, and 3 in skin, which suggest that targeting these subunits with pharmacological agents may have different and more pronounced effects on mechanosensitivity in the viscera. Findings of both positive and negative effects of ASIC mutations on mechanosensitivity suggest a complexity in the way they contribute to mechanotransduction. It is therefore unlikely that ASICs function simply as individual mechanically gated cation channels, and in some cases they may in fact dampen the mechanotransduction process. This would be the case for ASIC2 in colonic afferents and for ASIC1a in all populations of visceral afferents, because in both instances mechanosensitivity was increased in null mutant mice. This negative modulatory or "dampening" role is probably a result of existence of all three ASIC subtypes as heteromultimers, in which each member contributes directly or indirectly to mechanotransduction. ASIC1a clearly appears to make little if any direct contribution to mechanotransduction, because without it mechanosensitivity is universally increased in visceral afferents, suggesting that the heteromultimeric mechanotransducer becomes more efficient. ASIC3 appears to make a positive contribution in most cases, whereas the role of ASIC2 is interesting in its capacity to influence mechanosensitivity negatively in lower gut afferents and positively in upper gut afferents.

The way in which ASICs are tethered to other cellular components is critical in their function. The integral membrane protein stomatin (which is found in lipid/protein-rich microdomains) binds to ASIC1a, 2, and 3 subunits and can alter each of their functions, with strikingly different functional effects between subunits. Notably, stomatin has the most prominent effect on ASIC3, potently reducing acid-evoked currents (202). The question of how these acid-evoked currents relate to the differences observed with mechanical stimuli remains to be elucidated. However, this system is similar to a suggested model of mechanotransduction in *Caenorhabditis elegans* whereby MEC-2 (which shares a 65% identity and an 85% similarity to stomatin) functions to link MEC-4 and MEC-10 (related to ASICs) channels to the intracellular cytoskeleton and the extracellular matrix. Deformation of this system by mechanical stimuli is then thought to open the channel complex (203,204).

Recent evidence indicates that the capsaicin receptor TRPV1 may be involved in visceral mechanotransduction. A study of mechanosensitivity in TRPV1 wild-type and null mutant mice showed more directly that mechanotransduction was reduced in the knockout compared to the wild type. Additionally the TRPV1 antagonist capsazepine was effective in reducing mechanical responses in the wild-type—a response that was totally lost in TRPV1 null mutant mice (109).

The role $P2X_3$ plays in sensory signaling is evident in $P2X_3$ null mutant mice. These mice exhibit marked urinary bladder hyporeflexia, have reduced pain-related behavior in response to injection of ATP or formalin, and are unable to code the intensity of non-noxious "warming stimuli" (110,111). These results lead to the suggestion that the $P2X_3$ receptors are involved in mechanosensation. This mechanism is proposed to occur via ATP acting as the molecular messenger that is released from the epithelial cells in response to distension, and channels made of $P2X_3$ receptors detect ATP and trigger the neuronal pathway signaling bladder fullness (110,111,205). A similar mechanism has been proposed in the colon whereby ATP present in the colon is released by colorectal distension and that responses of pelvic distension sensitive afferents are inhibited by P2X receptor antagonists (123). This mechanism appears to have an enhanced role in mechanosensory transduction during inflammation as augmented distension-evoked sensory nerve responses are observed after application of ATP and α,β-meATP (206).

The involvement of a range of molecules in mechanotransduction may therefore take several forms—as direct mechanotransducers, as responders to local release of endogenous mediators by mechanical stimuli, or as modulators of cellular excitability.

CONCLUSIONS

It is becoming clear from the literature that visceral afferents represent a heterogeneous population of fibers that are individually tuned to detect distinct types of mechanical and or chemical stimuli by virtue of their location in the gastrointestinal tract. Different anatomical pathways may contain different classes of afferent fiber allowing for the specific detection and interpretation of certain stimuli. Moreover, the same class of afferent in different anatomical pathways is capable of responding with differing sensitivities, demonstrating the great detail in which mechanical and chemical events are signaled to the CNS.

REFERENCES

1. Camilleri M. Management of the irritable bowel syndrome. Gastroenterology 2001; 120:652–668.
2. Drossman D, Corazziari E, Talley N, Thompson W, Whitehead W. Rome II: a multinational consensus document on functional gastrointestinal disorders. Gut 1999; 45:1–81.
3. Hungin A, Whorwell P, Tack J, Mearin F. The prevalence, patterns and impact of irritable bowel syndrome: an international survey of 40,000 subjects. Aliment Pharmacol Ther 2003; 17:643–650.
4. Camilleri M, Choi MG. Review article: irritable bowel syndrome. Aliment Pharmacol Ther 1997; 11:3–15.
5. Jones J, Boorman J, Cann P, et al. British Society of Gastroenterology guidelines for the management of the irritable bowel syndrome. Gut 2000; 47(suppl 2):ii1–ii19.
6. Thompson WG, Heaton KW, Smyth GT, Smyth C. Irritable bowel syndrome in general practice: prevalence, characteristics, and referral. Gut 2000; 46:78–82.
7. Gralnek IM, Hays RD, Kilbourne A, Naliboff B, Mayer EA. The impact of irritable bowel syndrome on health-related quality of life. Gastroenterology 2000; 119:654–660.
8. Ragnarsson G, Bodemar G. Division of the irritable bowel syndrome into subgroups on the basis of daily recorded symptoms in two outpatients samples. Scand J Gastroenterol 1999; 34:993–1000.
9. Guilera M, Balboa A, Mearin F. Bowel habit subtypes and temporal patterns in irritable bowel syndrome: systematic review. Am J Gastroenterol 2005; 100:1174–1184.
10. Spiller R. Neuropathology of IBS? Gastroenterology 2002; 123:2144–2147.
11. Spiller RC. Irritable bowel syndrome. Br Med Bull 2005; 72:15–29.
12. Spiller R. Postinfectious irritable bowel syndrome (1). Gastroenterology 2003; 124:1662–1671.
13. Ritchie J. Pain from distention of the pelvic colon by inflating a balloon in the irritable bowel syndrome. Gut 1973; 6:105–112.
14. Naliboff BD, Munakata J, Fullerton S, et al. Evidence for two distinct perceptual alterations in irritable bowel syndrome. Gut 1997; 41:505–512.
15. Barbara G, Stanghellini V, De Giorgio R, et al. Activated mast cells in proximity to colonic nerves correlate with abdominal pain in irritable bowel syndrome. Gastroenterology 2004; 126: 693–702.
16. Lembo T, Munakata J, Mertz H, et al. Evidence for the hypersensitivity of lumbar splanchnic afferents in irritable bowel syndrome. Gastroenterology 1994; 107:1686–1696.
17. Verne GN, Himes NC, Robinson ME, et al. Central representation of visceral and cutaneous hypersensitivity in the irritable bowel syndrome. Pain 2003; 103:99–110.
18. Munakata J, Naliboff B, Harraf F, et al. Repetitive sigmoid stimulation induces rectal hyperalgesia in patients with irritable bowel syndrome. Gastroenterology 1997; 112:55–63.
19. Chadwick V, Chen W, Shu D, et al. Activation of the mucosal immune system in irritable bowel syndrome. Gastroenterology 2002; 122:1778–1783.
20. Dunlop S, Jenkins D, Neal K, Spiller R. Relative importance of enterochromaffin cell hyperplasia, anxiety, and depression in postinfectious IBS. Gastroenterology 2003; 125:1651–1659.
21. Wilhelmsen I. The role of psychosocial factors in gastrointestinal disorders. Gut 2000; 47(suppl 4): iv73–iv75.
22. Mayer EA, Naliboff BD, Chang L, Coutinho SV. V. Stress and irritable bowel syndrome. Am J Physiol Gastrointest Liver Physiol 2001; 280:G519–G524.
23. Schmulson M, Lee OY, Chang L, Naliboff B, Mayer EA. Symptom differences in moderate to severe IBS patients based on predominant bowel habit. Am J Gastroenterol 1999; 94:2929–2935.
24. Mayer EA. Psychological stress and colitis. Gut 2000; 46:595–596.
25. Mayer EA. The neurobiology of stress and gastrointestinal disease. Gut 2000; 47:861–869.
26. Emmanuel AV, Mason HJ, Kamm MA. Relationship between psychological state and level of activity of extrinsic gut innervation in patients with a functional gut disorder. Gut 2001; 49:209–213.

27. Berthoud HR, Patterson LM, Willing AE, Mueller K, Neuhuber WL. Capsaicin-resistant vagal afferent fibers in the rat gastrointestinal tract: anatomical identification and functional integrity. Brain Res 1997; 746:195–206.

28. Blackshaw LA, Gebhart GF. The pharmacology of gastrointestinal nociceptive pathways. Curr Opin Pharmacol 2002; 2:642–649.

29. Berthoud HR, Jedrezejewska A, Powley TL. Simultaneous labeling of vagal innervation of the gut and afferent projections form the visceral forebrain with DiI injected into the dorsal vagal complex in the rat. J Comp Neurol 1990; 301:65–79.

30. Baron R, Janig W, McLachlan EM. The afferent and sympathetic components of the lumbar spinal outflow to the colon and pelvic organs in the cat. III. The colonic nerves, incorporating an analysis of all components of the lumbar prevertebral outflow. J Comp Neurol 1985; 238:158–168.

31. Baron R, Janig W, McLachlan EM. The afferent and sympathetic components of the lumbar spinal outflow to the colon and pelvic organs in the cat. II. The lumbar splanchnic nerves. J Comp Neurol 1985; 238:147–157.

32. Baron R, Janig W, McLachlan EM. The afferent and sympathetic components of the lumbar spinal outflow to the colon and pelvic organs in the cat. I. The hypogastric nerve. J Comp Neurol 1985; 238:135–146.

33. Baron R, Janig W, Kollmann W. Sympathetic and afferent somata projecting in hindlimb nerves and the anatomical organization of the lumbar sympathetic nervous system of the rat. J Comp Neurol 1988; 275:460–468.

34. Baron R, Janig W. Afferent and sympathetic neurons projecting into lumbar visceral nerves of the male rat. J Comp Neurol 1991; 314:429–436.

35. Sengupta J, Gebhart G. The sensory innervation of the colon and its modulation. Curr Opin Gastroenterol 1998; 14:15–20.

36. Janig W, Koltzenburg M. Receptive properties of sacral primary afferent neurons supplying the colon. J Neurophysiol 1991; 65:1067–1077.

37. Janig W, Koltzenburg M. On the function of spinal primary afferent fibres supplying colon and urinary bladder. J Auton Nerv Syst 1990; 30(suppl):S89–S96.

38. Nadelhaft I, Vera PL. Neurons labelled after the application of tracer to the distal stump of the transected hypogastric nerve in the rat. J Auton Nerv Syst 1991; 36:87–96.

39. Ness TJ, Gebhart GF. Characterization of neurons responsive to noxious colorectal distension in the T13-L2 spinal cord of the rat. J Neurophysiol 1988; 60:1419–1438.

40. Hulsebosch CE, Coggeshall RE. An analysis of the axon populations in the nerves to the pelvic viscera in the rat. J Comp Neurol 1982; 211:1–10.

41. Traub RJ, Hutchcroft K, Gebhart GF. The peptide content of colonic afferents decreases following colonic inflammation. Peptides 1999; 20:267–273.

42. Keast J, de Groat W. Segmental distribution and peptide content of primary afferent neurons innervating the urogenital organs and colon of male rats. J Comp Neurol 1992; 319:615–623.

43. Robinson DR, McNaughton PA, Evans ML, Hicks GA. Characterization of the primary spinal afferent innervation of the mouse colon using retrograde labelling. Neurogastroenterol Motil 2004; 16:113–124.

44. Berthoud HR, Patterson LM, Neumann F, Neuhuber WL. Distribution and structure of vagal afferent intraganglionic laminar endings (IGLEs) in the rat gastrointestinal tract. Anat Embryol (Berl) 1997; 195:183–191.

45. Phillips RJ, Powley TL. Tension and stretch receptors in gastrointestinal smooth muscle: re-evaluating vagal mechanoreceptor electrophysiology. Brain Res Brain Res Rev 2000; 34:1–26.

46. Fox EA, Phillips RJ, Martinson FA, Baronowsky EA, Powley TL. Vagal afferent innervation of smooth muscle in the stomach and duodenum of the mouse: morphology and topography. J Comp Neurol 2000; 428:558–576.

47. Wang FB, Powley TL. Topographic inventories of vagal afferents in gastrointestinal muscle. J Comp Neurol 2000; 421:302–324.

48. Zagorodnyuk VP, Brookes SJ. Transduction sites of vagal mechanoreceptors in the guinea pig esophagus. J Neurosci 2000; 20:6249–6255.

49. Zagorodnyuk VP, Chen BN, Brookes SJ. Intraganglionic laminar endings are mechano-transduction sites of vagal tension receptors in the guinea-pig stomach. J Physiol 2001; 534:255–268.

50. Zagorodnyuk VP, Chen BN, Costa M, Brookes SJ. Mechanotransduction by intraganglionic laminar endings of vagal tension receptors in the guinea-pig oesophagus. J Physiol 2003; 553:575–587.

51. Berthoud HR, Blackshaw LA, Brookes SJ, Grundy D. Neuroanatomy of extrinsic afferents supplying the gastrointestinal tract. Neurogastroenterol Motil 2004; 16(suppl 1):28–33.

52. Neuhuber WL, Kressel M, Stark A, Berthoud HR. Vagal efferent and afferent innervation of the rat esophagus as demonstrated by anterograde DiI and DiA tracing: focus on myenteric ganglia. J Auton Nerv Syst 1998; 70:92–102.

53. Neuhuber W. Sensory vagal innervation of the rat esophagus and cardia. A light and electron microscopic anterograde tracing study. J Auton Nerv Syst 1987; 20:243–255.

54. Lynn PA, Olsson C, Zagorodnyuk V, Costa M, Brookes SJ. Rectal intraganglionic laminar endings are transduction sites of extrinsic mechanoreceptors in the guinea pig rectum. Gastroenterology 2003; 125:786–794.

55. Lynn PA, Zagorodnyuk VP, Hennig GW, Costa M, Brookes SJH. Mechanical activation of rectal intraganglionic laminar endings in the guinea pig distal gut. J Physiol (Lond) 2005; 564:589–601.
56. Zagorodnyuk VP, Lynn P, Costa M, Brookes SJH. Mechanisms of mechanotransduction by specialized low threshold mechanoreceptors in the guinea pig rectum. Am J Physiol Gastrointest Liver Physiol 2005; 289(3):G397–G406.
57. Olsson C, Costa M, Brookes SJ. Neurochemical characterization of extrinsic innervation of the guinea pig rectum. J Comp Neurol 2004; 470:357–371.
58. Berthoud HR, Powley TL. Vagal afferent innervation of the rat fundic stomach: morphological characterization of the gastric tesion receptor. J Comp Neurol 1992; 319:261–276.
59. Ward S, Bayguinov J, Won K, Grundy D, Berthoud H. Distribution of the vanilloid receptor (VR1) in the gastrointestinal tract. J Comp Neurol 2003; 465:121–135.
60. Clerc N, Mazzia C. Morphological relationships of choleragenoid horseradish peroxidase-labeled spinal primary afferents with myenteric ganglia and mucosal associated lymphoid tissue in the cat esophagogastric junction. J Comp Neurol 1994; 347:171–186.
61. Lewin GR, Moshourab R. Mechanosensation and Pain. J Neurobiol 2004; 61:30–44.
62. Koltzenburg M, Stucky CL, Lewin GR. Receptive properties of mouse sensory neurons innervating hairy skin. J Neurophysiol 1997; 78:1841–1850.
63. Cervero F. Sensory innervation of the viscera: peripheral basis of visceral pain. Physiol Rev 1994; 74:95–138.
64. Sengupta JN, Gebhart GF. Characterization of mechanosensitive pelvic nerve afferent fibers innervating the colon of the rat. J Neurophysiol 1994; 71:2046–2060.
65. Morrison JFB. Splanchnic slowly adapting mechanoreceptors with punctate receptove fields in the mesentery and the gastrointestinal tract of the cat. J Physiol 1973; 233:349–361.
66. Janig W, Koltzenburg M. The neural basis of consciously perceived sensations from the gut. In: Singer MV, Goebell H, eds. Nerves in the Gastrointestinal Tract. Lancester: MTP Press, 1989: 183–197.
67. Blumberg H, Haupt P, Janig W, Kohler W. Encoding of visceral noxious stimuli in the discharge patterns of visceral afferent fibres from the colon. Pflugers Arch 1983; 398:33–40.
68. Janig W, Haupt-Schade P, Kohler W. Afferent innervation of the colon: the neurophysiological basis for visceral sensation and pain. In: In: Basic and Clinical Aspects of Chronic Abdominal Pain. Amsterdam: Elsevier, 1993:71–86.
69. Sengupta JN, Gebhart GF. Mechanosensitive properties of pelvic nerve afferent fibers innervating the urinary bladder of the rat. J Neurophysiol 1994; 72:2420–2430.
70. Grundy D. What activates visceral afferents?. Gut 2004; 53:5ii–8ii.
71. Page AJ, Blackshaw LA. An in vitro study of the properties of vagal afferent fibres innervating the ferret oesophagus and stomach. J Physiol 1998; 512(Pt 3):907–916.
72. Page AJ, Martin CM, Blackshaw LA. Vagal mechanoreceptors and chemoreceptors in mouse stomach and esophagus. J Neurophysiol 2002; 87:2095–2103.
73. Haupt P, Janig W, Kohler W. Response pattern of visceral afferent fibres, supplying the colon, upon chemical and mechanical stimuli. Pflugers Arch 1983; 398:41–47.
74. Berthoud HR, Lynn PA, Blackshaw LA. Vagal and spinal mechanosensors in the rat stomach and colon have multiple receptive fields. Am J Physiol Regul Integr Comp Physiol 2001; 280: R1371–R1381.
75. Su X, Gebhart GF. Mechanosensitive pelvic nerve afferent fibers innervating the colon of the rat are polymodal in character. J Neurophysiol 1998; 80:2632–2644.
76. Lynn PA, Blackshaw LA. In vitro recordings of afferent fibres with receptive fields in the serosa, muscle and mucosa of rat colon. J Physiol 1999; 518(Pt 1):271–282.
77. Hicks GA, Coldwell JR, Schindler M, et al. Excitation of rat colonic afferent fibres by 5-HT(3) receptors. J Physiol 2002; 544:861–869.
78. Bahns E, Halsband U, Janig W. Responses of sacral visceral afferents from the lower urinary tract, colon and anus to mechanical stimulation. Pflugers Arch 1987; 410:296–303.
79. Ruhl A, Thewissen M, Ross H, Cleveland S, Frieling T, Enck P. Discharge patterns of intramural mechanoreceptive afferents during selective distension of the cat's rectum. Neurogastroenterol Motil 1998; 10:219–225.
80. Brierley SM, Jones RCW III, Gebhart GF, Blackshaw LA. Splanchnic and pelvic mechanosensory afferents signal different qualities of colonic stimuli in mice. Gastroenterology 2004; 127:166–178.
81. Bahr R, Bartel B, Blumberg H, Janig W. Secondary functional properties of lumbar visceral preganglionic neurons. J Auton Nerv Syst 1986; 15:141–152.
82. Bahr R, Bartel B, Blumberg H, Janig W. Functional characterization of preganglionic neurons projecting in the lumbar splanchnic nerves: neurons regulating motility. J Auton Nerv Syst 1986; 15:109–130.
83. Bessou P, Perl ER. Amovement receptor of the small intestine. J Physiol 1966; 182:404–426.
84. Brierley SM, Jones RCW III, Xu L, Gebhart GF, Blackshaw LA. Activation of splanchnic and pelvic colonic afferents by bradykinin in mice. Neurogastroenterol & Motility 2005; 17(6):854–862.
85. Brierley SM, Jones RCW III, Xu L, et al. Differential chemosensory function and receptor expression of splanchnic and pelvic colonic afferents in mice. J Physiol 2005; 567:267–281.

86. Kirkup AJ, Brunsden AM, Grundy D. Receptors and transmission in the brain-gut axis: potential for novel therapies. I. Receptors on visceral afferents. Am J Physiol Gastrointest Liver Physiol 2001; 280:G787–G794.

87. Blackshaw LA. Receptors and transmission in the brain-gut axis: potential for novel therapies. IV. GABA(B) receptors in the brain-gastroesophageal axis. Am J Physiol Gastrointest Liver Physiol 2001; 281:G311–G315.

88. Bueno L, Fioramonti J, Delvaux M, Frexinos J. Mediators and pharmacology of visceral sensitivity: from basic to clinical investigations. Gastroenterology 1997; 112:1714–1743.

89. Bueno L, Fioramonti J. Visceral perception: inflammatory and non-inflammatory mediators. Gut 2002; 51:19i–23i.

90. Bueno L, Fioramonti J, Garcia-Villar R. Pathobiology of visceral pain: molecular mechanisms and therapeutic implications. III. Visceral afferent pathways: a source of new therapeutic targets for abdominal pain. Am J Physiol Gastrointest Liver Physiol 2000; 278:G670–G676.

91. Grundy D, Winchester W. Molecular mechanisms in the control of gastrointestinal function. Curr Opin Pharmacol 2003; 3:S1–S4.

92. Cervero F, Laird JM. Role of ion channels in mechanisms controlling gastrointestinal pain pathways. Curr Opin Pharmacol 2003; 3:608–612.

93. Cervero F, Laird JM. Understanding the signaling and transmission of visceral nociceptive events. J Neurobiol 2004; 61:45–54.

94. Caterina MJ, Schumacher MA, Tominaga M, Rosen TA, Levine JD, Julius D. The capsaicin receptor: a heat-activated ion channel in the pain pathway. Nature 1997; 389:816–824.

95. Caterina MJ, Leffler A, Malmberg AB, et al. Impaired nociception and pain sensation in mice lacking the capsaicin receptor. Science 2000; 288:306–313.

96. Caterina MJ, Julius D. The vanilloid receptor: a Molecular Gateway to the Pain Pathway. Annu Rev Neurosci 2001; 24:487–517.

97. Davis JB, et al. Vanilloid receptor-1 is essential for inflammatory thermal hyperalgesia. Nature 2000; 405:183–187.

98. North RA. P2X3 receptors and peripheral pain mechanisms. J Physiol 2004; 554:301–308.

99. North RA. Molecular Physiology of P2X Receptors. Physiol Rev 2002; 82:1013–1067.

100. Berkley KJ, Robbins A, Sato Y. Functional differences between afferent fibers in the hypogastric and pelvic nerves innervating female reproductive organs in the rat. J Neurophysiol 1993; 69: 533–544.

101. Franz M, Mense S. Muscle receptors with group IV afferent fibres responding to application of bradykinin. Brain Res 1975; 92:369–383.

102. Messlinger K, Pawlak M, Schepelmann K, Schmidt RF. Responsiveness of slowly conducting articular afferents to bradykinin: effects of an experimental arthritis. Pain 1994; 59:335–343.

103. Mizumura K, Minagawa M, Tsujii Y, Kumazawa T. The effects of bradykinin agonists and antagonists on visceral polymodal receptor activities. Pain 1990; 40:221–227.

104. Shin J et al. Bradykinin-12-lipoxygenase-VR1 signaling pathway for inflammatory hyperalgesia. Proc Natl Acad Sci U S A 2002; 99:10150–10155.

105. Tjen ALSC, Pan HL, Longhurst JC. Endogenous bradykinin activates ischaemically sensitive cardiac visceral afferents through kinin B2 receptors in cats. J Physiol 1998; 510(Pt 2):633–641.

106. Brunsden AM, Grundy D. Sensitization of visceral afferents to bradykinin in rat jejunum in vitro. J Physiol 1999; 521(Pt 2):517–527.

107. Koltzenburg M, Kress M, Reeh PW. The nociceptor sensitization by bradykinin does not depend on sympathetic neurons. Neuroscience 1992; 46:465–473.

108. Neugebauer V, Schaible HG, Schmidt RF. Sensitization of articular afferents to mechanical stimuli by bradykinin. Pflugers Arch 1989; 415:330–335.

109. Rong W, Hillsley K, Davis JB, Hicks GA, Winchester WJ, Grundy D. Jejunal afferent nerve sensitivity in wild type and TRPV1 knockout mice. J Physiol (Lond) 2004; 560:867–881.

110. Souslova V, Cesare P, Ding Y, et al. Warm-coding deficits and aberrant inflammatory pain in mice lacking P2X3 receptors. Nature 2000; 407:1015–1017.

111. Cockayne DA et al. Urinary bladder hyporeflexia and reduced pain-related behaviour in P2X3-deficient mice. Nature 2000; 407:1011–1015.

112. Dai Y, Fukuoka T, Wang H, et al. Contribution of sensitized P2X receptors in inflamed tissue to the mechanical hypersensitivity revealed by phosphorylated ERK in DRG neurons. Pain 2004; 108: 258–266.

113. Yiangou Y, Facer P, Baecker PA, et al. ATP-gated ion channel P2X(3) is increased in human inflammatory bowel disease. Neurogastroenterol Motil 2001; 13:365–369.

114. Yiangou Y, Facer P, Dyer NHC, et al. Vanilloid receptor 1 immunoreactivity in inflamed human bowel. Lancet 2001; 357:1338–1339.

115. Yiangou Y, Facer P, Smith JAM, et al. Increased acid-sensing ion channel ASIC-3 in inflamed human intestine. Eu J Gastroenterol Hepatol 2001; 13:891–896.

116. Stadnicki A, Pastucha E, Nowaczyk G, et al. Immunolocalization and expression of kinin B1R and B2R receptors in human inflammatory bowel disease. Am J Physiol Gastrointest Liver Physiol 2005; 289:G361–G366.

117. Vulchanova L, Riedl MS, Shuster SJ, et al. Immunohistochemical study of the P2X2 and P2X3 receptor subunits in rat and monkey sensory neurons and their central terminals. Neuropharmacology 1997; 36:1229–1242.
118. Vulchanova L, Riedl MS, Shuster SJ, et al. P2X3 is expressed by DRG neurons that terminate in inner lamina II. Eu J Neurosci 1998; 10:3470–3478.
119. Barden JA, Bennett MR. Distribution of P2X purinoceptor clusters on individual rat dorsal root ganglion cells. Neurosci Lett 2000; 287:183–186.
120. Bradbury EJ, Burnstock G, McMahon SB. The expression of P2X3 purinoreceptors in sensory neurons: effects of axotomy and glial-derived neurotrophic factor. Mol Cell Neurosci 1998; 12:256–268.
121. Guo A, Vulchanova L, Wang J, Li X, Elde R. Immunocytochemical localization of the vanilloid receptor 1 (VR1): relationship to neuropeptides, the P2X3 purinoceptor and IB4 binding sites. Eu J Neurosci 1999; 11:946–958.
122. Petruska JC, Cooper BY, Gu JG, Rau KK, Johnson RD. Distribution of P2X1, P2X2, and P2X3 receptor subunits in rat primary afferents: relation to population markers and specific cell types. J Chem Neuroanat 2000; 20:141–162.
123. Wynn G, Rong W, Xiang Z, Burnstock G. Purinergic mechanisms contribute to mechanosensory transduction in the rat colorectum. Gastroenterology 2003; 125:1398–1409.
124. Chen CC, Akopian AN, Sivilottit L, Colquhoun D, Burnstock G, Wood JN. A P2X purinceptor expressed by a subset of sensory neurons. Nature 1995; 377:428–431.
125. Aoki Y, Takahashi Y, Ohtori S, Moriya H, Takahashi K. Distribution and immunocytochemical characterization of dorsal root ganglion neurons innervating the lumbar intervertebral disc in rats: a review. Life Sci 2004; 74:2627–2642.
126. Bardoni R, Goldstein PA, Lee CJ, Gu JG, MacDermott AB. ATP P2X receptors mediate fast synaptic transmission in the dorsal horn of the rat spinal cord. J Neurosci 1997; 17:5297–5304.
127. Burgard EC, Niforatos W, van Biesen T, et al. P2X receptor-mediated ionic currents in dorsal root ganglion neurons. J Neurophysiol 1999; 82:1590–1598.
128. Chen M, Gu J. A P2X receptor-mediated nociceptive afferent pathway to lamina I of the spinal cord. Mol Pain 2005; 1:4.
129. Grubb BD, Evans RJ. Characterization of cultured dorsal root ganglion neuron P2X receptors. Eu J Neurosci 1999; 11:149–154.
130. Petruska JC, Cooper BY, Johnson RD, Gu JG. Distribution patterns of different P2x receptor phenotypes in acutely dissociated dorsal root ganglion neurons of adult rats. Exper Brain Res 2000; 134:126–132.
131. Burnstock G. P2X receptors in sensory neurones. Br J Anaesth 2000; 84:476–488.
132. Kirkup AJ, Booth CE, Chessell IP, Humphrey PP, Grundy D. Excitatory effect of P2X receptor activation on mesenteric afferent nerves in the anaesthetised rat. J Physiol 1999; 520(Pt 2):551–563.
133. Page AJ, O'Donnell TA, Blackshaw LA. P2X purinoceptor-induced sensitization of ferret vagal mechanoreceptors in oesophageal inflammation. J physiol (lond) 2000; 523(Pt 2):403–411.
134. Brierley SM, Carter R, Jones CRW, et al. Differential chemosensory function and receptor expression of splanchnic and pelvic colonic afferents in mice. J Physiol 2005; 567:267–281.
135. Marceau F, Hess JF, Bachvarov DR. The B1 Receptors for Kinins. Pharmacol Rev 1998; 50:357–386.
136. Leeb-Lundberg LMF, Marceau F, Muller-Esterl W, Pettibone DJ, Zuraw BL. International Union of Pharmacology. XLV. Classification of the kinin receptor family: from molecular mechanisms to pathophysiological consequences. Pharmacol Rev 2005; 57:27–77.
137. Hall JM. Bradykinin receptors. Gen Pharmac 1997; 28:1–6.
138. Pan HL, Chen SR. Myocardial ischemia recruits mechanically insensitive cardiac sympathetic afferents in cats. J Neurophysiol 2002; 87:660–668.
139. Kajekar R, Proud D, Myers AC, Meeker SN, Undem BJ. Characterization of vagal afferent subtypes stimulated by bradykinin in guinea pig trachea. J Pharmacol Exp Ther 1999; 289:682–687.
140. Maubach KA, Grundy D. The role of prostaglandins in the bradykinin-induced activation of serosal afferents of the rat jejunum in vitro. J Physiol 1999; 515(Pt 1):277–285.
141. Bandell M, Story GM, Hwang SW, et al. Noxious cold ion channel TRPA1 is activated by pungent compounds and bradykinin. Neuron 2004; 41:849–857.
142. Clapham DE, Montell C, Schultz G, Julius D. International Union of Pharmacology. XLIII. Compendium of voltage-gated ion channels: transient receptor potential channels. Pharmacol Rev 2003; 55:591–596.
143. Caterina MJ, Julius D. Sense and specificity: a molecular identity for nociceptors. Curr Opin Neurobiol 1999; 9:525–530.
144. Tominaga M, Julius D. Capsaicin receptor in the pain pathway. Jap J Pharmacol 2000; 83:20–24.
145. Julius D, Basbaum AI. Molecular mechanisms of nociception. Nature 2001; 413:203–210.
146. McKemy DD, Neuhausser WM, Julius D. Identification of a cold receptor reveals a general role for TRP channels in thermosensation. Nature 2002; 416:52–58.
147. Jordt S-E, Julius D. Molecular basis for species-specific sensitivity to "hot" chili peppers. Cell 2002; 108:421–430.
148. Jordt SE, Tominaga M, Julius D. Acid potentiation of the capsaicin receptor determined by a key extracellular site. Proc Natl Acad Sci USA 2000; 97:8134–8139.

149. Tominaga M, Caterina MJ, Malmberg AB, et al. The cloned capsaicin receptor integrates multiple pain-producing stimuli. Neuron 1998; 21:531–543.

150. Hudson LJ, Bevan S, Wotherspoon G, Gentry C, Fox A, Winter J. VR1 protein expression increases in undamaged DRG neurons after partial nerve injury. Eur J Neurosci 2001; 13:2105–2114.

151. Hwang SJ, Min Oh J, Valtschanoff JG. Expression of the vanilloid receptor TRPV1 in rat dorsal root ganglion neurons supports different roles of the receptor in visceral and cutaneous afferents. Brain Res 2005; 1047:261–266.

152. Jordt S-E, McKemy DD, Julius D. Lessons from peppers and peppermint: the molecular logic of thermosensation. Curr Opin Neurobiol 2003; 13:487–492.

153. Holzer P. Neural injury, repair, and adaptation in the GI tract. II. The elusive action of capsaicin on the vagus nerve. Am J Physiol 1998; 275:G8–G13.

154. Bielefeldt K. Differential effects of capsaicin on rat visceral sensory neurons. Neuroscience 2000; 101:727–736.

155. Su X, Wachtel RE, Gebhart GF. Capsaicin sensitivity and voltage-gated sodium currents in colon sensory neurons from rat dorsal root ganglia. Am J Physiol 1999; 277:G1180–G1188.

156. Blackshaw LA, Page AJ, Partosoedarso ER. Acute effects of capsaicin on gastrointestinal vagal afferents. Neuroscience 2000; 96:407–416.

157. Longhurst JC, Kaufman MP, Ordway GA, Musch TI. Effects of bradykinin and capsaicin on endings of afferent fibers from abdominal visceral organs. Am J Physiol 1984; 247:R552–R559.

158. Sugiura T, Bielefeldt K, Gebhart GF. TRPV1 function in mouse colon sensory neurons is enhanced by metabotropic 5-hydroxytryptamine receptor activation. J Neurosci 2004; 24:9521–9530.

159. Chan C, Facer P, Davis J, et al. Sensory fibres expressing capsaicin receptor TRPV1 in patients with rectal hypersensitivity and faecal urgency. Lancet 2003; 361:385–391.

160. Kimball ES, Wallace NH, Schneider CR, D'Andrea MR, Hornby PJ. Vanilloid receptor 1 antagonists attenuate disease severity in dextran sulphate sodium-induced colitis in mice. Neurogastroenterol Motil 2004; 16:1–8.

161. Andrews PL, Davis CJ, Bingham S, Davidson HI, Hawthorn J, Maskell L. The abdominal visceral innervation and the emetic reflex: pathways, pharmacology, and plasticity. Can J Physiol Pharmacol 1990; 68:325–345.

162. Bearcroft CP, Perrett D, Farthing MJ. Postprandial plasma 5-hydroxytryptamine in diarrhoea predominant irritable bowel syndrome: a pilot study. Gut 1998; 42:42–46.

163. Spiller RC, Jenkins D, Thornley JP, et al. Increased rectal mucosal enteroendocrine cells, T lymphocytes, and increased gut permeability following acute Campylobacter enteritis and in post-dysenteric irritable bowel syndrome. Gut 2000; 47:804–811.

164. O'Sullivan M, Clayton N, Breslin NP, et al. Increased mast cells in the irritable bowel syndrome. Neurogastroenterol Motil 2000; 12:449–457.

165. Houghton LA, Atkinson W, Whitaker RP, Whorwell PJ, Rimmer MJ. Increased platelet depleted plasma 5-hydroxytryptamine concentration following meal ingestion in symptomatic female subjects with diarrhoea predominant irritable bowel syndrome. Gut 2003; 52:663–670.

166. Camilleri M, Northcutt AR, Kong S, Dukes GE, McSorley D, Mangel AW. Efficacy and safety of alosetron in women with irritable bowel syndrome: a randomised, placebo-controlled trial. Lancet 2000; 355:1035–1040.

167. Coates MD, Mahoney CR, Linden DR, et al. Molecular defects in mucosal serotonin content and decreased serotonin reuptake transporter in ulcerative colitis and irritable bowel syndrome. Gastroenterology 2004; 126:1657–1664.

168. Blackshaw LA, Grundy D. Effects of 5-hydroxytryptamine on discharge of vagal mucosal afferent fibres from the upper gastrointestinal tract of the ferret. J Auton Nerv Syst 1993; 45:41–50.

169. Hillsley K, Kirkup AJ, Grundy D. Direct and indirect actions of 5-hydroxytryptamine on the discharge of mesenteric afferent fibres innervating the rat jejunum. J Physiol 1998; 506(Pt 2):551–561.

170. Zhu JX, Zhu XY, Owyang C, Li Y. Intestinal serotonin acts as a paracrine substance to mediate vagal signal transmission evoked by luminal factors in the rat. J Physiol 2001; 530:431–442.

171. Zeitz KP, Guy N, Malmberg AB, et al. The 5-HT3 subtype of serotonin receptor contributes to nociceptive processing via a novel subset of myelinated and unmyelinated nociceptors. J Neurosci 2002; 22:1010–1019.

172. Danzebrink RM, Gebhart GF. Evidence that spinal 5-HT1, 5-HT2 and 5-HT3 receptor subtypes modulate responses to noxious colorectal distension in the rat. Brain Res 1991; 538:64–75.

173. McRoberts JA, Coutinho SV, Marvizon JC, et al. Role of peripheral N-methyl-D-aspartate (NMDA) receptors in visceral nociception in rats. Gastroenterology 2001; 120:1737–1748.

174. Sengupta JN, Petersen J, Peles S, Shaker R. Response properties of antral mechanosensitive afferent fibers and effects of ionotropic glutamate receptor antagonists. Neuroscience 2004; 125:711–723.

175. Page AJ, Young RL, Martin CM, et al. Metabotropic glutamate receptors inhibit mechanosensitivity in vagal sensory neurons. Gastroenterology 2005; 128:402–410.

176. Blackshaw LA, Staunton E, Lehmann A, Dent J. Inhibition of transient LES relaxations and reflux in ferrets by GABA receptor agonists. Am J Physiol 1999; 277:G867–G874.

177. Page AJ, Blackshaw LA. GABA(B) receptors inhibit mechanosensitivity of primary afferent endings. J Neurosci 1999; 19:8597–8602.

178. Smid SD, Young RL, Cooper NJ, Blackshaw LA. GABA(B)R expressed on vagal afferent neurones inhibit gastric mechanosensitivity in ferret proximal stomach. Am J Physiol Gastrointest Liver Physiol 2001; 281:G1494–G1501.

179. Staunton E, Smid SD, Dent J, Blackshaw LA. Triggering of transient LES relaxations in ferrets: role of sympathetic pathways and effects of baclofen. Am J Physiol Gastrointest Liver Physiol 2000; 279:G157–G162.

180. Sengupta JN, Medda BK, Shaker R. Effect of GABA(B) receptor agonist on distension-sensitive pelvic nerve afferent fibers innervating rat colon. Am J Physiol Gastrointest Liver Physiol 2002; 283:G1343–G1351.

181. Page AJ, Slattery JA, O'Donnell TA, Cooper NJ, Young RL, Blackshaw L. Modulation of gastro-oesophageal vagal afferents by galanin in mouse and ferret. J Physiol 2005; 563:809–819.

182. Hollenberg MD, Compton SJ. International Union of Pharmacology. XXVIII. Proteinase activated receptors. Pharmacol Rev 2002; 54:203–217.

183. Vergnolle N. Modulation of visceral pain and inflammation by protease-activated receptors. Br J Pharmacol 2004; 141:1264–1274.

184. Vergnolle N, Cellars L, Mencarelli A, et al. A role for proteinase-activated receptor-1 in inflammatory bowel diseases. J Clin Invest 2004; 114:1444–1456.

185. Kirkup A, Bunnett N, Grundy D. A proteinase-activated receptor subtype 2 (PAR-2) agonist stimulates mesenteric afferent nerve discharge. Gastroenterology 2000; 118:A173.

186. Amadesi S, Nie J, Vergnolle N, et al. Protease-activated receptor 2 sensitizes the capsaicin receptor transient receptor potential vanilloid receptor 1 to induce hyperalgesia. J Neurosci 2004; 24: 4300–4312.

187. Beyak MJ, Ramji N, Krol KM, Kawaja MD, Vanner SJ. Two TTX-resistant Na+ currents in mouse colonic dorsal root ganglia neurons and their role in colitis-induced hyperexcitability. Am J Physiol Gastrointest Liver Physiol 2004; 287:G845–G855.

188. Krempels K, Hunyady B, O'Carroll A, Mezey E. Distribution of somatostatin receptor messenger RNAs in the rat gastrointestinal tract. Gastroenterology 1997; 112:1948–1960.

189. Hasler W, Soudah H, Owyang C. Somatostatin analog inhibits afferent response to rectal distention in diarrhea-predominant irritable bowel patients. J Pharmacol Exp Ther 1994; 268:1206–1211.

190. Booth CE, Kirkup AJ, Hicks GA, Humphrey PP, Grundy D. Somatostatin sst(2) receptor-mediated inhibition of mesenteric afferent nerves of the jejunum in the anesthetized rat. Gastroenterology 2001; 121:358–369.

191. Gillespie PG, Walker RG. Molecular basis of mechanosensory transduction. Nature 2001; 413: 194–202.

192. Welsh MJ, Price MP, Xie J. Biochemical basis of touch perception: mechanosensory function of degenerin/epithelial Na+ channels. J Biol Chem 2002; 277:2369–2372.

193. Suzuki M, Mizuno A, Kodaira K, Imai M. Impaired pressure sensation in mice lacking TRPV4. J Biol Chem 2003; 278:22664–22668.

194. Corey DP et al. TRPA1 is a candidate for the mechanosensitive transduction channel of vertebrate hair cells. Nature 2004; 432:723–730.

195. Liedtke WB. TRPV4 plays an evolutionary conserved role in the transduction of osmotic and mechanical stimuli in live animals. J Physiol (Lond) 2005; 567:53–58.

196. Driscoll M, Chalfie M. The mec-4 gene is a member of a family of Caenorhabditis elegans genes that can mutate to induce neuronal degeneration. Nature 1991; 349:588–593.

197. Benson CJ, Xie J, Wemmie JA, et al. Heteromultimers of DEG/ENaC subunits form H+-gated channels in mouse sensory neurons. Proc Natl Acad Sci U S A 2002; 99:2338–2343.

198. Price MP et al. The mammalian sodium channel BNC1 is required for normal touch sensation. Nature 2000; 407:1007–1011.

199. Price MP, McIlwrath SL, Xie J, et al. The DRASIC cation channel contributes to the detection of cutaneous touch and acid stimuli in mice. Neuron 2001; 32:1071–1083.

200. Page AJ, Brierley SM, Martin CM, et al. The ion channel ASIC1 contributes to visceral but not cutaneous mechanoreceptor function. Gastroenterology 2004; 127:1739–1747.

201. Page A, Brierley SM, Martin CM, et al. Different contributions of ASIC channels 1a, 2 and 3 in gastrointestinal mechanosensory function. Gut 2005; 54(10):1408–1415.

202. Price MP, Thompson RJ, Eshcol JO, Wemmie JA, Benson CJ. Stomatin modulates gating of acid-sensing ion channels. J Biol Chem 2004; 279:53886–53891.

203. Tavernarakis N, Driscoll M. Molecular modeling of mechanotransduction in the nematode Caenorhabditis elegans. Annu Rev Physiol 1997; 59:659–689.

204. Chalfie M, Au M. Genetic control of differentiation of the caenorhabditis elegans touch receptor neurons. Science 1989; 243:1027–1033.

205. Cook SP, McCleskey EW. ATP, pain and a full bladder. Nature 2000; 407:951–952.

206. Wynn G, Ma B, Ruan HZ, Burnstock G. Purinergic component of mechanosensory transduction is increased in a rat model of colitis. Am J Physiol Gastrointest Liver Physiol 2004; 287:G647–G657.

6 Neurochemical and Molecular Basis of Peripheral Sensitization

Klaus Bielefeldt
Division of Gastroenterology, Hepatology and Nutrition, University of Pittsburgh Physicians, Pittsburgh, Pennsylvania, U.S.A.

INTRODUCTION

The terminals of sensory nerves express specialized molecules that transduce the energy of mechanical, thermal, or chemical stimuli into electrical signals, which may trigger one or several action potentials. These action potentials will propagate along the axon and cause transmitter release at the synapse with second order neurons, thereby initiating central processing of sensory information that may ultimately lead to conscious perception (Fig. 1). Studies performed in vivo and in vitro have demonstrated a significant plasticity of primary sensory neurons, which contributes to the development of hyperalgesia (peripheral sensitization) (1–5). This chapter will describe mechanisms of peripheral sensitization based on the functionally distinct steps from the stimulus-induced depolarization of the nerve terminal to the transmitter release at the presynaptic ending.

ION CHANNELS AS TRANSDUCERS
Molecular Sensors

Neurons express specialized membrane proteins, ion channels, which can be activated by mechanical (e.g., stretch), chemical (e.g., protons), and thermal stimuli (Fig. 1). Within the last decade, we have gained significant insight into the structure and function of these channels in somatic and—to a lesser degree—visceral afferents.

At least two distinct pathways have been identified that depolarize neurons in response to "mechanical stimulation." Sensory neurons express several members of the family of degenerins and the epithelial sodium channels, generally referred to as acid-sensitive ion channels (ASIC) because of their activation by protons. These channels also open in response to stretch, allowing sodium influx into the cell, which leads to depolarization. While they were initially identified because of their response to acid, these channels are expressed in specialized mechanoreceptors, and genetic deletion of these channels in mice leads to impaired touch sensation (6). In addition, stretch activates an inward current through nonselective, calcium-permeable cation channels. A member of the transient receptor potential (TRP) family of ion channels, TRP vanilloid receptor 4 (TRPV4), is a likely candidate for such a mechanosensitive channel because knockout mice display reduced sensitivity to pressure application (7). Interactions between the ion channel and cytoskeleton during stretch lead to channel opening without the need for other mediators. Mucosal stimulation of gastrointestinal or urinary epithelium also triggers the release of chemical signals from enteroendocrine or urothelial cells with serotonin [5-hydroxytryptamine (5-HT)] and adenosine triphosphate (ATP) as the most important signaling molecules (8,9). These, in turn, can directly bind to receptors located on the nerve terminals and activate afferent neurons. Experiments with knockout mice lacking the $P2X_3$ receptor, an ion channel activated by ATP, showed an impaired micturition reflex, demonstrating the important contribution of this sensory mechanism to mechanoreception (10,11).

Protons are a distinct *chemical stimulus* that can excite sensory neurons. The above-mentioned ASIC have initially been identified and cloned in primary sensory neurons (12). These currents are typically activated at pH values below 7.0 and desensitize with longer acid exposure. Compared to skin and muscle afferents, more neurons innervating the heart and stomach express acid-sensitive ion currents, raising the question whether they play a unique

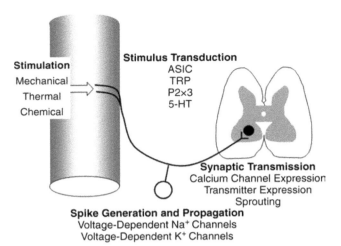

Figure 1 Signal transduction and transmission in sensory neurons. Stimulation gates ion channels at the sensory terminal leading to a depolarization and activation of action potentials. The action potential propagates along the axon and triggers transmitter release at the central terminal (synapse). *Abbreviations*: ASIC, acid-sensitive ion channels; TRP, transient receptor potential channels. 5-HT, 5-hydroxytryptamine.

role in visceral sensation, specifically in the detection of ischemia, which is associated with a pH drop due to lactate production (13). A second group of ion channels is also gated by protons. The best-described member is TRPV1, which was initially named capsaicin receptor because it is activated by the pungent vanilloid capsaicin (14). Compared to ASIC, significantly higher proton concentrations (pH < 6) are required for activation. This ion channel and other members of the TRP family also respond to *thermal stimulation*. Consistent with a role in heat sensation, knockout mice lacking TRPV1 showed defects in thermal sensation and heat hyperalgesia in models of inflammatory pain (15). Interestingly, these mice also have impaired micturition with bladder hyporeflexia, suggesting additional roles of this ion channel in visceral function (16). Nerve terminals expressing TRPV1 channels can be found in the mucosa of the gastrointestinal region, where they may contribute to responses to chemical and thermal stimuli (17,18).

Clinical Implications

The identification of ion channels important in nociception has led to the development of specific antagonists with the hope to block the initial step in the transduction of painful stimuli. While these agents have not yet moved into clinical practice, initial studies in animal models of human disease support the potential therapeutic value of this approach.

The concentration of such nociceptive channels may also allow targeted inhibition or even destruction of nerves triggering abnormal activity. This strategy is used successfully in patients with interstitial cystitis, where instillation of capsaicin or resifineratoxin, both activators of the TRPV1 channel, improve symptoms associated with a transient decrease in the density of nerve fibers within the bladder wall.

Modulation of Sensory Transducers

Ion channels such as ASICs or TRPV1 exhibit a graded response to appropriate stimuli, resulting in more frequent and/or longer openings with increasing stimulus intensity, thereby allowing more current flow. Under physiological conditions, the progressively stronger and more lasting depolarization will eventually exceed threshold, trigger action potentials, and, thereby, encode the stimulus intensity as spike frequency. Changes in the properties and/or number of mechano-, thermo- or chemosensitive ion channels can alter this stimulus response function and thus sensitize peripheral afferents.

As discussed above, two physiologically important stimuli, heat and protons, can activate TRPV1 channels. Both stimuli can cooperatively affect the channel, significantly shifting the stimulus-response function. For example, a drop in pH to about 6.4, which is in the range of values seen during prolonged ischemia or localized inflammation, triggers significant channel activity when the temperature rises to values close to the normal body temperature (19). Similarly, endogenous lipid mediators produced during inflammation, intracellular ATP, and changes in the concentration of phosphatidyl-inositides within the cell membrane can enhance the activity of TRPV1 channels by directly interacting with binding sites on the channel complex (20–23). These effects occur rapidly and do not require covalent modification of the channel, thus differing from modulation of ion channels through phosphorylation (see below), which is typically triggered by activation of G-protein–coupled receptors.

Signaling molecules implicated in nociception, such as bradykinin, 5-HT, and prostaglandins, can activate G-protein–coupled receptors, resulting in generation of second messengers within the cytosol. These in turn activate protein kinases, which will phosphorylate ion channels and other targets. This covalent modification of the channel protein significantly changes channel properties and, in the case of TRPV1 or ASIC, shifts their activation to lower temperatures and/or proton concentrations, respectively (24–26).

The covalent modulation of stimulus-transducing ion channels may play an especially important role in visceral pain, where mucosal stimulation triggers the release of mediators, primarily 5-HT and ATP, from enteroendocrine or urothelial cells, respectively (27–29). In addition to the activation of the ligand-gated 5-HT3 and P2X$_3$ receptors, these mediators may interact with metabotropic 5-HT and purinergic receptors, thereby sensitizing primary afferents. As shown in Figure 2, 5-HT decreased the threshold temperature for current activation in dorsal root ganglion neurons innervating the mouse colon. The resulting inward currents were sufficient to trigger action potential generation at the normal core body temperature. Recent studies reported an increase in enteroendocrine cells and enhanced 5-HT release from mucosal biopsies in subgroup of patients with irritable bowel syndrome (30,31). Considering the 5-HT effects described above, the resulting modulation of TRPV1 receptors may sensitize primary afferents and contribute to the hyperalgesia in these patients even in the absence of obvious inflammation.

Clinical Implications

The rapid effects of inflammatory mediators on ion channels sensitize neurons during inflammation. Blocking the formation and release of these substances through cyclo-oxygenase inhibitors reverses this process and decreases pain.

Serotonin plays a unique role in visceral sensation from the gastrointestinal tract. Serotonin release from enteroendocrine cells within the mucosa interacts with G-protein–coupled 5-HT receptors on afferent neurons and alters the properties of ion channels, including the TRPV1 receptor. Modulation of this heat- and proton-sensitive channel allows current flow and thus neuron activation at normal body temperatures, thereby contributing to symptoms in patients with functional diseases such as irritable bowel syndrome.

Expression and Insertion of Sensory Transducers

In addition to covalent and noncovalent modulation described above, the number of ion channels at the site of stimulus energy transduction (i.e., the nerve terminal) affects the current amplitude in response to stimulation. While nonexcitable cells regulate ion and water flux through insertion and retrieval of channels, the relative importance of this pathway in the regulation of neuron excitability remains unclear at this point (32–34). However, many studies have demonstrated the importance of changes in gene transcription and protein expression in peripheral sensitization in the context of visceral inflammation. Inflammation is associated with the production and release of mediators, which may acutely alter nerve properties as discussed above. Nerve growth factor (NGF) has attracted significant attention because the majority of nociceptive neurons express the high-affinity receptor for NGF, tyrosine kinase receptor A (Trka) (35,36). Increases in NGF have been reported during visceral inflammation in humans and in various animal models of visceral pain (37–42). Gene transfer of NGF into the bladder wall using an adenoviral vector system triggered bladder overactivity in the

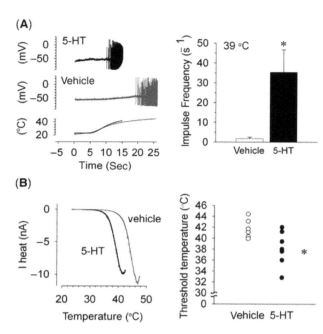

Figure 2 Serotonin sensitizes temperature responses in mouse colon afferents. (**A**) Current-clamp recordings show action potentials in response to temperature ramps after vehicle (*grey trace*) and 1 μM 5-HT (*black trace*). The action potential frequency at 39°C is summarized in the right panel. (**B**) Under voltage-clamp conditions, a temperature ramp triggers inward currents as shown for vehicle (*grey trace*) or 1 μM 5-HT (*black trace*). 5-HT shifts the threshold for current activation to lower temperatures as summarized in the right panel. *Abbreviation*: 5-HT, 5-hydroxy-tryptamine.

absence of inflammation, consistent with a sensitization of the micturition reflex (43). Conversely, immunoneutralization of NGF blunted nocifensive behavior in animals with experimentally induced gastric ulcers (44). While it is likely that multiple mechanisms contribute to these effects, NGF alters TRPV1 and ASIC-3 expression in primary sensory neurons (45,46). Consistent with a potential role of changes in channel expression in the pathogenesis of visceral hyperalgesia, patients with interstitial cystitis and rectal pain or fecal urgency have an increased density of TRPV1 immunoreactive fibers within the mucosa (18,47). Similar changes in channel expression have been described for other channels involved in sensory signal transduction (26,48,49).

Figure 3 schematically summarizes different mechanisms that alter properties and expression of one channel involved in nociception, TRPV1. Considering its activation by at least two distinct stimulus modalities, heat and protons, and its modulation by different signaling molecules, TRPV1 may play an important role in integrating potentially noxious stimuli and in the sensitization of peripheral neurons. This may be especially relevant for visceral afferents because TRPV1 channels are found in a higher number of sensory neurons and may contribute to the regulation of normal organ function (16,50,51). Future studies with recently developed selective, high-affinity antagonists will soon enable us to determine more directly the importance of this molecule as a therapeutic target (52,53).

Clinical Implications

Tissue injury and inflammation lead to the production and release of mediators that affect nerves by changing ion channel expression, thereby contributing to sensitization. This development of hyperalgesia can be blunted by antagonizing such mediators, such as nerve growth factor, or blocking their second messenger systems. While results obtained in animal experiments are promising, unwanted effects on other systems (e.g., immune function) have limited the use of this approach in humans.

Determinants and Modulation of Neuron Excitability

The previous section described mechanisms depolarizing nerve terminals in response to stimulation. Depending on stimulus intensity, this depolarization may exceed the threshold for action potential generation, triggering spikes, which will propagate along the axon.

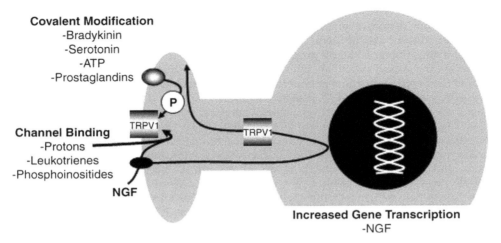

Figure 3 Mechanisms of altered stimulus transduction in nerve terminals. The heat- and proton-gated TRPV1 channel can be activated by lipid mediators interacting with the channel and covalently modulated through channel phosphorylation. In addition to rapid effects, activation of the NGF receptor triggers increase in TRPV1 gene transcription and enhances current responses through this channel. *Abbreviations*: NGF, nerve growth factor; ATP, adenosine triphosphate; TRPV1, transient receptor potential vanilloid receptor 1.

The threshold for action potential generation and the firing frequency depends on the rate, amplitude, and duration of the stimulus-induced depolarization ('receptor potential') and the neuron's electrophysiological response characteristics ('excitability'). These properties are subject to many modulating influences and thus contribute to peripheral sensitization.

Experimentally induced inflammation sensitizes primary afferent neurons (Fig. 4). This is at least in part due to inflammatory mediators, such as bradykinin or prostaglandin E2, which rapidly and reversibly alter the excitability of visceral sensory neurons, decreasing the threshold for action potential generation and/or increasing action potential frequency in response to a given stimulation (54,55). While inflammatory mediators contribute to these changes in vivo, the increase in excitability can be seen in vitro hours after neurons have been dissociated and cultured, suggesting that more lasting changes, i.e., alterations in gene expression, underlie this effect (56,57). A recent report indicates that this enhanced responsiveness of primary visceral afferents may persist for months after the complete resolution of the initiating inflammatory event (58). Several ion channels determine the excitability of primary sensory neurons. Their modulation through phosphorylation or dephosphorylation, and changes in their expression play an important role in peripheral sensitization.

Voltage-Sensitive Sodium Channels

Activation of "voltage-sensitive sodium channels" (VSSC) is responsible for the rapid upstroke of the action potential. Ten molecularly distinct pore-forming subunits (α-subunits) of VSSC have been identified and are generally referred to as Nav 1.1 to Nav 1.9 (59). The most striking difference between these channels is their sensitivity to the neurotoxin, tetrodotoxin (TTX). While nanomolar concentrations of TTX completely block sodium currents in neurons

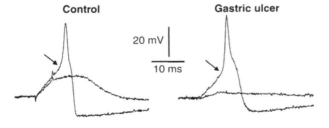

Figure 4 Experimental ulcers sensitize gastric sensory neurons. Superimposed voltage tracings show the response of gastric dorsal root ganglion neurons to depolarizing current injection. The arrow indicates the onset of the action potential.

within the central nervous system, a fraction of the voltage-sensitive sodium current in primary sensory neurons persists even in micromolar TTX concentrations. As shown in Figure 5, this TTX-resistant current activates and inactivates more slowly than the TTX-sensitive current. Because of the different kinetic properties, a significant contribution of TTX-resistant current prolongs the action potential. Interestingly, this TTX-resistant current is primarily found in small diameter, unmyelinated neurons (C-fibers), which are important in nociception (60,61). No selective blockers of TTX-resistant sodium channels are currently available to directly test their importance in pain sensation. Therefore, two complementary approaches employed genetic manipulations, decreasing or eliminating Nav1.8 expression using antisense oligodeoxynucleotides or knockout mice, which led to a blunted response to noxious mechanical stimulation or inflammatory pain (62,63). Conversely, experimental models of visceral inflammation and pain are associated with an increase in TTX-resistant sodium currents (Fig. 5). While these results all point at a central role of TTX-resistant sodium currents in nociception, functional changes are not restricted to this sodium channel. In addition, the properties of TTX-sensitive sodium channels are altered with a shift in the voltage-dependence of activation to less depolarized potentials and a faster recovery from inactivation. The increase in channel expression, changes in voltage-dependence, and recovery kinetics together will lower the threshold for action potential generation and contribute to higher spike frequencies (64–66).

Two primary mechanisms have been described that alter sodium currents in primary sensory neurons: covalent modulation through phosphorylation and changes in channel expression. Phosphorylation of the pore-forming channel subunit shifts the voltage dependence of activation to more negative potentials (67). Several inflammatory mediators activate protein kinases, which then in turn phosphorylate sodium channels (68–70). As discussed above, 5-HT may play a unique role as a chemical mediator within the gastrointestinal tract, considering its functions as a physiological signal that is released from enteroendocrine cells upon mechanical or chemical stimulation. Interestingly, activation of metabotropic 5-HT receptors enhances TTX-resistant sodium currents in primary afferent neurons (71,72). While it remains unclear whether 5-HT similarly affects all visceral afferent neurons (73), this mechanism may contribute to peripheral sensitization.

The expression of sodium channels appears to be regulated by target-derived factors produced by cells within the vicinity of sensory endings. Axotomy, which deprives the neuron of these signals, decreases sodium channel expression and reduces excitability (74–76). Conversely, signals released during inflammation increase sodium channel expression, thereby contributing to peripheral sensitization (77). As already discussed above, NGF is one of these target-derived signals and is involved in the regulation of sodium channel expression. Administration of NGF to the cut end of the axon prevents the decrease in Nav1.8

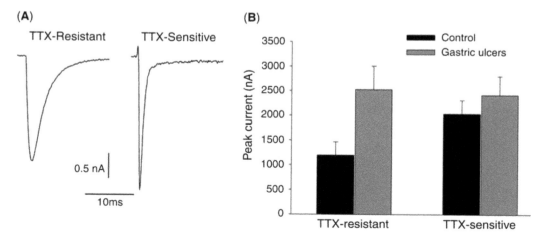

Figure 5 Sodium channels in visceral sensory neurons. (**A**) Gastric sensory neurons express TTX-resistant (*left panel*) and TTX-sensitive (*right panel*) sodium currents. (**B**) Experimental ulcers increase the peak of TTX-resistant but not TTX-sensitive sodium currents in gastric sensory neurons. *Abbreviation*: TTX, tetrodotoxin.

expression observed after axotomy (78). Similarly, addition of NGF increases TTX-resistant sodium currents in cultured sensory neurons, while NGF depletion using neutralizing antibodies decreases sodium currents (40,79).

Most of the experiments investigating the role of VSSC focused on the pore-forming α subunit of the channel complex. However, several associated proteins have been identified that modulate channel insertion into the membrane and channel function. In the case of VSSC, three different β subunits can coassemble with the α subunit and significantly increase peak amplitude and alter kinetics of sodium currents (80). Injury and inflammation differentially affect the expression of these associated subunits, which may lead to some of the functional changes observed (81).

While many studies support the importance of VSSC in pain syndromes, the translation of this information into new therapies has been slow. Several anticonvulsive and antiarrhythmic agents block VSSC and have been used to treat patients with chronic pain syndromes (82,83). Moreover, some peripherally active κ opioid agonists and tricyclic antidepressants cause a use-dependent inhibition of sodium currents, which may contribute to their effectiveness in visceral pain syndromes (84–86). However, the lack of selectivity with cardiac and neurological side effects limits the utility of these agents in pain management.

Clinical Implications

Patients with painful neuromas have abnormal expression of voltage-sensitive sodium channels. Similar changes in sodium channel expression have been identified in animal models of gastrointestinal diseases associated with pain. Patients with neuromas or neuropathic pain often benefit from anticonvulsive drugs, many of which block sodium channels. A similar mechanism may contribute to the effect of tricyclic antidepressants or opioid agonists, both of which are effective in patients with chronic visceral pain.

Voltage-Sensitive Potassium Channels

Opening of voltage-sensitive potassium channels and the related calcium-dependent potassium channels is responsible for the repolarizing phase of the action potential. Especially, the calcium-dependent potassium channels remain active even after return of the membrane potential to its baseline, and are the basis of the often long-lasting afterhyperpolarization, which is associated with a significant decrease in excitability following the action potential. Eighteen distinct voltage-sensitive potassium channels belonging to four families have been cloned. Compared to sodium channels, the structure–function relationship of potassium channels is more complex because four proteins combine into a homo- or hetero-oligomeric complex to form the channel pore (87,88). This picture is further confounded by associated β subunits that modulate channels properties. The expression pattern of potassium channel provides some clues about their role in the sensation of pain with one channel subunit, Kv1.4, preferentially expressed in primary sensory neurons that are positive for neurochemical markers associated with nociception (89). More direct information comes from experiments with knockout animals. Consistent with the role of potassium channels in repolarization, neurons lacking Kv1.1, a rapidly inactivating potassium channel, respond with prolonged bursts of action potentials when stimulated (90). Such enhanced responses may contribute to the hyperalgesia seen in Kv1.1-deficient mice during heat stimuli and inflammation (91).

Same as VSSC, potassium channels are modulated by inflammatory mediators. However, while prostaglandins enhance sodium channel activity, they decrease potassium currents, both of which will increase excitability (92). In addition to this rapid modulation through inflammatory mediators, experimental models of visceral inflammation and pain are associated with a lasting decrease in potassium currents due to changes in channel expression (Fig. 6). This change primarily involves the rapidly activating and inactivating potassium current (A current) (50,64,93). Pharmacologic inhibition of this A current significantly increases excitability. Consistent with these results, neurons obtained from animals with visceral inflammation showed a decrease in the transient potassium current, had a lower

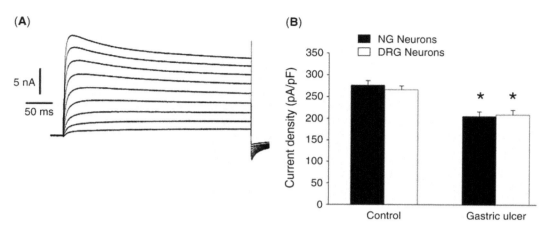

Figure 6 Potassium currents in visceral inflammation. (**A**) Superimposed current tracings triggered by stepwise depolarization of a gastric dorsal root ganglion neuron show transient and sustained potassium currents. (**B**) Ulceration decreases the transient current in gastric nodose and dorsal root ganglion neurons. *Abbreviations*: NG, nodose ganglion; DRG, dorsal root ganglion.

threshold for action potential generation, and responded with higher spike frequencies during prolonged stimulation (57).

Several potassium channels also contribute to the resting membrane potential. Modulation or loss of these channels increases excitability and is associated with seizures and cardiac arrhythmias, disorders associated with an increase in excitability (94). While hyperexcitability is also the hallmark of peripheral sensitization, the role of these channels in pain is less clear. Recently, KCNQ2 and KCNQ3 channels have been identified in primary sensory neurons. Pharmacologic activators of these channels blunted responses to afferent stimulation and inhibited pain behavior during chronic inflammation (95). While still untested in the clinical arena, the use of such potassium channel openers may provide novel options for analgesic therapy.

Clinical Implications

Development of hyperalgesia is associated with a decrease of potassium currents. Considering the importance of these channels in determining the resting membrane potential and neuron excitability, activators of potassium channels or enhancers of their expression are potentially interesting targets for treatment of chronic pain syndromes. While limited experimental evidence supports this concept, the widespread expression of these channels and their complex pharmacological properties still require extensive preclinical studies before this approach can be tested in humans.

Voltage-Sensitive Calcium Channels

Voltage-sensitive calcium channels (VSCC) are activated during depolarization and allow the influx of calcium, thereby contributing to depolarization. The current flux generated by the movement of this divalent ion is relatively small compared to sodium and potassium currents. However, calcium is not only a charge carrier; it also functions as a second messenger within cells, opening calcium-dependent ion channels, triggering neurotransmitter release in presynaptic terminals and activating calcium-dependent enzymes within the cytosol. Ten molecularly distinct pore-forming calcium channel subunits have been described (96). Based on electrophysiological properties, these can be differentiated into high- or low-threshold VSCC, both of which can be found in visceral sensory neurons. The high-threshold VSCC can be separated into L, N, P/Q, and R type currents based on their pharmacological properties. The N and P/Q type calcium currents are blocked by ω-conotoxin GIVA and ω-agatoxin, respectively. Both toxins significantly inhibit synaptic transmission within the spinal cord demonstrating the importance of these channels in transmitter release (97). Genetic deletion or pharmacologic inhibition of VSCC blunts pain responses in experimental animals, which is at least in part due to the decreased transmitter release within the spinal cord (98–101). Conversely, hypersensitivity induced by gastric inflammation is associated with a shift in the voltage-dependence of activation to less depolarized potentials, which may enhance transmitter release and contribute to the development of visceral hypersensitivity (Fig. 7).

Activation of opioid receptors on primary afferent neurons inhibits VSCC and may thus modulate transmitter release (102,103). Initial results point at differences between cutaneous and visceral afferents with κ- rather than μ- or δ-opioid agonists primarily affecting VSCC in colon sensory neurons (104). Considering the possible use of peripherally acting agents without the typical adverse effects of traditional opioids, these findings may open up important therapeutic options.

VSCC are comprised of different proteins that form a multimeric complex, which—in the case of high-threshold VSCC—includes the pore-forming α subunit, an intracellular β subunit, and a large α2δ subunit. The interactions between these proteins are functionally very important as illustrated by the genetic deletion of the β3 subunit, which alters the voltage-dependence of calcium currents in dorsal root ganglion neurons and blunts responses to inflammatory pain (105). Nerve injury is associated with an increase in the expression of this α2δ subunit (106). Interestingly, this subunit binds the anticonvulsive agent gabapentin, which inhibits VSCC (107). This effect may underlie the finding that gabapentin can improve neuropathic pain and may be beneficial in the treatment of visceral hyperalgesia (108–110).

Clinical Implications

The calcium ion carries a charge and contributes to the depolarization during the opening of voltage-sensitive calcium channels. It also functions as a second messenger and triggers transmitter release. Clinically used calcium channel blockers interact with L-type calcium channels, which do not play a significant role in fast synaptic transmission. However, gabapentin, an anticonvulsive drug, binds an accessory calcium channel subunit, leading to a lower expression of calcium channels on the cell surface and, thereby, to a decrease in excitability. This mechanism may be responsible for the reported beneficial effects in patients with neuropathic pain.

SYNAPTIC TRANSMISSION

When the action potential invades the presynaptic terminal, VSCC open and allow calcium influx, which triggers the fusion of transmitter vesicles with the cell membrane and release of neurotransmitter. The exocytic transmitter release is steeply dependent on the intracellular calcium concentration (111). Therefore, increases in calcium currents due to changes in channel properties or expression during inflammation may enhance transmitter release. In addition, proteins regulating the fusion of vesicles with the presynaptic membrane are subject to modulation and can increase or decrease transmitter release. While this presynaptic facilitation is an important mechanism for memory formation and learning, its relevance in the development of hyperalgesia remains unknown (112).

Glutamate is the main transmitter within the spinal cord and—in the case of the vagus—the nucleus of the solitary tract (113,114). In many nerve terminals, glutamate coexists with neuropeptides, which are stored in larger vesicles that appear dense in electron microscopic images (115). Substance-P plays a unique role in this context because it is primarily found in unmyelinated C fibers. Chemical ablation of these nerve fibers with the neurotoxin capsaicin blunts responses to painful stimuli, pointing at an important role of substance-P–containing neurons in nociception (116,117). Consistent with this assumption, innocuous stimulation generally does not trigger substance-P release, while noxious stimuli or visceral inflammation cause the release of this transmitter (118). Conversely, substance-P antagonists or knockout mice deficient in substance-P or its receptor exhibit blunted responses to painful visceral stimulation (119–122). Inflammation rapidly activates the transcription of substance-P and other neurotransmitters in primary sensory neurons, which may affect synaptic transmission

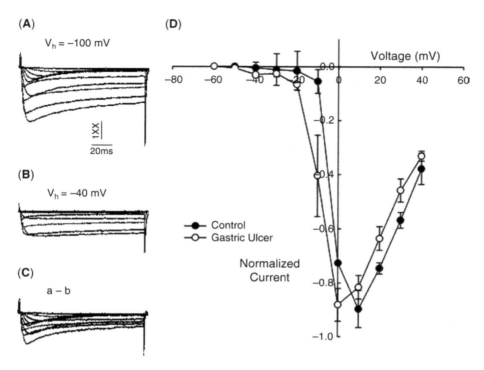

Figure 7 Calcium currents in visceral inflammation. The left panel shows families of calcium currents triggered by stepwise depolarization between −100 mV (**A**) and −40 mV (**B**). The digital subtraction reveals a transient component activated by hyperpolarization (**C**). The current-voltage relationship demonstrates that calcium currents activate at more native potentials in nodose neurons obtained from animals with gastric ulcerations (**D**).

(123–125). Combined with other changes such as enhanced neuron excitability and calcium influx into the presynaptic terminal, the altered transmitter expression may contribute to the increased activation of substance-P–receptors in the spinal cord (118,126). In addition, previously silent synapses can become active and sprouting of nerve terminals after injury or inflammation may establish new connections in the spinal cord (127–130). Many of these newly formed synapses convey information about innocuous stimuli onto neurons within regions involved in nociception (lamina I or II of the spinal cord), thus providing a potential mechanism for the development of allodynia (Fig. 8).

Clinical Implications

Peptide transmitters such as substance-P- or calcitonin-gene–related peptide, play an important role in synaptic transmission of nociceptive information from first- to second-order neuron in the spinal cord. Selective antagonists have been developed to block this information transfer. While effective in animal experiments, initial human studies did not show significant analgesic properties of these agents.

Central terminations of primary afferent neurons sprout in the rostrocaudal axis within the spinal cord in response to injury and inflammation. This mechanism may contribute to the wider pain referral area in patients with chronic visceral pain syndromes.

NERVE-IMMUNE INTERACTIONS AND PERIPHERAL SENSITIZATION

The previous sections described how inflammatory mediators modulate the function of sensory neurons. However, neurons also affect immune cells, many of which express receptors for neuropeptides such as substance-P, calcitonin-gene–related peptide (CGRP), or

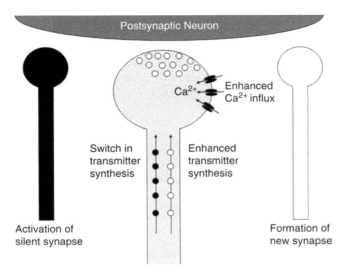

Figure 8 Presynaptic mechanisms of altered synaptic transmission in nociceptive signaling. Inflammation increases calcium currents, which will enhance transmitter release. This can be associated with changes in transmitter expression. Silent synapses may become active or sprouting of central nerve terminals may lead to the formation of new synapses.

somatostatin (131–134). Therefore, release of these peptides from nerve terminals can attract and/or activate immune cells, thereby contributing to the inflammatory response (neurogenic inflammation) (135,136). A family of G-protein–coupled receptors, the protease-activated receptors (PAR), demonstrates the potential importance of this cross talk between sensory neurons and immune cells. In addition to inflammatory mediators, immune cells release proteases such as cathepsin G or tryptase into the interstitial space. These enzymes cleave the N terminal of PAR, thereby releasing a small peptide that activates the G-protein. PAR-2 receptors are expressed on extrinsic and intrinsic visceral sensory neurons (137,138). Activation of these receptors triggers an increase in intracellular calcium and release of neurotransmitters, which interact with mast cells and other immune cells, leading to protease release and further proteolytic activation of PAR-2 receptors. Considering the high concentration of proteases within the pancreas, this pathway may play an especially important role in pain development during pancreatic diseases (139). However, PAR-2 may play a role in other areas because it can be activated by mast cells, which are found in close proximity to nerves and release tryptase (140,141). Consistent with such a more general role of PAR-2 activation, the PAR-2–activating peptide enhanced responses to colorectal distension in rats (142).

> ***Clinical Implications***
> Close proximity between nerves and immune cells as well as shared signaling pathways demonstrate the importance of interactions between the nervous and the immune system. The recently characterized PAR-2 receptor plays a special role in this context because it is found on primary afferent neurons, can be activated by mast cell tryptase, and triggers hyperalgesia, making it an interesting target for drug development.

PERIPHERAL SENSITIZATION AND VISCERAL PAIN SYNDROMES

The current understanding of mechanisms of peripheral sensitization is largely derived from studies examining the effects of injury or inflammation on visceral afferents. Most patients with chronic visceral pain, such as irritable bowel syndrome, nonulcer dyspepsia or interstitial cystitis, do not have signs of inflammation, raising questions about the relevance of these findings. While the definition of such functional diseases excludes active inflammation, up to one-third of patients with such functional disorders mentioned a precipitating infection or other insult (31,143,144). Interestingly, pelvic afferents demonstrated increased excitability up to two months after complete resolution of colitis in rats (58). Rectal pain and urgency were associated with an increase in the density of TRPV1 immunoreactive nerve fibers within the mucosa (18). These initial results suggest that persistent changes in visceral afferents are involved in the pathogenesis of visceral hyperalgesia and may be important targets in the treatment of visceral pain syndromes.

REFERENCES

1. Ozaki N, Gebhart GF. Characterization of mechanosensitive splanchnic nerve afferent fibers innervating the rat stomach. Am J Physiol 2001; 281:G1449–G1459.
2. Ozaki N, Sengupta JN, Gebhart GF. Mechanosensitive properties of gastric vagal afferent fibers in the rat. J Neurophysiol 1999; 82:2210–2220.
3. Gebhart GF, Su X, Joshi S, Ozaki N, Sengupta JN. Peripheral opioid modulation of visceral pain. Ann N Y Acad Sci 2000; 909:41–50.
4. Page AJ, O'Donnell TA, Blackshaw LA. P2X purinoceptor-induced sensitization of ferret vagal mechanoreceptors in oesophageal inflammation. J Physiol (Lond) 2000; 523:403–411.
5. Brunsden AM, Grundy D. Sensitization of visceral afferents to bradykinin in rat jejunum in vitro. J Physiol (Lond) 1999; 521:517–527.
6. Welsh MJ, Price MP, Xie J. Biochemical basis of touch perception: mechanosensory function of degenerin/epithelial Na+ channels. J Biol Chem 2002; 277:2369–2372.
7. Suzuki M, Mizuno A, Kodaira K, Imai M. Impaired Pressure Sensation in Mice Lacking TRPV4. J Biol Chem 2003; 278:22664–22668.
8. Gershon MD. Review article: roles played by 5-hydroxytryptamine in the physiology of the bowel. Aliment Pharmacol Therap 1999; 13(suppl 2):15–30.
9. Burnstock G. Purine-mediated signalling in pain and visceral perception. Trends Pharmacol Sci 2001; 22:182–188.
10. Cockayne DA, Hamilton SG, Zhu QM, et al. Urinary bladder hyporeflexia and reduced pain-related behaviour in P2X3-deficient mice. Nature 2000; 407:1011–1015.
11. Vlaskovska M, Kasakov L, Rong W, et al. P2X3 knock-out mice reveal a major sensory role for urothelially released ATP. J. Neurosci. 2001; 21:5670–5677.
12. Waldmann R, Bassilana F, de Weille J, Champigny G, Heurteaux C, Lazdunski M. Molecular cloning of a non-inactivating proton-gated Na+ channel specific for sensory neurons. J Biol Chem 1997; 272:0975–22854.
13. Benson CJ, Eckert SP, McCleskey EW. Acid-evoked currents in cardiac sensory neurons: a possible mediator of myocardial ischemic sensation. Circ Res 1999; 84:921–928.
14. Caterina MJ, Schumacher MA, Tominaga M, Rosen TA, Levine JD, Julius D. The capsaicin receptor: a heat-activated ion channel in the pain pathway. Nature 1997; 389:816–824.
15. Caterina MJ, Leffler A, Malmberg AB, et al. Impaired nociception and pain sensation in mice lacking the capsaicin receptor. Science 2000; 288:306–313.
16. Birder LA, Nakamura Y, Kiss S, et al. Altered urinary bladder function in mice lacking the vanilloid receptor TRPV1. Nature Neuroscience 2002:856–860.
17. Patterson LM, Zheng H, Ward SM, Berthoud HR. Vanilloid receptor (VR1) expression in vagal afferent neurons innervating the gastrointestinal tract. Cell Tissue Res 2003; 311:277–287.
18. Chan CLH, Facer P, Davis JB, et al. Sensory fibres expressing capsaicin receptor TRPV1 in patients with rectal hypersensitivity and faecal urgency. Lancet 2003; 361:385–391.
19. Tominaga M, Caterina MJ, Malmberg AB, et al. The cloned capsaicin receptor integrates multiple pain producing stimuli. Neuron 1998; 21:531–543.
20. Hwang SW, Cho H, Kwak J, et al. Direct activation of capsaicin receptors by products of lipoxygenases: endogenous capsaicin-like substances. Proc Natl Acad Sci 2000; 97:6155–6716.
21. Kwak J, Wang MH, Hwang SW, Kim TY, Lee SY, Oh U. Intracellular ATP increases capsaicin-activated channel activity by interacting with nucleotide-binding domain. J. Neurosci. 2000; 20:8298–8304.
22. Chuang HH, Prescott ED, Kong H, et al. Bradykinin and nerve growth factor release the capsaicin receptor from PtdIns (4,5) P2-mediated inhibition. Nature 2001; 411:957–962.
23. Di Marzo V, Blumberg PM, Szallasi A. Endovanilloid signaling in pain. Curr Opin Neurobiol 2002; 12:372–379.
24. Premkumar LS, Qi Z-H, Van Buren J, Raisinghani M. Enhancement of potency and efficacy of NADA by PKC-mediated phosphorylation of vanilloid receptor. J Neurophysiol 2004; 91: 1442–1449.
25. Tominaga M, Wada M, Masu M. Potentiation of capsaicin receptor activity by metabotropic ATP receptors as a possible mechanism for ATP-evoked pain and hyperalgesia. Proc Natl Acad Sci 2001; 98:6951–6956.

26. Voilley N, de Weille J, Mamet J, Lazdunski M. Nonsteroid anti-inflammatory drugs inhibit both the activity and the inflammation-induced expression of acid-sensing ion channels in nociceptors. J Neurosci 2001; 21:8026–8033.
27. Birder LA, Barrick SR, Roppolo JR, et al. Feline interstitial cystitis results in mechanical hypersensitivity and altered ATP release from bladder urothelium. Am J Physiol Renal Physiol 2003; 285:F423–F429.
28. Kim M, Javed NH, Yu JG, Christofi F, Cooke HJ. Mechanical stimulation activates Galphaq signaling pathways and 5-hydroxytryptamine release from human carcinoid BON cells. J Clin Invest 2001a; 108:1051–1059.
29. Pan H, Gershon MD. Activation of intrinsic afferent pathways in submucosal ganglia of the guinea pig small intestine. J Neurosci 2000; 20:3295–3309.
30. Spiller RC, Jenkins D, Thornley JP, et al. Increased rectal mucosal enteroendocrine cells, T lymphocytes and increased gut permeability following acute campylobacter enteritis and in post-dysenteric irritable bowel syndrome. Gut 2000; 47:804–811.
31. Spiller RC. Postinfectious irritable bowel syndrome. Gastroenterology 2003; 124:1662–1671.
32. Snyder PM. The epithelial Na+ channel: cell surface insertion and retrieval in Na+ homeostasis and hypertension. Endocr Rev 2002; 23:258–275.
33. Kleizen B, Braakman I, de Jonge HR. Regulated trafficking of the CFTR chloride channel. Eu J Cell Biol 2000; 79:544–556.
34. Cayouette S, Lussier MP, Mathieu E-L, Bousquet SM, Boulay G. Exocytotic insertion of TRPC6 channel into the plasma membrane upon gq protein-coupled receptor activation. J Biol Chem 2004; 279:7241–7246.
35. Mendell LM, Albers KM, Davis BM. Neurotrophins, nociceptors, and pain. Microsc Res Tech 1999; 45:252–261.
36. Shu XQ, Mendell LM. Neurotrophins and hyperalgesia. Proc Natl Acad of Sci U S A 1999; 96: 7693–7696.
37. di Mola FF, Friess H, Zhu ZW, et al. Nerve growth factor and Trk high affinity receptor (TrkA) gene expression in inflammatory bowel disease. Gut 2000; 46:670–679.
38. Friess H, Zhu ZW, di Mola FF, et al. Nerve growth factor and its high-affinity receptor in chronic pancreatitis. Ann Surg 1999; 230:615–624.
39. Vizzard MA. Changes in urinary bladder neurotrophic factor mRNA and NGF protein following urinary bladder dysfunction. Exp Neurol 2000a; 161:273–284.
40. Bielefeldt K, Ozaki N, Gebhart GF. Role of nerve growth factor in modulation of gastric afferent neurons in the rat. Am J Physiol 2003; 284:G499–G507.
41. Toma H, Winston J, Micci MA, Shenoy M, Pasricha PJ. Nerve growth factor expression is upregulated in the rat model of L-arginine-induced acute pancreatitis. Gastroenterology 2000; 119:1373–1381.
42. Lowe EM, Anand P, Terenghi G, Williams-Chestnut RE, Sinicropi DV, Osborne JL. Increased nerve growth factor levels in the urinary bladder of women with idiopathic sensory urgency and interstitial cystitis. Br J Urol 1997; 79:572–577.
43. Lamb K, Gebhart GF, Bielefeldt K. Increased nerve growth factor expression triggers bladder overactivity. J Pain 2004; 5:150–156.
44. Lamb K, Kang YM, Gebhart GF, Bielefeldt K. Nerve growth factor and gastric hyperalgesia in the rat. Neurogastroenterol Motil 2003a; 15:355–361.
45. Winston J, Toma H, Shenoy M, Pasricha PJ. Nerve growth factor regulates VR-1 mRNA levels in cultures of adult dorsal root ganglion neurons. Pain 2001; 89:181–186.
46. Mamet J, Lazdunski M, Voilley N. How nerve growth factor drives physiological and inflammatory expressions of acid-sensing ion channel 3 in sensory neurons. J Biol Chem 2003; 278:48907–48913.
47. Brady CM, Apostolidis AN, Harper M, et al. Parallel changes in bladder suburothelial vanilloid receptor TRPV1 and pan-neuronal marker PGP9.5 immunoreactivity in patients with neurogenic detrusor overactivity after intravesical resiniferatoxin treatment. BJU Int 2004; 93:770–776.
48. Yiangou Y, Facer P, Smith JAM, et al. Increased acid-sensing ion channel ASIC-3 in inflamed human intestine. Eur J Gastroenterol Hepatol 2001; 13:891–896.
49. Mamet J, Baron A, Lazdunski M, Voilley N. ProInflammatory mediators, stimulators of sensory neuron excitability via the expression of acid-sensing ion channels. J Neurosci 2002; 22:10662–10670.
50. Yoshimura N, Seki S, Erickson KA, Erickson VL, Hancellor MB, Groat WCd. Histological and electrical properties of rat dorsal root ganglion neurons innervating the lower urinary tract. J Neurosci 2003; 23:4355–4361.
51. Robinson DR, McNaughton PA, Evans ML, Hicks GA. Characterization of the primary spinal afferent innervation of the mouse colon using retrograde labelling. Neurogastroenterol Motil 2004; 16:113–124.
52. Jaggar SI, Scott HCF, James IF, Rice ASC. The capsaicin analogue SDZ249–665 attenuates the hyperreflexia and referred hyperalgesia associated with inflammation of the rat urinary bladder. Pain 2001; 89:229–235.
53. Pomonis JD, Harrison JE, Mark L, Bristol DR, Valenzano KJ, Walker K. N-(4-Tertiarybutylphenyl)-4-(3-cholorphyridin-2-yl)tetrahydropyrazine –1 (2H)-carbox-amide (BCTC), a Novel, orally effective

vanilloid receptor 1 antagonist with analgesic properties: II. in vivo characterization in rat models of inflammatory and neuropathic pain. J Pharmacol Exp Ther 2003; 306:387–393.

54. Gold MS, Traub RJ. Cutaneous and colonic rat drg neurons differ with respect to both baseline and PGE2-induced changes in passive and active electrophysiological properties. J Neurophysiol 2004; 91:2524–2531.

55. Oh EJ, Weinreich D. Bradykinin decreases K+ and increases Cl- conductances in vagal afferent neurones of the guinea pig. J Physiol (Lond) 2004; 558:513–526.

56. Moore BA, Stewart TMR, Hill C, Vanner SJ. TNBS ileitis evokes hyperexcitability and changes in ionic membrane properties of nociceptive DRG neurons. Am J Physiol Gastrointest Liver Physiol 2002; 282:G1045–G1051.

57. Yoshimura N, deGroat WC. Increased excitability of afferent neurons innervating rat urinary bladder after chronic bladder inflammation. J. Neurosci. 1999; 19:4644–4653.

58. Lin C, Al-Chaer ED. Long-term sensitization of primary afferents in adult rats exposed to neonatal colon pain. Brain Res 2003; 971:73–82.

59. Goldin AL, Barchi RL, Caldwell JH, et al. Nomenclature of voltage-gated sodium channels. Neuron 2000; 28:365–368.

60. Akopian AN, Sivilotti L, Wood JN. A tetrodotoxin-resistant voltage-gated sodium channel expressed by sensory neurons. Nature 1996; 379:257–262.

61. Djouhri L, Fang X, Okuse K, Wood JN, Berry CM, Lawson S. The TTX-resistant sodium channel Nav1.8 (SNS/PN3): expression and correlation with membrane properties in rat nociceptive primary afferent neurons. J Physiol (Lond) 2003; 550(3):739–752.

62. Akopian AN, Souslova V, England S, et al. The tetrodotoxin-resistant sodium channel SNS has a specialized function in pain pathways. Nature Neuroscience 1999; 2:541–548.

63. Yoshimura N, Seki S, Novakovic SD, et al. The involvement of the tetrodotoxin-resistant sodium channel nav1.8 (pn3/sns) in a rat model of visceral pain. J Neurosci 2001; 21:8690–8696.

64. Stewart TM, Beyak MJ, Vanner SJ. Ileitis modulates potassium and sodium currents in guinea pig dorsal root ganglia neurons. J Physiol 2003; 552(3):797–807.

65. Bielefeldt K, Ozaki N, Gebhart GF. Mild gastritis alters voltage-sensitive sodium currents in gastric sensory neurons in rats. Gastroenterology 2002; 122:752–761.

66. Bielefeldt K, Ozaki N, Gebhart GF. Experimental ulcers alter voltage-sensitive sodium currents in rat gastric sensory neurons. Gastroenterology 2002; 122:394–405.

67. Dascal N, Lotan I. Activation of protein kinase C alters voltage dependence of a Na+ channel. Neuron 1991; 6:165–175.

68. Gold MS, Levine JD, Correa AM. Modulation of TTX-R INa by PKC and PKA and their role in PGE2-induced sensitization of rat sensory neurons in vitro. Journal of Neuroscience 1998; 18:10345–10355.

69. Gold MS, Reichling DB, Shuster MJ, Levine JD. Hyperalgesic agents increase a tetrodotoxin-resistant Na+ current in nociceptors. Proc Natl Acad Sci 1996; 93:1108–1112.

70. Gold MS, Zhang L, Wrigley DL, Traub RJ. Prostaglandin E2 modulates TTX-R INa in rat colonic sensory neurons. J Neurophysiol 2002; 88:1512–1522.

71. d'Alcantara P, Cardenas LM, Swillens S, Scroggs RS. Reduced Transition between Open and Inactivated Channel States Underlies 5HT Increased INa+ in Rat Nociceptors. Biophys J 2002; 83:21.

72. Cardenas CG, Del Mar LP, Cooper BY, Scroggs RS. 5HT4 receptors couple positively to tetrodotoxin-insensitive sodium channels in a subpopulation of capsaicin-sensitive rat sensory neurons. J Neurosci 1997; 17:7181–7189.

73. Su X, Wachtel RE, Gebhart GF. Capsaicin sensitivity and voltage-gated sodium currents in colon sensory neurons from rat dorsal root ganglia. Am J Physiol 1999; 277:G1180-G1188.

74. Lancaster E, Oh EJ, Weinreich D. Vagotomy decreases excitability in primary vagal afferent somata. J Neurophysiol 2001; 85:247–253.

75. Lancaster E, Weinreich D. Sodium currents in vagotomized primary afferent neurones of the rat. J Physiol (Lond) 2001; 536:445–458.

76. Dib-Hajj S, Black JA, Felts P, Waxman SG. Down-regulation of transcripts for Na channel alpha-SNS in spinal sensory neurons following axotomy. Proc Natl Acad Sci U S A 1996; 93:14950–14954.

77. Oyelese AA, Rizzo MA, Waxman SG, Kocsis JD. Differential effects of NGF and BDNF on axotomy-induced changes in GABA(A)-receptor-mediated conductance and sodium currents in cutaneous afferent neurons. J Neurophysiol 1997; 78:1–42.

78. Leffler A, Cummins TR, Dib-Hajj SD, Hormuzdiar WN, Black JA, Waxman SG. GDNF and NGF reverse changes in repriming of TTX-sensitive Na+ currents following axotomy of dorsal root ganglion neurons. J Neurophysiol 2002; 88:650–658.

79. Fjell J, Cummins TR, Fried K, Black JA, Waxman SG. In vivo NGF deprivation reduces SNS expression and TTX-R sodium currents in IB4-negative DRG neurons. J Neurophysiol 1999; 81:803–810.

80. Hanlon MR, Wallace BA. Structure and function of voltage-dependent ion channel regulatory subunits. Biochemistry 2002; 41:2886–2894.

81. Blackburn-Munro G, Fleetwood-Walker SM. The sodium channel auxiliary subunits [beta]1 and [beta]2 are differentially expressed in the spinal cord of neuropathic rats. Neuroscience 1999; 90:153–164.

82. Pugsley MK, Yu EJ, McLean TH, Goldin AL. Blockade of neuronal sodium channels by the antiepileptic drugs phenytoin, carbamazepine and sodium valproate. Proc Western Pharmacol Soc 1999; 42:105–108.

83. Erichsen HK, Hao J-X, Xu X-J, Blackburn-Munro G. A comparison of the antinociceptive effects of voltage-activated Na+ channel blockers in two rat models of neuropathic pain. Eu J Pharmacol 2003; 458:275–282.

84. Su X, Joshi SK, Kardos S, Gebhart GF. Sodium channel blocking actions of the kappa -opioid receptor agonist U50,488 contribute to its visceral antinociceptive effects. J Neurophysiol 2002; 87: 1271–1279.

85. Bielefeldt K, Ozaki N, Whiteis C, Gebhart GF. Amitriptyline inhibits voltage-sensitive sodium currents in rat gastric sensory neurons. Digest Dis Sci 2002b; 47:959–966.

86. Joshi SK, Lamb K, Bielefeldt K, Gebhart GF. Arylamide k-opioid receptor agonist produce a tonic- and use-dependent block of tetrodotoxin-sensitive and -resistant sodium currents in colon sensory neurons. J Pharmacol Exp Therap 2003; 307:367–372.

87. Jan LY, Jan YN. Cloned potassium channels from eukaryotes and prokaryotes. Ann Rev Neurosci 1997; 20:91–123.

88. Pongs O. Voltage-gated potassium channels: from hyperexcitability to excitement. FEBS Letters 1999; 452:1–35.

89. Rasband MN, Park EW, Vanderah TW, Lai J, Porreca F, Trimmer JS. Distinct potassium channels on pain-sensing neurons. PNAS 2001; 98:13373–13378.

90. Zhou L, Messing A, Chiu SY. Determinants of Excitability at Transition Zones in Kv1.1-Deficient Myelinated Nerves. J Neurosci 1999; 19:5768–5781.

91. Clark JD, Tempel BL. Hyperalgesia in mice lacking the Kv1.1 potassium channel gene. Neuroscience Letters 1998; 251:121–124.

92. Jiang X, Zhang YH, Clark JD, Tempel BL, Nicol GD. Prostaglandin e2 inhibits the potassium current in sensory neurons from hyperalgesic kv1.1 knockout mice. Neuroscience 2003; 119:5–72.

93. Dang K, Bielefeldt K, Gebhart GF. Modulation of potassium currents in a model of gastric hyperalgesia. Am J Physiol 2004; 286:G573–G579.

94. Robbins J. Kcnq potassium channels: physiology, pathophysiology, and pharmacology. Pharmacol Therap 2001; 90:1–19.

95. Passmore GM, Selyanko AA, Mistry M, et al. KCNQ/M currents in sensory neurons: significance for pain therapy. J Neurosci 2003; 23:7227–7236.

96. Catterall WA, Striessnig J, Snutch TP, Perez-Reyes E. International union of pharmacology. XL. compendium of voltage-gated ion channels: calcium channels. Pharmacol Rev 2003; 55:579–581.

97. Heinke B, Balzer E, Sandkuhler J. Pre- and postsynaptic contributions of voltage-dependent Ca2+ channels to nociceptive transmission in rat spinal lamina I neurons. Eur J Neurosci 2004; 19:103–111.

98. Kim C, Jun K, Lee T, et al. Altered nociceptive response in mice deficient in the [alpha]1b subunit of the voltage-dependent calcium channel. Mol Cell Neurosci 2001b; 18:235–245.

99. Saegusa H, Kurihara T, Zong S, et al. Altered pain responses in mice lacking alpha 1E subunit of the voltage-dependent Ca2+ channel. Proc Natl Acad Sci 2000; 97:7132–7674.

100. Saegusa H, Matsuda Y, Tanabe T. Effects of ablation of N- and R-type Ca2+ channels on pain transmission. Neuroscience Research 2002; 43:1–7.

101. Horvath G, Brodacz B, Holzer-Petsche U. Role of calcium channels in the spinal transmission of nociceptive information from the mesentery. Pain 2001; 93:5–41.

102. Moises H, Rusin K, Macdonald R. Mu- and kappa-opioid receptors selectively reduce the same transient components of high-threshold calcium current in rat dorsal root ganglion sensory neurons. J Neurosci 1994; 14:5903–5916.

103. Acosta CG, Lopez HS. delta Opioid receptor modulation of several voltage-dependent Ca2+ currents in rat sensory neurons. J Neurosci 1994; 14:5903–5916.

104. Su X, Wachtel RE, Gebhart GF. Inhibition of calcium currents in rat colon sensory neurons by K- but not mu- or delta-opioids. J Neurophysiol 1998; 80:3112–3119.

105. Murakami M, Fleischmann B, De Felipe C, et al. Pain perception in mice lacking the beta 3 subunit of voltage-activated calcium channels. J Biol Chem 2002; 277:40342–40351.

106. Newton RA, Bingham S, Case PC, Sanger GJ, Lawson SN. Dorsal root ganglion neurons show increased expression of the calcium channel á2ä-1 subunit following partial sciatic nerve injury. Mol Brain Res 2001; 95:1–8.

107. Gee NS, Brown JP, Dissanayake VUK, Offord J, Thurlow R, Woodruff GN. The novel anticonvulsant drug, gabapentin (neurontin), binds to the alpha(2)[image] subunit of a calcium channel. J Biol Chem 1996; 271:5768–5776.

108. Diop L, Raymond F, Fargeau H, Petoux F, Chovet M, Doherty AM. Pregabalin (CI-1008) inhibits the trinitrobenzene sulfonic acid-induced chronic colonic allodynia in the rat. J Pharmacol Exp Ther 2002; 302:1013–1022.

109. Eutamene H, Coelho A-M, Theodorou V, et al. Antinociceptive effect of pregabalin in septic shock-induced rectal hypersensitivity in rats. J Pharmacol Exp Ther 2000; 295:162–167.

110. Luo ZD, Calcutt NA, Higuera ES, et al. Injury type-specific calcium channel alpha 2delta -1 subunit up-regulation in rat neuropathic pain models correlates with antiallodynic effects of gabapentin. J Pharmacol Exp Ther 2002; 303:1199–1205.

111. Heidelberger R, Heinemann C, Neher E, Matthews G. Calcium dependence of the rate of exocytosis in a synaptic terminal. Nature 1994; 371:513–515.

112. Geppert M, Sudhof TC. RAB3 and synaptotagmin: the yin and yang of synaptic membrane fusion. Ann Rev Neurosci 1998; 21:5–95.

113. Schneider S, Perl E. Comparison of primary afferent and glutamate excitation of neurons in the mammalian spinal dorsal horn. J Neurosci 1988; 8:2062–2073.

114. Zhuo H, Ichikawa H, Helke CJ. Neurochemistry of the nodose ganglion. Prog Neurobiol 1997; 52: 79–107.

115. Kupfermann I. Functional studies of cotransmission. Physiol Rev 1991; 71:783–732.

116. Ness TJ, Randich A, Gebhart GF. Further behavioral evidence that colorectal distension is a 'noxious' visceral stimulus in rats. Neurosci Lett 1991; 131:113–116.

117. Lamb K, Kang YM, Gebhart GF, Bielefeldt K. Gastric inflammation triggers hypersensitivity to acid in awake rats. Gastroenterology 2003b:126.

118. Honore P, Kamp EH, Rogers SD, Gebhart GF, Manyth RW. Activation of lamina 1 spinal cord neurons that express the substance P receptor in visceral nociception and hyperalgesia. J Pain 2002; 3:3–11.

119. Chien C-T, Yu H-J, Lin T-B, Lai M-K, Hsu S-M. Substance P via NK1 receptor facilitates hyperactive bladder afferent signaling via action of ROS. Am J Physiol Renal Physiol 2003; 284:F840–F851.

120. Laird JM, Olivar T, Roza C, De Felipe C, Hunt SP, Cervero F. Deficits in visceral pain and hyperalgesia of mice with a disruption of the tachykinin NK1 receptor gene. Neuroscience 2000; 98: 345–352.

121. Zimmer A, Zimmer AM, Baffi J, et al. Hypoalgesia in mice with a targeted deletion of the tachykinin 1 gene. Proc Natl Acad Sci 1998; 95:2630–2635.

122. De Felipe C, Herrero JF, O'Brien JA, et al. Altered nociception, analgesia and aggression in mice lacking the receptor for substance P Nature 1998; 392:394–397.

123. Fischer A, McGregor GP, Saria A, Philippin B, Kummer W. Induction of tachykinin gene and peptide expression in guinea pig nodose primary afferent neurons by allergic airway inflammation. J Clin Invest 1996; 98:2284–2291.

124. Bulling DGS, Kelly D, Bond S, McQueen DS, Seckl JR. Adjuvant-induced joint inflammation causes very rapid transcription of CGRP genes in innervating sensory ganglia. J Neurochem 2001; 77: 372–382.

125. Vizzard MA. Up-regulation of pituitary adenylate cyclase-activating polypeptide in urinary bladder pathways after chronic cystitis. J Comp Neurol 2000; 420:335–348.

126. Honore P, Menning PM, Rogers SD, et al. Spinal substance P receptor expression and internalization in acute, short-term, and long-term inflammatory pain states. J Neurosci 1999; 19:7670–7678.

127. Li P, Zhuo M. Silent glutamatergic synapses and nociception in mammalian spinal cord. Nature 1998; 393:695–698.

128. Nakatsuka T, Park J-S, Kumamoto E, Tamaki T, Yoshimura M. Plastic changes in sensory inputs to rat substantia gelatinosa neurons following peripheral inflammation. Pain 1999; 82:9–47.

129. Furue H, Katafuchi T, Yoshimura M. Sensory processing and functional reorganization of sensory transmission under pathological conditions in the spinal dorsal horn. Neurosci Res 2004; 48: 361–368.

130. Baba H, Doubell TP, Woolf CJ. Peripheral Inflammation Facilitates Abeta Fiber-Mediated Synaptic Input to the Substantia Gelatinosa of the Adult Rat Spinal Cord. J Neurosci 1999; 19:859–867.

131. Goode T, O'Connell J, Sternini C, et al. Substance P (neurokinin-1) receptor is a marker of human mucosal but not peripheral mononuclear cells: molecular quantitation and localization. J Immunol 1998; 161:2232–2240.

132. Saban R, Gerard NP, Saban MR, Nguyen N-B, DeBoer DJ, Wershil BK. Mast cells mediate substance P-induced bladder inflammation through an NK1 receptor-independent mechanism. Am J Physiol Renal Physiol 2002a; 283:F616-F629.

133. Theodorou V, Fioramonti J, Bueno L. Integrative neuroimmunology of the digestive tract. Veter Res 1996; 27:427–442.

134. Bracci-Laudiero L, Aloe L, Buanne P, et al. NGF modulates CGRP synthesis in human B-lymphocytes: a possible anti-inflammatory action of NGF? J Neuroimmunol 2002; 123:8–65.

135. Saban MR, Saban R, Hammond TG, et al. LPS-sensory peptide communication in experimental cystitis. Am J Physiol Renal Physiol 2002b; 282:F202-F210.

136. Steinhoff M, Vergnolle N, Young SH, et al. Agonists of proteinase-activated receptor 2 induce inflammation by a neurogenic mechanism. Nature Medicine 2000; 6:151–158.

137. Vergnolle N, Bunnett NW, Sharkey KA, et al. Proteinase-activated receptor-2 and hyperalgesia: A novel pain pathway. Nature Medicine 2001; 7:821–826.

138. Gao C, Liu S, Hu HZ, et al. Serine proteases excite myenteric neurons through protease-activated receptors in guinea pig small intestine. Gastroenterology 2002; 123:1554–1564.

139. Hoogerwerf WA, Zou L, Shenoy M, et al. The proteinase-activated receptor 2 is involved in nociception. J Neurosci 2001; 21:9036–9042.

140. Stead RH, Tomioka M, Quinonez G, Simon GT, Felten SY, Bienenstock J. Intestinal mucosal mast cells in normal and nematode-infected rat intestines are in intimate contact with peptidergic nerves. Proc Natl Acad Sci U S A 1987; 84:2975–2979.

141. Vergnolle N. Modulation of visceral pain and inflammation by protease-activated receptors. Br J Pharmacol 2004; 141:1264–1274.
142. Coelho A-M, Vergnolle N, Guiard B, Fioramonti J, Bueno L. Proteinases and proteinase-activated receptor 2: a possible role to promote visceral hyperalgesia in rats. Gastroenterology 2002; 122:1035–1047.
143. Tack J, Demedts I, Dehondt G, et al. Clinical and pathophysiological characteristics of acute-onset functional dyspepsia. Gastroenterology 2002; 122:1738–1747.
144. Thornley JP, Jenkins D, Neal K, Wright T, Brough T, Spiller RC. Relationship of Campylobacter toxigenicity In vitro to the development of postinfectious irritable bowel syndrome. J Infect Dis 2001; 184:606–609.

7 | Spinal Mechanisms of Visceral Pain and Sensitization

Richard J. Traub

Department of Biomedical Sciences and Research Center for Neuroendocrine Influences on Pain, University of Maryland Dental School, Baltimore, Maryland, U.S.A.

INTRODUCTION

Humans experience a range of sensations arising from the abdominal viscera. Nonpainful sensations such as a feeling of satiety, gas, and the urge to defecate are part of everyday life. The stimuli that evoke these sensations are limited to a few organs in the gastrointestinal (GI) tract and occur with little concern by the individual. In contrast, the perception of pain arising from noxious stimulation of the viscera, for example, cramps due to acute noxious stimuli or hyperalgesia coincident with irritable bowel syndrome (IBS), can have a profound effect on an individual's quality of life. An understanding of the mechanisms underlying spinal processing of acute and chronic visceral stimuli is essential to develop further therapies for the treatment of visceral pain.

Visceral pain, regardless of the originating tissue, tends to have the following common characteristics (1,2): (i) initially it is poorly localized and diffuse, most often perceived as pain along the midline of the trunk; (ii) as the stimulus increases in intensity or duration, pain is more distinctly referred to somatic tissue; (iii) stimulation at the site where the pain is referred may be perceived as sensitized or hyperalgesic, although there is no pathology in the somatic tissue; and (iv) intense visceral stimuli evoke nonspecific or whole body motor responses, strong autonomic responses, and strong affective responses. Unlike somatic pain, visceral pain is inescapable. Reflexes may function to orient the individual to a more comfortable position, but there is no withdrawal reflex to escape the source of the pain.

The study of the mechanisms underlying these conditions lags behind such inquiry from somatic structures, in part because somatic tissue is much more readily accessible than are visceral structures. Furthermore, what is considered a noxious stimulus for somatic tissue may not be painful when applied to the viscera. Cutting, crushing, and burning of the intestines or colon fails to evoke pain [see reference to Lennander (1901) in Ref. 3].

Of stimuli that can evoke visceral pain (hollow organ distention, inflammation, ischemia, smooth muscle contraction, traction on mesentery, and distention of the capsule of solid organs), hollow organ distention and inflammation are the easiest to model. Inflating a balloon inside a hollow organ evokes transient pain in the absence of tissue damage and several substances injected into the lumen of organs induce inflammation and hyperalgesia. However, many clinical visceral pain conditions of the GI tract are considered functional bowel disorders. There are no indications of pathology associated with these diseases, though there is hyperalgesia (4). Most investigators use noxious stimuli such as colorectal distention (CRD) applied to healthy organs or inflammation to model or approximate these diseases in order to investigate underlying mechanisms that contribute to visceral pain. Only recently have models approximating these clinical conditions been reported (5,6).

Experimental evidence supports both peripheral and central mechanisms in the etiology of visceral pain and hyperalgesia. Furthermore, when compared to somatic pain, there are many similarities, but some obvious differences in the anatomy, physiology, and pharmacology of viscerosensory processing. This chapter will review the role of spinal cord processing underlying visceral pain and hyperalgesia. The discussion will center on pain arising from the GI tract, but references to other organs will be included as appropriate.

VISCERAL AFFERENT ORGANIZATION CONTRIBUTING TO VISCERAL PAIN AND HYPERALGESIA

Several features of the innervation and central projection of visceral afferent fibers, which are unique to the viscera, underlie the way information is processed in the spinal cord contributing to visceral pain and hyperalgesia.

Dual Innervation

Unlike somatic tissue, the viscera are unique. They are dually innervated by primary afferents that project to separate regions of the neuraxis and appear to contribute to different aspects of visceral pain and hyperalgesia (7–12). These afferent fibers project in the same nerves as sympathetic and parasympathetic efferent fibers, but similar to somatic primary afferents, have their cell bodies in the dorsal root ganglia (and nodose ganglia for vagal afferents).

The esophagus to the middle of the transverse colon is innervated by primary afferents in the vagus nerve (parasympathetic pathway) that project centrally to the nucleus of the solitary tract and primary afferents in the splanchnic nerves (sympathetic pathway) that project centrally to the thoracic spinal cord segments. The distal bowel (transverse, descending, sigmoid colon and rectum) is innervated by primary afferents in the pelvic nerve (parasympathetic pathway), which project centrally to the sacral spinal cord and primary afferents in the least and lumbar splanchnic nerves, which project centrally to the lower thoracic/upper lumbar spinal cord (Fig. 1) (8,11,13–15).

This dual innervation holds true for other organ systems as well: cardiovascular and respiratory organs are innervated by vagal and splanchnic afferents (17), and urinary and reproductive organs are innervated by pelvic and splanchnic (hypogastric) afferents (7,18–21). The role of this dual innervation remains unclear. Most indications are that the splanchnic innervation conveys nociception and the vagal/pelvic pathways subserve homeostatic functions. However, recent studies elucidated below suggest this simple dichotomy of function is much more complex.

Divergence of Visceral Afferents in the Spinal Cord

In addition to the dual innervation of viscera by sensory afferent fibers, the central projection and terminal arborization of these visceral afferent fibers are highly divergent compared to somatic afferents. Somatic afferents project to well-defined regions within the dorsal horn (Fig. 2A) (22–26). Small diameter myelinated and unmyelinated fibers, most of which are associated with nociceptors, terminate in the superficial dorsal horn and to a lesser extent in

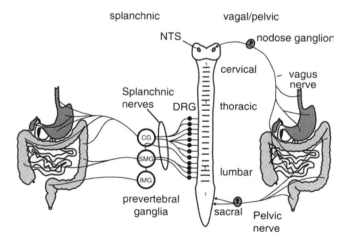

Figure 1 The sensory innervation of the gastrointestinal tract. The splanchnic afferent innervation is shown on the left, the vagal/pelvic afferent innervation is shown on the right. The splanchnic afferent nerves have cell bodies in the thoracolumbar dorsal root ganglia (DRG) and project centrally through the dorsal roots into the spinal cord. The vagal/pelvic afferents that innervate the esophagus to the middle of the transverse colon project in the vagus nerve with cell bodies in the nodose ganglia. These afferents project centrally to the nucleus tractus solitarius. Pelvic afferents innervating the lower bowel have cell bodies in the lumbosacral DRG and project centrally into the lumbosacral spinal cord. *Source*: From Ref. 16.

(A)

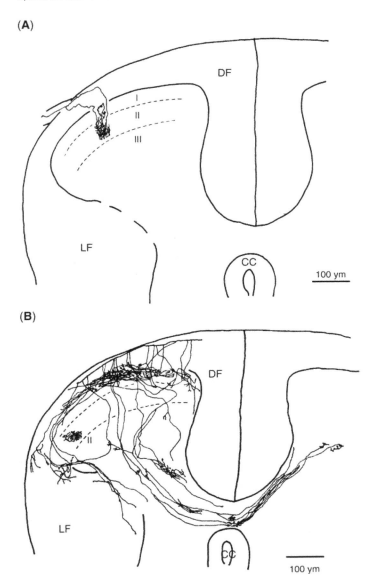

(B)

Figure 2 (**A**) The central projection of a single somatic C polymodal nociceptor shown in the transverse plane. The image is collapsed into two dimensions from a serial reconstruction of an intracellularly labeled primary afferent fiber. Note the limited mediolateral and dorsoventral extent of the terminal arborization. The rostrocaudal extent of the arborization was approximately 500 μm. (**B**) The central projection of a visceral afferent fiber shown in the transverse plane. The image is collapsed into two dimensions as in A. This afferent projected at least 15 mm in the rostrocaudal direction sending at least 14 collateral branches into the grey matter. These collaterals formed the terminal arborization that extends across the superficial dorsal horn, down into the deep dorsal horn and across the midline to the contralateral dorsal horn. *Source*: From Ref. 22.

lamina V and VI, while larger diameter low threshold fibers terminate in lamina III and IV (27,28). Intracellular recording and labeling individual afferent fibers further reveal rostrocaudal projections extending two to three segments with terminal arborizations restricted in the mediolateral and dorsoventral planes. This mediolateral specificity helps define the somatotopic map. Thus, precise localization of external stimuli to the body surface can be determined. Visceral afferent fibers, in contrast, have an extensive terminal arborization in the spinal cord that extends rostrocaudally for 5 to 10 segments and covers the mediolateral and dorsoventral extent of the dorsal horn. Horseradish peroxidase applied to the pelvic nerve or splanchnic nerve labels bundles of fibers terminating in the superficial dorsal horn, lamina

V and VI, and the dorsal gray commissure (29–32). Labeled fibers project in Lissauer's tract four to five segments rostrally and many segments caudally. Intra-axonal labeling of visceral afferent fibers provides greater detail of their central projection (22). A single afferent fiber projects into the superficial dorsal horn, the deep dorsal horn, and across the dorsal gray commissure to the contralateral side (Fig. 2B). The medial and lateral paths taken by branches of a single afferent fiber correspond to the medial and lateral collateral pathways reported in whole nerve studies. This extremely divergent terminal arborization of visceral afferent fibers likely contributes to the poor localization of visceral pain.

REFERRED PAIN AND HYPERALGESIA: CONVERGENCE OF THE SOMATIC AND VISCERAL BODY
Visceral Pain Is Referred to Somatic Structures

The initial perception of pain from the viscera is described as diffuse pain along the midline of the trunk (3,2). It is poorly localized relative to the originating tissue. This likely results from the divergent central projection of visceral afferent fibers synapsing with scores of dorsal horn neurons in many segments. As the pain intensifies, it is more clearly referred to somatic tissue. It is perceived as originating from the area of the body that is innervated by somatic primary afferent fibers which project in the same dorsal roots as the visceral afferent fibers innervating the affected organ. One likely cause is convergence of the somatic afferent projection and the visceral afferent projection onto the same dorsal horn neurons: Ruch's convergence-projection theory (33). According to this hypothesis, dorsal horn neurons (or higher in the brain) usually respond to somatic stimuli and rarely respond to stimuli from visceral tissue. Upon persistent afferent input evoked by visceral stimulation, activity in this neuronal circuit is interpreted as arriving over somatic primary afferents and the pain is perceived as originating in somatic tissue (Fig. 3).

Referred pain is generally confined to one or a few dermatomes/myotomes and appears relatively constant with respect to a particular organ. For example, referred pain from angina pectoris is generally perceived in the left arm, shoulder, and jaw. Likewise, referred pain from an inflamed appendix is generally perceived in the right lower quadrant of the abdomen. This hypothesis, however, is inconsistent with the extensively divergent central projection of visceral afferents, which would predict referred pain over a larger portion of the trunk. Because the referred pain is restricted to a few dermatomes, additional factors likely function to confine the region of referred pain. When this balance is disturbed, referred pain is perceived over a larger area and is more intense. For example, the expanded area of referred pain and hyperalgesia in IBS patients (35).

Animal studies support viscerosomatic convergence as a mechanism underlying referred pain (Fig. 3). It is estimated that greater than 90% of dorsal horn neurons that respond to visceral stimuli have somatic receptive fields. Dorsal horn neurons in the lower lumbar/sacral spinal segments that respond to stimulation of the colon/rectum, bladder, or reproductive organs respond to stimulation of the skin and/or muscle of the hindlimbs, pelvic belly, and perianal area (36–42). Indeed, colonic inflammation in mice evokes withdrawal from mechanical stimuli applied to the lower abdomen at lower thresholds than noninflamed mice, suggesting that animals experience referred pain and hyperalgesia (43).

Likewise, dorsal horn neurons in the thoracic spinal cord that respond to visceral stimulation have convergent somatic receptive fields on the trunk (44–49). The location of the somatic receptive field illustrates two points: first, it is what would be expected based on the location of the dorsal horn neuron with respect to the somatotopic map in the spinal cord. This provides direct support for the hypothesis that referred pain results from convergence of somatic and visceral afferents onto the same dorsal horn neurons. Second, it also points to another paradox in spinal processing. As mentioned previously, the viscera receive dual afferent innervation. In the case of the descending colon and rectum, this is provided by the pelvic nerve projecting to the lumbosacral spinal cord (sacral in man) and the hypogastric/lumbar colonic nerves projecting to the thoracolumbar spinal cord. Experimental balloon distention of the colon and rectum in volunteers evokes referred pain in the sacral dermatomes consistent with input from the pelvic nerve (34,35). Likewise, in rats, sacral dorsal horn neurons that respond to CRD have somatic receptive fields corresponding to sacral dermatomes. However, the thoracolumbar segments receive colonic afferent input via the hypogastric/lumbar colonic

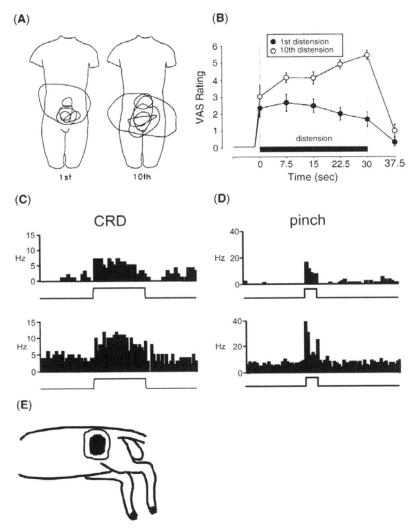

Figure 3 (**A**) and (**B**) Volunteers reported the area of referred pain (**A**) and the pain intensity (**B**) during the 1st and 10th trial of CRD. By the 10th distention, the area of referred pain expanded and the intensity increased, suggesting central sensitization. *Source*: Reprinted from Ref. 34. (**C–E**) Sensitization of a visceroceptive dorsal horn neuron that may underlie visceral hypersensitivity and referred pain. (**C**) the response to noxious CRD before (*top*) and following (*bottom*) colonic inflammation. The response of the cell increased slightly in addition to the significant increase in spontaneous activity. (**D**) The response to pinch of the convergent somatic receptive field before (*top*) and following (*bottom*) colonic inflammation. Because the inflammation was confined to the colon, the somatic primary afferents would not be sensitized. Therefore, the increase in the response to pinch following inflammation must result from central sensitization of the dorsal horn neuron. (**E**) the size of the convergent receptive field before (*black*) and after (outlined) colonic inflammation. Surrounding the original receptive field (*black*) is an area innervated by primary afferents that directly or indirectly connect to the dorsal horn neuron, but have subliminal input incapable of producing action potentials. When the neuron becomes sensitized, the subliminal input now reaches threshold to evoke action potentials, expanding the size of the receptive field. *Abbreviation*: CRD, colorectal distention.

nerves. Dorsal horn neurons in these segments have somatic receptive fields on the trunk, separate from the sacral neuron receptive fields. It would then be expected that referred pain should also be perceived as originating in the trunk. This does not occur in normal volunteers, but the area of referred pain expands into the lower abdomen following repetitive colonic distention (Fig. 3A) (34). In contrast, in patients with a functional bowel disorder or an inflammatory bowel disease, referred pain is perceived in the lower abdomen and thorax, as well as in the pelvic area (35). This dermatomal organization of referred pain suggests that acute colorectal pain is processed in the spinal cord segments receiving pelvic nerve afferent input and that following injury or disease, additional processing occurs in the spinal segments receiving afferent input over the hypogastric/lumbar colonic nerves (10).

Alternatively, there may be an interaction between visceral and somatic afferent fibers, which alters somatic sensitivity. Inflammation of the uterus induces localized plasma extravasation in the lower abdomen, demarcating the area of referred pain (50). Several mechanisms have been proposed to account for these data, but the most likely is that visceral afferent fibers project into the spinal cord and induce an antidromically propagating dorsal root reflex in somatic afferent fibers that produce localized neurogenic inflammation in the skin (51). This localized neurogenic inflammation may sensitize nearby somatic afferent fibers evoking a somatic hyperalgesia resulting from a visceral stimulus.

Viscerovisceral Convergence

Mechanistically, viscerovisceral convergence is similar to viscerosomatic convergence. The extensive divergence of the visceral afferent fibers in the spinal cord results in primary afferents that innervate different viscera converging onto a single dorsal horn neuron (37,52–55). This may result in stimulation of two viscera exciting the same dorsal horn neuron (Fig. 4A) or stimulation of one viscus, through interneurons, inhibiting a dorsal horn neuron while stimulation of another organ excites the same neuron (Fig. 4B).

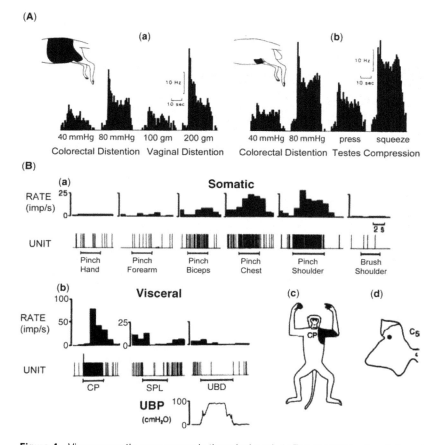

Figure 4 Viscerosomatic convergence in the spinal cord. **A**: Two examples of excitatory viscerovisceral convergence. In (**a**), the cell is excited by colorectal distention and vaginal distension. In (**b**), the cell is excited by colorectal distention and testes compression. In both cases, the visceral afferents project in the pelvic nerve and the convergent somatic receptive field corresponds to the area expected based on the location of the neuron in the spinal cord. *Source*: Reprinted from Ref. (56). **B**: Viscerovisceral-somatic convergence producing excitation and inhibition. The neuron was excited by pinch to the chest and shoulder (**a**). Cardiopulmonary afferent stimulation (CP in **b**) was excitatory, but splanchnic nerve stimulation (**b**) and urinary bladder stimulation (**b**) inhibited the neuron. This illustrates that viscera can differentially modulate dorsal horn neuronal activity in a complex pattern. *Source*: Reprinted from Ref. 54.

Because the dorsal horn neuron cannot distinguish the source of the afferent input, there is confusion as to the site of the initial stimulus contributing to poor localization. The consequences of these viscerovisceral interactions are more profound than that of the referred somatic pain. Viscerovisceral interactions can produce inflammation in normal visceral tissue (via the dorsal root reflex) and can increase pain originating in other viscera (e.g., endometriosis increases pain from ureteral stones) (57).

Referred Hyperalgesia Arising from Normal Somatic Tissue

As visceral afferent input increases over time, it sensitizes dorsal horn neurons inducing a state of hyperexcitability or central sensitization. At this point, convergent somatic input onto sensitized dorsal horn neurons evokes greater responses than normal. For example, the response to pinch increases and cells may start responding to innocuous somatic stimuli (Fig. 3D). In addition, the size of the somatic receptive field of individual dorsal horn neurons increases as normally subliminal input becomes capable of exciting the dorsal horn neuron (Fig. 3E). Ultimately, this is manifest as a decrease in the threshold to evoke a reflex response to thermal or mechanical stimuli applied within the area of referred pain: referred hyperalgesia (43).

MEASUREMENT OF EXPERIMENTAL VISCERAL PAIN AND HYPERALGESIA

In the GI tract, hollow organ distention occurs orad to an obstruction produced by a tumor or disease-induced motility disorders (e.g., ganglionic megacolon). In the genitourinary tract, distention of the ureter occurs during passage of a stone, resulting in severe abdominal pain. Hollow organ distention produced by a balloon placed in the lumen of an organ mimics these natural stimuli and is used to examine mechanisms underlying the processing of visceral pain. In addition, several compounds (e.g., mustard oil, capsaicin, turpentine, acid, and zymosan) injected into the lumen of hollow organs induce inflammation and increase the magnitude of the response to distention resulting in visceral hyperalgesia.

Visceromotor Response

The visceromotor response is a whole body motor reflex to an acute visceral stimulus (Fig. 5). During distention of a hollow organ, muscles of the abdomen, trunk, and limbs contract. The magnitude of the electromyogram recorded from these muscles is positively correlated with the stimulus intensity providing a readily quantifiable measure of the response to distention in an awake or lightly anesthetized animal. This visceromotor response is commonly used to study responses to distention or stimulation of hollow visceral organs including the colon (58–64), bladder (65), uterine–cervix/vagina (66–69), and ureter (70,71). Following inflammation, the magnitude of the visceromotor response increases: visceral hyperalgesia. Pharmacological (e.g., opioids or *N*-methyl-D-aspartate (NMDA) receptor antagonists) or surgical intervention that attenuates the perception of pain attenuates the magnitude of the visceromotor response, further supporting the validity of this end point as a measure of visceral pain and hyperalgesia.

Functional Anatomy

An anatomical correlate to the increase in the visceromotor response is an increase in Fos expression in the spinal cord. Fos is the protein product of the immediate-early gene *c-fos*. Constitutive expression of Fos is very low in the spinal cord, but noxious visceral stimulation of the colon, bladder, uterus, or ureter, (72–79) as well as innocuous visceral stimulation (78–80) induces spinal Fos expression. Fos is mostly expressed in the superficial and deep dorsal horn, and lamina X consistent with the termination of visceral afferent fibers and the location of visceroceptive dorsal horn neurons. Following inflammation of the colon (81,82), bladder (83–89) or ureter (90,91) Fos expression is further increased, suggesting an increase in neuronal activity due to inflammation that correlates with the increase in behavioral responses.

Because the viscera are dually innervated, noxious visceral stimulation-induced Fos expression in multiple segments of the spinal cord would be expected. This, however, is not the case. Repetitive hollow organ distention of the esophagus, stomach, or colon induces Fos expression in segments receiving vagal (esophagus and stomach) or pelvic (colon) afferents,

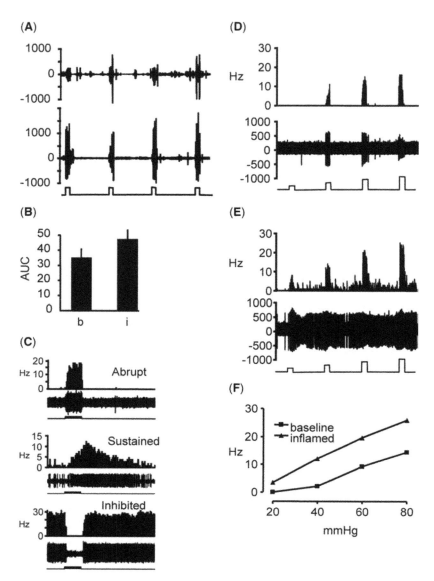

Figure 5 Visceral hyperalgesia and central sensitization. (**A**) Electromyogram (EMG) traces illustrating abdominal muscle contraction in response to noxious colorectal distention and visceral hyperalgesia (the visceromotor response). EMG electrodes were chronically implanted in the external oblique muscle. The top trace shows the baseline response to repeated colorectal distention as indicated in the bottom line. The middle trace shows the increase in response (hyperalgesia) following colonic inflammation by intrarectal injection of mustard oil. (**B**) The mean response from the four distentions in (**A**) quantifying the increase in the magnitude of the visceromotor response (b, baseline; i, inflamed). (**C**) Examples of the response of dorsal horn neurons to colorectal distention. Three types of responses are shown. In each case, the top panel is the peristimulus time histogram and the middle panel is a record of an extracellular recording. Colorectal distention is indicated by the black bar. Abrupt neurons are phase locked to the stimulus. Sustained neurons have a prolonged after discharge. Inhibited neurons have a high rate of spontaneous activity and are inhibited during distention. (**D, E, F**) The response of a dorsal horn neuron to graded intensities of colorectal distention before (**D**) and after (**E**) colonic inflammation with mustard oil. In (**D**) and (**E**), the top trace shows the rate histogram for the response of the neuron to graded intensities of colorectal distention (marked by bottom trace). The middle trace shows the microelectrode recording. (**F**) The stimulus response function showing the increase in the magnitude of the response at each distention pressure following colonic inflammation-central sensitization.

but not spinal splanchnic afferent input (77,92–94). Esophageal and gastric distention induce Fos expression in the nucleus of the solitary tract via vagal afferent input. Very little Fos is expressed in the thoracic spinal segments receiving splanchnic input. Likewise, CRD induces Fos in the lumbosacral spinal cord receiving pelvic nerve input, but very little in the thoracolumbar spinal

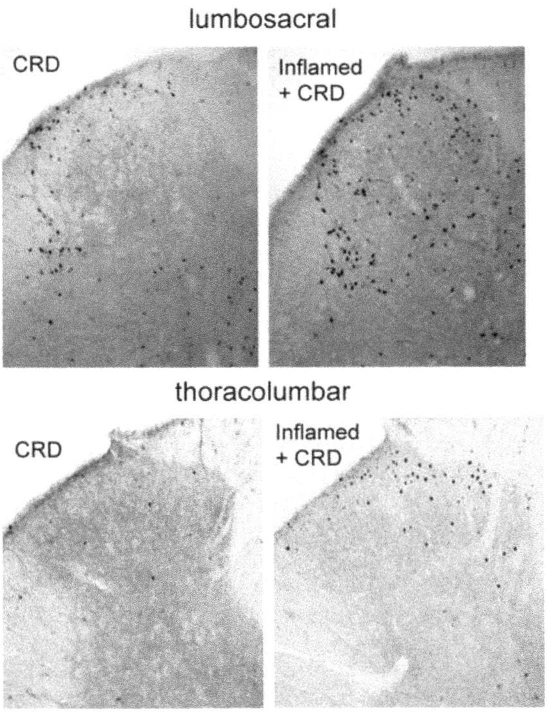

lumbosacral

thoracolumbar

Figure 6 Photomicrographs of CRD-induced Fos expression. In the lumbosacral spinal cord, Fos is induced by CRD and expression is upregulated following colonic inflammation. In contrast, there is little distention-induced Fos expression in the thoracolumbar spinal cord, but colonic inflammation induces Fos and expression is further increased following inflammation plus distention. *Abbreviation*: CRD, colorectal distention.

cord receiving splanchnic afferent input. However, following inflammation, Fos is upregulated in multiple regions of the spinal cord. For example, following colonic inflammation there is a significant increase in Fos expression in the thoracolumbar spinal cord as well as in the lumbosacral spinal cord (Fig. 6) (82). Because Fos expression is indicative of neuronal activity, the induction of Fos in the thoracolumbar spinal cord following colonic inflammation suggests that inflammation increases thoracolumbar spinal activity that is manifest as expansion of the area of referred pain and visceral hyperalgesia.

Physiology of Dorsal Horn Neurons Responding to Visceral Stimulation

Extracellular single unit recordings from neurons in the spinal dorsal horn indicate three general categories of responses (abrupt, sustained, inhibited) to stimulation of visceral organs. The organs studied include the esophagus (47,48,95), stomach (96), gall bladder (97,98), ureter (49,99), bladder (42,55,100) and descending colon/rectum (8,37–39,41,101–118) Although the terminology used to describe responses of these neurons to a distending stimulus differs, response profiles are fundamentally similar for all organs studied, suggesting some constant in the way the nervous system processes innocuous and noxious stimuli from the viscera.

The most extensively studied neurons are those that respond to distention of the colon and rectum. Abrupt neurons (also called short latency-abrupt, short lasting–abrupt) begin firing at the onset of the distention stimulus and cease firing at the cessation of the stimulus (Fig. 5C). Overall, the proportion of Abrupt neurons ranges from 40% to 75% of lumbosacral dorsal horn neurons that respond to CRD.

Sustained neurons (short latency–sustained, long-lasting excitatory) constitute 0% to 50% of visceroceptive dorsal horn neurons. These cells begin to discharge at the onset of the stimulus, but do not reach a peak discharge until 10 to 20 seconds after the start of the stimulus (the stimulus duration is 20 second). At the cessation of the distention, Sustained neurons maintain an after discharge that ranges from five to several hundred seconds (Fig. 5C). The large discrepancy in the relative proportion of these neurons, at least with respect to the colon, is due to the segmental location of recording in the dorsal horn. Sustained neurons constitute 30% to 50% of the visceroceptive dorsal horn neurons in the lumbosacral spinal cord, but less than 5% of the neurons in the thoracolumbar spinal cord of intact rats (117).

Neurons inhibited by a visceral stimulus form a third group of visceroceptive neurons. These neurons have a high rate of spontaneous activity that decreases during distention, generally in an intensity dependent manner (Fig. 5C). Inhibited neurons constitute up to 40% of the visceroceptive neuronal population, depending on the spinal segment of recording. In the thoracolumbar spinal cord for example, approximately 40% of the neurons that respond to CRD are inhibited while this value is closer to 10% in the lumbosacral spinal cord (116,117).

Additional response profiles to hollow organ distention have been described by various investigators. These additional types of neurons either have longer onset latencies or transiently increase or decrease firing at the cessation of the stimulus.

The role of these different types of neurons in the processing of hollow organ distention is uncertain. It was suggested that sustained neurons are better suited for signaling colorectal nociception because the response threshold is greater than that for Abrupt neurons (41). Furthermore, lidocaine, clonidine, morphine, and κ opioid receptor agonists are more potent against Sustained neurons than Abrupt neurons (119–121). Following colonic inflammation in male rats, the response of Sustained neurons increases, while the response of Abrupt neurons decreases (117,122). In contrast, the discharge pattern of Abrupt neurons is similar to the discharge pattern of colonic primary afferents and the visceromotor response. Furthermore, in female rats, estrogen replacement following ovariectomy increases colorectal sensitivity as measured by an increase in the magnitude of the visceromotor response. This is mirrored by an increase in the magnitude of the response of Abrupt neurons, but not in Sustained neurons (105,123). These data make a compelling argument for a role for both neuronal subtypes in processing colorectal pain and hyperalgesia and suggest that the relative contribution of each subtype is dependent on a number of factors.

The location of dorsal horn neurons responding to visceral stimulation can be marked by electrolytically lesioning the recording site with the microelectrode or injecting a marker dye through the electrode. Although either strategy lacks precision, it is possible to localize the recording site to the superficial dorsal horn or deeper lamina of the dorsal horn as well as its mediolateral location. Neurons that respond to visceral stimulation are located in the superficial dorsal horn, deep dorsal horn, and around the central canal in lamina X (8,41,47,95, 102,112). These locations correspond to sites of primary afferent termination and match the locations of Fos induced by visceral stimulation. There does not appear to be a correlation between the response to visceral stimulation and location in the dorsal horn as there is with respect to somatic stimuli. Abrupt and Sustained neurons responding to stimulation of different visceral tissues are intermixed in the superficial and deep lumbosacral dorsal horn.

Response of Visceroceptive Dorsal Horn Neurons to Inflammation

Visceroceptive dorsal horn neurons have heterogeneous responses to organ inflammation. In male rats, the response of Abrupt neurons to CRD increases in the thoracolumbar spinal cord, but decreases in the lumbosacral spinal cord. In contrast, the response of Sustained neurons in the lumbosacral spinal cord increases (there are only a few Sustained neurons in the thoracolumbar spinal cord) (42,115,117,124). Other investigators, however, report in comparable populations of lumbosacral neurons (Abrupt neurons), increasing responses following colonic inflammation in male (36) or female rats (125) or no change in the response of abrupt neurons following inflammation in intact female rats, but increasing responses following ovariectomy and subsequent estrogen replacement (123).

Viscerosomatic Inhibition

Patients with IBS or other disorders with visceral hypersensitivity report referred somatic hypersensitivity in the dermatomes where referred pain is perceived. However, outside the area of referred pain, as long as there is not a codiagnosis of another ailment such as fibromyalgia, patients report normal or hyposensitivity to noxious (electric and mechanical) somatic stimuli (4,126–131). In contrast, thermal stimulation is more painful in IBS patients compared to controls, although this cutaneous hypersensitivity decreases as the site of stimulation moves away from the region of referred pain (132). In healthy volunteers, slow ramp CRD inhibits the RIII nocifensive reflex in both the arm and leg although the fast ramp distention facilitates the reflex in the leg (133). These data suggest that acute or chronic colorectal pain can modulate somatic sensitivity to noxious stimuli.

Viscerosomatic inhibition (also called nocigenic inhibition or counterirritation) can be modeled in animal studies. Pelvic nerve stimulation in the rat inhibits the withdrawal response to noxious pinch of the foot (134). Noxious stimulation of the colon or urinary bladder inhibits populations of dorsal horn neurons in the cervical and upper thoracic spinal segments that respond to thoracic somatic and/or visceral stimuli (135–137). Additionally, CRD inhibits the response of dorsal horn neurons in the lumbar spinal cord to thermal stimulation of the hindpaw (136) and inhibits the tail flick reflex in lightly anesthetized rats (138). Colonic inflammation also inhibits paw withdrawal from noxious thermal stimuli (139,140). These studies suggest that noxious stimulation of pelvic viscera can inhibit sensory neuron processing of somatic stimuli and somatic reflexes evoked outside the presumptive region of referred pain comparable to the somatic hyposensitivity in IBS patients.

PHARMACOLOGY OF SPINAL PROCESSING OF VISCERAL PAIN
Excitatory Amino Acid Receptors and Visceral Pain

It is generally accepted that the excitatory amino acid α-amino-3-hydroxy-5-methylisoxazole-4-propionic acid (AMPA) receptors, but not NMDA receptors, are involved in signaling acute noxious and innocuous somatic stimuli in the spinal cord. Following persistent noxious stimulation (inflammation following injury and neuropathic injury), a cascade of events including activation of signal transduction pathways, protein kinases and phosphatases, and NMDA receptor activation induce central sensitization and hyperalgesia (141,142).

In contrast to somatic stimuli, experimental data support a role for NMDA receptor activity in addition to AMPA receptor activity in spinal processing of acute innocuous and noxious visceral stimuli. NMDA receptor antagonists attenuate the pressor response evoked by noxious ureter distention, but have no effect on the pressor response evoked by noxious somatic stimulation (143). Likewise, NMDA receptor antagonists attenuate changes in mean arterial pressure and the visceromotor response to urinary bladder distention (65) and behavioral responses to vaginal–cervical stimulation (144). The visceromotor response evoked by transient noxious and innocuous CRD is attenuated by NMDA receptor antagonists (38,64, 79,145). Interestingly, the dose of the NMDA receptor antagonist DL-2-amino-5-phosphono-pentanoic acid that produces approximately 50% attenuation of the visceromotor response to noxious CRD completely attenuates acquisition of avoidance behavior to the same stimulus (64).

Intrathecal administration of the agonist NMDA, at doses that do not evoke caudally directed biting and scratching behavior (an indication of spontaneous pain), facilitates neuronal and behavioral responses to noxious CRD (108,109). However, the response to innocuous colonic stimuli is not affected.

At the cellular level, noxious and innocuous CRD-induced Fos expression in dorsal horn neurons is attenuated by the NMDA receptor antagonist, MK-801 (64,79). The efficacy of MK-801 is greater for noxious stimuli compared to that of innocuous stimuli (79), but NMDA receptor antagonists attenuate dorsal horn neuronal responses to noxious and innocuous CRD with equal efficacy (38). Additionally, the antinociceptive effect of NMDA receptor antagonists is similar for Abrupt and Sustained neurons. Likewise, NMDA receptor antagonists attenuate neuronal responses to acute bladder distention (146) in the rat and CRD in the cat (143,147).

Antagonists that act at the AMPA glutamate receptor also attenuate neuronal responses to CRD (39,101,110,147). However, when different populations of neurons are examined, a greater proportion of Sustained neurons are modulated compared to Abrupt neurons, although the magnitude of the attenuation is greater in the Abrupt neurons (39).

Following injury, visceral tissue, like somatic tissue, becomes inflamed. In addition, disease states, with or without inflammation, produce visceral hyperalgesia (i.e., IBS) (4). Under these conditions, spinal processing of visceral stimuli is similar to somatic stimuli. Like somatic hyperalgesia, visceral hyperalgesia is also NMDA and AMPA receptor mediated. NMDA and AMPA receptor antagonists attenuate visceromotor responses evoked by stimulation of the inflamed colon (148–150). In models of bladder irritation or inflammation, NMDA receptor antagonists attenuate Fos expression (151,152) and behavioral responses (153,154) and inflammation-induced pancreatic hyperalgesia is attenuated by NMDA receptor antagonists (155,156).

Several signal transduction pathways contribute to central sensitization and hyperalgesia. The study of the role of these mechanisms in modulating visceral pain lags behind that for somatic pain. Nevertheless, these mechanisms are starting to be examined. Src, a member of the Src-family of nonreceptor tyrosine kinases, phophorylates the NMDA receptor to increase activity. Inhibition of Src attenuates inflammatory somatic pain (157,158). Preliminary studies indicate Src inhibitors attenuate colonic hyperalgesia, but not acute visceral pain (unpublished observations). Activation of the mitogen-activated protein kinase pathway, downstream from NMDA receptor activation, also mediates visceral hyperalgesia. Colonic inflammation induces spinal extracellular signaling–related kinase-1 and -2 (ERK1/2) activation (159). Inhibition of ERK1/2 activation by a MEK inhibitor attenuates referred hyperalgesia, supporting a role for ERK activation in visceral pain.

Even though acute visceral stimuli are considered transient, visceral stimuli do last for seconds or tens of seconds. Noxious stimuli might then produce sufficient afferent input to activate NMDA receptors, perhaps initiating a mild form of central sensitization without significant tissue injury. Indeed, repetitive innocuous CRD induces Fos expression in the spinal cord (78), which is attenuated by NMDA receptor antagonists (79), suggesting induction of spinal plasticity.

Clinically, NMDA receptor antagonists attenuate acute and inflammatory esophageal pain (160,161) but are less effective as analgesics to somatic pain, supporting the experimental animal data. In contrast, NMDA receptor antagonists failed to attenuate pain from gastric distention (162,163), but did decrease adverse sensations from nonpainful gastric distention.

Neurokinin Receptors

Substance P is expressed in a greater percentage of visceral afferent fibers than somatic afferent fibers (164). This suggests that tachykinins may contribute to viscerosensory processing. Inflammation of the colon or bladder increases neurokinin-1 (NK1) receptor expression in the gut wall, colonic afferent fibers, and spinal dorsal horn neurons (165,166) and concomitantly decreases substance P expression in primary afferents (11). NK1 receptor internalization in spinal dorsal horn neurons increases following CRD of the normal and inflamed colon (167). However, parasitic gastric inflammation decreases NK1 receptor expression in the spinal cord, and increases substance P expression in dorsal root ganglia (168).

Consistent with an upregulation of NK1 receptor activity, spinal administration of NK1 receptor antagonists generally attenuate the visceromotor response evoked from distention of the inflamed colon (169–171) or in acutely stressed rats (172) and visceral hyperalgesia is attenuated in NK1 receptor knockout mice (173). Likewise, spinally administered NK3 receptor antagonists attenuate the visceromotor response (171,174).

In contrast to a decidedly spinal site of action, peripherally, but not spinally administered NK2 receptor antagonists attenuate the visceromotor response to CRD (40,171,175).

Opioids

Opioids constitute a major class of analgesic to treat visceral pain. Experimentally, within the types of pain discussed in this chapter, studies have focused on two sites of action for opioids, the periphery and the spinal cord. Systemic administration of μ or κ opioid receptor agonists attenuates responses to noxious stimulation of the colon, bladder, and uterine–cervix. Administration of naloxone methiodide, which does not cross the blood–brain barrier, indicates separate sites of action for μ and κ agonists. Systemic morphine attenuates the visceromotor response evoked by CRD of the inflamed and noninflamed colon (59,62,176–178), bladder (179,180), uterine–cervix distention (69,181,182), ureter (183) and stomach (184) as well as referred pain from colonic inflammation (43). Systemically administered μ and κ opioid receptor agonists attenuate Fos expression, dorsal horn neuronel activity, and the visceromotor response evoked by colorectal distention in rats and mice (110,185-187,191). Both peripheral and spinal sites of action are indicated for μ agonists. However, a peripheral site of action is controversial since activity in decentralized pelvic nerve primary afferents was not attenuated by systemic morphine (186,188) but the effects of systemic morphine on the CRD-evoked visceromotor response was dose-dependently reversed by naloxone methiodide and the peripherally acting μ opioid agonist loperamide attenuated the visceromotor response (191). Conversely, intrathecal administration of morphine dose-dependently attenuated the visceromotor response evoked by CRD (189–191) and the response of dorsal horn neurons to CRD was attenuated by intraspinal administration of morphine (101). Intrathecal morphine attenuates cyclophosphamide-induced interstitial cystitis (21). Of particular note is that morphine directed at the L1-L2 and L6-S1 spinal segments had an additive effect, suggesting pain from bladder inflammation is processed in multiple regions of the spinal cord.

In contrast to a spinal site of action for morphine and other μ and delta opioid agonists, κ agonists have a peripheral site of action. Systemic, but not intrathecal, κ agonists attenuate visceral pain (190,192,193) and κ agonists attenuate pelvic nerve responses to CRD (188,194).

These findings support the hypothesis that IBS patients may have an altered central release of endogenous opioids in response to visceral stimulation (195,196). The μ opioid receptor agonist fentanyl dose-dependently increased perception thresholds to colon distension in both healthy control subjects and IBS patients with a greater relative efficacy in IBS patients than in normal subjects.

GONADAL HORMONE MODULATION OF VISCERAL PAIN

The preponderance of evidence suggests that females are more sensitive to pain than males and several chronic pain syndromes including IBS, fibromyalgia, and temporomandibular disorders are more prevalent in women than in men (197–199). Furthermore, nociceptive thresholds are lowest and pain responses highest during periods of elevated estrogen (199–204), strongly suggesting that sex hormones modulate pain sensation.

Several labs have demonstrated that gonadal hormones modulate behavioral responses to noxious visceral stimuli and there is a large body of evidence that estrogen increases nociceptive sensitivity. From most studies it cannot be determined where the gonadal hormones are exerting their influence, be it peripherally or centrally, and a full discussion of this topic is beyond the scope of this chapter. There are, however, a few studies indicating hormonally mediated nociceptive plasticity is spinally mediated. Dorsal horn neurons express estrogen receptors (ERs) (205–207), providing an anatomical framework for estrogen modulation of viscerosensory processing at the level of the dorsal horn. Additionally, the cytostolic estrogen receptor (ER) concentration in the spinal cord is positively correlated with the serum estrogen concentration (208), further suggesting that estrogen can increase nociceptive sensitivity by modulating activity in dorsal horn neurons. Indeed, it was recently demonstrated that spinal aromatase converts testosterone to estrogen and increases sensitivity to noxious somatic stimuli (209). CRD induces Fos expression in spinal neurons that coexpress ER (unpublished observations) and the threshold for the visceromotor response to CRD is lowest when estrogen levels peak during proestrus (210,211). In complementary studies, ovariectomy decreased behavioral and dorsal horn neuronal responses to CRD. These responses were restored to levels observed in intact female rats by estrogen replacement, suggesting estrogen is pronociceptive (105). This estrogen-induced hypersensitivity may be partially mediated by increased activity at NMDA receptors. ER α colocalizes with the NMDA receptor in dorsal horn neurons (unpublished) and estrogen decreases the potency of NMDA receptor antagonists in attenuating the visceromotor response to CRD (150).

Estrogen also contributes to sex differences in opioid analgesia. Systemic morphine attenuates the CRD-evoked visceromotor response in male rats with a greater potency than in intact female rats (191). In the female rat, this sex difference correlates with the plasma estrogen concentration because ovariectomy increases the potency and subsequent estrogen replacement decreases the potency (Ji et al., submitted). In addition, estrogen decreases the potency of morphine in attenuating reflex responses to uterine–cervix distention although estrogen does not modulate the response itself (181,182).

CONCLUSIONS AND A HYPOTHESIS

Clearly, peripheral and spinal processing mediates visceral pain and hyperalgesia. But, what is the evidence that central sensitization and the dual innervation of the internal organs contribute to spinal processing of visceral pain? Healthy volunteers report that the area of referred pain and the magnitude of the pain sensation increase following repetitive CRD (34). In experimental animals, repetitive CRD does not sensitize colonic primary afferents (212), yet there is an initial sensitization of the visceromotor response (62), and an upregulation of Fos expression in the absence of colonic inflammation (78), suggesting repetitive visceral afferent activity evokes central changes. More importantly, somatic primary afferents are not injured, even during colonic inflammation. Therefore, any change in the response of dorsal horn neurons to somatic stimulation must be due to central sensitization.

What is the role of the dual innervation? IBS patients report increased colorectal sensitivity and referred pain expanding into thoracic dermatomes innervated by splanchnic spinal nerves suggesting segments receiving this dual afferent input differentially contribute to spinal processing of visceral pain. Likewise, animal studies show differential activation of spinal segments receiving hypogastric/lumbar splanchnic and pelvic nerve afferent input (10). Data from our lab suggest that the pelvic nerve inhibits the thoracolumbar spinal cord processing of colorectal input (116). Thoracolumbar dorsal horn neurons are thus less responsive to CRD than lumbosacral neurons, and a significantly greater percentage are inhibited by CRD. Colonic inflammation induces central sensitization, increasing spinal dorsal horn neuron excitability, and reducing inhibition of thoracolumbar visceroceptive neurons. Similarly, if the pelvic nerve is cut, there is an increase in the excitability and a decrease in inhibition of thoracolumbar visceroceptive neurons. These data point to complex modulation of the spinal processing of visceral input with pelvic nerve afferent input inhibiting or dampening spinal processing of lumbar splanchnic nerve afferent input to the thoracolumbar spinal cord (213). This likely functions to reduce the overall level of spinal excitability to acute colorectal stimuli. Colonic inflammation can override this inhibitory process. It is possible then, that this inhibitory circuit is attenuated in patients with functional bowel disorders, leading to increased spinal excitability and visceral hyperalgesia.

REFERENCES

1. Cervero F, Laird JM. Visceral pain. Lancet 1999; 353:2145–2148.
2. Giamberardino MA. Visceral hyperalgesia. In: Devor M, Rowbotham MC, Wiesenfeld-Hallin Z, eds. Proceedings of the 9th World Congress on Pain. Seattle: IASP Press, 2000:523–550.
3. Bonica JJ. The Management of Pain. 2nd ed. Philadelphia: Lea & Febiger, 1990.
4. Ritchie J. Pain from distention of the pelvic colon by inflating a balloon in the irritable colon syndrome. Gut 1973; 14:125–132.
5. Al-Chaer ED, Kawasaki M, Pasricha PJ. A new model of chronic visceral hypersensitivity in adult rats induced by colon irritation during postnatal development. Gastroenterology 2000; 119:1276–1285.
6. Coutinho SV, Plotsky PM, Sablad M, et al. Neonatal maternal separation alters stress-induced responses to viscerosomatic nociceptive stimuli in rat. Am J Physiol Gastrointest Liver Physiol 2002; 282:G307–G316.
7. Berkley KJ, Robbins A, Sato Y. Afferent fibers supplying the uterus in the rat. J Neurophysiol 1988; 59:142–163.
8. Ness TJ, Gebhart GF. Characterization of neurons responsive to noxious colorectal distention in the T13-L2 spinal cord of the rat. J Neurophysiol 1988; 60:1419–1438.
9. Steinman JL, Carlton SM, Willis WD. The segmental distribution of afferent fibers from the vaginal cervix and hypogastric nerve in rats. Brain Res 1992; 575:25–31.
10. Traub RJ. Evidence for thoracolumbar spinal cord processing of inflammatory, but not acute colonic pain. Neuroreport 2000; 11:2113–2116.
11. Traub RJ, Hutchcroft K, Gebhart GF. The peptide content of colonic afferents decreases following colonic inflammation. Peptides 1999; 20:267–273.
12. Vera PL, Nadelhaft I. Afferent and sympathetic innervation of the dome and the base of the urinary bladder of the female rat. Brain Res Bull 1992; 29:651–658.
13. Baron R, Janig W. Afferent and sympathetic neurons projecting into lumbar visceral nerves of the male rat. J Comp Neurol 1991; 314:429–436.
14. Christianson JA, Traub RJ, Davis BM. Differences in spinal distribution and neurochemical phenotype of colonic afferents in mouse and rat. J Comp Neurol 2005; 494: 246–259.
15. Dutsch M, Eichhorn U, Worl J, et al. Vagal and spinal afferent innervation of the rat esophagus: a combined retrograde tracing and immunocytochemical study with special emphasis on calcium-binding proteins. J Comp Neurol 1998; 398:289–307.
16. Blackshaw LA, Gebhart GF. The pharmacology of gastrointestinal nociceptive pathways. Curr Opin Pharmacol 2002; 2:642–649.
17. Malliani A, Lombardi F, Pagani M. Sensory innervation of the heart. In: Cervero F, Morrison JFB, eds. Visceral Sensation. Progress in Brain Research. Amsterdam: Elsevier, 1986:39–48.
18. Andersson KE. Bladder activation: afferent mechanisms. Urology 2002; 59:43–50.
19. Berkley KJ, Robbins A, Sato Y. Functional differences between afferent fibers in the hypogastric and pelvic nerves innervating female reproductive organs in the rat. J Neurophysiol 1993; 69:533–544.
20. Kawatani M, Takeshige C, De Groat WC. Central distribution of afferent pathways from the uterus of the cat. J Comp Neurol 1990; 302:294–304.
21. Meen M, Coudore-Civiale MA, Eschalier A, et al. Involvement of hypogastric and pelvic nerves for conveying cystitis induced nociception in conscious rats. J Urol 2001; 166:318–322.

22. Sugiura Y, Terui N, Hosoya Y. Difference in distribution of central terminals between visceral and somatic unmyelinated (C) primary afferent fibers. J Neurophysiol 1989; 62:834–840.
23. Brown AG. Organization in the spinal cord. Berlin: Springer-Verlag, 1981.
24. Light AR, Perl ER. Spinal termination of functionally identified primary afferent neurons with slowly conducting myelinated fibers. J Comp Neurol 1979; 186:133–150.
25. Sugiura Y, Terui N, Hosoya Y, et al. Quantitative analysis of central terminal projections of visceral and somatic unmyelinated (C) primary afferent fibers in the guinea pig. J Comp Neurol 1993; 332: 315–325.
26. Sugiura Y, Lee CL, Perl ER. Central projections of identified, unmyelinated (C) afferent fibers innervating mammalian skin. Science 1986; 234:358–361.
27. Light AR, Perl ER. Reexamination of the dorsal root projection to the spinal dorsal horn including observations on the differential termination of coarse and fine fibers. J Comp Neurol 1979; 186: 117–131.
28. Swett JE, Woolf CJ. The somatotopic organization of primary afferent terminals in the superficial laminae of the dorsal horn of the rat spinal cord. J Comp Neurol 1985; 231:66–77.
29. Cervero F, Connell LA. Distribution of somatic and visceral primary afferent fibres within the thoracic spinal cord of the cat. J Comp Neurol 1984; 230:88–98.
30. Morgan C, Nadelhaft I, De Groat WC. The distribution of visceral primary afferents from the pelvic nerve to Lissauer's tract and the spinal gray matter and its relationship to the sacral parasympathetic nucleus. J Comp Neurol 1981; 201:415–440.
31. Nadelhaft I, Roppolo J, Morgan C, et al. Parasympathetic preganglionic neurons and visceral primary afferents in monkey sacral spinal cord revealed following application of horseradish peroxidase to pelvic nerve. J Comp Neurol 1983; 216:36–52.
32. Nadelhaft I, Booth AM. The location and morphology of preganglionic neurons and the distribution of visceral afferents from the rat pelvic nerve: a horseradish peroxidase study. J Comp Neurol 1984; 226:238–245.
33. Ruch TC. Visceral sensation and referred pain. In: Fulton JF, ed. Howell's Textbook of Physiology. Philadelphia: WB Saunders, 1946:385–401.
34. Ness TJ, Metcalf AM, Gebhart GF. A psychophysiological study in humans using phasic colonic distention as a noxious visceral stimulus. Pain 1990; 43:377–386.
35. Bernstein CN, Niazi N, Robert M, et al. Rectal afferent function in patients with inflammatory and functional intestinal disorders. Pain 1996; 66:151–161.
36. Al-Chaer ED, Westlund KN, Willis WD. Sensitization of postsynaptic dorsal column neuronal responses by colon inflammation. Neuroreport 1997; 8:3267–3273.
37. Berkley KJ, Hubscher CH, Wall PD. Neuronal responses to stimulation of the cervix, uterus, colon, and skin in the rat spinal cord. J Neurophysiol 1993; 69:545–556.
38. Ji Y, Traub RJ. Spinal NMDA receptors contribute to neuronal processing of acute noxious and non-noxious colorectal stimulation in the rat. J Neurophysiol 2001; 86:1783–1791.
39. Ji Y, Traub RJ. Differential effects of spinal CNQX on two populations of dorsal horn neurons responding to colorectal distention in the rat. Pain 2002; 99:217–222.
40. Laird JM, Olivar T, JA, et al. Responses of rat spinal neurons to distension of inflamed colon: role of tachykinin NK2 receptors. Neuropharmacology 2001; 40:696–701.
41. Ness TJ, Gebhart GF. Characterization of neuronal responses to noxious visceral and somatic stimuli in the medial lumbosacral spinal cord of the rat. J Neurophysiol 1987; 57:1867–1892.
42. Ness TJ, Castroman P. Evidence for two populations of rat spinal dorsal horn neurons excited by urinary bladder distension. Brain Res 2001; 923:147–156.
43. Laird JM, Martinez-Caro L, Garcia-Nicas E, et al. A new model of visceral pain and referred hyperalgesia in the mouse. Pain 2001; 92:335–342.
44. Ammons WS, Girardot MN, Foreman RD. T2-T5 spinothalamic neurons projecting to medial thalamus with viscerosomatic input. J Neurophysiol 1985; 54:73–89.
45. Blair RW, Weber RN, Foreman RD. Characteristics of primate spinothalamic tract neurons receiving viscerosomatic convergent inputs in T3-T5 segments. J Neurophysiol 1981; 46:797–811.
46. Cervero F, Laird JM, Pozo MA. Selective changes of receptive field properties of spinal nociceptive neurones induced by noxious visceral stimulation in the cat. Pain 1992; 51:335–342.
47. Euchner-Wamser I, Sengupta JN, Gebhart GF, et al. Characterization of responses of T2-T4 spinal cord neurons to esophageal distension in the rat. J Neurophysiol 1993; 69:868–883.
48. Qin C, Chandler MJ, Foreman RD. Esophagocardiac convergence onto thoracic spinal neurons: comparison of cervical and thoracic esophagus. Brain Res 2004; 1008:193–197.
49. Roza C, Laird JM, Cervero F. Spinal mechanisms underlying persistent pain and referred hyperalgesia in rats with an experimental ureteric stone. J Neurophysiol 1998; 79:1603–1612.
50. Wesselmann U, Lai J. Mechanisms of referred visceral pain: uterine inflammation in the adult virgin rat results in neurogenic plasma extravasation in the skin. Pain 1997; 73:309–317.
51. Sluka KA, Rees H, Westlund KN, et al. Fiber types contributing to dorsal root reflexes induced by joint inflammation in cats and monkeys. J Neurophysiol 1995; 74:981–989.
52. Berkley KJ, Guilbaud G, Benoist JM, et al. Responses of neurons in and near the thalamic ventrobasal complex of the rat to stimulation of uterus, cervix, vagina, colon, and skin. J Neurophysiol 1993; 69:557–568.

53. Brennan TJ, Oh UT, Hobbs SF, et al. Urinary bladder and hindlimb afferent input inhibits activity of primate T2-T5 spinothalamic tract neurons. J Neurophysiol 1989; 61:573–588.

54. Hobbs SF, Chandler MJ, Bolser DC, et al. Segmental organization of visceral and somatic input onto C3-T6 spinothalamic tract cells of the monkey. J Neurophysiol 1992; 68:1575–1588.

55. Qin C, Foreman RD. Viscerovisceral convergence of urinary bladder and colorectal inputs to lumbosacral spinal neurons in rats. Neuroreport 2004; 15:467–471.

56. Ness TJ, Gebhart GF. Visceral pain: a review of experimental studies. Pain 1990; 41:167–234.

57. Giamberardino MA, Berkley KJ, Affaitati G, et al. Influence of endometriosis on pain behaviors and muscle hyperalgesia induced by a ureteral calculosis in female rats. Pain 2002; 95:247–257.

58. Gschossmann JM, Adam B, Liebregts T, et al. Effect of transient chemically induced colitis on the visceromotor response to mechanical colorectal distension. Eur J Gastroenterol Hepatol 2002; 14:1067–1072.

59. Kamp EH, Jones RC III, Tillman SR, et al. Quantitative assessment and characterization of visceral nociception and hyperalgesia in mice. Am J Physiol Gastrointest Liver Physiol 2003; 284: G434–G444.

60. Morteau O, Hachet T, Caussette M, et al. Experimental colitis alters visceromotor response to colorectal distension in awake rats. Dig Dis Sci 1994; 39:1239–1248.

61. Morteau O, Julia V, Eeckhout C, et al. Influence of 5-HT3 receptor antagonists in visceromotor and nociceptive responses to rectal distension before and during experimental colitis in rats. Fundam Clin Pharmacol 1994; 8:553–562.

62. Ness TJ, Gebhart GF. Colorectal distention as a noxious visceral stimulus: physiologic and pharmacologic characterization of pseudoaffective responses in the rat. Brain Res 1988; 450:153–169.

63. Palecek J, Willis WD. The dorsal column pathway facilitates visceromotor responses to colorectal distention after colon inflammation in rats. Pain 2003; 104:501–507.

64. Traub RJ, Zhai QZ, Ji Y, et al. NMDA receptor antagonists attenuate noxious and nonnoxious colorectal distention-induced Fos expression and the visceromotor reflex. Neurosci 2002; 113: 205–211.

65. Castroman PJ, Ness TJ. Ketamine, an *N*-methyl-d-aspartate receptor antagonist, inhibits the reflex responses to distension of the rat urinary bladder. Anesthesiology 2002; 96:1401–1409.

66. Berkley KJ, Wood E, Scofield SL, et al. Behavioral responses to uterine or vaginal distension in the rat. Pain 1995; 61:121–131.

67. Cason AM, Samuelsen CL, Berkley KJ. Estrous changes in vaginal nociception in a rat model of endometriosis. Horm Behav 2003; 44:123–131.

68. Du D, Eisenach JC, Ririe DG, et al. The antinociceptive effects of spinal cyclooxygenase inhibitors on uterine cervical distension. Brain Res 2004; 1024:130–136.

69. Sandner-Kiesling A, Eisenach JC. Pharmacology of opioid inhibition to noxious uterine cervical distension. Anesthesiology 2002; 97:966–971.

70. Giamberardino MA, Valente R, de Bigontina P, et al. Artificial ureteral calculosis in rats: behavioural characterization of visceral pain episodes and their relationship with referred lumbar muscle hyperalgesia. Pain 1995; 61:459–469.

71. Giamberardino MA, Affaitati G, Valente R, et al. Changes in visceral pain reactivity as a function of estrous cycle in female rats with artificial ureteral calculosis. Brain Res 1997; 774:234–238.

72. Chinapen S, Swann JM, Steinman JL, et al. Expression of c-fos protein in lumbosacral spinal cord in response to vaginocervical stimulation in rats. Neurosci Lett 1992; 145:93–96.

73. Fitch GK, Patel KP, Weiss ML. Increased renal interstitial hydrostatic pressure causes c-fos expression in the rat's spinal cord dorsal horn. Brain Res 1997; 753:340–347.

74. Lanteri-Minet M, Isnardon P, De Pommery J, et al. Spinal and hindbrain structures involved in visceroception and visceronociception as revealed by the expression of Fos, Jun and Krox-24 proteins. Neuroscience 1993; 55:737–753.

75. Palecek J, Paleckova V, Willis WD. Fos expression in spinothalamic and postsynaptic dorsal column neurons following noxious visceral and cutaneous stimuli. Pain 2003; 104:249–257.

76. Tong C, Ma W, Shin SW, et al. Uterine cervical distension induces cFos expression in deep dorsal horn neurons of the rat spinal cord. Anesthesiology 2003; 99:205–211.

77. Traub RJ, Herdegen T, Gebhart GF. Differential expression of c-Fos and c-Jun in two regions of the rat spinal cord following noxious colorectal distention. Neurosci Lett 1993; 160:121–125.

78. Traub RJ, Pechman P, Iadarola MJ, et al. Fos-like proteins in the lumbosacral spinal cord following noxious and non-noxious colorectal distention in the rat. Pain 1992; 49:393–403.

79. Zhai QZ, Traub RJ. The NMDA receptor antagonist MK-801 attenuates c-Fos expression in the lumbosacral spinal cord following repetitive noxious and nonnoxious colorectal distention. Pain 1999; 83:321–329.

80. Birder LA, De Groat WC. Induction of c-fos expression in spinal neurons by nociceptive and nonnociceptive stimulation of LUT. Am J Physiol 1993; 265:R326–R333.

81. Miampamba M, Sharkey KA. c-Fos expression in the myenteric plexus, spinal cord and brainstem following injection of formalin in the rat colonic wall. J Auton Nerv Syst 1999; 77:140–151.

82. Traub RJ, Murphy AZ. Colonic inflammation induces Fos expression in the thoracolumbar spinal cord increasing activity in the spinoparabrachial pathway. Pain 2002; 95:93–102.

83. Birder LA, De Groat WC. Increased c-fos expression in spinal neurons after irritation of the lower urinary tract in the rat. J Neurosci 1992; 12:4878–4889.
84. Callsen-Cencic P, Mense S. Increased spinal expression of c-Fos following stimulation of the lower urinary tract in chronic spinal cord-injured rats. Histochem Cell Biol 1999; 112:63–72.
85. Cruz F, Avelino A, Coimbra A. Desensitization follows excitation of bladder primary afferents by intravesical capsaicin, as shown by c-fos activation in the rat spinal cord. Pain 1996; 64:553–557.
86. Dinis P, Charrua A, Avelino A, et al. Intravesical resiniferatoxin decreases spinal c-fos expression and increases bladder volume to reflex micturition in rats with chronic inflamed urinary bladders. BJU Int 2004; 94:153–157.
87. Ding YQ, Qin BZ, Li JS, et al. Induction of c-fos-like protein in the spinoparabrachial tract-neurons locating within the sacral parasympathetic nucleus in the rat. Brain Res 1994; 659:283–286.
88. Lanteri-Minet M, Bon K, De Pommery J, et al. Cyclophosphamide cystitis as a model of visceral pain in rats: model elaboration and spinal structures involved as revealed by the expression of c-Fos and Krox-24 proteins. Exp Brain Res 1995; 105:220–232.
89. Vizzard MA. Alterations in spinal cord Fos protein expression induced by bladder stimulation following cystitis. Am J Physiol Regul Integr Comp Physiol 2000; 278:R1027–R1039.
90. Aloisi A, Ceccarelli I, Affaitati G, et al. c-Fos expression in the spinal cord of female rats with artificial ureteric calculosis. Neurosci Lett 2004; 361:212–215.
91. Avelino A, Cruz F, Coimbra A. Sites of renal pain processing in the rat spinal cord. A c-fos study using a percutaneous method to perform ureteral obstruction. J Auton Nerv Syst 1997; 67:60–66.
92. Martinez V, Wang L, Mayer E, et al. Proximal colon distention increases Fos expression in the lumbosacral spinal cord and activates sacral parasympathetic NADPHd-positive neurons in rats. J Comp Neurol 1998; 390:311–321.
93. Traub RJ, Lim F, Sengupta J, et al. Differential c-Fos staining of second order neurons in the spinal cord and NTS receiving "sympathetic" and "parasympathetic" afferent input from viscera in the rat. Neurosci Lett 1994; 180:71–75.
94. Traub RJ, Sengupta JN, Gebhart GF. Differential c-fos expression in the nucleus of the solitary tract and spinal cord following noxious gastric distention in the rat. Neuroscience 1996; 74:873–884.
95. Qin C, Chandler MJ, Jou CJ, et al. Responses and afferent pathways of C1-C2 spinal neurons to cervical and thoracic esophageal stimulation in rats. J Neurophysiol 2004; 91:2227–2235.
96. Qin C, Chandler MJ, Miller KE, et al. Responses and afferent pathways of C(1)-C(2) spinal neurons to gastric distention in rats. Auton Neurosci 2003; 104:128–136.
97. Ammons WS, Blair RW, Foreman RD. Responses of primate T1-T5 spinothalamic neurons to gallbladder distension. Am J Physiol 1984; 247:R995–R1002.
98. Cervero F. Noxious intensities of visceral stimulation are required to activate viscerosomatic multireceptive neurons in the thoracic spinal cord of the cat. Brain Res 1982; 240:350–352.
99. Laird JM, Roza C, Cervero F. Spinal dorsal horn neurons responding to noxious distension of the ureter in anesthetized rats. J Neurophysiol 1996; 76:3239–3248.
100. Hobbs SF, Oh UT, Brennan TJ, et al. Urinary bladder and hindlimb stimuli inhibit T1-T6 spinal and spinoreticular cells. Am J Physiol 1990; 258:R10–R20.
101. Al-Chaer ED, Lawand NB, Westlund KN, et al. Pelvic visceral input into the nucleus gracilis is largely mediated by the postsynaptic dorsal column pathway. J Neurophysiol 1996; 76:2675–2690.
102. Al-Chaer ED, Lawand NB, Westlund KN, et al. Visceral nociceptive input into the ventral posterolateral nucleus of the thalamus: a new function for the dorsal column pathway. J Neurophysiol 1996; 76:2661–2674.
103. Bernard JF, Huang GF, Besson JM. The parabrachial area: electrophysiological evidence for an involvement in visceral nociceptive processes. J Neurophysiol 1994; 71:1646–1660.
104. Greenwood-Van Meerveld B, Johnson AC, Foreman RD, et al. Attenuation by spinal cord stimulation of a nociceptive reflex generated by colorectal distention in a rat model. Auton Neurosci 2003; 104:17–24.
105. Ji Y, Murphy AZ, Traub RJ. Estrogen modulates the visceromotor reflex and responses of spinal dorsal horn neurons to colorectal stimulation in the rat. J Neurosci 2003; 23:3908–3915.
106. Katter JT, Dado RJ, Kostarczyk E, et al. Spinothalamic and spinohypothalamic tract neurons in the sacral spinal cord of rats. II. Responses to cutaneous and visceral stimuli. J Neurophysiol 1996; 75:2606–2628.
107. Kawasaki M, Al Chaer ED. Intradermal capsaicin inhibits lumbar dorsal horn neuronal responses to colorectal distention. Neuroreport 2003; 14:985–989.
108. Kolhekar R, Gebhart GF. Modulation of spinal visceral nociceptive transmission by NMDA receptor activation in the rat. J Neurophysiol 1996; 75:2344–2353.
109. Kolhekar R, Gebhart GF. NMDA and quisqualate modulation of visceral nociception in the rat. Brain Res 1994; 651:215–226.
110. Kozlowski CM, Bountra C, Grundy D. The effect of fentanyl, DNQX and MK-801 on dorsal horn neurones responsive to colorectal distension in the anaesthetized rat. Neurogastroenterol Motil 2000; 12:239–247.
111. Miranda A, Peles S, Rudolph C, et al. Altered visceral sensation in response to somatic pain in the rat. Gastroenterology 2004; 126:1082–1089.

112. Ness TJ, Gebhart GF. Characterization of superficial T13-L2 dorsal horn neurons encoding for colorectal distention in the rat: comparison with neurons in deep laminae. Brain Res 1989; 486: 301–309.
113. Peles S, Miranda A, Shaker R, et al. Acute nociceptive somatic stimulus sensitizes neurons in the spinal cord to colonic distension in the rat. J Physiol 2004; 560:291–302.
114. Qin C, Greenwood-Van Meerveld B, Foreman RD. Visceromotor and spinal neuronal responses to colorectal distension in rats with aldosterone onto the amygdala. J Neurophysiol 2003; 90:2–11.
115. Wang G, Traub RJ. Differential response properties of thoracolumbar and lumbosacral visceroceptive dorsal horn neurons in the rat. Soc Neurosci abstr 2003; 63:9.
116. Wang G, Traub RJ. Pelvic neurectomy alters the response of thoracolumbar dorsal horn neurons to colonic stimulation. Soc Neurosci 2004; 286:5.
117. Wang G, Traub RJ. Differential processing of noxious colonic input by thoracolumbar and lumbosacral dorsal horn neurons. J Neurophysiol 2005; 94:3788–3794.
118. Zhang HQ, Al Chaer ED, Willis WD. Effect of tactile inputs on thalamic responses to noxious colorectal distension in rat. J Neurophysiol 2002; 88:1185–1196.
119. Ness TJ. Intravenous lidocaine inhibits visceral nociceptive reflexes and spinal neurons in the rat. Anesthesiology 2000; 92:1685–1691.
120. Ness TJ, Gebhart GF. Differential effects of morphine and clonidine on visceral and cutaneous spinal nociceptive transmission in the rat. J Neurophysiol 1989; 62:220–230.
121. Omote K, Kawamata M, Iwasaki H, et al. Effects of morphine on neuronal and behavioural responses to visceral and somatic nociception at the level of spinal cord. Acta Anaesthesiol Scand 1994; 38:514–517.
122. Ness TJ, Gebhart GF. Inflammation enhances reflex and spinal neuron responses to noxious visceral stimulation in rats. Am J Physiol Gastrointest Liver Physiol 2001; 280:G649–G657.
123. Ji Y, Tang B, Traub RJ. The effects of estrogen and progesterone on behavioral and neuronal responses to colorectal distention following colonic inflammation in the rat. Pain 2005; 117:433–442.
124. Ness TJ, Gebhart GF. Acute inflammation differentially alters the activity of two classes of rat spinal visceral nociceptive neurons. Neurosci Lett 2000; 281:131–134.
125. Olivar T, Cervero F, Laird JM. Responses of rat spinal neurones to natural and electrical stimulation of colonic afferents: effect of inflammation. Brain Res 2000; 866:168–177.
126. Chang L, Munakata J, Mayer EA, et al. Perceptual responses in patients with inflammatory and functional bowel disease. Gut 2000; 47:497–505.
127. Cook IJ, van Eeden A, Collins SM. Patients with irritable bowel syndrome have greater pain tolerance than normal subjects. Gastroenterology 1987; 93:727–733.
128. Mertz H, Naliboff B, Munakata J, et al. Altered rectal perception is a biological marker of patients with irritable bowel syndrome. Gastroenterology 1995; 109:40–52.
129. Munakata J, Naliboff B, Harraf F, et al. Repetitive sigmoid stimulation induces rectal hyperalgesia in patients with irritable bowel syndrome [published erratum appears in Gastroenterology 1997; 113(3):1054], Gastroenterology 1997; 112, 55–63.
130. Rössel P, Drewes AM, Petersen P, et al. Pain produced by electric stimulation of the rectum in patients with irritable bowel syndrome: further evidence of visceral hyperalgesia. Scand J Gastroenterol 1999; 34:1001–1006.
131. Whitehead WE, Holtkotter B, Enck P, et al. Tolerance for rectosigmoid distention in irritable bowel syndrome. Gastroenterology 1990; 98:1187–1192.
132. Verne GN, Robinson ME, Price DD. Hypersensitivity to visceral and cutaneous pain in the irritable bowel syndrome. Pain 2001; 93:7–14.
133. Bouhassira D, Sabate JM, Coffin B, et al. Effects of rectal distensions on nociceptive flexion reflexes in humans. Am J Physiol Gastrointest Liver Physiol 1998; 275:G410–G417.
134. Cueva-Rolon R, Gomez LE, Komisaruk BR, et al. Inhibition of withdrawal responses by pelvic nerve electrical stimulation. Brain Res 1995; 679:267–273.
135. Chandler MJ, Qin C, Zhang J, et al. Differential effects of urinary bladder distension on high cervical projection neurons in primates. Brain Res 2002; 949:97–104.
136. Ness TJ, Gebhart GF. Interactions between visceral and cutaneous nociception in the rat. II. Noxious visceral stimuli inhibit cutaneous nociceptive neurons and reflexes. J Neurophysiol 1991; 66:29–39.
137. Qin C, Chandler MJ, Foreman RD. Effects of urinary bladder distension on activity of T3-T4 spinal neurons receiving cardiac and somatic noxious inputs in rats. Brain Res 2003; 971:210–220.
138. Zhuo M, Gebhart GF. Inhibition of a cutaneous nociceptive reflex by a noxious visceral stimulus is mediated by spinal cholinergic and descending serotonergic systems in the rat. Brain Res 1992; 585:7–18.
139. Kalmari J, Pertovaara A. Colorectal distension-induced suppression of a nociceptive somatic reflex response in the rat: modulation by tissue injury or inflammation. Brain Res 2004; 1018:106–110.
140. Traub RJ, Wang G. Colonic inflammation decreases thermal sensitivity of the forepaw and hindpaw in the rat. Neurosci Lett 2004; 359:81–84.
141. Millan MJ. The induction of pain: an integrative review. Prog Neurobiol 1999; 57:1–164.
142. Woolf CJ, Salter MW. Neuronal plasticity: increasing the gain in pain. Science 2000; 288:1765–1769.

143. Olivar T, Laird JM. Differential effects of *N*-methyl-D-aspartate receptor blockade on nociceptive somatic and visceral reflexes. Pain 1999; 79:67–73.

144. Caba M, Komisaruk BR, Beyer C. Analgesic synergism between AP5 (an NMDA receptor antagonist) and vaginocervical stimulation in the rat. Pharmacol Biochem Behav 1998; 61:45–48.

145. Gaudreau GA, Plourde V. Involvement of *N*-methyl-aspartate (NMDA) receptors in a rat model of visceral hypersensitivity. Behav Brain Res 2004; 150:185–189.

146. Castroman PJ, Ness TJ. Ketamine, an *N*-methyl-d-aspartate receptor antagonist, inhibits the spinal neuronal responses to distension of the rat urinary bladder. Anesthesiology 2002; 96:1410–1419.

147. Song XJ, Zhao ZQ. Involvement of NMDA and non-NMDA receptors in transmission of spinal visceral nociception in cat. Zhongguo Yao Li Xue Bao 1999; 20:308–312.

148. Coutinho SV, Meller ST, Gebhart GF. Intracolonic zymosan produces visceral hyperalgesia in the rat that is mediated by spinal NMDA and nonNMDA receptors. Brain Res 1996; 736:7–15.

149. Ide Y, Maehara Y, Tsukahara S, et al. The effects of an intrathecal NMDA antagonist (AP5) on the behavioral changes induced by colorectal inflammation with turpentine in rats. Life Sci 1997; 60:1359–1363.

150. Traub RJ, Ji Y, Kovalenko M. Estrogen alters sensitivity of the visceromotor reflex to NMDA receptor antagonists in the rat. IASP 10th World Congress on Pain. 2002, 287.

151. Birder LA, De Groat WC. The effect of glutamate antagonists on c-fos expression induced in spinal neurons by irritation of the lower urinary tract. Brain Res 1992; 580:115–120.

152. Kakizaki H, Yoshiyama M, De Groat WC. Role of NMDA and AMPA glutamatergic transmission in spinal c-fos expression after urinary tract irritation. Am J Physiol 1996; 270:R990–R1006.

153. Rice AS, McMahon SB. Pre-emptive intrathecal administration of an NMDA receptor antagonist (AP-5) prevents hyper-reflexia in a model of persistent visceral pain. Pain 1994; 57:335–340.

154. Meen M, Coudore-Civiale MA, Parry L, et al. Involvement of *N*-methyl-d-aspartate receptors in nociception in the cyclophosphamide-induced vesical pain model in the conscious rat. European Journal of Pain 2002; 6:307–314.

155. Lu Y, Vera-Portocarrero LP, Westlund KN. Intrathecal coadministration of D-APV and morphine is maximally effective in a rat experimental pancreatitis model. Anesthesiology 2003; 98:734–740.

156. Vera-Portocarrero LP, Lu Y, Westlund KN. Nociception in persistent pancreatitis in rats: effects of morphine and neuropeptide alterations. Anesthesiology 2003; 98:474–484.

157. Yu XM, Askalan R, Keil GJ, et al. NMDA channel regulation by channel-associated protein tyrosine kinase Src. Science 1997; 275:674–678.

158. Guo W, Zou S, Guan Y, et al. Tyrosine phosphorylation of the NR2B subunit of the NMDA receptor in the spinal cord during the development and maintenance of inflammatory hyperalgesia. J Neurosci 2002; 22:6208–6217.

159. Galan A, Cervero F, Laird JM. Extracellular signaling-regulated kinase-1 and -2 (ERK 1/2) mediate referred hyperalgesia in a murine model of visceral pain. Brain Res Mol Brain Res 2003; 116:126–134.

160. Willert R, Woolf C, Hobson A, et al. The development and maintenance of human visceral pain hypersensitivity is dependent on the *N*-methyl-d-aspartate receptor. Gastroenterology 2004; 126:683–692.

161. Strigo IA, Duncan GH, Catherine Bushnell M, et al. The effects of racemic ketamine on painful stimulation of skin and viscera in human subjects. Pain 2005; 113:255–264.

162. Kuiken SD, Lei A, Tytgat GNJ, et al. Effect of the low-affinity, noncompetitive *N*-methyl-d-aspartate receptor antagonist dextromethorphan on visceral perception in healthy volunteers. Aliment Pharmacol Ther 2002, 16, 1955–1962.

163. Kuiken SD, van den Berg SJ, Tytgat GN, et al. Oral S(+)-ketamine does not change visceral perception in health. Dig Dis Sci 2004; 49:1745–1751.

164. Perry MJ, Lawson SN. Differences in expression of oligosaccharides, neuropeptides, carbonic anhydrase and neurofilament in rat primary afferent neurons retrogradely labeled via skin, muscle or visceral nerves. Neuroscience 1998; 85:293–310.

165. Ishigooka M, Zermann DH, Doggweiler R, et al. Spinal NK1 receptor is upregulated after chronic bladder irritation. Pain 2001; 93:43–50.

166. Palecek J, Paleckova V, Willis WD. Postsynaptic dorsal column neurons express NK1 receptors following colon inflammation. Neuroscience 2003; 116:565–572.

167. Honore P, Kamp EH, Rogers SD, et al. Activation of lamina I spinal cord neurons that express the substance P receptor in visceral nociception and hyperalgesia. J Pain 2002; 3:3–11.

168. De Giorgio R, Barbara G, Blennerhassett P, et al. Intestinal inflammation and activation of sensory nerve pathways: a functional and morphological study in the nematode infected rat. Gut 2001; 49:822–827.

169. Greenwood-Van Meerveld B, Gibson MS, Johnson AC, et al. NK1 receptor-mediated mechanisms regulate colonic hypersensitivity in the guinea pig. Pharmacol Biochem Behav 2003; 74:1005–1013.

170. Okano S, Ikeura Y, Inatomi N. Effects of tachykinin NK1 receptor antagonists on the viscerosensory response caused by colorectal distention in rabbits. J Pharmacol Exp Ther 2002; 300:925–931.

171. Gaudreau GA, Plourde V. Role of tachykinin NK1, NK2 and NK3 receptors in the modulation of visceral hypersensitivity in the rat. Neurosci Lett 2003; 351:59–62.

172. Schwetz I, Bradesi S, McRoberts JA, et al. Delayed stress-induced colonic hypersensitivity in male Wistar rats: role of neurokinin-1 and corticotropin-releasing factor-1 receptors. Am J Physiol Gastrointest Liver Physiol 2004; 286:G683–G691.

173. Laird JM, Olivar T, Roza C, et al. Deficits in visceral pain and hyperalgesia of mice with a disruption of the tachykinin NK1 receptor gene. Neuroscience 2000; 98:345–352.

174. Kamp EH, Beck DR, Gebhart GF. Combinations of neurokinin receptor antagonists reduce visceral hyperalgesia. J Pharmacol Exp Ther 2001; 299:105–113.

175. Julia V, Morteau O, Bueno L. Involvement of neurokinin 1 and 2 receptors in viscerosensitive response to rectal distension in rats. Gastroenterology 1994; 107:94–102.

176. Friedrich AE, Gebhart GF. Modulation of visceral hyperalgesia by morphine and cholecystokinin from the rat rostroventral medial medulla. Pain 2003; 104:93–101.

177. Diop L, Raymond F, Fargeau H, et al. Pregabalin (CI-1008) inhibits the trinitrobenzene sulfonic acid-induced chronic colonic allodynia in the rat. J Pharmacol Exp Ther 2002; 302:1013–1022.

178. Messaoudi M, Desor D, Grasmück V, et al. Behavioral evaluation of visceral pain in a rat model of colonic inflammation. Neuroreport 1999; 10:1137–1141.

179. Castroman P, Ness TJ. Vigor of visceromotor responses to urinary bladder distension in rats increases with repeated trials and stimulus intensity. Neurosci Lett 2001; 306:97–100.

180. Boucher M, Meen M, Codron JP, et al. Cyclophosphamide-induced cystitis in freely-moving conscious rats: behavioral approach to a new model of visceral pain. J Urol 2000; 164:203–208.

181. Sandner-Kiesling A, Eisenach JC. Estrogen reduces efficacy of [mu]-but not [kappa]-opioid agonist inhibition in response to uterine cervical distension. Anesthesiology 2002; 96:375–379.

182. Shin SW, Eisenach JC. Intrathecal morphine reduces the visceromotor response to acute uterine cervical distension in an estrogen-independent manner. Anesthesiology 2003; 98:1467–1471.

183. Roza C, Laird JM. Pressor responses to distension of the ureter in anaesthetised rats: characterisation of a model of acute visceral pain. Neurosci Lett 1995; 198:9–12.

184. Rouzade ML, Fioramonti J, Bueno L. A model for evaluation of gastric sensitivity in awake rats. Neurogastroenterol Motil 1998; 10:157–163.

185. Traub RJ, Stitt S, Gebhart GF. Attenuation of c-Fos expression in the rat lumbosacral spinal cord by morphine or tramadol following noxious colorectal distention. Brain Res 1995; 701:175–182.

186. Sengupta JN, Snider A, Su X, et al. Effects of kappa opioids in the inflamed rat colon. Pain 1999; 79:175–185.

187. Larsson M, Arvidsson S, Ekman C, et al. A model for chronic quantitative studies of colorectal sensitivity using balloon distension in conscious mice-effects of opioid receptor agonists. Neurogastroenterol Motil 2003; 15:371–381.

188. Sengupta JN, Su X, Gebhart GF. Kappa, but not mu or delta, opioids attenuate responses to distention of afferent fibers innervating the rat colon. Gastroenterology 1996; 111:968–980.

189. Friedrich AE, Gebhart GF. Effects of spinal cholecystokinin receptor antagonists on morphine antinociception in a model of visceral pain in the rat. J Pharmacol Exp Ther 2000; 292:538–544.

190. Danzebrink RM, Green SA, Gebhart GF. Spinal mu and delta, but not kappa, opioid-receptor agonists attenuate responses to noxious colorectal distension in the rat. Pain 1995; 63:39–47.

191. Ji Y, Murphy AZ, Traub RJ. Sex differences in morphine induced analgesia of visceral pain are supraspinally and peripherally mediated. Am J Physiol 2006.

192. Joshi SK, Su X, Porreca F, et al. kappa-Opioid receptor agonists modulate visceral nociception at a novel, peripheral site of action. J Neurosci 2000; 20:5874–5879.

193. Sandner-Kiesling A, Pan HL, Chen SR, et al. Effect of kappa opioid agonists on visceral nociception induced by uterine cervical distension in rats. Pain 2002; 96:13–22.

194. Su X, Sengupta JN, Gebhart GF. Effects of kappa opioid receptor-selective agonists on responses of pelvic nerve afferents to noxious colorectal distension. J Neurophysiol 1997; 78:1003–1012.

195. Lembo T, Naliboff BD, Matin K, et al. Irritable bowel syndrome patients show altered sensitivity to exogenous opioids. Pain 2000; 87:137–147.

196. Spiller R. Pharmacotherapy: non-serotonergic mechanisms. Gut 2002; 51:i87–i90.

197. Berkley KJ. Sex differences in pain. Behav Brain Sci 1997; 20:371–380.

198. Unruh AM. Gender variations in clinical pain experience. Pain 1996; 65:123–167.

199. Riley JL3, Robinson ME, Wise EA, et al. Sex differences in the perception of noxious experimental stimuli: a meta-analysis. Pain 1998; 74:181–187.

200. Riley JL3, Robinson ME, Wise EA, et al. A meta-analytic review of pain perception across the menstrual cycle. Pain 1999; 81:225–235.

201. Fillingim RB, Maixner W, Kincaid S, et al. Sex differences in temporal summation but not sensory-discriminative processing of thermal pain. Pain 1998; 75:121–127.

202. Fillingim RB, Maixner W, Girdler SS, et al. Ischemic but not thermal pain sensitivity varies across the menstrual cycle. Psychosom Med 1997; 59:512–520.

203. Drury RA, Gold RM. Differential effects of ovarian hormones on reactivity to electric footshock in the rat. Physiol Behav 1978; 20:187–191.

204. Kayser V, Berkley KJ, Keita H, et al. Estrous and sex variations in vocalization thresholds to hind-paw and tail pressure stimulation in the rat. Brain Res 1996; 742:352–354.

205. Amandusson A, Hermanson O, Blomqvist A. Estrogen receptor-like immunoreactivity in the medullary and spinal dorsal horn of the female rat. Neurosci Lett 1995; 196:25–28.

206. Papka RE, Storey-Workley M, Shughrue PJ, et al. Estrogen receptor-alpha and beta-immunoreactivity and mRNA in neurons of sensory and autonomic ganglia and spinal cord. Cell Tissue Res 2001; 304:193–214.
207. Williams SJ, Papka RE. Estrogen receptor-immunoreactive neurons are present in the female rat lumbosacral spinal cord. J Neurosci Res 1996; 46:492–501.
208. Williams SJ, Chung K, Om AS, et al. Cytosolic estrogen receptor concentrations in the lumbosacral spinal cord fluctuate during the estrous cycle. Life Sci 1997; 61:2551–2559.
209. Evrard HC, Balthazart J. Rapid Regulation of pain by estrogens synthesized in spinal dorsal horn neurons. J Neurosci 2004; 24:7225–7229.
210. Sapsed-Byrne S, Ma DQ, Ridout D, et al. Estrous cycle phase variations in visceromotor and cardiovascular responses to colonic distension in the anesthetized rat. Brain Res 1996; 742:10–16.
211. Holdcroft A, Sapsed-Byrne S, Ma D, et al. Sex and oestrous cycle differences in visceromotor responses and vasopressin release in response to colonic distention in male and female rats anesthetized with halothane. Br J Anaesth 2000; 85:907–910.
212. Sengupta JN, Gebhart GF. Characterization of mechanosensitive pelvic nerve afferent fibers innervating the colon of the rat. J Neurophysiol 1994; 71:2046–2060.
213. Wall PD, Hubscher CH, Berkley KJ. Intraspinal modulation of neuronal responses to uterine and cervix stimulation in rat L1 and L6 dorsal horn. Brain Res 1993; 622:71–78.

8 Animal Models of Visceral Pain

David R. Robinson and G. F. Gebhart
Center for Pain Research, University of Pittsburgh, Pittsburgh, Pennsylvania, U.S.A.

INTRODUCTION
Visceral Pain

Visceral pain is the most common form of pain produced by disease, but the mechanisms that underlie it have been studied considerably less than those involved in nonvisceral, somatic pain. Here, we review some of the more pertinent models of abdominal and visceral pain, following a general introduction to the neuroanatomy of visceral pain and the use of animal models in pain paradigms.

The Neuroanatomy of Visceral Pain

While Chapter 4 provides a review of the neuroanatomy of visceral pain, a basic understanding is advantageous when considering the models presented here. We therefore begin with a brief overview of the basic afferent innervation of the viscera.

The visceral organs are innervated by extrinsic afferent nerves that run alongside the sympathetic and parasympathetic nervous systems, but are not part of these efferent pathways (however, they are referred to by the name of the respective autonomic nerve, e.g., pelvic afferent). Most visceral afferent fibers are pseudounipolar spinal afferents that travel through prevertebral ganglia and terminate in the spinal cord (eventually projecting indirectly to various thalamic and other supraspinal nuclei) with cell bodies in the dorsal root ganglia. A smaller proportion of afferent fibers terminate in the nucleus tractus solitarius (in the brainstem) with cell bodies in the nodose ganglia (vagal afferents). Less than 10% of the total spinal afferent input is visceral (1); however, this is compensated by the greater intersegmental spread of visceral nerve terminals within the spinal cord.

Vagal afferent fibers are principally involved in the transmission of physiological events, but accumulating evidence suggests they can also contribute to visceral pain transmission, principally chemonociception. Indeed, vagal afferents can activate neurons in the spinothalamic tract (at least in high cervical spinal levels), which could provide sensory input to pain pathways (2), and vagal afferents are well known for their modulatory roles in nociceptive processing (3). Relevant to the consideration of abdominal pain mechanisms, vagal afferents, unlike the spinal afferent system, do not converge onto second-order neurons that also receive nonvisceral input.

Additional afferent systems are also involved in the transmission of pain from the viscera. For example, the rectum and distal colon are innervated by intestinofugal and rectospinal afferents. The former have cell bodies in enteric ganglia that project back to synapse on postganglionic efferent neurons in prevertebral ganglia, whereas the latter project from their cell bodies in the gut wall directly to the spinal cord, probably traveling through dorsal roots. One of the roles of intestinofugal fibers is to detect volume; rectospinal fibers may contribute directly to high threshold (and therefore perhaps nociceptive) mechanosensory input to central processing pathways. Rectospinal fibers may also act as second-order neurons to transmit impulses from a number of intrinsic afferent neurons, although the intrinsic innervation of the viscera is not discussed here.

Visceral vs. Somatic Pain

In contrast to the somatic system (a misleading term since the viscera are certainly of the body), relatively little is known about the mechanisms of visceral pain sensation. We do know, however, that whereas some characteristics are shared between the visceral and nonvisceral (somatic) systems, there are also significant differences. Therefore, results from experiments on somatic tissue cannot automatically be assumed to correlate with the visceral organs. The major features (4) that differentiate visceral from nonvisceral pain are as follows:

1. *Visceral pain is not evoked from all viscera*: A large portion of the viscera is innervated by afferents and their receptive endings that convey purely regulatory, or at least non-noxious, information, and many forms of (presumed) noxious stimulation do not produce a conscious sensation of discomfort or pain in the viscera.
2. *Visceral pain is not always linked to tissue injury*: Acute colonic pain, for example, can be evoked by colonic distension without any associated tissue damage, whereas cutting or crushing of the colon does not reliably evoke pain.
3. *Visceral pain is referred to other locations*: This, alongside the following observations, is related to the convergence of visceral and nonvisceral pathways onto second-order neurons in the spinal cord. Angina, for example, is referred to the upper left shoulder and left arm.
4. *Visceral pain is diffuse and poorly localized*: The proportion of visceral to nonvisceral afferents is low; thus each unit must represent a larger receptive field in the viscera compared to an equivalent unit in skin, muscle, or joint. Viscerovisceral convergence (e.g., colon and bladder) onto the same second-order spinal cord neurons also contributes to the poor localization of visceral pain.
5. *Visceral pain is accompanied by motor and autonomic reflexes*: Primary afferent neurons innervating the viscera possess axon collaterals that synapse with autonomic system secretory and motor neurons in prevertebral ganglia. Moreover, the emotional component of undefined visceral pain, such as chest pain, is typically greater than that associated with skin, muscle, or joint insult.

The Use of Animal Models for the Study of Visceral Pain

The study of visceral pain has been considerably advanced by the use of both human (5) and nonhuman animal models. The latter, although not directly reflecting specific disease mechanisms, nevertheless provide a valuable insight into pain mechanisms, and models have been developed specifically to address different aspects and processes that contribute, for example, to acute visceral pain, visceral hypersensitivity, and visceral hyper-reflexia. Many different animals have been used for the development of visceral pain models, but we concentrate on rodents in this review.

How is "Pain", Measured in an Animal Model?

Pain, of course, is a subjective human experience, and so it is more appropriate to refer to nonhuman animal models as nocifensive or nociceptive. By this, we mean that although the sensory receptors (nociceptors) and the neural encoding and processing of noxious stimuli are present in animals (and function as they do in humans), the affective and cognitive features that define human pain are missing. Semantics aside, because noxious stimuli commonly act to warn all animals, and responses are often marked and similar (e.g., muscular contraction and withdrawal), we consider here the two alike.

As indicated above, stimuli that are noxious to somatic structures (i.e., those that damage or threaten to damage) are not reliably so in the viscera. Instead, hollow organ distension, traction on the mesentery, ischemia, inflammation, and chemical stimuli are adequate, in the context proposed by Sherrington, for the activation of visceral nociceptors. To evaluate pain in an animal model, a suitably measured variable must be chosen that correlates with the pain evoked by a given stimulus. Candidates are numerous and range from pseudaffective responses such as vasomotor, visceromotor, and respiratory reflexes, to the expression of intermediate-early genes such as *c-fos* in the dorsal horn of the spinal cord or brainstem. Typically, contractile responses of the abdominal muscles are recorded using mechanical (force transduction equipment) or electrophysiological [electromyography (EMG)] methods. It should be noted, however, that anesthesia will affect pseudaffective responses (6). More invasive in vivo electrophysiological techniques such as recording from primary afferent neurons, the dorsal horn neurons upon which they synapse, or the dorsal roots in which they travel, can be employed, which may result in a more detailed assessment.

So, what evidence is the most important with which to characterize an animal model as painful? Certainly, behavioral responses, where the experimental method allows, will give a sound indication of an aversive, "painful" experience, but in the absence of such a readout, other factors should be considered. Histological analysis will give an indication of a tissue insult that may lead to a painful pathology [e.g., inflammation, which may also be assessed by the detection of myeloperoxidase (MPO) activity]. But this is certainly not a definitive (or causative) measure of pain. For example, dextran sodium sulphate (DSS)-induced colitis produces marked inflammation, but no colonic hypersensitivity in at least two different strains of mouse (7). The electrophysiological recording of nerve bundles or individual neurons can be informative regarding peripheral pain mechanisms, but even here we cannot be certain of their direct relevance to pain in the absence of a behavioral correlate. One can record from neuronal populations that are believed to carry nociceptive information (e.g., based on the presence of certain receptors and peptides, or by diameter and conduction velocity), but even then we rely upon two assumptions: (i) these neurons are truly nociceptive and (ii) their activation would, indeed, be painful (i.e., their input is not prohibited from reaching central pain generation areas by one or more "gate" mechanisms). Some of these limitations may be improved by the pharmacological testing of models using (behaviorally) well-defined analgesics such as morphine. Dose-dependent inhibition of presumed pain-indicating responses to a particular test gives confidence that this may, indeed, represent a painful experience should the animal have been able to express the response behaviorally.

Pain Stimuli in Animal Models

Models of visceral pain can be implemented using a variety of stimuli: chemical, developmental, electrical, environmental, infectious, mechanical, surgical, and thermal, or by genetic means. In the field of visceral pain research, thermal stimuli have not been extensively studied as the basis of animal models, and electrical stimulation of either isolated nerves or organs should be used with caution; such stimuli are not specific to visceral modalities (especially considering their convergence with somatic pain systems), cannot be considered natural, and do not involve any neural change that might be expected in conditions that manifest with visceral pain. These two methods aside, we have incorporated as many different approaches as possible into this review, which is organized by visceral system, and then by organ, beginning with those in the thorax and traveling distally to the genitourinary organs.

THE CARDIOPULMONARY SYSTEM
The Heart

Human angina (angina pectoris), a painful (or uncomfortable) visceral sensation, is transmitted through cardiac primary afferent neurons to the central nervous system. Angina is the result of ischemic episodes, i.e., any situation in which there is an insufficient supply of oxygen to the myocardium for its metabolic demands. This has been exploited in a wide range of species to produce animal models of cardiac ischemia, using chemical and surgical methods. Chemical approaches are based on reports of increased concentrations of bradykinin (BK) or adenosine in sinus blood after experimental coronary artery occlusion. For example, one study reported pseudaffective responses in dogs, following intracoronary injection of acetylcholine, BK, 5-hydroxytryptamine (5-HT), histamine, or K^+ (potassium chloride) (8), although it is unclear how relevant any one chemical individually might relate to clinical angina. In the case of BK, human studies have shown that intracoronary injection will result in pain that is reported as both different to (9), and indistinguishable from (10), the ischemic pain normally experienced by study participants. Consequently, a study was instigated in our laboratory to investigate the effects of coadministration of a number of algogenic substances (BK, acetylcholine, adenosine, histamine, 5-HT, and prostaglandin E_2) into the pericardial sac of awake rats (11). Those animals that received the algogenic mixture showed a quicker establishment of passive avoidance behavior than those animals that received BK alone, saline, or the mixture without BK. This suggests that the mixture was aversive, but there is a paucity of behavioral data in the current literature to support such models as useful visceral pain models.

A logical and widely used model of cardiac pain is that of coronary artery occlusion, because myocardial ischemia is the major factor that leads to angina. Coronary artery occlusion is a procedure that, in the rat, can be achieved by either complete or partial ligation of the left descending coronary artery. Despite what is a relatively simple technique, such models result in a high initial mortality rate (typically 40–60%), a large variation in the size of any resultant myocardial infarction, and only a proportion of rats with an infarction will actually develop apparent heart failure. This said, angina is not experienced by all (or even most) patients in the clinic, even in the presence of severe coronary artery damage/disease; angina can also be seen in patients who exhibit no sign of coronary artery disease. Furthermore, as with chemical models, there is a lack of published studies showing that these models actually result in behaviors that can be interpreted as pain. This is not to say that pseudaffective responses, attributed to pain, have not been reported in animal models of coronary artery occlusion; however, it is possible that these responses were artifactual, and due to the mechanical manipulation of the vessel, inflammation of the area, and too short a period between surgery and experimentation, or all three (12).

The Lungs

Pain and discomfort are the only sensations that can be evoked following direct stimulation of the respiratory system, but the lung is reportedly insensitive to pain (13). It is acknowledged, however, that inhalation of ammonia or other irritants leads to discomfort, if not pain, in humans, and studies have documented the chemosensitivity of lung afferents (14) and of spinal dorsal horn neurons receiving input from the respiratory system (Fig. 1) (15). Aside from these and other electrophysiological studies, there are no reliable animal models.

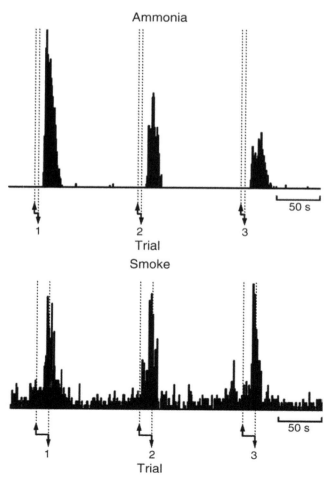

Figure 1 Lower airway irritants activate spinal cord neurons. Examples of thoracic spinal cord neuron responses to repetitive stimulation of the lower airways by 100% ammonia (*upper panel*) or high-tar, high-nicotine smoke (*lower panel*). Onset and termination of stimuli are represented by upward- and downward-pointing arrows, respectively, and dotted lines. Responses from two different thoracic spinal cord neurons are shown. Not shown here is that these neurons received convergent cutaneous and esophageal inputs, emphasizing an important characteristic of visceral pain. *Source*: From Ref. 15.

THE GASTROINTESTINAL TRACT
The Esophagus

Distension of the hollow visceral organs is commonly employed to study pain processing from these sites; the esophagus is no exception. Esophageal distension in the anesthetized rat evokes pseudoaffective responses including pressor (heart rate and arterial blood pressure) responses concomitant with the stimulus (16). These effects are dependent upon the location of the distension: Significantly greater cardiovascular responses are found in the lower and middle esophagus compared to upper areas (16), suggesting that the lower esophagus should be considered for experiments using such a model. This distension stimulus is administered by the injection of water into a spherical balloon (typically for 20–30 seconds) that is inserted into the distal esophagus under anesthesia following cannulation of the carotid or femoral artery (for measurement of blood pressure and heart rate). Tracheal cannulation ensures a clear airway. These factors mean that such experiments cannot be carried out in free-moving animals; therefore behavioral testing is not possible (but psychophysical studies are often performed in humans who can voluntarily swallow a balloon). As an interesting aside, evidence exists for a significant convergence of esophageal and cardiac afferent pathways (17). For example, patients often perceive (referred) esophageal and cardiac pain in a very similar manner. This phenomenon is not restricted to the esophagus and the heart; thus, one should not necessarily assume that behaviors observed from similar experiments are affecting just one organ or neural pathway.

The Stomach

Gastric pain is most often modeled using distension, chemical challenge, or both, of the stomach. Many different chemicals have been used to produce gastric damage, the most common of these employed in animal models of visceral sensory transduction being hydrochloric acid or acetic acid. Intragastric administration (using a feeding tube) of hydrochloric acid, at a concentration that will induce *c-fos* expression in the brainstem (0.5 M), causes writhing movements indicative of a noxious visceral insult with a peak response approximately 45 minutes after administration (18). Even so, only 42% (15 of 36) of rats that received the acid infusion responded in this way (a figure reported to be similar to the incidence of pain produced in humans following infusion of hydrochloric acid onto symptomatic peptic ulcers).

Following the publication of methods by which acetic acid could be used to produce gastric ulceration (19,20) came the development of the "kissing ulcer" (21,22). This ulceration model involves the surgical exposure of the rat stomach (under anesthesia) and the brief (45 seconds) infusion of 60% acetic acid into a restricted area of the fundus. The animals recover, but will develop ulcers on the anterior and posterior walls of the stomach within three days (Fig. 2A) (22). Rats with kissing ulcers demonstrate a significantly enhanced visceromotor response to gastric distension (measured using surgically implanted EMG electrodes in the *acromiotrapezius* muscle; distension balloons were implanted at the same time) for two weeks after the procedure (23). This enhanced response will remain up to 60 days following injection of 20% acetic acid into the stomach wall (Fig. 2) (24).

High distension pressures alone will also produce pain-like behaviors (and EMG activity recordings from the neck muscles) in rats, the threshold of which can be increased following morphine administration (25). In a comparative study of the EMG responses seen during gastric distension from different muscles (abdominal: *rectus abdominus* and *obliquus externus*; neck: *acromiotrapezius* and *sternomastoideus*; back: *spinotrapezius*), the most vigorous responses were seen in the *acromiotrapezius* muscles (24). EMG responses are graded with the distension pressure, relatively stable, and reproducible at time points beyond, and including, three days after electrode implantation (24). Rats that experience gastric distension will rapidly learn passive avoidance behavior (they will not step down from a platform if they receive a 100 mmHg gastric distension as they do so; without the distension stimulus, they will readily step down from the platform), providing further evidence that this stimulus is painful.

The Small Intestine

Distension [and resection (26)] of the ileum, jejunum [including traction of the mesentery (27)], and duodenum has been described in rodents; for the purposes of this review, we shall

(A)

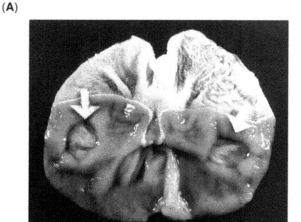

(B)

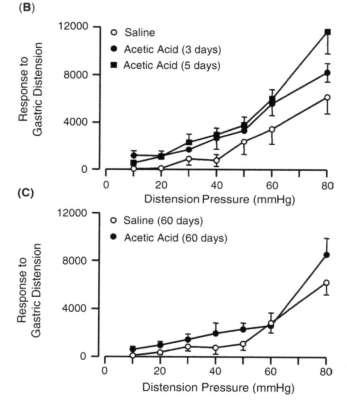

(C)

Figure 2 Acetic acid produces gastric ulcers in the rat. Kissing ulcers (**A**), induced in a rat three days after intraluminal application of 60% acetic acid. Arrows indicate round ulcers on the posterior and anterior walls. Using a different method (injection of 20% acetic acid into the stomach wall), the visceromotor response to gastric distension is significantly enhanced from three days (**B**) to 60 days (**C**) after acetic acid treatment ($p < 0.05$). *Source*: (**A**) From Ref. 22; (**B**) Redrawn and adapted from Ref. 24.

concentrate on just one—the duodenum. As described by Colburn et al. (28), a balloon catheter is surgically inserted into the duodenum through the stomach and exteriorized at the base of the skull. The animal is allowed to recover following closure of the incisions, and testing is initiated 5 to 14 days later. Inflation of the balloon results in writhing behaviors, the score of which (higher scores relating to pain-like behavior) increases with increasing distension volume (28,29) and are dose-dependently inhibited by morphine (28). Passive avoidance testing also provides behavioral evidence that duodenal distension in the rat is aversive (30,31).

The response to distension of the viscera is often assessed in restrained or lightly anesthetized animals using chronically implanted EMG electrodes in the abdominal wall. This method has been modified to allow the study of duodenal distension-evoked responses in the freely moving rat (30,31). Abdominal EMG electrodes and an arterial catheter (tunneled through the femoral artery to the aorta) are connected to a telemetry transmitter, and EMG, blood pressure, and heart rate are recorded simultaneously before, during, and after duodenal distension. Nijsen et al. report a volume-dependent increase in the EMG activity, blood pressure, and heart rate; morphine inhibited the EMG increases during distension (30). A similar method has been used to examine the cardiovascular response to distensions lasting both 5 and 20 seconds (31).

The Pancreas

Experimental models of pancreatic pain have focused almost exclusively on the chemical initiation of pancreatitis. One such model involves the intraperitoneal injection of rats with 20% L-arginine twice at an interval of one hour (32). This model produces an increase in sensitivity to mechanical stimulation of the upper abdomen (lower threshold to probing with von Frey filaments), indicative of referred pain, during the first week (33). The same model produces an increase in EMG activity (and, therefore, abdominal contractions) of the abdominal muscles that correlates with the severity of pancreatic inflammation and the expression of *c-fos* in the thoracolumbar spinal cord (34). This, and similar, models have an advantage over many of the others we review here in that surgical manipulation is not required, thus avoiding any possible complication arising from tissue damage or manipulation. Pancreatitis can also be induced in rats by the injection of $8\,mg\,kg^{-1}$ dibutyltin dichloride (dissolved in two parts ethanol and then mixed with three parts glycerol) into the tail vein (35). Treated rats show hypersensitivity to abdominal probing with von Frey filaments and significantly shorter withdrawal latencies for thermal stimuli at three and seven days (and one day in the case of thermal stimulation) following initiation of pancreatitis (36). These responses were dose-dependently inhibited by morphine treatment.

An alternative method to introduce chemicals into the pancreas is the surgical cannulation of the common bile (biliopancreatic) duct (37). Studies show that introduction of capsaicin or agonists for the proteinase-activated receptor 2 (trypsin or its selective activating peptide) will produce increased EMG activity in the *acromiotrapezius* muscle (38). Administration of the hapten 2,4,6-trinitrobenzenesulfonic acid (TNBS) (see section "The Large Intestine, Rectum, and Anus" for more information) in the same manner (37) will produce referred abdominal mechanical sensitivity for as long as six weeks postinstillation, and rats show significant hypersensitivity to all forces of von Frey filament tested (2.75–120 mN) three weeks after instillation (Fig. 3) (39).

An extension of these intraductal delivery models is the intraperitoneal injection of the Cholecystokinin analogue caerulein (to accelerate the contraction of the bile system) alongside infusion of a bile salt, glycodeoxycholic acid, into the pancreas. Pancreatitis [described as moderately severe; (40)] develops after 12 hours, and experimental animals show significantly reduced activity (40,41), a measure that has been used to grade visceral pain.

The Liver and the Gall Bladder

There are a number of rodent models for human liver and gall bladder diseases such as hepatic porphyria and cholelithiasis; however, we are unaware of any studies that have quantified any painful component of these.

The Large Intestine, Rectum, and Anus

Colorectal distension (CRD) is the most widely used model of organ distension, and has been characterized in both the rat (6) and the mouse (42,43). This method reproducibly generates painful responses in both animals and humans as the result of a natural visceral stimulus, and is minimally invasive: a balloon or similar device can be inserted anally. Such techniques produce acute pain and can be combined with intracolonic treatment with chemicals that produce insult or inflammation such as acetic acid. Normally, the responses to CRD are recorded using electrodes that have been implanted in the abdominal muscle a week or so before measuring responses to distension. These electrodes allow the study of the visceromotor response in the absence of anesthesia: the electrical contractile activity of the muscles in response to a painful (or painless) distension.

(A)

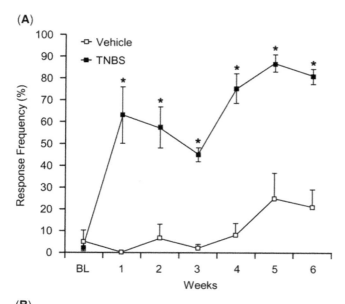

(B)

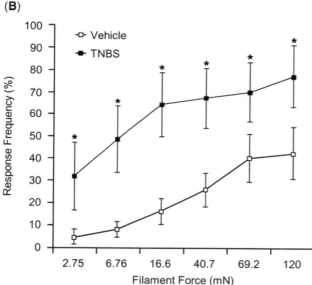

Figure 3 TNBS-induced pancreatitis produces referred muscle hypersensitivity. These panels show the response frequency (percentage of positive responses) to mechanical stimulation of the abdomen with von Frey-like monofilaments. Panel **A** reports the responses to a 40.7 mN filament before (BL), and up to six weeks following induction of pancreatitis (*$p < 0.001$), while panel **B** shows the responses to all filaments tested three weeks after induction of pancreatitis (*$p < 0.05$). Although omitted here for clarity of presentation, baseline response frequencies were similar to those recorded for the vehicle and were significantly different from the TNBS treatment data for responses to filaments of 6.76 mN and greater. *Abbreviation*: TNBS, 2, 4, 6-trinitrobenzenesulfonic acid. *Source*: Redrawn from Ref. 39.

One of the postulated risk factors for irritable bowel syndrome (IBS), a key symptom of which is visceral pain, is acute transient infection, and this has been applied to animal models. Such infectious stimuli as that produced by the nematode *Nippostrongylus brasiliensis* or *Trichinella spiralis* result in hypermotility, hypersecretion, and intestinal inflammation. This is accompanied by increased visceral sensitivity and is used as a chronic model, because these effects can be seen after the inflammation has resolved, although effects may be related more directly to the jejunum rather than the colon (44). If an insult such as an infection is experienced by neonatal animals, it may induce a sensitization that can significantly affect nociceptive processing in adults, and this is the theoretical basis of animal models involving developmental stimuli. Indeed, both mechanical and chemical neonatal colonic irritation in rats have been reported to produce visceral hypersensitivity in adults (45). Furthermore, environmental changes during neonatal life can have similar effects. For example, separation of rat pups from their mothers for 180 minutes on each of postnatal days 2 to 14 results in increased EMG output in response to CRD compared to nonhandled litters (46). Similar studies show exaggeration of the immune response and long-term changes in the colonic epithelial barrier of these animals (47). These effects may be the result of increased anxiety, another stimulus that can reproduce some IBS symptoms in adult rats following partial restraint (48) and other experimental stressors (49).

Genetic models have been used with some success to examine visceral pain. For example, the Wistar Kyoto rat (a high-anxiety strain) exhibits significantly more colonic hypersensitivity than other strains, including the commonly used Sprague Dawley rat strain (50). Specific transgenic models have been produced with intestinal inflammation, results that have been used to propose the pathophysiology of inflammatory bowel disease (IBD). Such genetic models include the knockout of genes such as that for the anti-inflammatory cytokine interleukin-10, which results in increased cytokine production by T_H1 lymphocytes and chronic enterocolitis with some IBD-like symptoms (51).

Finally, chemical stimuli are perhaps the most diverse group of stimuli. Most of these will generate a state of colonic hypersensitivity (e.g., to balloon distension) by inducing inflammation. While intraperitoneal injection of substances is unreliable (and questionably ethical) for visceral pain studies (52,53), localized intracolonic application of compounds such as acetic acid (54), antibiotics (55), butyrate (56), capsaicin (57), DSS (58), glycerol (59), mustard oil (60), TNBS (61), turpentine (62), or zymosan (63) will either directly produce pain-like behaviors (e.g., capsaicin and mustard oil) or induce inflammation. These compounds are either used to study their acute effects (recording within minutes or hours of instillation) or to produce long-lasting, persistent, visceral hypersensitivity (days or even months after instillation), depending upon the agent.

It is beyond the scope of this review to give a detailed account of each of these models; however, we shall discuss two: one inflammatory (TNBS) and one without colonic inflammation (butyrate). TNBS is used routinely in many laboratories for the study of behavioral, biochemical, pathological, and electrophysiological changes in rodents. Initially developed in the rat, the TNBS model of colitis (in which colon inflammation and symptoms develop that are frequently associated with human IBD) has since been documented in the mouse (64,65). TNBS (also known as picrylsulfonic acid), as a hapten, is not itself immunogenic, but can become so when combined with larger carrier molecules. It is therefore incapable of producing any immune reaction alone and so is coadministered with a "barrier-breaking" compound, ethanol, to produce acute colonic mucosal damage (66) and increased MPO activity (42). The MPO activity in a given tissue is a measure of neutrophil infiltration, and therefore an index of inflammation, supported by both macro- and microscopic histology. This combination therefore enables both entry and immunogenicity of TNBS instilled into the colon, leading to the introduction of intestinal bacterial flora into the colon wall and macrophage activation. These macrophages will secrete a number of cytokines that result in a T_H1-dominant cascade. Alterations in the mucosal serotonergic system are also present. For example, downregulation of the 5-HT reuptake transporter increases the amount of 5-HT available to depolarize the peripheral terminals of both intrinsic and extrinsic primary afferent neurons, probably by activation of $5-HT_3$ receptors. This is by no means an exhaustive account of proposed mechanisms; further details can be found in the literature (67,68).

Previous studies document that TNBS produces colon inflammation and colon hypersensitivity in rats (69–71), and we are now assessing the behavioral characteristics of this model in mice (Robinson and Gebhart, unpublished). TNBS colitis in mice is normally initiated by the intracolonic instillation, via the rectum, of the hapten (in our experience, mortality is negligible at doses up to $10\,mg\,mL^{-1}$) dissolved in ethanol (typically 25–50%) under light anesthesia. Alternatively, the mixture has been injected into the colon during laparotomy (72). Typically, colonic inflammation and elevated MPO activity are seen a few days following instillation of TNBS. Animals can, however, exhibit colonic hypersensitivity after the resolution of this inflammation, as measured by visceromotor response to distension (Fig. 4). This may therefore be an interesting model for the study of postinflammatory hyperalgesia.

A new, noninflammatory model (no mucosal damage or detectable MPO activity was observed) of visceral hypersensitivity was recently described by Bourdu et al. (56). This model uses twice-daily intracolonic instillation of butyrate solution (1 mL of 8–1000 mM; 200 mM was selected as the most appropriate concentration) over three days. Treated rats show a significantly decreased threshold for CRD-evoked pain behaviors and greater pain score (rated 0–5) than rats treated intracolonically with saline. Referred cutaneous hyperalgesia, measured using von Frey filaments to probe the lumbar abdomen, was present up to 12 days after

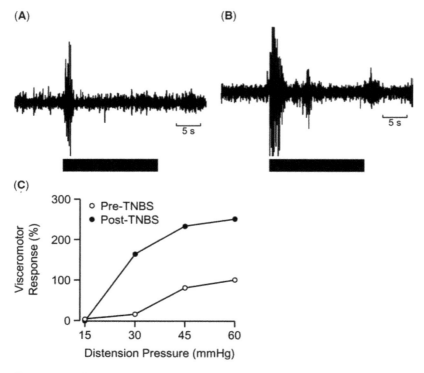

Figure 4 TNBS can produce colonic hypersensitivity in the mouse. The upper two panels show electromyographic recordings [visceromotor response (VMR)] in response to a 20-second colorectal distension (*black bar*) before (**A**) and seven days after (**B**) intracolonic installation of TNBS. Panel *C* shows the VMR recorded at four different distending pressures (15, 30, 45, and 60 mmHg for 10 seconds) before (○) and after (●) TNBS, revealing increased responses after colon inflammation (i.e., colonic hypersensitivity). Data are standardized to the 60 mmHg distending pressure measured before TNBS instillation. Data in all panels are taken from the same animal. *Source*: D.R. Robinson and G.F. Gebhart, unpublished data.

butyrate treatment (200 mM concentration). All these effects were significantly more pronounced in female rats (Fig. 5), a feature of this model that, in conjunction with the lack of visible intestinal inflammation, referred nonvisceral hypersensitivity, and colorectal hypersensitivity, may make it particularly relevant in the study of IBS. Intracolonic administration of butyrate has also been reported to prolong TNBS-induced hypersensitivity in rats (73).

THE GENITOURINARY TRACT
The Renal System

Probably the most intense of pains experienced by humans is that resulting from nephrolithiasis (kidney stones), which can be reproduced with some symptomatic accuracy in rats. With any pain model, but especially those of a potentially severe nature, the ethical implications should be addressed. A stimulus that cannot be terminated by either the experimenter or animal (e.g., by escape or an operant response) is of particular concern, and a factor that is more common in visceral than somatic pain models due to the nature of the pain. With this in mind, a number of models have been introduced to replicate nephrolithiasis, one of which is the introduction of artificial ureteral calculosis in the rat—the surgical formation of an artificial kidney stone in the ureter. Such a model was presented by Giamberardino et al. (74), and involves the injection of 20 μL dental resin cement solution into the upper-third of one ureter. The cement will harden and block the ureter, resulting in a marked hyperalgesia that is accompanied by visceral pain–related behavior (Fig. 6) not seen in sham-operated rats or rats submitted to a permanent ligature of one ureter (74,75). The threshold for vocalization to

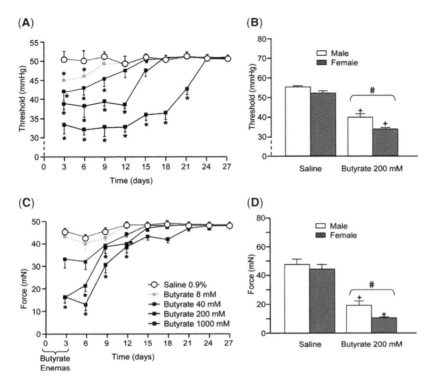

Figure 5 (*See color insert*) Intracolonic butyrate produces enhanced colonic sensitivity and referred hypersensitivity in the rat. The effect of six (twice daily) intracolonic infusions of 1 mL saline or butyrate solution (8, 40, 200, or 1000 mM) on the pressure thresholds inducing a specific behavior following colorectal distension (**A**), and on forces exerted by application of von Frey filaments to the lumbar abdominal skin required to induce a reaction (**C**). These effects are significantly enhanced in female compared to male rats (**B** and **D**). *Source*: From Ref. 56.

electrical stimulation of the *obliquus externus* muscle is decreased as the number and duration of visceral episodes increases (75). This observation may be used as a correlate of referred pain, a phenomenon that is often found in human visceral pain disorders, as is the finding that ureteral pain sensitivity varies with the estrous cycle in both humans and rats with nephrolithiasis (76). These similarities add weight to the rationale for the use of such an animal model. (It is important to note, however, that rodent vocalizations at ultrasonic frequencies are better related to painful experiences than those vocalizations at frequencies within the human aural range.) However, while useful for behavioral analysis of visceral pain, this model is not ideal for the study of neuronal activation, as the precise time at which the experimental stone forms is unknown.

An alternative model is the percutaneous ureteral obstruction model, proposed by Avelino et al. (77). Following a low-midline abdominal incision (under halothane anesthesia), a knot is loosely tied around one ureter using nylon, the ends of which are exteriorized before the wound is closed, and the animal allowed to recover. Eight days later (a time point at which spinal *c-fos* expression, evoked by the surgical procedure, is completely gone (77), and thus only the effect of the ureteral obstruction is understudy). The ends of the nylon thread can be pulled to ligate the ureter. Rats that have undergone this procedure show pain-like behavior, but only after the knot has been pulled tight (77). Note, however, that previous studies that employed an ureteral ligature found no significant muscle hyperalgesia as determined by the vocalization threshold to stimulation of the *obliquus externus* muscle (74).

The pain produced from models such as these (especially from ureteral ligation) may result from distension of the ureter central to the ligation or the renal pelvis. Distension pressures greater than 25 mmHg in the rat produce cardiovascular pseudoaffective responses likely to represent painful experiences (78), a claim strengthened by the observation that pressor responses to ureter distension are significantly, and dose-dependently, reduced following

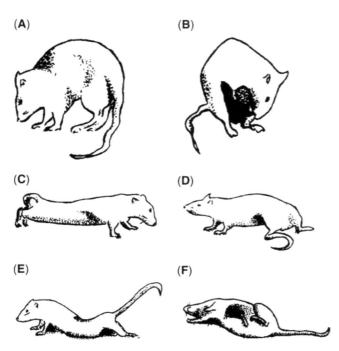

Figure 6 Behavioral phases of a visceral episode. Rats with implanted ureteral stones present graded visceral behavioral episodes as reported by Giamberardino et al. (75). These behavioral manifestations consisted of: (**A**) hump-backed position; (**B**) licking of the lower abdomen, the left flank, or both; (**C**) contraction of the left oblique musculature with inward moving of the hind limb; (**D**) stretching of the body; (**E**) squashing of the lower abdomen against the floor; (**F**) supine position with left hind limb adducted and compressed against the abdomen. *Source*: From Ref. 75.

intravenous morphine (78). Again, this model is not appropriate for behavioral studies of ureter-evoked visceral pain, as the animals are both anesthetized and under neuromuscular block. Distension of the renal pelvis in anesthetized rats produces a depressor response (a decrease in blood pressure that is restored following cessation of the distension stimulus) that is reversed by morphine administration (79).

Rather than inserting an artificial kidney stone into the ureter, other models have been developed to promote the "natural" formation of Ca^{2+} stones. The rat model of calcium oxalate nephrolithiasis (the hyperoxaluric rat, hyperoxaluria being excessive urinary excretion of oxalate, and calcium oxalate stones are the most common in clinical nephrolithiasis) involves the inclusion of 1% ethylene glycol in the drinking water and the subsequent formation of calcium oxalate deposits in the proximal tubules of the kidney (80). Enhanced calcium oxalate deposition was reported in animals given ethylene glycol while on a Mg^{2+}-deficient diet (80,81). A subsequent study used ethylene glycol with 1% ammonium chloride to produce nephrolithiasis, and this group have published the experimental conditions required to achieve different phases of calcium oxalate nephrolithiasis (82). Alternatively, there is a genetic model of hypercalciuria (excessive urinary calcium excretion), a condition that is common in patients with calcium oxalate nephrolithiasis, known as the genetic hypercalciuric rat. Hypercalciuria occurs spontaneously in a small population of rats (83), and these rats can be inbred to establish an experimental colony (84). Unfortunately, however, there are no behavioral data to indicate whether these animals exhibit behaviors suggestive of visceral pain.

Recently, two new rat models of calcium oxalate nephrolithiasis have been reported: the first, an example of a surgical intervention—small-bowel resection (85); the second, pharmacological—using a selective cyclooxygenase 2 inhibitor (86). Both these models also involve dietary modification, and it will be interesting to see if these models exhibit behavioral pain responses.

The Bladder

The most common form of bladder pain in the clinic is that caused by infection, resulting in cystitis, although overdistension of the bladder in acute urinary retention is also very painful. These two mechanisms have been employed in the design of rodent models of bladder pain, using direct distension of the bladder, or instillation of chemical or infectious agents. Environmental stressors have also been used, as stress is known to exacerbate symptoms in human disease.

Ness et al. demonstrated reliable pressor and visceromotor responses during distension of the bladder in anesthetized rats that were inhibited dose-dependently by intravenous morphine or lidocaine (87). The authors did, in addition, point out that sex differences and estrous phase will alter the variability of results—something to consider during the experimental planning phase. Distension involves the catheterization of the bladder, either intrauretherally (females) or via a small abdominal incision (males); these two methods did not alter the results obtained (87). For the study of phasic distension, compressed air is blown into the bladder through the catheter until the required distension pressure is reached, and simultaneous recordings taken from surgically implanted electrodes in the abdominal muscle (for visceromotor responses), and from cannulae in the jugular vein (heart rate) and carotid artery (blood pressure). Increasing the number of distensions performed was noted to increase the robustness of the recorded responses. Saline can be used in place of compressed air if a slow volume-controlled distension is required. Given the increasing interest in genetic manipulations of the mouse, this model has subsequently been characterized in mice, with similar results (88). As with the rat model, visceromotor responses were reproducible and attenuated by (subcutaneous) morphine; however, heart rate and respiratory responses may not be optimal pseudaffective responses with which to gauge the painful responses in this species.

The induction of cystitis, using the prodrug cyclophosphamide, is a common model of choice for assessing bladder hyper-reflexia and hypersensitivity; intraperitoneal cyclophosphamide administration results in the accumulation of its toxic metabolites (mostly acrolein) in the urine, which produce bladder irritation and inflammation. This model has the advantage that it does not require surgery, and appears to be similar to human visceral pain: cyclophosphamide-induced cystitis in humans is also painful. The behavioral effects of this model have been characterized in both rats (89) and mice (90) and show dose-related increases in pain-related behavior score (although the nature of the behaviors differed to a certain degree between species) that was reversed, again in a dose-dependent manner, by morphine. Rats and mice required one-time dosages of $\geq 100 \, \mathrm{mg \, kg^{-1}}$ cyclophosphamide to produce an increase in behavioral score compared to controls, although this was not significantly so in mice; $300 \, \mathrm{mg \, kg^{-1}}$ was required (89,90). Administration of cyclophosphamide in lower, divided doses over the course of days produces bladder hypersensitivity with reduced bladder inflammation/hemorrhagic cystitis (Lamb and Gebhart, unpublished). It should also be noted that there is a significantly faster onset of behavioral score in female rats compared to their male counterparts, although both sexes plateau to the same value (91).

The direct intravesicular application of inflammatory agents such as acetic acid, acetone, capsaicin, croton oil, mustard oil, turpentine, and xylene has been employed as an alternative strategy to investigate bladder pain in rodents. McMahon and Abel (92) investigated the effects of turpentine (25%), mustard oil (2.5%), and croton oil (2%) instilled into the bladder via the urethra. They report a number of different observations that accompanied an inflammatory response: increased protein extravasation, bladder hyper-reflexia, and patterns of somatic pain behavior resembling referred visceral hyperalgesia, among others. The authors conclude by recommending the use of turpentine as the preferred agent. First demonstrated in decerebrate rats, this model has since been modified for use in anesthetized and unanesthetized animals. Intravesicular instillation of xylene produces behavioral responses in the rat indicative of visceral pain (including evidence that the pain is referred to related somatic dermatomes) that are abolished following pelvic ganglionectomy and by prior administration of subcutaneous morphine (93,94). In this model, a narrow tube is chronically implanted into the bladder lumen under anesthesia and one end exteriorized to allow xylene administration (300 µL of 30%) 24 hours later.

Escherichia coli is the cause of the majority of urinary tract infections in humans, and intravesicular infusion of lipopolysaccharide from this bacteria, has been studied as a potential animal model of painful bladder inflammation. This, as with polyinosinic-polycytidylic acid (a synthetic ribonucleic acid) or xylene, produces inflammation in the rat bladder for at least seven days and a concomitant decrease of substance P within the bladder (95). Since substance P is involved in nociception, and xylene produces behavioral responses consistent with the presentation of visceral pain, these models may also be considered relevant for use in pain research.

There also exist rodent models that employ environmental stress to instigate bladder pain. An example is the use of restraint stress, which results in the activation of three-quarters of bladder mast cells (96), but since such studies are yet to be validated in behavioral pain models, we shall not dwell upon them here. Note, however, that environmental stress likely affects many systems and can produce other visceral complications, such as those described above for the large intestine.

The Uterus

Animal models for the study of uterine pain have focused on either distension or inflammatory protocols, although there appear to be significantly fewer studies in the current literature compared to, for example, the colon or bladder. Uterine inflammation in the anesthetized rat can be achieved by the introduction of 10% mustard oil into one uterine horn through an implanted catheter (97). A modification of this model enabled its behavioral characterization, and involved the tight ligation of one uterine horn followed by the injection of mustard oil into the lumen, with the rats subsequently allowed to recover (98). Observation of the rats over the following seven days revealed abnormal behavior similar to that reported for the ureteral calculosis model (among others) described above, in the majority (11 of 14) of rats. No sham-operated controls showed these behaviors. Muscle hypersensitivity of the lower back and flanks (a referred pain perhaps comparable to pelvic pain seen in patients) that remained after the extinction of abnormal behavior was recorded in two-thirds (six of nine) of animals studied with abnormal behavior following mustard oil instillation.

As with a number of the organ systems discussed in this chapter, distension is also used as a method to invoke uterine pain. This can be achieved by implanting, under anesthesia, a balloon (approximately 5 mm long and 1.5 mm wide) and its attached catheter into the right uterine horn of a rat. The catheter is then secured in place, and the end exteriorized (99). The balloon can be filled with water to various volumes, calibrated for each animal individually while under anesthesia. Berkley et al. used an operant response, the escape response to a noxious tail pinch, to assess the behavioral responses to uterine distensions, and found that, similar to the uterine inflammation model above, only about three-quarters (17 of 23) of the animals responded to distension (99). However, for these 17 animals, their probability of presenting an escape response increased with the distension volume. The authors point out that the magnitude of uterine distension required to elicit responses is beyond the range of any natural event, at least in nonpregnant or parturient animals; thus it is not clear how appropriate this model may be as a clinical correlate of uterine pain.

Endometriosis, while not exclusively an uterine phenomenon, is a common clinical disorder that is often accompanied by severe dysmenorrhea (painful menstruation), painful defecation, chronic pelvic pain, and dyspareunia (pain during sexual intercourse), and thus is relevant to this discussion. It is characterized by the growth of uterine tissue outside of the uterus and has been modeled in both the rat (100) and the mouse (101), although behavioral data is only currently available in the rat (102). One uterine horn is removed surgically from animals and placed in culture medium at 37°C, where it is cut into equal-sized fragments (three to six, depending upon species and laboratory), each of which is then sutured to a blood vessel in the mesentery of the small intestine, lower abdominal wall, ovary, or all three (note that autotransplants to the abdominal wall rarely produce cysts, and only small ones when they do). Following wound closure, the animal is allowed to recover. In all (five) rats that developed cysts resulting from this procedure, escape responses to vaginal distension were significantly increased postsurgery versus presurgery (102). This indication of the development of vaginal hypersensitivity was not seen in sham controls that received autotransplantation of fat, not uterine horn tissue.

The Vagina

Distension of the vaginal canal in a manner similar to that used for the uterus results in a robust and reproducible response, with the added advantage that surgical implantation of the balloon is not required; a lubricated balloon is inserted into the vaginal canal, ensuring it cannot touch the cervix even when fully inflated (99). Rats can detect low vaginal distension pressures (cf. the uterus, above), and the direct relationship between escape response probability and distension volume (99) indicates that this protocol is a useful model of visceral pain. It also suggests that both nonnoxious and noxious stimuli can be experienced, perhaps similar to that described above for organs such as the colon.

Vaginal hypersensitivity can often result from loss of ovarian function in women, and the laboratory of Berkley and coworkers have taken the same behavioral protocol described for vaginal distension (escape behavior, above) and combined it with ovariectomy to propose a rat model for the study of dyspareunia associated with ovarian function loss (103). This model appears to produce vaginal hypersensitivity in the majority, but not all, of the rats investigated, which is reversed by estrogen replacement and unaffected by the surgical manipulations associated with ovariectomy.

The Testes

We are currently unaware of any rodent models of testicular pain—indeed, there are very few models in any animal. There does exist, however, a surgical model of equine nociception, castration, in which an altered electroencephalogram is reported under anesthesia (104), and electrophysiological study of the spermatic nerve innervation of the dog testis (105) reveals that these visceral afferent fibers, such as those that innervate other viscera, are polymodal in character.

CLOSING NOTES

This is not intended to be an exhaustive account of every visceral pain model currently known; however this has been written to show the diversity of different approaches taken to further investigate the mechanisms that underlie human visceral pain–producing conditions. The purpose of developing animal models such as those we describe here is, ultimately, to further our knowledge of the processes and mechanisms of visceral pain and visceral hypersensitivity that characterize human disease, and develop strategies to treat the pain and hypersensitivity. An animal model should, therefore, exhibit symptoms that reliably match some or all of those in the human disorder—not just in appearance, but insofar as possible also in severity, temporal resolution, and response to current therapies. This is particularly difficult in diseases for which the underlying cause is unknown (e.g., functional disorders such as IBS), but the creation of models to study processes, mediators, and molecules contributing to an underlying characteristic of the disease or syndrome (i.e., visceral hypersensitivity) may lead to new hypotheses and avenues of possibility that, with further research, help to point the way forward. As we have discussed, the validity of any one particular animal model must be assessed in relation to the purpose for which it is being used; it is important for the experimenter to choose the most appropriate model according to the aims of their investigation, keeping in mind the ethical implications of any such study.

REFERENCES

1. Cervero F, Connell LA, Lawson SN. Somatic and visceral primary afferents in the lower thoracic dorsal root ganglia of the cat. J Comp Neurol 1984; 228(3):422–431.
2. Chandler MJ, Zhang J, Foreman RD. Vagal, sympathetic and somatic sensory inputs to upper cervical (C1-C3) spinothalamic tract neurons in monkeys. J Neurophysiol 1996; 76(4):2555–2567.
3. Randich A, Gebhart GF. Vagal afferent modulation of nociception. Brain Res Brain Res Rev 1992; 17(2):77–99.
4. Cervero F. Visceral pain–central sensitisation. Gut 2000; 47(suppl 4):iv56–iv57.
5. Drewes AM, Gregersen H, Arendt-Nielsen L. Experimental pain in gastroenterology: a reappraisal of human studies. Scand J Gastroenterol 2003; 38(11):1115–1130.
6. Ness TJ, Gebhart GF. Colorectal distension as a noxious visceral stimulus: physiologic and pharmacologic characterization of pseudaffective reflexes in the rat. Brain Res 1988; 450(1–2):153–169.
7. Larsson MH, Rapp L, Lindström E. Effect of DSS-induced colitis on visceral sensitivity to colorectal distension in mice. Neurogastroenterol Motil 2006; 18(2):144–152.

8. Guzman F, Braun C, Lim RKS. Visceral pain and the pseudaffective response to intra-arterial injection of bradykinin and other algesic agents. Arch Int Pharmacodyn Ther 1962; 136(3–4):353–384.
9. Schaefer S, Valente RA, Laslett LJ, Longhurst JC. Cardiac reflex effects of intracoronary bradykinin in humans. J Investig Med 1996; 44(4):160–167.
10. Gaspardone A, Crea F, Tomai F, et al. Effect of acetylsalicylate on cardiac and muscular pain induced by intracoronary and intra-arterial infusion of bradykinin in humans. J Am Coll Cardiol 1999; 34(1):216–222.
11. Euchner-Wamser I, Meller ST, Gebhart GF. A model of cardiac nociception in chronically instrumented rats: behavioral and electrophysiological effects of pericardial administration of algogenic substances. Pain 1994; 58(1):117–128.
12. Meller ST, Gebhart GF. A critical review of the afferent pathways and the potential chemical mediators involved in cardiac pain. Neuroscience 1992; 48(3):501–524.
13. Cervero F. Sensory innervation of the viscera: peripheral basis of visceral pain. Physiol Rev 1994; 74(1):95–138.
14. Undem BJ, Chuaychoo B, Lee MG, Weinreich D, Myers AC, Kollarik M. Subtypes of vagal afferent C-fibres in guinea-pig lungs.
    J Physiol 2004; 556(Pt 3):905–917.
15. Hummel T, Sengupta JN, Meller ST, Gebhart GF. Responses of T2-4 spinal cord neurons to irritation of the lower airways in the rat. Am J Physiol 1997; 273(3 Pt 2):R1147–R1157.
16. Loomis CW, Yao D, Bieger D. Characterization of an esophagocardiovascular reflex in the rat. Am J Physiol 1997; 272(6 Pt 2):R1783–R1791.
17. Jou CJ, Farber JP, Qin C, Foreman RD. Convergent pathways for cardiac - and esophageal-somatic motor reflexes in rats. Auton Neurosci 2002; 99(2):70–77.
18. Schuligoi R, Jocič M, Heinemann Á, Schöninkle E, Pabst MA, Holzer P. Gastric acid-evoked c-fos messenger RNA expression in rat brainstem is signaled by capsaicin-resistant vagal afferents. Gastroenterology 1998; 115(3):649–660.
19. Takagi K, Okabe S, Saziki R. A new method for the production of chronic gastric ulcer in rats and the effect of several drugs on its healing. Jpn J Pharmacol 1969; 19(3):418–426.
20. Okabe S, Roth JL, Pfeiffer CJ. A method for experimental, penetrating gastric and duodenal ulcers in rats. Observations on normal healing. Am J Dig Dis 1971; 16(3):277–284.
21. Okabe S, Tsukimi Y, Nishimura H. A new and simple method to produce gastric ulcers, chemical antrectomy and corpectomy in rats (acetic acid ulcer, type III). Digestion 1991; 49(suppl 1):47.
22. Tsukimi Y, Okabe S. Validity of kissing gastric ulcers induced in rats for screening of antiulcer drugs. J Gastroenterol Hepatol 1994; 9(suppl 1):S60–S65.
23. Kang YM, Lamb K, Gebhart GF, Bielefeldt K. Experimentally induced ulcers and gastric sensory-motor function in rats. Am J Physiol Gastrointest Liver Physiol 2005; 288(2):G284–G291.
24. Ozaki N, Bielefeldt K, Sengupta JN, Gebhart GF. Models of gastric hyperalgesia in the rat. Am J Physiol Gastrointest Liver Physiol 2002; 283(3):G666–G676.
25. Rouzade ML, Fioramonti J, Buéno L. A model for evaluation of gastric sensitivity in awake rats. Neurogastroenterol Motil 1998; 10(2):157–163.
26. Gillingham MB, Clark MD, Dahly EM, Krugner-Higby LA, Ney DM. A comparison of two opioid analgesics for relief of visceral pain induced by intestinal resection in rats. Contemp Top Lab Anim Sci 2001; 40(1):21–26.
27. Holzer-Petsche U, Brodacz B. Traction on the mesentery as a model of visceral nociception. Pain 1999; 80(1–2):319–328.
28. Colburn RW, Coombs DW, Degnan CC, Rogers LL. Mechanical visceral pain model: chronic intermittent intestinal distention in the rat. Physiol Behav 1989; 45(1):191–197.
29. Feng Y, Cui M, Al-Chaer ED, Willis WD. Epigastric antinociception by cervical dorsal column lesions in rats. Anesthesiology 1998; 89(2):411–420.
30. Nijsen MA, Ongenae NG, Coulie B, Meulemans AL. Telemetric animal model to evaluate visceral pain in the freely moving rat. Pain 2003; 105(1–2):115–123.
31. Stam R, van Laar TJ, Wiegant VM. Physiological and behavioural responses to duodenal pain in freely moving rats. Physiol Behav 2004; 81(1):163–169.
32. Takács T, Czakó L, Jármay K, Farkas G Jr, Mándi Y, Lonovics J. Cytokine level changes in L-arginine-induced acute pancreatitis in rat. Acta Physiol Hung 1996; 84(2):147–156.
33. Winston JH, Toma H, Shenoy M, et al. Acute pancreatitis results in referred mechanical hypersensitivity and neuropeptide up-regulation that can be suppressed by the protein kinase inhibitor k252a. J Pain 2003; 4(6):329–337.
34. Wick EC, Hoge SG, Grahn SW, et al. Transient receptor potential vanilloid 1, calcitonin gene-related peptide, and substance P mediate nociception in acute pancreatitis. Am J Physiol Gastrointest Liver Physiol 2006; 290(5).
35. Sparmann G, Merkord J, Jäschke A, et al. Pancreatic fibrosis in experimental pancreatitis induced by dibutyltin dichloride. Gastroenterology 1997; 112(5):1664–1672.
36. Vera-Portocarrero LP, Lu Y, Westlund KN. Nociception in persistent pancreatitis in rats: effects of morphine and neuropeptide alterations. Anesthesiology 2003; 98(2):474–484.

37. Puig-Diví V, Molero X, Salas A, Guarner F, Guarner L, Malagelada JR. Induction of chronic pancreatic disease by trinitrobenzene sulfonic acid infusion into rat pancreatic ducts. Pancreas 1996; 13(4):417–424.
38. Hoogerwerf WA, Shenoy M, Winston JH, Xiao SY, He Z, Pasricha PJ. Trypsin mediates nociception via the proteinase-activated receptor 2: a potentially novel role in pancreatic pain. Gastroenterology 2004; 127(3):883–891.
39. Winston JH, He ZJ, Shenoy M, Xiao SY, Pasricha PJ. Molecular and behavioral changes in nociception in a novel rat model of chronic pancreatitis for the study of pain. Pain 2005; 117(1–2): 214–222.
40. Zhang L, Zhang X, Westlund KN. Restoration of spontaneous exploratory behaviors with an intrathecal NMDA receptor antagonist or a PKC inhibitor in rats with acute pancreatitis. Pharmacol Biochem Behav 2004; 77(1):145–153.
41. Houghton AK, Kadura S, Westlund KN. Dorsal column lesions reverse the reduction of homecage activity in rats with pancreatitis. Neuroreport 1997; 8(17):3795–3800.
42. Kamp EH, Jones RC III, Tillman SR, Gebhart GF. Quantitative assessment and characterization of visceral nociception and hyperalgesia in mice. Am J Physiol Gastrointest Liver Physiol 2003; 284(3):G434–G444.
43. Larsson M, Arvidsson S, Ekman C, Bayati A. A model for chronic quantitative studies of colorectal sensitivity using balloon distension in conscious mice—effects of opioid receptor agonists. Neurogastroenterol Motil 2003; 15(4):371–381.
44. McLean PG, Picard C, Garcia-Villar R, Moré J, Fioramonti J, Buéno L. Effects of nematode infection on sensitivity to intestinal distension: role of tachykinin NK2 receptors. Eur J Pharmacol 1997; 337(2–3):279–282.
45. Al-Chaer ED, Kawasaki M, Pasricha PJ. A new model of chronic visceral hypersensitivity in adult rats induced by colon irritation during postnatal development. Gastroenterology 2000; 119(5): 1276–1285.
46. Coutinho SV, Plotsky PM, Sablad M, et al. Neonatal maternal separation alters stress-induced responses to viscerosomatic nociceptive stimuli in rat. Am J Physiol Gastrointest Liver Physiol 2002; 282(2):G307–G316.
47. Barreau F, Ferrier L, Fioramonti J, Buéno L. Neonatal maternal deprivation triggers long term alterations in colonic epithelial barrier and mucosal immunity in rats. Gut 2004; 53(4):501–506.
48. Williams CL, Villar RG, Peterson JM, Burks TF. Stress-induced changes in intestinal transit in the rat: a model for irritable bowel syndrome. Gastroenterology 1988; 94(3):611–621.
49. Morrow NS, Garrick T. Effects of intermittent tail shock or water avoidance on proximal colonic motor contractility in rats. Physiol Behav 1997; 62(2):233–239.
50. Gunter WD, Shepard JD, Foreman RD, Myers DA, Greenwood-Van Meerveld B. Evidence for visceral hypersensitivity in high-anxiety rats. Physiol Behav 2000; 69(3):379–382.
51. Kühn R, Löhler J, Rennick D, Rajewsky K, Müller W. Interleukin-10-deficient mice develop chronic enterocolitis. Cell 1993; 75(2):263–274.
52. Gebhart GF, Ness TJ. Central mechanisms of visceral pain. Can J Physiol Pharmacol 1991; 69(5): 627–634.
53. Ness TJ. Models of visceral nociception. ILAR J 1999; 40(3):119–128.
54. MacPherson BR, Pfeiffer CJ. Experimental production of diffuse colitis in rats. Digestion 1978; 17(2):135–150.
55. Verdú EF, Bercik P, Verma-Gandhu M, et al. Specific probiotic therapy attenuates antibiotic induced visceral hypersensitivity in mice. Gut 2006; 55(2):182–190.
56. Bourdu S, Dapoigny M, Chapuy E, et al. Rectal instillation of butyrate provides a novel clinically relevant model of noninflammatory colonic hypersensitivity in rats. Gastroenterology 2005; 128(7):1996–2008.
57. Laird JMA, Martinez-Caro L, Garcia-Nicas E, Cervero F. A new model of visceral pain and referred hyperalgesia in the mouse. Pain 2001; 92:335–342.
58. Okayasu I, Hatakeyama S, Yamada M, Ohkusa T, Inagaki Y, Nakaya R. A novel method in the induction of reliable experimental acute and chronic ulcerative colitis in mice. Gastroenterology 1990; 98(3):694–702.
59. Botella A, Fioramonti J, Eeckhout C, Buéno L. Intracolonic glycerol induces abdominal contractions in rats: role of 5-HT3 receptors. Fundam Clin Pharmacol 1998; 12(6):619–623.
60. Al-Chaer ED, Westlund KN, Willis WD. Potentiation of thalamic responses to colorectal distension by visceral inflammation. Neuroreport 1996; 7(10):1635–1639.
61. Morris GP, Beck PL, Herridge MS, Depew WT, Szewczuk MR, Wallace JL. Hapten-induced model of chronic inflammation and ulceration in the rat colon. Gastroenterology 1989; 96(3):795–803.
62. Ness TJ, Gebhart GF. Inflammation potentiates responses to colorectal distension in the rat. Abstr Soc Neurosci 1989; 15:847.
63. Coutinho SV, Meller ST, Gebhart GF. Intracolonic zymosan produces visceral hyperalgesia in the rat that is mediated by spinal NMDA and non-NMDA receptors. Brain Res 1996; 736(1–2):7–15.
64. Beagley KW, Black CA, Elson CO. Strain differences in susceptibility to TNBS-induced colitis. Gastroenterology 1991; 100(5 Part 2):A560.

65. Chin KW, Barrett KE. Mast cells are not essential to inflammation in murine model of colitis. Dig Dis Sci 1994; 39(3):513–525.

66. Wallace JL, Whittle BJR, Boughton-Smith NK. Prostaglandin protection of rat colonic mucosa from damage induced by ethanol. Dig Dis Sci 1985; 30(9):866–876.

67. Keates AC, Castagliuolo I, Cruickshank WW, et al. Interleukin 16 is up-regulated in Crohn's disease and participates in TNBS colitis in mice. Gastroenterology 2000; 119(4):972–982.

68. Mizoguchi A, Mizoguchi E, Bhan AK. Immune networks in animal models of inflammatory bowel disease. Inflamm Bowel Dis 2003; 9(4):246–259.

69. Morteau O, Hachet T, Caussette M, Buéno L. Experimental colitis alters visceromotor response to colorectal distension in awake rats. Dig Dis Sci 1994; 39(6):1239–1248.

70. Fioramonti J, Gaultier E, Toulouse M, Sanger GJ, Buéno L. Intestinal anti-nociceptive behaviour of NK3 receptor antagonism in conscious rats: evidence to support a peripheral mechanism of action. Neurogastroenterol Motil 2003; 15(4):363–369.

71. Messaoudi M, Desor D, Grasmück V, Joyeux M, Langlois A, Roman FJ. Behavioral evaluation of visceral pain in a rat model of colonic inflammation. Neuroreport 1999; 10(5):1137–1141.

72. Beyak MJ, Ramji N, Krol KM, Kawaja MD, Vanner SJ. Two TTX-resistant Na+ currents in mouse colonic dorsal root ganglia neurons and their role in colitis-induced hyperexcitability. Am J Physiol Gastrointest Liver Physiol 2004; 287(4):G845–G855.

73. Tarrerias AL, Millecamps M, Alloui A, et al. Short-chain fatty acid enemas fail to decrease colonic hypersensitivity and inflammation in TNBS-induced colonic inflammation in rats. Pain 2002; 100(1–2):91–97.

74. Giamberardino MA, Vecchiet L, Albe-Fessard D. Comparison of the effects of ureteral calculosis and occlusion on muscular sensitivity to painful stimulation in rats. Pain 1990; 43(2):227–234.

75. Giamberardino MA, Valente R, de Bigontina P, Vecchiet L. Artificial ureteral calculosis in rats: behavioural characterization of visceral pain episodes and their relationship with referred lumbar muscle hyperalgesia. Pain 1995; 61(3):459–469.

76. Giamberardino MA, Affaitati G, Valente R, Iezzi S, Vecchiet L. Changes in visceral pain reactivity as a function of estrous cycle in female rats with artificial ureteral calculosis. Brain Res 1997; 744(1–2):234–238.

77. Avelino A, Cruz F, Coimbra A. Sites of renal pain processing in the rat spinal cord. A c-fos study using a percutaneous method to perform ureteral obstruction. J Auton Nerv Syst 1997; 67(1–2):60–66.

78. Roza C, Laird JMA. Pressor responses to distension of the ureter in anaesthetised rats: characterisation of a model of acute visceral pain. Neurosci Lett 1995; 198(1):9–12.

79. Brasch H, Zetler G. Caerulein and morphine in a model of visceral pain. Effects on the hypotensive response to renal pelvis distension in the rat. Naunyn Schmiedebergs Arch Pharmacol 1982; 319(2):161–167.

80. Rushton HG, Spector M, Rodgers AL, Hughson M, Magura CE. Developmental aspects of calcium oxalate tubular deposits and calculi induced in rat kidneys. Invest Urol 1981; 19(1):52–57.

81. Rushton HG, Spector M. Effects of magnesium deficiency on intratubular calcium oxalate formation and crystalluria in hyperoxaluric rats. J Urol 1982; 127(3):598–604.

82. Yamaguchi S, Wiessner JH, Hasegawa AT, Hung LY, Mandel GS, Mandel NS. Study of a rat model for calcium oxalate crystal formation without severe renal damage in selected conditions. Int J Urol 2005; 12(3):290–298.

83. Favus MJ, Coe FL. Evidence for spontaneous hypercalciuria in the rat. Miner Electrolyte Metab 1979; 2:150–154.

84. Bushinsky DA, Favus MJ. Mechanism of hypercalciuria in genetic hypercalciuric rats. Inherited defect in intestinal calcium transport. J Clin Invest 1988; 82(5):1585–1591.

85. O'Connor RC, Worcester EM, Evan AP, et al. Nephrolithiasis and nephrocalcinosis in rats with small bowel resection. Urol Res 2005; 33(2):105–115.

86. Jeong BC, Park MY, Kwak C, Kim BS, Kim JI, Kim HH. An animal model of calcium oxalate urolithiasis based on a cyclooxygenase 2 selective inhibitor. Urol Res 2005; 33(6):453–459.

87. Ness TJ, Lewis-Sides A, Castroman P. Characterization of pressor and visceromotor reflex responses to bladder distention in rats: sources of variability and effect of analgesics. J Urol 2001; 165(3):968–974.

88. Ness TJ, Elhefni H. Reliable visceromotor responses are evoked by noxious bladder distention in mice. J Urol 2004; 171(4):1704–1708.

89. Boucher M, Meen M, Codron JP, Coudore F, Kemeny JL, Eschalier A. Cyclophosphamide-induced cystitis in freely-moving conscious rats: behavioral approach to a new model of visceral pain. J Urol 2000; 164(1):203–208.

90. Olivar T, Laird JMA. Cyclophosphamide cystitis in mice: behavioural characterisation and correlation with bladder inflammation. Eur J Pain 1999; 3(2):141–149.

91. Bon K, Lantéri-Minet M, Menétrey D, Berkley KJ. Sex, time-of-day and estrous variations in behavioral and bladder histological consequences of cyclophosphamide-induced cystitis in rats. Pain 1997; 73(3):423–429.

92. McMahon SB, Abel C. A model for the study of visceral pain states: chronic inflammation of the chronic decerebrate rat urinary bladder by irritant chemicals. Pain 1987; 28(1):109–127.

93. Abelli L, Conte B, Somma V, et al. The contribution of capsaicin-sensitive sensory nerves to xylene-induced visceral pain in conscious, freely moving rats. Naunyn Schmiedebergs Arch Pharmacol 1988; 337(5):545–551.
94. Abelli L, Conte B, Somma V, Maggi CA, Giuliani S, Meli A. A method for studying pain arising from the urinary bladder in conscious, freely-moving rats. J Urol 1989; 141(1):148–151.
95. Luber-Narod J, Austin-Ritchie T, Hollins C III, et al. Role of substance P in several models of bladder inflammation. Urol Res 1997; 25(6):395–399.
96. Spanos C, Pang X, Ligris K, et al. Stress-induced bladder mast cell activation: implications for interstitial cystitis. J Urol 1997; 157(2):669–672.
97. Wesselmann U, Lai J. Mechanisms of referred visceral pain: uterine inflammation in the adult virgin rat results in neurogenic plasma extravasation in the skin. Pain 1997; 73(3):309–317.
98. Wesselmann U, Czakanski PP, Affaitati G, Giamberardino MA. Uterine inflammation as a noxious visceral stimulus: behavioral characterization in the rat. Neurosci Lett 1998; 246(2):73–76.
99. Berkley KJ, Wood E, Scofield SL, Little M. Behavioral responses to uterine or vaginal distension in the rat. Pain 1995; 61(1):121–131.
100. Vernon MW, Wilson EA. Studies on the surgical induction of endometriosis in the rat. Fertil Steril 1985; 44(5):684–694.
101. Cummings AM, Metcalf JL. Induction of endometriosis in mice: a new model sensitive to estrogen. Reprod Toxicol 1995; 9(3):233–238.
102. Berkley KJ, Cason A, Jacobs H, Bradshaw H, Wood E. Vaginal hyperalgesia in a rat model of endometriosis. Neurosci Lett 2001; 306(3):185–188.
103. Bradshaw HB, Berkley KJ. Estrogen replacement reverses ovariectomy-induced vaginal hyperalgesia in the rat. Maturitas 2002; 41(2):157–165.
104. Murrell JC, Johnson CB, White KL, Taylor PM, Haberham ZL, Waterman-Pearson AE. Changes in the EEG during castration in horses and ponies anaesthetized with halothane. Vet Anaesth Analg 2003; 30(3):138–146.
105. Kumazawa T, Mizumura K. The polymodal receptors in the testis of dog. Brain Res 1977; 136(3):553–558.

9

Measuring Pain and Hyperalgesia in Persistent Pain Conditions with a Special Emphasis on Irritable Bowel Syndrome

Donald D. Price
Departments of Oral Surgery and Neuroscience, University of Florida Colleges of Dentistry, Public Health and Health Professions, and Medicine, and McKnight Brain Institute, Gainesville, Florida, U.S.A.

Michael E. Robinson
Department of Clinical and Health Psychology, University of Florida Colleges of Dentistry, Public Health and Health Professions, and Medicine, and McKnight Brain Institute, Gainesville, Florida, U.S.A.

G. Nicholas Verne
Department of Medicine, University of Florida Colleges of Dentistry, Public Health and Health Professions, and Medicine, and McKnight Brain Institute, Gainesville, Florida, U.S.A.

INTRODUCTION

The psychophysics of pain has an important role in the understanding of the neurophysiology of pain and for providing a scientific basis for modern methods of pain measurement and assessment. Psychophysical methods of sensory testing also have a pivotal role in understanding the mechanisms of pathophysiological pain wherein pain is an integral component of the disease itself and not merely a symptom. The main objective of this chapter is to explain how the combination of simple methods of direct scaling and sensory testing can be used to identify some of the mechanisms of pathophysiological pain. Indeed, this approach has long been anticipated in classical work on this subject (1). Psychophysical methods of direct scaling in combination with sensory tests of abnormal or enhanced pain mechanisms are useful in characterizing different types of persistent and intermittent pain conditions, including different types of neuropathic pain such as complex regional pain syndrome (CRPS), fibromyalgia pain, and irritable bowel syndrome (IBS) pain. In this chapter, we discuss human tests of pain responsiveness in patients with these conditions, with the aims of showing how such tests may be useful in characterizing hyperalgesia, allodynia, severity of pain states, and the mechanisms that serve them. This approach is likely to be useful in aiding diagnoses and ultimately matching treatments to pain syndromes.

GENERAL CONSIDERATIONS CONCERNING PAIN MEASUREMENT

All methods of pain measurement share a common goal of accurately representing the human pain experience. Threshold measures of pain sensitivity are limited in that they do not assess changes in pain sensitivity that may occur over a wide range of noxious stimulus intensities. Although it is recognized that multiple methods of sensory testing are useful, including threshold and discrimination measures, this chapter will focus on direct scaling methods because they have the capacity to assess a wide range of responses to threshold and suprathreshold intensities, a characteristic that is most relevant to clinical pain assessment.

Visual Analog Scales
Visual Analog Scales Satisfy Several Criteria for Optimum Pain Measurement
Direct scales include numerical rating scales (NRSs), verbal rating scales (VRSs), verbal descriptor scales, magnitude estimation, and visual analog scales (VASs). VAS has emerged as having psychometric properties that are superior to other pain scaling methods just mentioned because they fulfill multiple criteria for ideal pain measurement and assessment (2,3).

These criteria include ratio scale properties (4–7), high test–retest reliability and repeatability (8), the capacity to detect small differences (8), internally consistent measures of clinical and experimental pain (5,6,9), sensitivity to variables that increase or decrease pain (7,10), capacity to measure multiple dimensions of pain (5,6,9,11), strong correlation with measures of pain-related activity in the human brain (12), detection of individual differences in pain sensitivity (12), and in the case of mechanical or electronic VAS, simplicity and ease of use (2,13). Probably as a consequence of these characteristics, the VAS is the most commonly used single scale in human research studies of pain. For example, among 121 human studies that used single pain scales and that were published in Pain in 2004, 49% used VAS, 36% used NRSs, 8% used VRSs, and 6.6% used another type of rating scale. The latter category included three studies that used faces scales for children. Similar proportions are present in other years and other pain journals.

Advantages of Combining Visual Analog Scale Measures with Sensory Tests

It is not widely recognized that the VAS has measurement properties that are superior to other commonly used scales such as the NRS. Unlike VAS, the 11 point-NRS definitely does not have ratio scale properties and has no distinct zero point [Fig. 4 of Ref. 13]. Compared to VAS ratings, NRS ratings have been shown to be artificially higher for both clinical and experimental pain (13). The notion that NRS ratings can easily substitute for VAS ratings because they are highly correlated with each other is very misguided. For example, both are monotonic functions of heat stimulus intensity and are likely to be highly correlated, yet the 11 point-NRS stimulus–response curve is displaced above the VAS curve. Only the latter reflects accurate ratios or proportions of pain intensity and appears to have a true zero point (3,13). Given the superior psychometric characteristics of VAS, it is astonishing that NRS has been recommended over other pain scales, including VAS, in clinical research and practice (14,15). Because of their measurement advantages, studies that use mechanical VAS to conduct sensory tests on patients with neuropathic pain, fibromyalgia syndrome, and IBS pain are emphasized in this chapter. Special emphasis will be placed on measuring and characterizing IBS pain.

PSYCHOPHYSICAL CHARACTERIZATION OF PATHOPHYSIOLOGICAL PAIN

The psychophysical attributes of pain that relate to pathophysiological pain have been characterized using several measurement methods, including direct scaling methods. These include thresholds for pain, adaptation, noxious stimulus intensity–pain intensity relationships, discriminability, and temporal and spatial summation of suprathreshold pain. Here we focus on a few tests that we consider to be simple and yet the most useful in characterizing hyperalgesia and allodynia in pain patients, including neuropathic pain, fibromyalgia, and IBS patients. Responses to these tests have been useful in characterizing the variability in severity of these pain conditions and their central pathophysiological mechanisms.

Direct Ratings of Noxious Temperatures in Patients with Pathophysiological Pain
Testing Heat Hyperalgesia in Complex Regional Pain Syndrome Patients

A reliable and valid test of heat allodynia and hyperalgesia consists of patients rating pain intensity on VAS in response to a range of cutaneous heat stimuli that includes those above and below normal pain threshold, evoked by either immersion of a hand or foot into heated water baths or ramp-and-hold contact heat stimuli delivered to the skin in different body areas. Ramp-and-hold heat stimuli have two distinct advantages. They can be adapted to predominately stimulate A-delta (2–10°C/sec) or C (<2°C/sec) heat sensitive nociceptors (16). The latter is more directly relevant to persistent clinical pain. The second is that they can be applied to many places on the body surface, both proximal and distal to sources of ongoing pain (e.g., hand and forearm of CRPS patients whose pain includes these areas).

Examples of heat-induced hyperalgesia are shown in Figure 1, which presents data from a CRPS patient (17). CRPS, formerly termed reflex sympathetic dystrophy, is characterized by regional pain (spontaneous and evoked) and other sensory changes following a physically traumatic event and the pain is associated with changes in skin color, skin temperature, abnormal sweating, edema, and sometimes motor abnormalities (18). When tested with ramp-and-hold heat stimuli, CRPS patients often though not always rate this experimental pain as

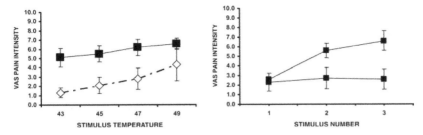

Figure 1 Pain intensity (visual analog scale) ratings of a patient who had both heat-induced hyperalgesia (*left graph*) and temporal summation of mechanical allodynia (*right graph*) to repeated von Frey filament stimulation. Note that temporal summation occurred with stimuli delivered one per three seconds but not one per 5 seconds (*right graph*).

much more intense when the stimuli are applied to skin areas proximal to the spontaneously painful body regions. These enhanced perceptions of pain occurred throughout a wide range of five second stimulus intensities (43–49°C) presented in random order. However, the differences between the patients' normal responses to pain, obtained from stimuli delivered to homologous contralateral nonpathological zones, and abnormal responses to pain, obtained from stimuli delivered to pathological zones, were greatest toward the lower end of the stimulus range, 43°C to 45°C, as exemplified in Figure 1. This pattern of increased responsiveness is remarkably similar to that obtained for C-polymodal nociceptive afferents and for human ratings of heat-induced pain after heat-induced injury of the skin (19,20).

Both in the case of CRPS and skin injury, the hyperalgesia is likely to be dynamically maintained by tonic input from primary nociceptive afferents, particularly C-nociceptive afferents (21). However, in the case of CRPS, tonic input is more likely to be related to peripheral ectopic foci of peripheral nerve axons because the skin is not injured. Based on the curves presented in Figure 1, it is also likely that the thermal threshold for pain was lowered in this patient thereby reflecting heat allodynia. Cold allodynia also has been shown to be a common characteristic of CRPS patients (19).

Heat Allodynia and Hyperalgesia in Fibromyalgia Patients

There are pain conditions that, unlike CRPS described above, are characterized by diffuse pains and hyperalgesia over large areas of body. The ability to use the same patients as their own control in establishing hyperalgesia and allodynia is therefore more challenging in these patient populations. An alternative approach is to compare their ratings of experimental heat stimuli to groups of age- and sex-matched control subjects.

For example, heat hyperalgesia has been shown to be a prevalent characteristic of fibromyalgia (22–25). Fibromyalgia is a common disease, prevalent in approximately 2% to 10% of the general population and it occurs predominately in females (26). The pathogenesis of fibromyalgia is unknown, although abnormal concentration of central nervous system (CNS) neuropeptides and alterations of the hypothalamic-pituitary-adrenal axis have been described (27,28). Fibromyalgia is a chronic pain syndrome, characterized by generalized pain, tender points, disturbed sleep, and pronounced fatigue. Pain in fibromyalgia is consistently felt in the musculature and may be related to sensitization of CNS pain pathways. Fibromyalgia patients also have heat allodynia/hyperalgesia when tested with ramp-and-hold skin temperatures, as shown in Figure 2 (3). However, unlike CRPS patients, fibromyalgia and IBS patients are more likely to have diffuse pain within many body areas. Thus, their heat hyperalgesia/ allodynia has been established by comparing their pain ratings to those of age- and sex-matched control subjects (Fig. 2).

Temporal Summations of Second Pain in Normal Control Subjects and Fibromyalgia Patients
Second Pain

A brief noxious stimulus, such as a heat tap at 51°C or percutaneous electrical stimulation of A and C axons, can evoke two distinct pain sensations called, "first" and "second" pain (22,29–31). First pain is usually an immediate sharp sensation, whereas second pain occurs

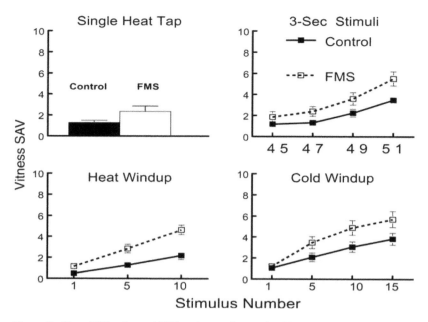

Figure 2 Mean VAS ratings of FMS and normal control subjects to single heat taps (*top left*), graded three-second heat stimuli (*top right*), repeated thenar heat taps (*bottom left*), and repeated cold taps (*bottom right*). *Abbreviations*: VAS, visual analog scale. *Source*: From Ref. 3.

about a second later and can be a dull, throbbing, or burning sensation depending on the type of stimulus used to evoke it. Second pain often lingers well beyond the brief stimulus that evokes it. VAS scaling methods have been used to analyze the temporal summation found in second pain (30,31). Examples of temporal summation of second pain in normal subjects and fibromyalgia patients are shown in Figure 2. These examples include responses to repeated heat and cold taps, both of which evoke reliable temporal summation. Among normal pain-free subjects, C-fiber–evoked second pain increases in intensity whenever the interstimulus interval is three seconds or less but does not change when the interstimulus interval is five seconds or greater. This slow temporal summation occurs even when the stimulus moves from spot to spot during the train of heat pulses, and even after total blockade of the peripheral impulses in the A axons necessary for first pain (29,30). Temporal summation of second pain usually results in a continuous burning pain after several stimuli and this burning pain often continues for several seconds after termination of the stimuli. This "after-sensation" has long been noted to be a common feature of pain evoked by stimulation of C nociceptive afferent neurons (1,22,24). Temporal summation of second pain reflects early mechanisms that lead to central sensitization, secondary hyperalgesia, and persistent pain states. For example, dorsal horn neurons show temporal summation or "windup" in response to repeated C-fiber stimulation (32,33). There are numerous parallels between "windup" and temporal summation of second pain and there is considerable evidence that enhanced second pain reflects activation of N-methyl-D-aspartate (NMDA) receptors as well as intracellular mechanisms of sensitization in the spinal dorsal horn (6,31,34).

Enhanced Second Pain Summation in Fibromyalgia Patients
In comparison to normal control subjects, fibromyalgia patients respond to repeated heat taps with enhanced slow temporal summation and more prolonged after-sensations, as shown in Figure 2 (3,22,25,35). Summation also occurs at a lower stimulus frequency (i.e., 0.2 Hz) in fibromyalgia patients, similar to that in patients with temporomandibular joint disease (36). Furthermore, once it occurs, enhanced second pain can be maintained by very low frequencies of stimulation in fibromyalgia but not in normal control subjects (24). This characteristic is parallel to that of "windup" of dorsal horn neuronal responses (32). Once "windup" occurs and reaches a plateau, only very low frequencies (e.g., one C-fiber volley every 10 seconds) are

required to maintain enhanced responsiveness. The enhanced responsiveness is accompanied by expanded receptive fields of dorsal horn neurons, which reflect a condition wherein a given cutaneous stimulus (e.g., 45°C) activates more dorsal horn neurons than would otherwise occur (32). All of these changes are likely to be integral to early mechanisms of central sensitization, allodynia and secondary hyperalgesia.

Relationships Between Temporal Summation of Second Pain and Clinical Pain
Some aspects of temporal summation of second pain appear integrally related to patients' ongoing clinical pain. For example, enhanced ratings of aftersensations that occur after temporal summation are salient predictors of fibromyalgia patients' ratings of clinical pain, accounting for 27% of the variance in ratings of clinical pain (23). Tender point count and pain-related emotions accounted for about 22% of the remaining variance. The approach of using controlled stimuli to characterize the basis for allodynia and hyperalgesia as well as the severity of patients' ongoing "spontaneous" clinical pain is one that has been applied to several types of pain conditions, including fibromyalgia, IBS, and CRPS.

It is also important to recognize that characteristics of temporal summation of second pain just described have been observed in several different laboratories using different methods. Temporal summation of second pain occurs in response to repeated cutaneous electric shocks before and after blockade of myelinated axons (29). It occurs in response to repeated brief heat pulses of 51°C or repeated 53°C heat taps to the skin (6,30,31,36,37). Similar to heat pulses or taps, temporal summation occurs with repetitive stimulation of muscle nociceptive afferents and is greatly enhanced in fibromyalgia (23,34). Both muscle- and heat-induced temporal summation can be reduced by NMDA receptor antagonists such as dextromethorphan (34). However it is more evident that heat-induced temporal summation reflects secondary hyperalgesia in fibromyalgia patients because fibromyalgia patients do not report ongoing burning pain from the skin and they have areas of heat hyperalgesia that are remote from body areas reported as painful (22,23,34). Temporal summation also occurs with repetitive stimulation of visceral nociceptive afferents (38).

Tests of Mechanical Allodynia
A-Beta and High-Threshold Mechanical Allodynia
Studies of neuropathic pain patients have shown pathological conditions characterized by zones of skin in which heat hyperalgesia is present in some patients, and larger zones in which mechanical hyperalgesia and/or allodynia is present in all or most patients (17,21,37). Two distinct types of mechanical allodynia have been characterized in neuropathic pain patients. The first is termed low threshold A-beta allodynia (17,37). Its presence is based on several lines of evidence. First, it occurs in response to electrical stimulation of the lowest threshold axons in nerves supplying the pathological zone. Second, it occurs in response to very gentle mechanical stimuli. Third, it is abolished by blockade of the largest fastest conducting axons within nerves (21). Finally, it has a reaction time consistent with conduction in myelinated afferents (21). It is also commonly characterized by the fact that moving stimuli or stimulus onset or offset is more painful than static mechanical stimuli (17,37). The other type of mechanical allodynia is characterized by evidence that A-beta afferents do not seem to be involved (see above) and that more intense but normally painless stimuli are required to evoke pain. For example, 15 to 600 g von Frey filament stimuli, which are well above threshold for A-beta primary mechanoreceptive afferents but are rarely painful under normal circumstances, evoke pain when applied to the pathological zones of these patients. This type of mechanical allodynia is termed high threshold and it may well be mediated by activation of nociceptive afferents under conditions that normally do not produce pain.

Abnormal Triggering of Temporal Summation by Primary Mechanoreceptive Neurons
Regardless of whether the mechanical allodynia is A-beta or high threshold, it often has characteristics similar to pains evoked by unmyelinated C nociceptive afferents described above for second pain (6). Thus, repeated brief mechanical stimulation of allodynic patients often evokes slow temporal summation of burning pain, as shown in Figure 1 (*right panel*). For some CRPS patients, slow temporal summation of burning pain occurs when gentle mechanical stimuli or electrical stimulation of A-beta afferents are applied at rates of once per three

seconds. For other patients, slow temporal summation occurs only with more intense but normally nonpainful mechanical stimuli. Still other patients do not exhibit slow temporal summation with these types of repetitive mechanical stimuli. Both mechanical allodynia and slow temporal summation of allodynia are completely or nearly completely reversed by anesthetic blockade of sympathetic ganglia in some CRPS patients, indicating that these sensory abnormalities can sometimes be dynamically maintained by sympathetic efferent activity, presumably activity that induces continuous input over nociceptive afferents. Slow temporal summation of mechanical allodynia, particularly that induced by stimulation of A-beta afferents, is abnormal because such types of stimuli neither evoke pain in pain-free subjects nor in CRPS patients when such stimuli are delivered to homologous contralateral pain-free zones. In fact, A-beta afferent stimulation even at extremely high frequencies does not evoke pain in normal human subjects (39). Therefore, A-beta mechanical allodynia and abnormal slow temporal summation of mechanical allodynia may represent an exaggeration and/or abnormal triggering of physiological mechanisms that already exist in normal pain-free individuals. Such mechanisms can be demonstrated in the latter by temporal summation of experimentally induced second pain, as described earlier. Thus, under some pathological conditions after nerve injury or nerve dysfunction, A-beta input may somehow gain access to and trigger the same temporal summation mechanisms normally activated by C afferent stimulation. In other pathological conditions, sensitized nociceptors themselves are likely to be the direct proximal cause of the slow temporal summation of mechanical allodynia.

Relationships of Temporal Summation of Mechanical Allodynia to Severity of Clinical Pain

Regardless of the exact mechanisms by which temporal summation of allodynia is generated, the phenomenon is likely to be at least part of the basis for CRPS patients' ongoing "spontaneous" pain. It has been suggested that temporal summation of A-beta allodynia provides at least part of the basis for ongoing background pain in neuropathic pain patients (17). This relationship could occur if continuous input from A-beta low threshold afferents (evoked in the normal course of mechanical stimulation from walking, sitting, or even contact with clothes) activated slow temporal summation of a type of burning, aching, or throbbing pain that built up slowly and dissipated slowly over time. This possibility was explicitly tested in a group of 31 CRPS patients by comparing intensities of ongoing pain between 10 patients who demonstrated slow temporal summation with 17 who did not (17). The former had significantly higher intensities of ongoing pain (mean $= 7.02$ on visual analog pain scale) than the latter (mean $= 4.04$ on visual analog pain scale; $p < .001$). Therefore, exaggerated or abnormally triggered mechanisms of slow temporal summation are likely to form at least part of the basis of persistent pain that usually occurs in CRPS patients.

TESTING VISCERAL AND CUTANEOUS HYPERALGESIA IN IRRITABLE BOWEL SYNDROME PATIENTS
Visceral Hyperalgesia in Irritable Bowel Syndrome Patients
Evidence for Visceral Hyperalgesia in Irritable Bowel Syndrome

Tests similar to those described above for CRPS and fibromyalgia patients also have been used to characterize pain in IBS. IBS is one of the most common disorders seen by gastroenterologists. Patients classically present with chronic abdominal pain associated with an alteration in bowel habits. It is now well accepted that the majority of patients with IBS demonstrate enhanced perception of balloon distension of the rectum (Fig. 3, *left panel*). This visceral hypersensitivity is manifested by increased intensity of sensations, lowered thresholds for visceral pain, and/or exaggerated viscerosomatic referral in comparison to control subjects (40–42). Visceral hypersensitivity is a biological marker of IBS (41).

Is Hyperalgesia Limited to the Gut in Irritable Bowel Syndrome?

The first studies to investigate visceral sensitivity in IBS concluded that enhanced sensitivity in IBS was limited to the gut (43–46). Interestingly, two prior studies have examined cutaneous pain in IBS patients using electrocutaneous stimulation (43,44). In one study, 13 patients with Crohn's disease, 13 control subjects, and 12 patients with IBS had electrodes positioned on the

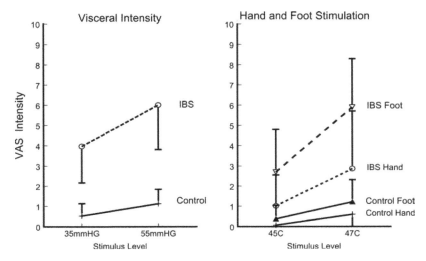

Figure 3 IBS patients' and normal control subjects' M-VAS pain intensity ratings of rectal distension pressures of 35 and 55 mmHg (*left panel*) and of thermal stimulation of the hand and foot (*right panel*). Note that patients with IBS rate pain intensity much higher than controls ($p < 0.001$) at both temperatures and skin sites. Values are represented as means $\pm$ SD, $n = 12$ IBS patients, 17 controls. *Abbreviations*: VAS, visual analog scale; IBS, irritable bowel syndrome. *Source*: From Ref. 40.

skin of their hands (44). Touch threshold, defined as the current just detectable by the subject, and pain threshold, defined as the current at which the subject first described the stimulus as painful, were significantly higher in both IBS and Crohn's disease, compared to normal subjects. A later study compared somatic transcutaneous electrical nerve stimulation in 17 patients with IBS and 15 healthy controls (43). The perception threshold and threshold for discomfort were both higher in the IBS subjects than controls. A possible limitation common to both studies is that the thresholds for perception and discomfort to electrical stimulation may not have necessarily involved stimulation of nociceptive receptors. Thresholds for detection of electric shock and discomfort thresholds may be below that required to activate nociceptive receptors (11). Furthermore, tactile input and perception are inhibited by nociceptive input. This may account for the higher thresholds in IBS patients if, unlike control subjects, they have ongoing visceral nociceptive input.

Thus, less agreement has been reached with regard to secondary cutaneous hyperalgesia in IBS patients (40,47–51). One study suggests that IBS patients exhibit cutaneous hypersensitivity only when they have fibromyalgia as a comorbid condition (48). However, some investigators have acquired evidence that patients with IBS but without other chronic pain conditions including fibromyalgia have both visceral hypersensitivity and cutaneous hypersensitivity in response to experimental stimuli (40,47,51). A number of these studies have compared results of both clinically relevant painful rectal distension and painful cutaneous heat stimulation in IBS patients with age- or sex-matched normal control subjects (40,49,51).

Evidence of Heat Hyperalgesia in Irritable Bowel Syndrome
Evidence from Human Irritable Bowel Syndrome Patients
The first study to show large magnitudes of heat hyperalgesia in IBS patients compared VAS ratings of pain intensity and unpleasantness in response to rectal distension and cutaneous thermal stimuli in 12 patients with IBS but without fibromyalgia and in 17 healthy controls (40). Using methods similar to those of other investigators (41,42), phasic distension of the rectum (870 mL/min) to constant pressure plateaus of 35 and 55 mmHg for 30 seconds each were performed, followed by a 60-second interstimulus rest at a resting pressure of 5 mmHg. Cutaneous (heat) sensitivity was tested by asking each subject to immerse his/her right hand (up to the level of the wrist) or right foot (up to the level of the right malleolus) in a circulating, heated, water bath at random temperatures of 45°C and 47°C for 20 seconds each with a five-minute rest between each stimulus.

Similar to previous studies (41,42,45), Verne et al. showed increased visceral perception to phasic rectal distension in IBS patients as compared with control (40). IBS patients rated both rectal distension pressures (35 and 55 mmHg) as more intense and unpleasant compared with controls (Fig. 3, *left panel*). These same IBS patients also rated cutaneous heat pain in the foot as much more intense and unpleasant in comparison to control subjects, thereby demonstrating secondary cutaneous heat hyperalgesia (Fig. 3, *right panel*). Heat hyperalgesia also was present in the hand of these patients (Fig. 3, *right panel*).

A limitation of this study, however, is that all the subjects were female. Thus, it is possible that cutaneous heat hyperalgesia may not be representative of other IBS populations. This limitation was explicitly addressed in a second study of male IBS patients who were veterans that had Gulf War syndrome, a very different population than those of the first study (49). Using the same experimental methodology and experimental design (e.g., ratings of male patients were statistically compared to male control subjects of similar age), this study demonstrated large magnitudes of both visceral and cutaneous heat hyperalgesia. Similar to female IBS patients, heat hyperalgesia was present in both the foot and the hand. Studies of female and male IBS patients were followed by a third study of IBS patients, including both male and female subjects, whose brains were scanned with functional magnetic resonance imaging (52). In comparison to age- and sex-matched control subjects, IBS patients had both visceral and cutaneous heat hyperalgesia that was accompanied by corresponding increased activation of brain regions involved in pain processing, including thalamus, somatosensory areas 1 and 2, insular cortex, anterior cingulate cortex, and prefrontal cortical areas (52). Thus, IBS patients had increased pain-related activation within an entire network of brain areas, including those involved in early levels of afferent processing such as the thalamus (52). In all three studies, the cutaneous hyperalgesia was pronounced in the lower extremity (foot), yet present in the upper extremity (hand) to a lesser extent (40,49,51). In combination, these results suggest that patients with IBS have visceral hyperalgesia and secondary cutaneous hyperalgesia that is distributed over widespread regions of the body, yet optimally expressed in lumbosacral dermatomes. This conclusion is further supported by observations that many IBS patients exhibit a number of extraintestinal pain symptoms such as back pain, migraine headaches, heartburn, dyspareunia, and muscle pain consistent with central hyperalgesic mechanisms (53,54). Similar to other pain conditions that likely depend on peripheral impulse input, such as CRPS, postherpetic neuralgia, and fibromyalgia, IBS patients may develop widely distributed hyperalgesia, possibly related to chronic peripheral nociceptive input from the rectum and colon.

Evidence of Secondary Cutaneous Hyperalgesia in Animal Models of Irritable Bowel Syndrome

The body distribution of hyperalgesia in IBS is consistent with widespread patterns of spinal hyperexcitability observed in animal models of IBS (55). In particular, it has been found that experimentally induced colon irritation in neonatal rats led to enhanced rectal sensitivity when the rats become adults (55). Rectal hypersensitivity is present in these adult rats despite the absence of identifiable peripheral pathology, similar to human IBS patients. Another similarity to human IBS patients was that these rats also displayed hypersensitivity to both rectal distension and cutaneous noxious stimuli (55). Finally, dorsal horn pain-related neurons of these rats also showed enhanced impulse responses to these stimuli. We have recently found similar results in another animal model of IBS (56).

Neural Mechanisms of Hyperalgesia in Irritable Bowel Syndrome
Three Possible General Mechanisms Underlying Hyperalgesia

These studies of animal models of IBS clearly point to a spinal mechanism, consistent with the observation that IBS patients have enhanced responses to visceral and cutaneous stimuli throughout the pain matrix of the brain (including thalamus). However, based on the evidence presented so far, it is not entirely clear the extent to which these enhanced responses are the result of (i) a facilitating mechanism confined within the brain, (ii) a spinal sensitization maintained by tonic impulse input from the rectum and/or colon, or (iii) a mechanism of descending facilitation from the brain to the spinal cord and/or gut. The first few neuroimaging studies to compare IBS with normal controls' brain responses to visceral stimulation produced mixed results that are difficult to interpret, including reduced anterior cingulate cortex (ACC) responses in IBS patients and increased responses in a limited number of regions in IBS patients (57–59). The enhancement in regions such as rostral ACC and prefrontal cortical areas provides limited support for the idea that enhanced pain in IBS is the result of cognitive enhancement rather than enhancement of activity in ascending pathways to the brain. Abnormally enhanced responses in ACC and prefrontal areas would be consistent with a cognitive enhancement mechanism (57). However, as described above, later studies found that IBS patients showed enhanced brain activations within multiple pain processing areas, including those at early levels of pain processing (51,60). These studies used higher numbers of subjects and possibly improved methods of brain imaging. Most critically, the results of later imaging studies are consistent with studies of animal models of IBS that show enhanced responses at the spinal cord level (55). Nevertheless, these three alternative mechanisms—tonic peripheral impulse input, descending facilitation, and intracerebral enhancement are not mutually exclusive and we need tests to determine the relative contribution of these general factors.

Testing Peripheral Sources of Secondary Hyperalgesia in Irritable Bowel Syndrome Patients

A test of the role of tonic peripheral impulse input is suggested by a model of neuropathic pain, in which ongoing afferent input from a peripheral source maintains altered central processing that accounts for spontaneous pain, allodynia, hyperalgesia, and other motor abnormalities (21). In their study, the potential role of ongoing afferent input was demonstrated in CRPS patients. Peripheral anesthetic blockade of nociceptive input from a few critical foci effectively abolished both spontaneous and elicited pain and cold/mechanoallodynia within widespread body regions in these patients, including regions that were remote from these critical foci. A similar reversal occurs with sympathetic blocks in some CRPS patients (37,61). Given the presence of widespread zones of hyperalgesia in neuropathic pain, fibromyalgia, and IBS patients, it is possible that hyperalgesia of these of patients is maintained to some extent by tonic impulse input from nociceptive and/or non-nociceptive primary afferent neurons.

Thus, the results of studies just described suggest that a similar experiment could be carried out in the case of IBS patients. If visceral hyperalgesia and secondary cutaneous hyperalgesia are dynamically maintained by tonic input from the rectum and/or colon, then local anesthesia of one or more of these visceral structures should reduce these forms of hyperalgesia. Our recent study tested the hypothesis that local anesthetic blockade of peripheral visceral nociceptive input reduces both visceral and cutaneous secondary hyperalgesia in IBS patients (51). This hypothesis was tested by administering controlled rectal distension and cutaneous heat stimuli before and after rectal administration of either lidocaine jelly or saline jelly in a double-blind crossover basis in IBS patients. The comparison was ideal because subjects cannot subjectively distinguish the two agents.

In comparison to saline placebo, lidocaine jelly completely normalized not only rectal hyperalgesia, as shown in Figure 4 (*left panel*), but also hyperalgesia to heat stimuli applied to the foot. This was not the result of systemic absorption of lidocaine, because significant blood levels were not detected during the 50-minute experimental session and most of the effects were present five minutes after treatment. Thus, tonic impulse input from the rectum appears to dynamically maintain not only primary hyperalgesia from the rectum/colon but also the secondary hyperalgesia that is spatially remote from the peripheral source of impulse input. One likely mechanism is that tonic input from the rectum/colon sensitizes spinal cord neurons that have viscerosomatic convergence, a mechanism additionally supported by animal studies described above.

Testing Central Sources of Hyperalgesia in Irritable Bowel Syndrome: Placebo and Nocebo Effects

The study just discussed was conducted as a standard clinical trial where patients were given an informed consent form, which stated that they "may receive an active pain reducing medication or an inert placebo agent" (52). In this study, there was a significant pain-relieving effect of rectal lidocaine as compared to rectal placebo ($p < 0.001$), and there was a significant pain-relieving effect of rectal placebo as compared to the natural history condition (Fig. 4, *left panel*). Taking into consideration previous meta-analyses showing enhanced placebo effects in experimental studies compared to clinical trials (63), a second study was carried out, which was almost identical to the first study. The one difference was that in the second study the patients

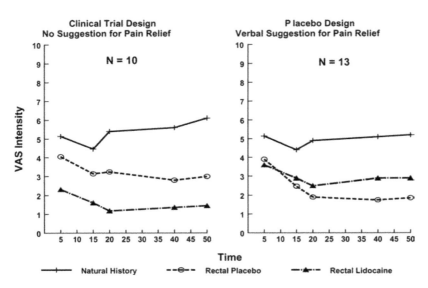

Figure 4 (*Left panel*): Visual analog scale pain intensity ratings during rectal distension (35 mmHg). Three separate trials were performed: natural history, rectal placebo, and rectal lidocaine. This study was conducted with a standard clinical trial design, without suggestions for analgesia. Values are represented as mean ± SD, $n = 10$ IBS patients. (*Right panel*) Results of a second study wherein a verbal suggestion for analgesia was added. Note that unlike the first study, the placebo effect was large as that of lidocaine. *Source*: From Ref. 62.

were told "the agent you have just been given is known to significantly reduce pain in some patients" at the onset of each treatment condition (rectal placebo and rectal lidocaine) (62). As shown in Figure 4 (*right panel*), a much larger placebo analgesic effect was found in the second study and the magnitude of placebo analgesia was so high (an effect size 2.0, Cohen's d) that there was no longer a significant difference between the magnitude of rectal lidocaine and rectal placebo. Hence, these two studies indicate that by adding an overt suggestion for pain relief, it is possible to increase the magnitude of placebo analgesia to a level that matches that of an active agent. It is important to recognize that these effects reflect antihyperalgesic effects, because both rectal lidocaine and placebo suggestions normalize the primary and secondary hyperalgesia and do not eliminate all pain from balloon distension. In fact, pain ratings of IBS patients after placebo or lidocaine are like those of normal control subjects (51,52,64).

   Although lidocaine jelly potently reduced experimentally evoked pain in IBS patients for at least 50 minutes (52); one can question whether rectal application of lidocaine jelly can directly reduce ongoing abdominal pain in these patients, especially if the area of gastrointestinal abnormality includes the colon. Thus, a double-blind, crossover trial on 10 IBS patients was conducted to determine whether administration of intrarectal (300 mg) lidocaine in jelly form could ameliorate the ongoing abdominal pain associated with IBS (65). All of the patients that participated had intermittent left lower quadrant pain and diarrhea. Each patient participated in two sessions in which saline jelly (placebo) and lidocaine jelly were administered on a double-blind, crossover basis. Patients participated in these sessions at a time when their ongoing pain was at least three on a 0 to 10 VAS. In comparison to placebo saline jelly, lidocaine jelly significantly decreased abdominal pain for at least four hours, as shown in Figure 5. These results are understandable if the rectum is a major source of tonic afferent input that sustains widespread visceral hyperalgesia, similar to the critical foci that sustain widespread hyperalgesia/allodynia in CRPS patients (21).

Is There a Synergistic Interaction Between Peripheral Impulse Input and Central Facilitation?

An important and surprising conclusion from comparing the studies just described is that primary and secondary hyperalgesia can be nearly completely normalized by either removing the source of tonic peripheral impulse input (i.e., local rectal anesthesia) or removing a source of facilitation within the CNS. The latter can be associated with placebo and nocebo influences

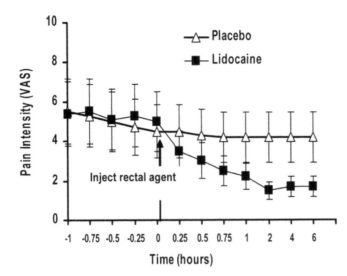

Figure 5 Results showing the therapeutic effects of 300 mg intrarectal lidocaine jelly as compared to intrarectal placebo saline jelly in 10 patients with abdominal pain associated with IBS. Vertical bars are standard deviations. These agents were administered on a double-blind basis. Each data point is the mean pain rating of the group. The vertical arrow at 0 indicates the time of intrarectal administration of placebo jelly or lidocaine jelly. *Abbreviations*: VAS, visual analog scale.

and therefore with mental events. These phenomena may be integrally related to hypervigilance, level of somatic focus, or other factors related to emotional regulation. The relationship of negative affect to pain conditions is well documented in the literature (66). In nearly all published reports, the presence of negative mood is associated with higher levels of pain. Induction of negative mood has also been shown to be related to pain report and pain behavior, with some specificity to the type of emotion induced (67–70). Interventions or instructional sets that reduce negative emotion also reduce pain report (62,71). Our work in IBS patients indicates that the magnitude of placebo analgesia is related to changes in expectations of pain (and anxiety), desire for pain relief, and somatic focus (72). That hyperalgesia can be completely normalized by either reducing a peripheral source of tonic impulse input or removing CNS facilitation is puzzling. It may be the case that there exists a synergistic interaction between peripheral and central factors, such that the removal of either factor alone is sufficient to normalize the hyperalgesia. If a type of synergistic interaction generalizes to other hyperalgesic states or pain conditions, it may have large implications for understanding how to assess the relative contribution of peripheral and central factors in persistent pain conditions as well as conceptualizing mind–body relationships.

Taken together, the combination of research studies of human IBS patients and studies of rats within experimentally induced delayed colitis strongly suggests a mechanism wherein both primary visceral hyperalgesia and secondary widespread cutaneous hyperalgesia are dynamically maintained by tonic impulse input from the colon and/or rectum. The secondary hyperalgesia is likely to be at least partly related to sensitization of spinal cord dorsal horn neurons and in this respect may be similar to other persistent pain conditions such as fibromyalgia and CRPS. A major source of evidence for this explanation is derived by the use of carefully controlled sensory tests in human patients, often in combination with pharmacological manipulations (e.g., intrarectal lidocaine) or brain imaging.

CONCLUSIONS AND FUTURE IMPLICATIONS

The combination of direct scaling techniques and sensory tests serves to characterize the severity of persistent and intermittent pain conditions such as CRPS, fibromyalgia, and IBS as well as at least part of the pathophysiological basis for these conditions. Thus, such tests help characterize these pain conditions and thereby aid in diagnoses. Perhaps even more important is the potential capacity for such tests to provide a strategy of matching treatments to mechanisms. For example, temporal summation of A-beta allodynia may be mediated by NMDA receptor mechanisms. If this is the case and if this type of allodynia is present in some but not all CRPS patients (37% in the study described above), then a clinical trial of a NMDA receptor blocker might detect a clinical benefit only if patients had been carefully examined for the presence of this particular sensory abnormality. In another example, evoked pains that radiate (i.e., shooting pain) may be particularly responsive to treatment with anticonvulsants. Sensory tests may also be used in combination with local anesthetic blocks to identify peripheral sources of tonic impulse input that sustain neuropathic and other types of pain conditions. An obvious example is that of using lidocaine patches to treat postherpetic neuralgia. This same principle may be used to treat IBS (52).

REFERENCES

1. Noordenbos W. Pain. Amsterdam: Elsevier, 1959.
2. Gracely RH, Dubner R. Pain assessment in humans—a reply to Hall. Pain 1981; 11(1):109–120.
3. Price DD et al. Enhanced temporal summation of second pain and its central modulation in fibromyalgia patients. Pain 2002; 99(1–2):49–59.
4. Myles PS et al. The pain visual analog scale: is it linear or nonlinear? Anesth Analg 1999; 89(6): 1517–1520.
5. Price DD et al. The validation of visual analogue scales as ratio scale measures for chronic and experimental pain. Pain 1983; 17(1):45–56.
6. Price DD et al. The N-methyl-d-aspartate receptor antagonist dextromethorphan selectively reduces temporal summation of second pain in man. Pain 1994; 59(2):165–174.
7. Price DD, Riley JL, Wade JB. Psychophysical approaches to the measurement of the dimensions and stages of pain. In: Turk DC, Melzack R, eds. Handbook of Pain Measurement. New York: The Guilford Press, 2001:115–134.
8. Rosier EM, Iadarola MJ, Coghill RC. Reproducibility of pain measurement and pain perception. Pain 2002; 98(1–2):205–216.
9. Price DD, Harkins SW. The combined use of visual analogue scales and experimental pain in providing standardized measurement of clinical pain. Clin J Pain 1987; 3:1–8.
10. Price DD et al. A simultaneous comparison of fentanyl's analgesic effects on experimental and clinical pain. Pain 1986; 24(2):197–203.
11. Price DD. Psychological Mechanisms of Pain and Analgesia. Seattle: IASP Press, 1999.
12. Coghill RC, McHaffie JG, Yen YF. Neural correlates of interindividual differences in the subjective experience of pain. Proc Natl Acad Sci USA 2003; 100(14):8538–8542.
13. Price DD et al. A comparison of pain measurement characteristics of mechanical visual analogue and simple numerical rating scales. Pain 1994; 56(2):217–226.
14. Dworkin RH et al. Core outcome measures for chronic pain clinical trials: IMMPACT recommendations. Pain 2005; 113(1–2):9–19.
15. Jensen MP, Karoly P. Self-report scales and procedures for assessing pain in adults. In: Turk DC, Melzack R, eds. Handbook of Pain Assessment. New York: The Guilford Press, 2001:135–151.
16. Yeomans DC, Proudfit HK. Nociceptive responses to high and low rates of noxious cutaneous heating are mediated by different nociceptors in the rat: electrophysiological evidence. Pain 1996; 68(1):141–150.
17. Price DD, Long S, Huitt C. Sensory testing of pathophysiological mechanisms of pain in patients with reflex sympathetic dystrophy. Pain 1992; 49(2):163–173.
18. Janig W, Stanton-Hicks M. Reflex sympathetic dystrophy: a reappraisal. Seattle: IASP Press, 1996.
19. Campbell JN, Raja SN, Meyer RA. Painful sequelae of nerve injury. In: Dubner R, Gebhart GF, Bond MR, eds. Pain Research and Clinical Management. New York: Elsevier, 1988:135–143.
20. Meyer RA, Campbell JN. Myelinated nociceptive afferents account for the hyperalgesia that follows a burn to the hand. Science 1981; 213(4515):1527–1529.
21. Gracely RH, Lynch SA, Bennett GJ. Painful neuropathy: altered central processing maintained dynamically by peripheral input. Pain 1992; 51(2):175–194.
22. Staud R et al. Abnormal sensitization and temporal summation of second pain (wind-up) in patients with fibromyalgia syndrome. Pain 2001; 91(1–2):165–175.
23. Staud R et al. Ratings of experimental pain and pain-related negative affect predict clinical pain in patients with fibromyalgia syndrome. Pain 2003; 105(1–2):215–222.
24. Staud R et al. Maintenance of windup of second pain requires less frequent stimulation in fibromyalgia patients compared to normal controls. Pain 2004; 110(3):689–696.
25. Vierck CJ Jr et al. The effect of maximal exercise on temporal summation of second pain (windup) in patients with fibromyalgia syndrome. J Pain 2001; 2(6):334–344.
26. Wolfe F, Cathey MA. Prevalence of primary and secondary fibrositis. J Rheumatol 1983; 10(6): 965–968.
27. Griep EN, Boersma JW, de Kloet ER. Altered reactivity of the hypothalamic-pituitary-adrenal axis in the primary fibromyalgia syndrome. J Rheumatol 1993; 20(3):469–474.
28. Russell IJ et al. Elevated cerebrospinal fluid levels of substance P in patients with the fibromyalgia syndrome. Arthritis Rheum 1994; 37(11):1593–1601.
29. Price DD. Characteristics of second pain and flexion reflexes indicative of prolonged central summation. Exp Neurol 1972; 37(2):371–387.

30. Price DD et al. Peripheral suppression of first pain and central summation of second pain evoked by noxious heat pulses. Pain 1977; 3(1):57–68.
31. Vierck CJ Jr et al. Characteristics of temporal summation of second pain sensations elicited by brief contact of glabrous skin by a preheated thermode. J Neurophysiol 1997; 78(2):992–1002.
32. Li J, Simone DA, Larson AA. Windup leads to characteristics of central sensitization. Pain 1999; 79(1):75–82.
33. Mendell LM, Wall PD. Responses of single dorsal cord cells to peripheral cutaneous unmyelinated fibres. Nature 1965; 206:97–99.
34. Staud R et al. Effects of the NMDA receptor antagonist dextromethorphan on temporal summation of pain are similar in fibromyalgia patients and normal controls. J Pain 2005; 6(5):323–332.
35. Merritt AM et al. Evaluation of method to experimentally induce colic in horses and the effects of acupuncture applied at the Guan-yuan-shu (similar to BL-21) acupoint. Am J Vet Res 2002; 66(5): 897–906.
36. Maixner W et al. Sensitivity of patients with painful temporomandibular disorders to experimentally evoked pain: evidence for altered temporal summation of pain. Pain 1998; 76(1–2):71–81.
37. Price DD, Bennett GJ, Rafii A. Psychophysical observations on patients with neuropathic pain relieved by a sympathetic block. Pain 1989; 36(3):273–288.
38. Arendt-Nielsen L. Induction and assessment of experimental pain from human skin, muscle, and viscera. In: Jensen TS, Turner JA, Wiesenfeld-Hallin Z, eds. Proceedings of the 8th World Congress on Pain. Seattle: IASP Press, 1997:393.
39. Collins WF, Nulsen FE, Randt CT. Relation of peripheral nerve fiber size and sensation in man. Arch Neurol (Chic) 1960; 3:381–385.
40. Verne GN, Robinson ME, Price DD. Hypersensitivity to visceral and cutaneous pain in the irritable bowel syndrome. Pain 2001; 93(1):7–14.
41. Mertz H et al. Altered rectal perception is a biological marker of patients with irritable bowel syndrome. Gastroenterology 1995; 109(1):40–52.
42. Naliboff BD et al. Evidence for two distinct perceptual alterations in irritable bowel syndrome. Gut 1997; 41(4):505–512.
43. Accarino AM, Azpiroz F, Malagelada JR. Selective dysfunction of mechanosensitive intestinal afferents in irritable bowel syndrome. Gastroenterology 1995; 108(3):636–643.
44. Cook IJ, van Eeden A, Collins SM. Patients with irritable bowel syndrome have greater pain tolerance than normal subjects. Gastroenterology 1987; 93(4):727–733.
45. Whitehead WE et al. Tolerance for rectosigmoid distention in irritable bowel syndrome. Gastroenterology 1990; 98(5 Pt 1):1187–1192.
46. Zighelboim J et al. Visceral perception in irritable bowel syndrome. Rectal and gastric responses to distension and serotonin type 3 antagonism. Dig Dis Sci 1995; 40(4):819–827.
47. Bouin M et al. Pain hypersensitivity in patients with functional gastrointestinal disorders: a gastro-intestinal-specific defect or a general systemic condition?. Dig Dis Sci 2001; 46(11):2542–2548.
48. Chang L et al. Differences in somatic perception in female patients with irritable bowel syndrome with and without fibromyalgia. Pain 2000; 84(2–3):297–307.
49. Dunphy RC et al. Visceral and cutaneous hypersensitivity in Persian Gulf War veterans with chronic gastrointestinal symptoms. Pain 2003; 102(1–2):79–85.
50. Gupta V, Sheffield D, Verne GN. Evidence for autonomic dysregulation in the irritable bowel syndrome. Dig Dis Sci 2002; 47(8):1716–1722.
51. Verne GN et al. Central representation of visceral and cutaneous hypersensitivity in the irritable bowel syndrome. Pain 2003; 103(1–2):99–110.
52. Verne GN et al. Reversal of visceral and cutaneous hyperalgesia by local rectal anesthesia in irritable bowel syndrome (IBS) patients. Pain 2003; 105(1–2):223–230.
53. Mayer EA, Raybould HE. Role of visceral afferent mechanisms in functional bowel disorders. Gastroenterology 1990; 99(6):1688–1704.
54. Mayer EA, Gebhart GF. Basic and clinical aspects of visceral hyperalgesia. Gastroenterology 1994; 107(1):271–293.
55. Al Chaer ED, Kawasaki M, Pasricha PJ. A new model of chronic visceral hypersensitivity in adult rats induced by colon irritation during postnatal development. Gastroenterology 2000; 119(5): 1276–1285.
56. Zhou Q et al. Visceral somatic convergence in TNBS induced colitis in rats, J Pain 2005; 7(4):330.
57. Mertz H et al. Regional cerebral activation in irritable bowel syndrome and control subjects with painful and nonpainful rectal distention. Gastroenterology 2000; 118(5):842–848.
58. Naliboff BD et al. Cerebral activation in patients with irritable bowel syndrome and control subjects during rectosigmoid stimulation. Psychosom Med 2001; 63(3):365–375.
59. Silverman DH, Phelps ME. Evaluating dementia using PET: how do we put into clinical perspective what we know to date?. J Nucl Med 2000; 41(11):1929–1932.
60. Yuan YZ et al. Functional brain imaging in irritable bowel syndrome with rectal balloon-distention by using fMRI. World J Gastroenterol 2003; 9(6):1356–1360.
61. Price DD et al. Analysis of peak magnitude and duration of analgesia produced by local anesthetics injected into sympathetic ganglia of complex regional pain syndrome patients. Clin J Pain 1998; 14(3):216–226.

62. Vase L et al. The contributions of suggestion, desire, and expectation to placebo effects in irritable bowel syndrome patients. An empirical investigation. Pain 2003; 105(1–2):17–25.

63. Vase L, Riley JL III, Price DD. A comparison of placebo effects in clinical analgesic trials versus studies of placebo analgesia. Pain 2002; 99(3):443–452.

64. Verne GN, Price DD. Irritable bowel syndrome as a common precipitant of central sensitization. Curr Rheumatol Rep 2002; 4(4):322–328.

65. Verne GN, Sen A, Price DD. Intrarectal lidocaine is an effective treatment for abdominal pain associated with diarrhea-predominant irritable bowel syndrome. J Pain 2005; 6(8):493–496.

66. Robinson ME, Riley JL. Negative emotion in pain. In: Gatchel R, Turk D, eds. Psychosocial Factors in Pain. New York: Guilford Press, 1998.

67. Ploghaus A et al. Exacerbation of pain by anxiety is associated with activity in a hippocampal network. J Neurosci 2001; 21(24):9896–9903.

68. Rhudy JL, Meagher MW. Fear and anxiety: divergent effects on human pain thresholds. Pain 2000; 84(1):65–75.

69. Rhudy JL, Meagher MW. Negative affect: effects on an evaluative measure of human pain. Pain 2003; 104(3):617–626.

70. Zelman DC et al. The effects of induced mood on laboratory pain. Pain 1991; 46(1):105–111.

71. McCracken LM, Gross RT. The role of pain-related anxiety reduction in the outcome of multidisciplinary treatment for chronic low back pain: preliminary results. J Occup Rehabil 1998; 8:179–189.

72. Vase L et al. The contributions of changes in expected pain levels and desire for pain relief to placebo analgesia. In: Price DD, Bushnell MC, eds. Psychological Methods of Pain Control: Basic Science and Clinical Perspectives. Seattle, WA: IASP Press, 2004:207–232.

10 Mechanisms of Visceral Sensitization in Humans

Abhishek Sharma and Q. Aziz

Department of Gastrointestinal Science, University of Manchester, Hope Hospital, Salford, U.K.

BACKGROUND

Chronic episodic pain is the commonest presenting complaint in functional gastrointestinal disorders (FGD) such as functional dyspepsia, irritable bowel syndrome (IBS), and noncardiac chest pain (NCCP). These conditions are characterized by recurrent, unexplained symptoms for which extensive investigations often fail to identify a cause. FGD are among the most common medical conditions seen in primary care as well as gastroenterology clinics. Symptoms often lead to recurrent attendances in hospital, poor patient satisfaction, and significant morbidity. Health care costs are estimated to be around $34 billion in the seven largest western economies (1,2). Despite intense research, our understanding of the mechanisms of pain in these patients remains far from complete.

Understanding the mechanisms leading to the development and maintenance of visceral pain requires an appreciation of the neuroanatomical structures and neurophysiological processes involved, and these have been previously described. It is important to appreciate that the complex physiological processes involved in pain transmission from the gut to the brain are highly dynamic and subject to change depending on the stresses imposed by the internal or external environment. As a result, pain transmission is modifiable, and as will be discussed, this may be relevant to the symptoms of chronic pain in FGD patients.

THE MODULATION OF PAIN PERCEPTION

In the presence of tissue inflammation or injury, the nervous system has evolved certain mechanisms to upregulate pain transmission. The ability to enhance pain transmission to the brain in these situations is important from an evolutionary perspective, as in such situations heightened bodily awareness can alter behavior to aid in the protection of injured sites and in the promotion of healing. Furthermore, learning and memory facilitate the future avoidance of adverse external stimuli, thereby conveying advantages that ensure the "survival of the fittest." If this enhanced pain transmission or awareness persists long after the initial insult, then aberrant or maladaptive physiological or psychological behavior may result.

VISCERAL HYPERSENSITIVITY

Although FGD patients show marked heterogeneity in their clinical presentation and response to treatment, common features have become apparent, as our knowledge of these disorders has increased. It was documented over 30 years ago by Ritchie that recto-sigmoid balloon distension was perceived as painful at lower volumes in IBS patients than in controls (3). This heightened pain sensitivity to experimental gut stimulation, a phenomenon known as visceral hypersensitivity, has been repeatedly demonstrated in patients with FGD. For instance, hypersensitivity to intraesophageal balloon distension has been reported in patients with NCCP as compared to controls, which was independent of esophageal tone and motility (4). In addition, hypersensitivity to intragastric balloon distension has been demonstrated in patients with functional dyspepsia as compared to controls, with them reporting higher scores for nausea, bloating, and pain (5). This visceral hypersensitivity does not appear to be site specific to the syndrome suspected, as Trimble et al. have shown heightened sensitivity to rectal distension in patients with both IBS and functional dyspepsia, with both groups of patients being hypersensitive to esophageal distensions (6). This latter finding, when taken with the fact that these patients often have enlarged referral patterns of their visceral pain to somatic structures, suggests a more generalized sensory disturbance (7,8).

Visceral hypersensitivity is thought to play an important role in the development of chronic pain in these patients; however, what causes and maintains this hypersensitivity is still poorly understood. A review of the possible biological factors that may be involved in modulating visceral pain sensitivity will now be presented, following which evidence for their involvement in FGD will be discussed.

Neuronal Sensitization

Research in somatic pain hypersensitivity has suggested that both peripheral and central mechanisms can increase nociceptive transmission following inflammation or injury to tissues (9), and these will be briefly outlined.

Peripheral Sensitization

During tissue injury and inflammation, peripheral nociceptor terminals are exposed to a mixture of immune and inflammatory mediators such as prostaglandins, leukotrienes, serotonin, histamine, cytokines, neurotrophic factors, and reactive metabolites (10,11). These chemicals can act on peripheral nociceptor terminals and alter synaptic function by modifying either the release of neurotransmitters from presynaptic terminals or transmitter responsiveness on the postsynaptic membrane. This modifiable synaptic activity has been termed "synaptic plasticity," and is an essential feature of the nervous system allowing it to adapt to adverse stimuli. Depending on the synapse and frequency, intensity and duration of activity, both increases (facilitation, potentiation, or sensitization) and decreases (habituation, depression, or desensitization) can be induced (12).

Inflammatory mediators act on G-protein–coupled or tyrosine kinase receptors expressed on nociceptor terminals leading to the activation of intracellular signalling pathways, which in turn upregulate the sensitivity and excitability of the nociceptor terminal through the phosphorylation of receptors and ion channels. For example, after inflammation, bradykinin induces activation of protein kinase C, which in turn sensitizes sodium channels (such as the voltage-gated Na^+ channel Na_V 1.8) and the vanilloid receptor TRPV1. This latter receptor is directly activated by noxious temperature (42–53°C), hydrogen ions and capsaicin (13). A number of other receptors and their mediators have been identified, such as the neurokinin receptors (e.g., NK1), which are responsive to substance P, the purinergic receptor $P2X_3$, which is activated by chemical mediators such as adenosine triphosphate (ATP), the acid sensitive ion channel (ASIC) receptors which are sensitive to hydrogen ions, and the nonselective cation channels (NSCCs) sensitive to capsaicin, ATP, and serotonin. Numerous intracellular signalling pathways and messengers such as cyclic-adenosine monophosphate (cAMP) interact to convert the information from these receptors into alterations in cellular activity (Fig. 1) (14).

This inflammatory mediator-induced reduction in the transduction threshold of nociceptor primary afferents has been termed "peripheral sensitization," and is believed to cause pain hypersensitivity at the site of injury or inflammation, resulting in a heightened awareness of subsequent painful stimuli (*primary hyperalgesia*), and the perception of innocuous stimuli as being painful (*primary allodynia*) (9,15). A good example of this is the increased heat pain sensitivity after sunburn where warm water applied to the affected area feels burning hot.

Such peripheral mechanisms have been implicated in animal models of post-injury gut dysfunction. For instance, animal studies in mice with ongoing intestinal contractile dysfunction following resolved gut infection have demonstrated the persistence of local inflammatory mediators such as cyclooxygenase-2 (16,17), and inflammatory mediators when instilled into the rat colon can sensitize the response of pelvic afferent nerve fibers to subsequent colonic distension (18).

Central Sensitization

As mentioned, peripheral injury of primary afferent sensory neurons can be associated with peripheral sensitization. Also, recruitment of previously silent nociceptive neurons can occur which remain active after the injury heals. The increase in nociceptive information arriving at the spinal cord from these peripheral sites can enhance the excitability of dorsal horn neurons,

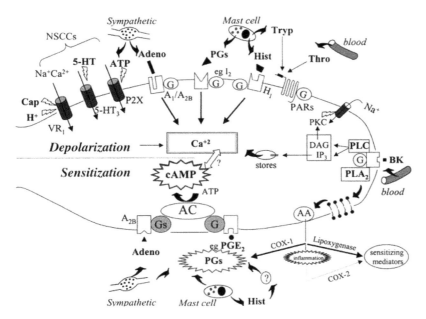

Figure 1 (*See color insert*) The potential receptor mechanisms mediating depolarization and sensitization of visceral afferent neurons. Inflammatory mediators can be released from a variety of cell types present around the afferent nerve terminal such as mast cells, sympathetic varicosities, and blood vessels. Adenosine, histamine, and tryptase bind to G protein–coupled receptors while serotonin (5-HT), ATP, and capsaicin can activate NSCCs. This leads to a Ca^{2+} dependent modulation of ion channel activity. Second messenger systems such as cAMP couple the signals from these receptors to alterations in cellular function, thus mediating sensitization. Adenosine and PGE_2 can generate cAMP directly via G protein–coupled stimulation of AC. Histamine however may act indirectly through generation of prostaglandins. *Abbreviations*: COX, cyclooxygenase; DAG, diacylglycerol; IP_3, inositol triphosphate; PARs, protease-activated receptors; PLC, phospholipase C; PLA_2, phospholipase A_2; PKC, protein kinase C; cAMP, cyclic adenosine monophosphate; ATP, adenosine triphosphate; NSCCs, nonselective cation channels; AC, adenyl cyclase; PGE2, prostaglandin E2; 5-HT, 5-hydroxytryptamine. *Source*: Adapted from Ref. 14.

through a variety of integrated mechanisms (Fig. 2). The central terminals of primary afferent neurons release a number of neurotransmitters including glutamate, substance P, prostaglandin E2 (PGE2), and brain-derived neurotrophic factor (BDNF). Increased levels of glutamate due to peripheral sensitization result in a removal of the magnesium ion block of the *N*-methyl-D-aspartate (NMDA) receptor and its subsequent activation (19). Glutamate also binds to ionotropic amino-methylene-phosphonic acid (AMPA) receptors and metabotropic glutamate receptors. Substance P binds to NK1 receptors, BDNF to tyrosine kinase B receptors, and PGE2 to endogenous prostanoid receptors on the postsynaptic membrane. A rise in intracellular postsynaptic calcium (Ca^{2+}) levels triggers the activation of second messenger systems including cAMP, protein kinases A and C, and Ca^{2+}-calmodulin-dependent protein kinase II (20). These kinases as well as tyrosine kinase Src phosphorylate AMPA and NMDA receptors, resulting in a further potentiation in their activity. The further release of nitric oxide and arachidonic acid (from cyclooxygenase-2 induction) potentiate presynaptic glutamate and prostaglandin release, respectively, thereby driving the cascade forward by a positive feedback loop.

This phenomenon has been termed "central sensitization" and is believed to be responsible for the pain hypersensitivity that occurs in surrounding healthy tissues (secondary hyperalgesia, or allodynia). Central sensitization is characterized by a decrease in threshold and an increase in response duration and magnitude to noxious stimuli and an expansion of the mechanosensitive receptive field of dorsal horn neurons (22). Both peripheral sensitization and central sensitization are the major mechanism in the development of neuropathic pain.

In animal models of cutaneous hypersensitivity, alterations in dorsal horn neuronal activity can be produced by peripheral tissue injury. Indeed, Jinks et al. demonstrated in anesthetized rats an expansion of the mechanical receptive field area of dorsal horn neurons after intracutaneous microinjection of histamine. Histamine evoked a dose-related increase in firing

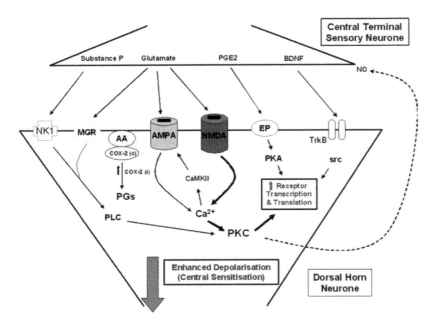

Figure 2 The potential receptor mechanisms underlying the development of central sensitization. Peripheral sensitization results in an increased afferent barrage to neurons in the spinal dorsal horn. A number of neurotransmitters and mediators are released from the central terminals of primary afferents, which upregulate neuronal activity in postsynaptic neurons and facilitate transmission of the nociceptive information. *Abbreviations*: PGE2, prostaglandin E2; BDNF, brain-derived neurotrophic factor; NK1, neurokinin 1; MGR, metabotropic glutamate receptor; AA, arachidonic acid; COX-2, cyclooxygenase-2; AMPA, amino-methylene-phosphonic acid; NMDA, *N*-methyl-D-aspartate; EP, endogenous prostanoid; TrkB, tyrosine kinase B; PKA, protein kinase A; PKC, protein kinase C; PG, prostaglandin; CAMKII, Ca^{2+}-calmodulin-dependent protein kinase II; PLC, phospholipase C. *Source*: Adapted from Ref. 21.

rate as well as a dose-dependent expansion in mean receptive field area of dorsal horn neurons that was prevented by NMDA receptor antagonists (23). A number of animal studies have highlighted the important role of the NMDA receptor in mediating central sensitization and behavioral hyperalgesia after peripheral tissue inflammation/injury (24,25). Human studies have also confirmed the role of the NMDA receptor in mediating central sensitization, and its prevention and attenuation by NMDA receptor antagonism have been demonstrated not only in somatic tissues but also in the viscera (26–30).

Spinal and Supra-Spinal Modulation of Pain Perception

Working with rats and using simple withdrawal reflexes as pain measures, Reynolds (31) showed that stimulation of a specific region of the midbrain periaqueductal gray (PAG) inhibited behavioral responses to noxious stimulation, giving rise to the term "stimulation produced analgesia." Stimulation of these sites inhibited responses of spinal neurons to noxious stimuli suggesting that the brain could modulate spinal activity. The PAG receives direct inputs from the hypothalamus and from the limbic forebrain, including several regions of the frontal neocortex and the central nucleus of the amygdala (Fig. 3). The PAG controls nociceptive transmission by means of connections through neurons in the rostral ventromedial medulla (RVM) and the dorsolateral pontine tegmentum (DLPT). These two regions project through the spinal cord dorsolateral funiculus and selectively target the dorsal horn laminae that accommodate nociceptive relay neurons. This circuit can therefore selectively modulate nociceptive transmission by its anatomical proximity to primary afferent nociceptor terminals and dorsal horn neurons that respond to noxious stimulation.

Some neurons in the dorsal horn of the spinal cord are strongly inhibited when a noxious stimulus is applied to any part of the body, distinct from their excitatory receptive fields. This phenomenon was termed "diffuse noxious inhibitory controls" (DNIC) (33). DNIC refers to a neurophysiological mechanism that underlies the long-established clinical phenomenon of counter-irritation, in which application of an acute aversive stimulus provides temporary

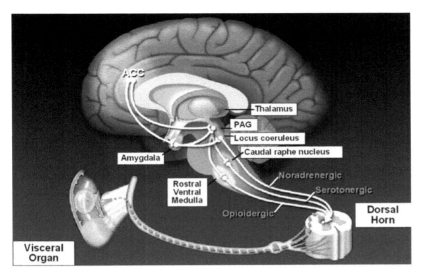

Figure 3 (*See color insert*) The principal components of descending pain modulatory pathways, which are activated in response to a painful visceral stimulus such as noxious balloon distension of the colon. Ponto-medullary networks including the PAG, rostral ventral medulla, and the raphe nuclei are modulated by inputs from the ACC, amygdala, and other cortical regions. The major descending pain inhibitory pathways are mediated via the opioidergic, serotonergic, and noradrenergic systems. These pathways modulate pain transmission at the level of the dorsal horn of the spinal cord. *Abbreviations*: PAG, periaqueductal gray; ACC, anterior cingulate cortex. *Source*: From the AGA gastroenterology teaching project (GTP). *Source*: American Gastroenterological Association, Baltimore, Maryland, U.S.A.

relief of chronic and recurrent pain (34). DNIC paradigms typically involve measurement of the nociceptive threshold for a "test" stimulus before, during, and after application of a second noxious "conditioning" stimulus to an anatomically remote area of the body. The RIII reflex is one such paradigm, and is a polysynaptic spinal reflex elicited by electrical stimulation of a sensory nerve and recorded from a flexor muscle in the ipsilateral limb. The threshold and amplitude of the RIII reflex are closely related to those of the concomitant cutaneous sensations evoked by electrical stimulation (35).

DNIC are not observed in patients with complete transection of the spinal cord (36), or specific medullary lesions, but are observed in patients with thalamic lesions (37). It has therefore been proposed that DNIC are triggered by ascending spinoreticular fibers, with the medullary reticular formation playing a crucial role in the subsequent descending modulation of spinal pain transmission (37).

Several neurotransmitters and their receptors are known to be involved in descending pain-inhibitory and pain-facilitatory pathways. The opioid system has been extensively described and investigations have largely focused on the μ-opioid receptor due to the powerful analgesic action of its widely used ligand morphine. This receptor is ubiquitous in the central nervous system (CNS) sites involved in pain modulation, such as the hypothalamus, amygdala, insular cortex, PAG, DLPT, RVM, and spinal cord dorsal horn (38,39). Behavioral responses to noxious stimulation can be attenuated by the administration of μ-opioid receptor agonists at these sites and disruption of RVM neurons that project to the spinal cord dorsal horn reduces the analgesic effects of morphine. There is evidence that opioid-mediated pain modulatory mechanisms operate in humans as naloxone has been reported to enhance experimental and postoperative pain in humans who have not received exogenous opioids (40,41).

Apart from opioid systems of pain modulation, norepinephrine (NE)-mediated and 5-hydroxytryptamine (5-HT)-mediated mechanisms of spinal and supraspinal pain modulation also exist and have been extensively described (42). The RVM contains the nucleus raphe magnus (NRM), and serotonergic neurons in this site demonstrate immunohistochemical FOS reactivity (a marker of noxious activity) following formalin injection and noxious heat stimulation of the hindpaw in the rat (43). Furthermore, Oatway et al. (44) recently demonstrated that ondansetron significantly attenuated mechanical allodynia in a rat model of spinal cord injury, whereas administration of a 5-HT3 receptor agonist exacerbated pain behavior.

In addition, treatment with 5,7-dihydroxytryptamine (which depletes endogenous 5-HT) eliminated the antiallodynic effect of ondansetron in spinal cord injury rats, further supporting the role of endogenous 5-HT in these pain behaviors through activation of 5-HT3 receptors.

Psychological Modulation of Pain Processing

Perception of visceral sensation is mediated at a cortical level and is therefore influenced by cognitive mechanisms such as stress, attention, and anxiety. Attention to gastrointestinal (GI) stimuli has been shown to increase their perception (45), and there is evidence that psychological mechanisms such as anxiety play a role in modulating visceral sensory perception (46).

Stress can be defined as an intrinsic or extrinsic disturbing force that threatens to disturb the homeostasis of an organism, and can be either real (physical) or perceived (psychological) (47,48). Stressors can be thought of as being internal ("interoceptive"—such as infection or inflammation), or external ("exteroceptive"—psychological) (49). They evoke an adaptive response, which serves to stabilize the internal environment of the organism and ensure its survival. The ability to defend homeostasis through change has been referred to as *allostasis* (50) and involves a number of neurobiological systems such as the hypothalamic–pituitary– adrenal (HPA) axis and autonomic nervous system (ANS). In healthy individuals, these physiological response systems are rapidly turned on and off to synchronize the stress response to the duration of stressor, thereby limiting the exposure time of the organism to the altered internal environment associated with it (49).

Stress can exert central effects that modulate both pain processing and perception. An organism's response to stress is generated by a network of integrative brain structures, in particular, subregions of the hypothalamus (paraventricular nucleus), amygdala, and PAG. These structures receive input from visceral and somatic afferents and from cortical structures, such as the medial prefrontal cortex (PFC), and subregions of the ACC and insula (51–53). This network provides outputs to the pituitary and pontomedullary nuclei [such as the locus coeruleus (LC) and raphe nuclei], which in turn mediate the neuroendocrine and autonomic output to the body, respectively (51,52). This central stress circuitry is under feedback control via ascending monoaminergic projections from these brain stem nuclei (Fig. 3), in particular serotonergic (raphe nuclei) and noradrenergic (including LC) nuclei, and via circulating glucocorticoids, which exert an inhibitory control via central glucocorticoid receptors located in the medial PFC and hippocampus. This complex network of brain structures modulates stress responses through an effector system referred to as the "emotional motor system," the main output components of which are the ANS, the HPA axis, endogenous pain modulatory systems, and ascending aminergic pathways (49).

Animal studies have shown that the responsiveness of these physiological systems and the ability to adapt can be altered by adverse early-life events, and that this seems to increase the organism's susceptibility to the negative effects of stress in later life. Al-Chaer et al. demonstrated chronic visceral hypersensitivity in adult rats that were subjected to either mechanical or chemical colonic irritation in neonatal life. Colon hypersensitivity was present in the absence of any persisting peripheral pathology (54). Early-life events can permanently influence the development of central corticotropin-releasing hormone (CRH) systems, which, in turn, mediate the expression of behavioral/emotional, autonomic, and endocrine responses to stress. In rodent and nonhuman primate studies, maternal deprivation in infancy is associated with enhanced neural CRH gene expression and increased stress reactivity. In adulthood, these animals show greater activation of the HPA axis, sympatho-adrenomedullary systems, and central monoaminergic systems, and thus, greater vulnerability for stress-induced illness (55,56).

Modulation of Pain by the Autonomic Nervous System

There has been increasing evidence to suggest that the ANS may modulate visceral sensory perception, and sympathetically mediated mechanisms are implicated in several chronic pain syndromes (57,58). In addition, there are animal and human data supporting a vagally mediated inhibition of visceral nociceptive sensory inputs (59,60). Iovino et al. used lower body negative pressure (LBNP) to experimentally activate the sympathetic nervous system by inducing venous pooling in the lower extremities, and to determine the effects on the perception of intestinal stimulation (61). Using brief distending stimuli in the intestine, the effect of sympathetic activation by LBNP on sympathetically mediated intestinal relaxation and on vagally mediated gastric relaxation was measured by corresponding barostats. The effect of LBNP on perception of duodenal distension was also compared to the perception of somatic stimulation. It was found that sympathetic activation significantly heightened perception of intestinal distension without modifying perception of somatic stimuli (perception scores increased by 41% and 2%, respectively). Also, the reflex responses to duodenal distension significantly increased during sympathetic activation both in the stomach and in the intestine (relaxation increased by 91% and 69%, respectively, with $p < 0.05$ for both).

In human studies, the activity of the ANS in response to stress or pain has mainly been determined by analysis of heart rate variability (HRV) or skin conductance. Evaluation of skin conductance via the Galvanic skin response provides a measure of relative sympathetic activation (62), whereas that of HRV allows an approximation of relative sympathetic and parasympathetic dominance, and the extraction of vagal tone (63). The beat-to-beat variability in the heart rate provides a window through which the autonomic input to the sinoatrial node in the heart can be evaluated. Power spectral analysis of HRV reveals a low-frequency band (LF), ranging from 0.05 to 0.15 Hz, which is believed to be largely under sympathetic control. The high-frequency band (HF), ranging from 0.2 to 0.5 Hz, is associated with respiratory sinus arrhythmia and is believed to be under vagal control. Sympathovagal balance has been expressed by the LF/HF ratio as it is said to reflect the relative dominance of efferent modulation of sinoatrial activity (64). Although this technique is not without its criticisms, and these will be discussed later, it may be possible to determine the relative contributions of the ANS components in an individual's response profile to an external stimulus.

Modulation of Pain by the Hypothalamic–Pituitary–Adrenal Axis

The hypothalamus is sited at the base of the brain around the third ventricle and above the pituitary stalk, which leads down to the pituitary itself, carrying the hypophyseal portal blood supply. It contains vital centers for functions including appetite, thirst, thermal regulation, and the sleep cycle, and acts as an integrator of many neuroendocrine inputs to control the release of pituitary hormone–releasing factors. Amongst other important influences, it plays a role in the circadian rhythm, menstrual cycle, and responses to stress, exercise, and mood. The pituitary gland is located in the sella turcica at the base of the brain and is around 1 cm in diameter and between 0.5 and 1 g in weight. CRH produced in the hypothalamus induces the release of adrenocorticotropin (ACTH) from specialized cells in the anterior pituitary. This in turn stimulates the release of cortisol from cells in the zona fasciculata and reticularis of the adrenal glands.

The HPA response to stress is a basic adaptive mechanism that modulates the metabolic and cardiovascular responses to it, whether it be acute stress or chronic. The CNS response to stress can modulate pain perception through the control of ANS outflow and activity of the HPA axis (49,65).

CRH has been implicated in the pathophysiology of anxiety. Centrally administered CRH produces several signs of increased anxiety and transgenic mice that overexpress CRH exhibit increased anxiogenic behavior; conversely, central administration of a CRH antagonist produces anxiolytic effects in the rat (66). These effects of CRH are thought to be mediated through actions of CRH on NE systems in the LC. The activity of the NE system has been observed to be increased during stress and anxiety in several animal species, and states of anxiety and fear appear to be associated with an increase in NE release in humans (67). There is anatomical evidence for direct synaptic contact between CRH terminals and dendrites of NE cells in the LC, and both acute and chronic stress increase CRH-like immunoreactivity in the LC (68). Stress increases the turnover of NE in terminal projection areas of the LC (69) and increases extracellular NE in the hippocampus (70). Projection sites of this LC–NE system include the medial PFC (71), PAG, hippocampus, hypothalamus, thalamus, and the nucleus tractus solitarius (NTS) (72,73). The LC has projections to areas such as the amygdala, known to process fear-relevant sensory stimuli, and to the medullary nucleus paragigantocellularis, which receives viscerosensory stimuli relayed by the NTS. Therefore, the LC is well positioned to integrate both external sensory and internal visceral information and influence a wide distribution of stress- and fear-related neural structures, including specific cortical areas.

During stress, the increased secretion of CRH and arginine vasopressin (AVP) into the hypophysial–portal system of the anterior pituitary enhances the synthesis and release of ACTH (Fig. 4), which can be demonstrated in both the cerebrospinal fluid and blood (74,75). Elevated ACTH content in blood, in turn, increases the synthesis and release of adrenal glucocorticoids, which act in synergy with catecholamines to produce lipolysis, glycogenolysis, and protein catabolism, resulting in increased blood glucose content, essentially providing a readily available energy source to aid in the stress response. The delivery of energy substrates is enhanced by increased blood flow as a result of glucocorticoid- and catecholamine-induced increases in cardiovascular tone. Prolonged exposure to elevated stress hormones, however, can present a risk. Glucocorticoids and catecholamines promote the suppression of anabolic processes, muscle atrophy, decreased sensitivity to insulin, and a risk of steroid-induced diabetes, hypertension, hyperlipidemia, hypercholesterolemia, arterial disease, amenorrhea, impotency, and the impairment of growth and tissue repair, as well as immunosuppression (76,77). Central CRH systems activate ascending serotonergic and noradrenergic pathways so that under conditions of threat, individuals become hypervigilant.

It is known that inflammatory cytokines, including tumor necrosis factor-α, interleukin-1, and interleukin-6, can stimulate the HPA axis (79,80). CRH is believed to be an important mediator of the central stress response, and indeed animal studies have demonstrated that experimentally induced stress in rats that alters gut motility in a similar pattern to that seen with stress in humans, can be mimicked by intracerebroventricular or intravenous administration of CRH and blocked by a CRH antagonist, α-helical CRH (81). Interestingly,

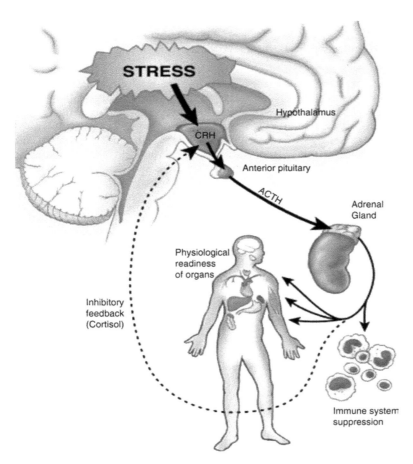

Figure 4   (*See color insert*) The functional anatomy of the hypothalamic-pituitary-adrenal axis. Stress stimulates release of CRH from the hypothalamus, which in turn stimulates the release of ACTH from the anterior pituitary. Cortisol released from the adrenal glands mediates the peripheral effects of this system whilst also providing feedback to higher centers. *Abbreviations*: CRH, corticotropin-releasing hormone; ACTH, adrenocorticotropic hormone. *Source*: Adapted from Ref. 78.

Gue et al. reported that both stress and the administration of CRH (either centrally or intraperitoneally) enhanced the number of abdominal cramps evoked by rectal distension in a rat model without affecting rectal compliance, suggesting a role of CRH in visceral hypersensitivity. These effects were also antagonized by α-helical CRH (82). This study also demonstrated that peripheral administration of doxantrazole, a mast cell stabilizer, suppressed stress and CRH-induced rectal hyperalgesia to rectal distension (82). It seems therefore that mast cell mediators are involved in the hypersensitivity response to rectal distension induced by stress. Previous studies have also highlighted the relationship between stress and colonic mast cell degranulation, and the fact that these effects can be reproduced by the administration of CRH (83); rather than, however, the mechanisms by which CRH modulates mast cell function are still unknown.

Modulation of Pain by Genotypic Profile

It has long been noted that some individuals are more sensitive to pain than others for a diverse range of noxious stimuli (84–86), some respond better to analgesics than others (87,88), and some individuals develop chronic pain syndromes after inflammation or injury whereas others do not. This variation is incompletely explained by environmental and cultural factors and research has therefore focused on the possible role of genetic factors. Inherited genetic variability, in the form of different DNA sequences in different individuals (their individual "genotype"), determines their individual biological traits (phenotype) via the pattern and quantities of proteins translated from active genes. Although environmental factors cannot alter the individual's genetic make-up, they can alter the pattern of transcription and translation resulting in altered protein expression, and ultimately cell function.

Certainly research on rodent populations has demonstrated large and heritable differences in both nociceptive and analgesic sensitivity, with genotypic differences being implicated in mediating basal pain sensitivity, the likelihood of developing neuropathic pain following neural injury, and in determining the sensitivity to pharmacological agents and endogenous antinociception (89,90). It is known that mice lacking the gene for TrkA, a tyrosine kinase receptor for nerve growth factor (NGF) have a loss of responsiveness to painful stimuli such as heat or pinpricks (91). NGF is important for the survival of embryonic sensory and sympathetic neurons. Patients with congenital insensitivity to pain with anhidrosis (CIPA) share phenotypic traits with TrkA knockout mice, and indeed Indo et al. recently demonstrated mutations in the Trk/NGF receptor gene in patients with CIPA (92). This suggests that mutations of certain genes may be involved in certain pain pathologies, particularly if they are important to the development of the nervous system.

VARIABILITY IN THE DEVELOPMENT OF SENSITIZED STATES

To determine whether peripheral sensitization and central sensitization can occur in healthy human viscera in response to injury/inflammation, a model was developed which has demonstrated that acid infusion localized to the distal esophagus can reduce subsequent pain thresholds to electrical stimulation at the site of the infusion compared to preacid baseline levels. After the acid infusion, a previously nonpainful stimulus is reported as painful demonstrating hypersensitivity at the site of infusion (93). This hypersensitivity is likely to be due to peripheral sensitization. Although continuous pH monitoring demonstrates no acid reflux into the proximal esophagus, a similar reduction in pain thresholds to electrical stimulation can be demonstrated at this site. This secondary hypersensitivity is believed to occur through the sensitization of spinal neurons (central sensitization), and indeed further work in our department has shown that this secondary esophageal hypersensitivity can be attenuated by both PGE2 receptor-1 (94) and NMDA receptor antagonists (Fig. 5) (26). These studies suggest that both peripheral and central sensitization can induce visceral hypersensitivity.

It has however been noted that around 20% of subjects fail to sensitize to esophageal acid infusion. Furthermore, there is a variation in the magnitude of response (reduction in pain threshold to acid infusion) between subjects to the order of 24%. Also, while most subjects will demonstrate reproducible sensitization to acid in repeated studies, around 14% will habituate to acid with diminishing sensitization to repeated acid infusions (95). Recent work in healthy subjects has shown that visceral pain thresholds inversely correlate with baseline anxiety scores (96). Whether the effect of anxiety in these subjects is to amplify pain responses through the effect of attention toward the visceral stimulation is unknown.

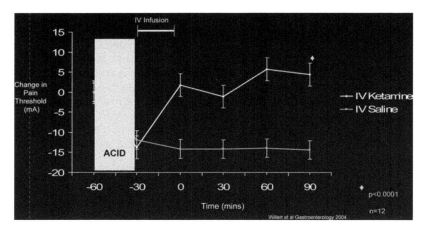

Figure 5 (*See color insert*) The effect of an *N*-methyl-D-aspartate receptor antagonist, ketamine, on proximal eso-phageal pain thresholds when given following a distal esophageal acid infusion. The acid causes a reduction in pain thresholds in the nonacid exposed proximal esophagus, demonstrating the development of visceral hypersensitivity, and this is reversed by ketamine. The hypersensitivity is not reversed by saline infusion. *Source*: Adapted from Ref. 26.

There may be phenotypic differences between subjects that determine their magnitude of sensitization and pain responsiveness after visceral injury. The biological factors involved in mediating visceral sensitization, particularly after injurious/inflammatory events, are incompletely understood, but may involve the systems previously discussed. It seems plausible that the complex interactions of these factors result in phenotypic traits that may determine patterns of postinjury gut sensitization. Identifying phenotypes may provide clues as to the mechanism of prolonged sensitization to inflammation/injury seen in FGD patients, and may lead to the identification of genotypic correlations. Evidence for the involvement of these factors in FGD will now be presented.

MECHANISMS OF VISCERAL SENSITIZATION IN FUNCTIONAL GASTROINTESTINAL DISORDER
Evidence for Peripheral Sensitization

It is known that at least a third of patients with FGD have a previous history of gut inflam-mation or injury in the form of gastroenteritis or surgery (97). Although the majority of patients with such gut injury recover, a proportion go on to develop chronic symptoms such as pain or bowel dysfunction, this subgroup being labeled as having postinfectious IBS (PI-IBS).

The environment of nociceptor terminals in the gut of some patients with IBS is likely to be altered given the increased number of inflammatory cells that have been demonstrated in these patients. Increased gut permeability and altered mucosal characteristics, such as increased numbers of rectal mucosal enteroendocrine cells and T lymphocytes that have been documented in subjects with PI-IBS suggest a role for these peripheral mechanisms in the vis-ceral hypersensitivity observed in these patients (98). Interleukin-1β (IL-1β) is an important modulator of the inflammatory process, and greater expression of IL-1β mRNA has been reported in patients with PI-IBS both during and after gastroenteritis compared to individuals who did not subsequently develop PI-IBS and controls (99). Furthermore, some recent prelimi-nary work has suggested that a proportion of IBS patients may be predisposed to prolonged inflammation due to reduced secretion of the counter inflammatory cytokines IL-10 and trans-forming growth factor-β. The frequency of the high producer alleles for both mediators was found to be significantly reduced in a proportion of IBS patients compared to controls. It was proposed that low secretors of these cytokines may be less efficient in down-regulating the response to inflammatory stimuli such as enteric infection (100).

Evidence for Central Sensitization

Although evidence for central sensitization is abundant in animal models of somatic and vis-ceral pain hypersensitivity (101–104), proving its role in patients with functional gut disorders has been more difficult, presumably due to technical and ethical reasons. Patients with IBS have been shown to demonstrate both visceral hyperalgesia to rectal balloon distension and cutaneous hyperalgesia to thermal stimulation over a broad rostral-caudal region yet most optimally expressed over lumbosacral dermatomes (105). It was suggested that this pattern of neural activity could be indicative of a widely distributed but topographically organized central hyperexcitability; however, hypervigilance or altered central descending inhibitory controls were also possible mechanisms. In addition, Sarkar et al. recently demonstrated exaggerated and prolonged viscero-visceral and viscerosomatic pain hypersensitivity after esophageal acid infusion in patients with NCCP compared to controls (93). Acid infusion in the distal esophagus resulted in a greater and prolonged fall in pain thresholds in the nonacid exposed proximal esophagus and chest wall, suggesting a central enhancement of nociceptive transmission. Furthermore, Munakata et al. showed that high pressure mechanical sigmoid stimulation induced the development of central sensitization in IBS patients compared to controls manifested by rectal hyperalgesia and increased viscerosomatic pain referral patterns (106). Whether this heightened sensory transmission is responsible for the prolonged visceral pain hypersensitivity in these disorders remains to be proven.

Evidence for Spinal and Supra-Spinal Pain Modulation

A number of animal and human studies have assessed the role of spinal nociceptive processes using DNIC paradigms. Recently, Coffin et al. assessed the spinal process of nociceptive signals in IBS patients by analyzing the effects of rectal distensions on electromyographic recordings of the somatic nociceptive flexion (RIII) reflex (107). They reported a significant progressive inhibition of the RIII reflex in healthy volunteers during slow ramp distension, with biphasic effects (facilitation and inhibition) observed during rapid distensions. In contrast, the RIII reflex was significantly facilitated in IBS patients during slow ramp distension and inhibitions induced by rapid distensions were significantly reduced, suggesting hyperexcitability of spinal nociceptive processes in a subgroup of IBS patients.

Mayer studied the perceptual responses to rectosigmoid distension in IBS patients and controls with functional brain imaging using $H_2^{15}O$ positron emission tomography and found that following a train of repetitive sigmoid distensions, control subjects demonstrated greater activation of the PAG and thalamic regions compared to IBS patients (108). This effect was seen both during actual rectal distension and the expectation of the stimulus, despite its absence. As has been outlined, the PAG is an important structure involved in the modulation of spinal pain processing, and the above finding suggests that a proportion of IBS patients have inadequate activation of brain regions involved with antinociception.

Evidence for Altered Psychological State

Certain stressful life events have been associated with both the onset and exacerbation of a number of disorders of the GI tract including FGD (109), PI-IBS (110), and inflammatory bowel disease (111). Anxiety, somatization, neuroticism, hypochondriasis, and preceding adverse life events have all been reported to increase the risk of developing IBS after gastroenteritis (110,112). Both early-life stress in the form of abuse and an acute episode of extreme stress in adult life such as rape have been suggested as important risk factors for the development of FGD (113,114).

A number of physiological and psychological theories have been proposed that might modulate the effects of anxiety and stress on pain sensitivity. Of the psychological theories, the *attributional* theory proposes that anxiety that has painful sensation as its focus (pain-relevant anxiety) will lead to heightened pain responses, whereas pain-irrelevant anxiety will reduce pain responses. The *attentional* theory proposes that the focus of attention can modulate pain responsiveness such that attention toward pain increases the pain experience whereas distraction can reduce it (115).

Brain-imaging studies have begun to address the possible neural mechanisms of hypersensitivity in IBS patients, and a common finding has been that compared to healthy controls, patients with IBS exhibit altered and/or enhanced activation of regions involved in pain processing, such as the ACC, thalamus, insula, and PFC, in response to experimental and anticipated rectal pain (116–118). Increases in anterior cingulate activity or prefrontal activity may reflect enhanced cerebral mechanisms related to cognitive evaluation and/or affect.

These findings raise the possibility that patients with FGD may pay more attention to GI events than normal subjects. However, other researchers have reported a reduction in activity of cortical structures including the ACC in IBS patients (119,120), highlighting both the variability in patient populations and the limitations of functional brain imaging paradigms.

Evidence for Autonomic Nervous System Dysfunction

A number of studies have addressed the role of the ANS in modulating visceral perception in FGD. Chen and Orr demonstrated enhanced sympathetic dominance to esophageal acid infusion in patients with gastroesophageal reflux disease (GERD), which appeared to be secondary to decreased vagal tone in these subjects (121). During acid infusion, there was a significant decrease in LF band power (a measure of sympathetic tone) in the control group, which was unchanged in the patient group, whereas the HF band power (a measure of vagal tone) was lower during all the infusion periods in the GERD group. The findings suggest the autonomic effects of acid infusion are different between healthy subjects and GERD patients. Indeed, the between-group comparisons did reveal a significant group difference during acid infusion, with GERD patients demonstrating a significantly larger LF/HF ratio compared with controls ($p < 0.05$). The healthy controls who had heartburn with acid infusion did not have a different LF/HF ratio from the controls who had no symptoms with acid infusion. These data seem to suggest that alterations in autonomic balance may play a role in modulating visceral sensation. The observed decrease in HF band power in the patient group (corresponding with a reduction in vagal tone) was proposed to be the cause of the increase in the LF/HF ratio; however, the ratio could also result from an increase in the LF band power (sympathetic component). This latter possibility was not borne out in the data, and therefore conflicts with the findings of Iovino et al. where increased sympathetic activity (albeit experimental) corresponded with heightened visceral sensitivity (61).

Increased sympathetic activity has been demonstrated in patients with IBS. Heitkemper et al. studied urinary catecholamine (NE and epinephrine) and cortisol levels in women diagnosed with IBS against women who reported similar symptoms but did not seek health care services and asymptomatic control women (122). Women with IBS had significantly higher urinary levels of all of these neuroendocrine indicators of arousal suggesting heightened sympathetic nervous system activation. Whether greater symptom distress in the IBS women resulted in increased sympathetic activation and health care seeking or the higher sympathetic activation increased pain perception leading to health care seeking is unclear. These investigators later demonstrated significantly lower parasympathetic tone and higher ANS balance in constipation-predominant compared to diarrhea-predominant subgroups of IBS but only when symptom severity scores were high. No difference was seen between IBS and control women, and between subgroups with IBS on autonomic function tests in the absence of severe symptoms, highlighting the importance of assessing symptom severity in these patients (123).

Diminished variability in heart rate and skin conductance has been demonstrated in anxiety, and these are likely to be due to the interaction of both the sympathetic and parasympathetic nervous systems. Piccirillo et al. demonstrated that healthy adults with higher anxiety scores have lower LF and HF power values, and demonstrate a higher LF/HF ratio compared to those that report lower anxiety scores on questionnaires (124). The significantly higher LF power suggested cardiac sympathetic hyperactivity. Other work has suggested that the variations in power spectral components in anxiety are associated with reduced vagal modulation of cardiac control (125). The mechanisms whereby anxiety can modulate the ANS, HPA axis, and eventually pain perception are incompletely understood, but this area of research is likely to gain interest due to their prevalence in FGD and the advancement of monitoring technologies.

Although much of the literature assessing the role of the ANS in various disorders involves power spectral analysis of HRV, the delineation into LF and HF band powers and the inference that the ratio of these two components can provide an idea of sympathovagal balance. This is controversial. The LF variability is a product of both sympathetic and parasympathetic influences on the heart, and as a result any change in LF power cannot be accurately taken as index of alterations in sympathetic cardiac control (126). The notion of sympathovagal balance has been questioned as its autonomic constructs are not always reciprocally controlled and can vary independently or demonstrate coactivation or coinhibition, particularly in the setting of stress and fear (127). HRV holds considerable promise for providing insights into the modulatory role of the ANS in health and disease, and for clarifying the relationship between psychological processes and observed physiological responses, but careful quantification and interpretation of data seems paramount.

Evidence for Hypothalamic–Pituitary–Adrenal Dysfunction

Human studies have demonstrated the effects of CRH and its antagonism, both in healthy subjects and in FGD. Fukudo et al. demonstrated that intravenous CRH induced greater abdominal symptoms, higher ACTH levels, and exaggerated gut motility in IBS patients compared to controls (128). This suggests a heightened sensitivity of the HPA axis in IBS patients, which may be at the hypothalamic-pituitary level as no significant difference was found between levels of cortisol response between the two groups. Peripheral administration of α-helical CRH has been shown to improve GI motility, visceral perception, and negative mood in response to gut stimulation in IBS patients, suggesting that CRH-signalling pathways play an important role in the pathophysiology of IBS. The precise site of action of intravenously administered CRH antagonists on GI function is unknown. Human studies have reiterated the findings of animal studies regarding the involvement of mast cells in the immunoregulatory response. Indeed, oral disodium chromoglycate has been shown to improve symptoms in selected subtypes of patients with diarrhea predominant IBS (129).

Conflicting results exist in the literature regarding the detection of humoral markers of the HPA axis in FGD. This is important, as assaying these various markers varies in expense, availability, and collection requirements with cortisol (plasma, salivary, or urinary) probably being the most favorable on all counts. Posserud et al. (130) examined the effects of mental stress on rectal distension thresholds in IBS patients and healthy controls. Thresholds increased during stress in controls but not in IBS patients; however, thresholds were lower in all groups after stress. Patients demonstrated higher stress ratings, higher ACTH content in blood during stress, and lower basal CRH content than controls. CRH content increased significantly during stress but did not in controls. No significant rise or group differences were seen in cortisol responses to stress. Other studies have demonstrated higher morning cortisol content in IBS patients both in the saliva (131) and in the urine (122), and different cortisol responses between IBS subgroups with elevated postprandial cortisol seen in diarrhea predominant IBS (132). Autonomic assessments in this latter study also suggested heightened postprandial sympathetic dominance and vagal withdrawal that correlated with increased symptoms in diarrhea predominant IBS (132).

Evidence for Genotypic Influences

Anecdotally, FGD appear to cluster in families, and recent research has confirmed these impressions. A large questionnaire-based same-sex twin pair study in Australia suggested a substantial proportion of the liability for FGD was under genetic control with a calculated heritability of 57%, and the remaining 43% being attributed to the individual's unique environment (133). A much larger questionnaire-based study by Levy et al. found a greater concordance for IBS in monozygotic versus dizygotic twins (17.2% vs. 8.4%, $p = 0.03$), supporting a genetic contribution to IBS (134); however, logistic regression analysis suggested that having a mother or father with IBS were independent predictors of IBS status ($p < 0.001$) and stronger predictors than having a twin with IBS. Therefore, although heredity certainly contributes to the development of IBS, social learning has an equal or greater influence.

Serotonin (5-HT) plays an important role in gut function and sensory signalling in the brain–gut axis. It is not only an important neurotransmitter in the enteric nervous system, stimulating both vagal and intrinsic (enteric) afferent fibers, but is also a signalling molecule participating in mucosal sensory transduction (135). Ninety-five percent of the 5-HT in the body is found in the GI tract where it is contained in enterochromaffin cells in the epithelial lining of the gut (90%) and in enteric neurons of the submucosal and myenteric plexuses (10%). The remaining 5% is found in the brain. There are seven subtypes of 5-HT receptors differentiated on the basis of structure and function (135). As a result of these features, it plays a pivotal role in initiating a wide range of intestinal responses and reflexes. The reuptake of 5-HT provides an adequate means of terminating its effects after it has exerted its synaptic action, and is mediated by the 5-HT transporter *SERT*. Deletion polymorphisms in SERT, producing short allelic variants, have been linked with diarrhea predominant IBS in women (136), and anxiety-related personality characteristics (137). Females homozygous for these short allelic variants have also been shown to demonstrate elevated behaviorally evoked heart rate reactivity (138). It is possible that these polymorphisms that reduce the efficacy of SERT as a transporter allow ongoing 5-HT–mediated effects at the synaptic junction, resulting in clinical consequences.

As mentioned earlier, sympathetic adrenergic dysfunction has been demonstrated in a subgroup of patients with IBS (122). Bharucha et al. compared the effects of saline (control) against clonidine (α_2-agonist), yohimbine (α_2-antagonist), phenylephrine (α_1-agonist), and ritodrine (β_2-agonist) on colonic motility, compliance, and sensation in healthy human volunteers (139). They demonstrated that clonidine reduced fasting colonic tone and phasic activity, increased colonic compliance, and markedly attenuated the perception of pain during colonic balloon distension, whereas yohimbine increased fasting colonic tone and enhanced colonic perception of pain. The other drugs tested showed no effects at the doses used which were said to be the maximal permissible in humans. These findings suggest a role for the α_2-adrenoceptor in modulating colonic motor and sensory function in the human GI tract.

Three human α_2-adrenoceptor subtypes have been identified: α_{2A}, α_{2B}, and α_{2C} (140). Prejunctional α_{2A} and α_{2C} adrenoceptor subtypes regulate the release of NE from sympathetic nerves through negative feedback at presynaptic nerve endings. Synaptic content of NE is modified by the NE transporter. Mutations in the NE transporter that reduce its efficacy in removing NE from the synapse could prolong the effects of NE, thereby resulting in a functional overstimulation of the sympathetic nervous system in response to physiological stimuli, possibly resulting in increased gut motility or enhanced sensory signalling. Recently, both SERT and α_2-adrenoceptor polymorphisms have been associated with high somatic symptom scores in FGD (141). As mentioned, anxiety and visceral hypersensitivity are both associated with FGD; however, whether these polymorphisms predict pain sensitivity to an adverse stimulus (such as esophageal acidification) is unknown.

Apart from abnormalities in reuptake transporters as described above, a role for underlying second messenger abnormalities has also been proposed. Holtmann et al. reported the association of functional dyspepsia with specific G-protein β3 subunit genotypes (142). G-proteins are heterotrimeric second messenger proteins that are essential in mediating cellular responses by coupling extracellular receptor activation to intracellular effector systems such as adenylcyclases and protein kinases (143). Approximately 80% of all known membrane receptors transduce their signals via heterotrimeric G-proteins. G-proteins are composed of different α, β, and γ subunit isoforms, the β-γ subunit forming a functional monomer. On receptor activation, both α and β-γ subunits dissociate from the receptor to then modulate a variety of intracellular effector systems. Dysfunction of these important second messenger systems could therefore alter intracellular signal transduction (142). A common C825T polymorphism has been described in the gene *GNB3* that encodes the β3 subunit of heterotrimeric G-proteins, which gives rise to 3 possible genotypes—CC, TC, or TT. The 825T allele of the TC or TT genotype is associated with alternative splicing of the gene and the formation of a truncated but functionally active splice variant (142). The 825T allele is associated with enhanced G-protein activation and increased cellular responses, and to that effect has been linked with enhanced α2-adrenoceptor–mediated coronary vasoconstriction in GNB3 825T allele carriers (144). Individuals who are homozygous 825C allele carriers (CC genotype) form much reduced quantities of the β3 splice variant and demonstrate reduced signal transduction responses. The GNB3 subunit has been proposed as a susceptibility factor for depression, and may predict the response to treatment with antidepressants (145). In addition, in vitro cellular studies have demonstrated the C825T allele to be associated with enhanced lymphocyte proliferation and chemotaxis (146).

SUMMARY

A proportion of patients with FGD can identify an adverse event that preceded the development of their symptoms, such as gastroenteritis or surgery. Recovery from such an insult varies and although the majority will recover without further consequences, a proportion may develop chronic unexplained pain. These latter subjects often display heightened pain sensitivity to experimental gut stimulation (visceral hypersensitivity). Understanding the

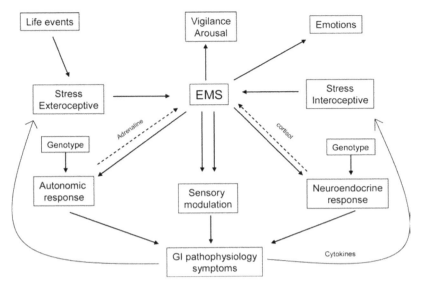

Figure 6 The potential factors that may interact with the EMS to govern an individual's visceral pain sensitivity. Stress, either exteroceptive (psychological) or interoceptive (such as infection or inflammation) can activate the EMS, and the resulting autonomic and neuroendocrine responses may modulate pain sensitivity. Dysfunction of these systems may be relevant in the pathophysiology of the visceral pain hypersensitivity seen in functional GI disorders. *Abbreviations*: EMS, emotional motor system; GI, gastrointestinal. *Source*: Adapted from Ref. 49.

phenotypic differences that determine a subject's response to a sensitizing stimulus could be the key to understanding why some patients develop visceral hypersensitivity in response to inflammation/injury while others do not. As this review suggests, an individual's phenotype is likely to be determined by a highly complex interplay between psychological, neurophysiological and hormonal systems, the response profiles of which may have a genetic basis (Fig. 6). For future studies, an integrated approach is required which incorporates an individual's psychological, neurophysiological, autonomic, endocrine, and genetic traits to identify phenotypes that may be at greater risk of developing sensitized states in response to gut inflammation or injury.

REFERENCES

1. Richter JE, Bradley LA, Castell DO. Esophageal chest pain: current controversies in pathogenesis, diagnosis, and therapy. Ann Intern Med 1989; 110(1):66–78.
2. Fullerton S. Functional digestive disorders (FDD) in the year 2000-economic impact. Eur J Surg Suppl 1998; 582:62–64.
3. Ritchie J. Pain from distension of the pelvic colon by inflating a balloon in the irritable colon syndrome. Gut 1973; 14(2):125–132.
4. Richter JE, Barish CF, Castell DO. Abnormal sensory perception in patients with esophageal chest pain. Gastroenterology 1986; 91(4):845–852.
5. Salet GA et al. Responses to gastric distension in functional dyspepsia. Gut 1998; 42(6):823–829.
6. Trimble KC et al. Heightened visceral sensation in functional gastrointestinal disease is not site-specific. Evidence for a generalized disorder of gut sensitivity. Dig Dis Sci 1995; 40(8):1607–1613.
7. Mertz H et al. Altered rectal perception is a biological marker of patients with irritable bowel syndrome. Gastroenterology 1995; 109(1):40–52.
8. Mertz H et al. Symptoms and visceral perception in severe functional and organic dyspepsia. Gut 1998; 42(6):814–822.
9. Treede RD et al. Peripheral and central mechanisms of cutaneous hyperalgesia. Prog Neurobiol 1992; 38(4):397–421.
10. Bueno L et al. Mediators and pharmacology of visceral sensitivity: from basic to clinical investigations. Gastroenterology 1997; 112(5):1714–1743.
11. Gebhart GF. Pathobiology of visceral pain: molecular mechanisms and therapeutic implications: IV. Visceral afferent contributions to the pathobiology of visceral pain. Am J Physiol Gastrointest Liver Physiol 2000; 278(6):834–838.

12. Mendell LM. Modifiability of spinal synapses. Physiol Rev 1984; 64(1):260–324.
13. Geppetti P, Trevisani M. Activation and sensitisation of the vanilloid receptor: role in gastrointestinal inflammation and function. Br J Pharmacol 2004; 141(8):1313–1320.
14. Kirkup AJ, Brunsden AM, Grundy D. Receptors and transmission in the brain-gut axis: potential for novel therapies. I. Receptors on visceral afferents. Am J Physiol Gastrointest Liver Physiol 2001; 280(5):787–794.
15. Torebjork HE, Lundberg LE, LaMotte RH. Central changes in processing of mechanoreceptive input in capsaicin-induced secondary hyperalgesia in humans. J Physiol Lond 1992; 448:765–780.
16. Barbara G, Vallance BA, Collins SM. Persistent intestinal neuromuscular dysfunction after acute nematode infection in mice. Gastroenterology 1997; 113(4):1224–1232.
17. Barbara G et al. Role of immunologic factors and cyclooxygenase 2 in persistent postinfective enteric muscle dysfunction in mice. Gastroenterology 2001; 120(7):1729–1736.
18. Su X, Gebhart GF. Mechanosensitive pelvic nerve afferent fibers innervating the colon of the rat are polymodal in character. J Neurophysiol 1998; 80(5):2632–2644.
19. Woolf CJ, Thompson SW. The induction and maintenance of central sensitization is dependent on N-methyl-D-aspartic acid receptor activation; implications for the treatment of post-injury pain hypersensitivity states. Pain 1991; 44(3):293–299.
20. Ji RR et al. Central sensitization and LTP: do pain and memory share similar mechanisms? Trends Neurosci 2003; 26(12):696–705.
21. Woolf CJ, Salter MW. Neuronal plasticity: increasing the gain in pain. Science 2000; 288(5472):1765–1768.
22. Woolf CJ. Somatic pain—pathogenesis and prevention. Br J Anaesth 1995; 75(2):169–176.
23. Jinks SL, Carstens E. Spinal NMDA receptor involvement in expansion of dorsal horn neuronal receptive field area produced by intracutaneous histamine. J Neurophysiol 1998; 79(4):1613–1618.
24. Ren K et al. The effects of a non-competitive NMDA receptor antagonist, MK-801, on behavioral hyperalgesia and dorsal horn neuronal activity in rats with unilateral inflammation. Pain 1992; 50(3):331–344.
25. Chaplan SR, Malmberg AB, Yaksh TL. Efficacy of spinal NMDA receptor antagonism in formalin hyperalgesia and nerve injury evoked allodynia in the rat. J Pharmacol Exp Ther 1997; 280(2):829–838.
26. Willert RP et al. The development and maintenance of human visceral pain hypersensitivity is dependent on the N-methyl-D-aspartate receptor. Gastroenterology 2004; 126(3):683–692.
27. Park KM et al. Effects of intravenous ketamine, alfentanil, or placebo on pain, pinprick hyperalgesia, and allodynia produced by intradermal capsaicin in human subjects. Pain 1995; 63(2):163–172.
28. Ilkjaer S et al. Effect of systemic N-methyl-D-aspartate receptor antagonist (ketamine) on primary and secondary hyperalgesia in humans. Br J Anaesth 1996; 76(6):829–834.
29. Andersen OK, Felsby S, Nicolaisen L, Bjerring P, Jensen TS, Arendt-Nielsen L. The effect of Ketamine on stimulation of primary and secondary hyperalgesia areas induced by capsaicin - a double blind placebo controlled, human experimental study. Pain 1996; 66:829–834.
30. Warncke T, Stubhaug A, Jorum E. Ketamine, an NMDA receptor antagonist, suppresses spatial and temporal properties of burn-induced secondary hyperalgesia in man: a double-blind, cross-over comparison with morphine and placebo. Pain 1997; 72:99–106.
31. Reynolds DV. Surgery in the rat during electrical analgesia induced by focal brain stimulation. Science 1969; 164(878):444–445.
32. Willert RP. Receptor mechanisms mediating human oesophageal pain hypersensitivity; PhD report 2005, University of Manchester. Adapted from Rainville P. Brain mechanisms of Pain Affect and Pain Modulation. In Current Opinion in Neurobiology 2002; 12:195–204.
33. Le Bars D, Dickenson AH, Besson JM. Diffuse noxious inhibitory controls (DNIC). I. Effects on dorsal horn convergent neurones in the rat. Pain 1979; 6(3):283–304.
34. Wand-Tetley JI. Historical methods of counter-irritation. Ann Phys Med 1956; 3(3):90–99.
35. Willer JC. Comparative study of perceived pain and nociceptive flexion reflex in man. Pain 1977; 3(1):69–80.
36. Roby-Brami A et al. An electrophysiological investigation into the pain-relieving effects of heterotopic nociceptive stimuli. Probable involvement of a supraspinal loop. Brain 1987; 110(Pt 6):1497–1508.
37. De Broucker T et al. Diffuse noxious inhibitory controls in man. Involvement of the spinoreticular tract. Brain 1990; 113(Pt 4):1223–1234.
38. Mansour A et al. Anatomy of CNS opioid receptors. Trends Neurosci 1988; 11(7):308–314.
39. Arvidsson U et al. Distribution and targeting of a mu-opioid receptor (MOR1) in brain and spinal cord. J Neurosci 1995; 15(5 Pt 1):3328–3341.
40. Levine JD et al. The narcotic antagonist naloxone enhances clinical pain. Nature 1978; 272(5656):826–827.
41. Pollo A et al. Response expectancies in placebo analgesia and their clinical relevance. Pain 2001; 93(1):77–84.
42. Millan MJ. Descending control of pain. Prog Neurobiol 2002; 66(6):355–474.
43. Suzuki R et al. Superficial NK1-expressing neurons control spinal excitability through activation of descending pathways. Nat Neurosci 2002; 5(12):1319–1326.

44. Oatway MA, Chen Y, Weaver LC. The 5-HT3 receptor facilitates at-level mechanical allodynia following spinal cord injury. Pain 2004; 110(1–2):259–268.
45. Accarino AM, Azpiroz F, Malagelada JR. Attention and distraction: effects on gut perception. Gastroenterology 1997; 113(2):415–422.
46. Ford MJ et al. Psychosensory modulation of colonic sensation in the human transverse and sigmoid colon. Gastroenterology 1995; 109(6):1772–1780.
47. Selye H. Stress and the general adaptation syndrome. Br Med J 1950; 4667:1383–1392.
48. Chrousos GP, Gold PW. The concepts of stress and stress system disorders. Overview of physical and behavioral homeostasis. JAMA 1992; 267(9):1244–1252.
49. Mayer EA. The neurobiology of stress and gastrointestinal disease. Gut 2000; 47(6):861–869.
50. Sterling PE, J Fisher S, et al. Handbook of Life Stress, Cognition and Health. New York, 1988: 629–649.
51. Sawchenko PE, Li H-Y, Ericsson A. Circuits and mechanisms governing hypothalamic responses to stress: a tale of two paradigms. In: Mayer EA, Saper CB, eds. The Biological Basis for Mind Body Interactions. Amsterdam: Elsevier Science, 2000:59–75.
52. Bandler R, Price JL, Keay KA. Brain mediation of active and passive emotional coping. In: Mayor EA, Saper CB, eds. The Biological Basis for Mind Body Interactions. Amsterdam: Elsevier Science, 2000:333–349.
53. Vogt BA, Sikes RW, Vogt LJ. Anterior cingulate cortex and the medial pain system. In: Vogt BA, Gabriel M, eds. Neurobiology of Cingulate Cortex and Limbic Thalamus: A Comprehensive Handbook. Boston: Birkhaeuser, 1993:313–344.
54. Al-Chaer ED, Kawasaki M, Pasricha PJ. A new model of chronic visceral hypersensitivity in adult rats induced by colon irritation during postnatal development. Gastroenterology 2000; 119(5): 1276–1285.
55. Meaney MJ et al. Early environmental regulation of forebrain glucocorticoid receptor gene expression: implications for adrenocortical responses to stress. Dev Neurosci 1996; 18(1–2):49–72.
56. Coplan JD et al. Persistent elevations of cerebrospinal fluid concentrations of corticotropin-releasing factor in adult nonhuman primates exposed to early-life stressors: implications for the pathophysiology of mood and anxiety disorders. Proc Natl Acad Sci USA 1996; 93(4):1619–1623.
57. Schott G. Visceral afferents: their contribution to sympathetic dependent' pain. Brain 1994; 117(2):397–413.
58. Green PG et al. Endocrine and vagal controls of sympathetically dependent neurogenic inflammation. Ann NY Acad Sci 1998; 840:282–288.
59. Randich A, Gebhart G. Vagal afferent modulation of nociception. Brain Res Rev 1992; 17:77–99.
60. Diop L et al. Role of vagal afferents in the antinociception produced by morphine and U-50,488H in the colonic pain reflex in rats. Eur J Pharmacol 1994; 257(1–2):181–187.
61. Iovino P et al. The sympathetic nervous system modulates perception and reflex responses to gut distention in humans. Gastroenterology 1995; 108(3):680–686.
62. Cacioppo JTTL, Berntson GG. Handbook of psychophysiology. 2nd ed. 2004.
63. Tougas G et al. Cardiac autonomic function and oesophageal acid sensitivity in patients with non-cardiac chest pain. Gut 2001; 49(5):706–712.
64. Baharav A et al. Fluctuations in autonomic nervous activity during sleep displayed by power spectrum analysis of heart rate variability. Neurology 1995; 45(6):1183–1187.
65. Dixon KE, Thorn BE, Ward LC. An evaluation of sex differences in psychological and physiological responses to experimentally-induced pain: a path analytic description. Pain 2004; 112(1–2):188–196.
66. Dunn AJ, Berridge CW. Physiological and behavioral responses to corticotropin-releasing factor administration: is CRF a mediator of anxiety or stress responses? Brain Res Brain Res Rev 1990; 15(2):71–100.
67. Charney DS, Bremner DJ, Redmond DE. Noradrenergic neural substrates for anxiety and fear: Clinical associations based on preclinical research. In: Kupfer FBD, ed. Psychopharmacology: The Fourth Generation of Progress. New York: Raven Press, 1995:387–395.
68. Chappell PB et al. Alterations in corticotropin-releasing factor-like immunoreactivity in discrete rat brain regions after acute and chronic stress. J Neurosci 1986; 6(10):2908–2914.
69. Korf J, Aghajanian GK, Roth RH. Increased turnover of norepinephrine in the rat cerebral cortex during stress: role of the locus coeruleus. Neuropharmacology 1973; 12(10):933–938.
70. Abercrombie ED, Keller RW Jr., Zigmond MJ. Characterization of hippocampal norepinephrine release as measured by microdialysis perfusion: pharmacological and behavioral studies. Neuroscience 1988; 27(3):897–904.
71. Kawahara H, Kawahara Y, Westerink BH. The role of afferents to the locus coeruleus in the handling stress-induced increase in the release of noradrenaline in the medial prefrontal cortex: a dual-probe microdialysis study in the rat brain. Eur J Pharmacol 2000; 387(3):279–286.
72. Van Bockstaele EJ, Colago EE, Aicher S. Light and electron microscopic evidence for topographic and monosynaptic projections from neurons in the ventral medulla to noradrenergic dendrites in the rat locus coeruleus. Brain Res 1998; 784(1–2):123–138.
73. Van Bockstaele EJ, Colago EE, Valentino RJ. Amygdaloid corticotropin-releasing factor targets locus coeruleus dendrites: substrate for the co-ordination of emotional and cognitive limbs of the stress response. J Neuroendocrinol 1998; 10(10):743–757.

74. Post RM et al. Peptides in the cerebrospinal fluid of neuropsychiatric patients: an approach to central nervous system peptide function. Life Sci 1982; 31(1):1–15.

75. Kling MA et al. Cerebrospinal fluid immunoreactive corticotropin-releasing hormone and adrenocorticotropin secretion in Cushing's disease and major depression: potential clinical implications. J Clin Endocrinol Metab 1991; 72(2):260–271.

76. Brindley DN, Rolland Y. Possible connections between stress, diabetes, obesity, hypertension and altered lipoprotein metabolism that may result in atherosclerosis. Clin Sci (Lond) 1989; 77(5): 453–461.

77. Munck A, Guyre PM, Holbrook NJ. Physiological functions of glucocorticoids in stress and their relation to pharmacological actions. Endocr Rev 1984; 5(1):25–44.

78. Fitch P. Recovering body and soul from PTSD. In American Massage Therapy Association 2000; 1:40–68.

79. Perlstein RS et al. Synergistic roles of interleukin-6, interleukin-1, and tumor necrosis factor in the adrenocorticotropin response to bacterial lipopolysaccharide in vivo. Endocrinology 1993; 132(3):946–952.

80. Sternberg EM et al. The stress response and the regulation of inflammatory disease. Ann Intern Med 1992; 117(10):854–866.

81. Williams CL et al. Corticotropin-releasing factor directly mediates colonic responses to stress. Am J Physiol 1987; 253(4 Pt 1):582–586.

82. Gue M et al. Stress-induced visceral hypersensitivity to rectal distension in rats: role of CRF and mast cells. Neurogastroenterol Motil 1997; 9(4):271–279.

83. Castagliuolo I et al. Acute stress causes mucin release from rat colon: role of corticotropin releasing factor and mast cells. Am J Physiol 1996; 271(5 Pt 1):884–892.

84. Clark JW, Bindra D. Individual differences in pain thresholds. Can J Psychol 1956; 10(2):69–76.

85. Woodrow KM et al. Pain tolerance: differences according to age, sex and race. Psychosom Med 1972; 34(6):548–556.

86. Wolff BB, Jarvik ME. Variations in cutaneous and deep somatic pain sensitivity. Can J Psychol 1963; 17:37–44.

87. Galer BS et al. Individual variability in the response to different opioids: report of five cases. Pain 1992; 49(1):87–91.

88. Portenoy RK, Foley KM, Inturrisi CE. The nature of opioid responsiveness and its implications for neuropathic pain: new hypotheses derived from studies of opioid infusions. Pain 1990; 43(3): 273–286.

89. Mogil JS et al. Heritability of nociception I: responses of 11 inbred mouse strains on 12 measures of nociception. Pain 1999; 80(1–2):67–82.

90. Mogil JS et al. Heritability of nociception II. Types of nociception revealed by genetic correlation analysis. Pain 1999; 80(1–2):83–93.

91. Smeyne RJ et al. Severe sensory and sympathetic neuropathies in mice carrying a disrupted Trk/NGF receptor gene. Nature 1994; 368(6468):246–249.

92. Indo Y et al. Mutations in the TRKA/NGF receptor gene in patients with congenital insensitivity to pain with anhidrosis. Nat Genet 1996; 13(4):485–488.

93. Sarkar S et al. Contribution of central sensitisation to the development of non-cardiac chest pain. Lancet 2000; 356(9236):1154–1159.

94. Sarkar S et al. The prostaglandin E2 receptor-1 (EP-1) mediates acid-induced visceral pain hypersensitivity in humans. Gastroenterology, 2003; 124(1):18–25.

95. Willert R. Receptor mechanisms mediating human oesophageal hypersensitivity. In: Gastrointestinal Sciences. Manchester: University of Manchester, 2005.

96. Worthen SF, Aziz Q, Hobson AR. Effect of anxiety on the sensory and perceptual characteristics of visceral and somatic sensation. Gut 2005; 54(suppl 2):19.

97. McKendrick MW, Read NW. Irritable bowel syndrome—post salmonella infection. J Infect 1994; 29(1):1–3.

98. Spiller RC et al. Increased rectal mucosal enteroendocrine cells, T lymphocytes, and increased gut permeability following acute Campylobacter enteritis and in post-dysenteric irritable bowel syndrome. Gut 2000; 47(6):804–811.

99. Gwee KA et al. Increased rectal mucosal expression of interleukin 1beta in recently acquired post-infectious irritable bowel syndrome. Gut 2003; 52(4):523–526.

100. Chan JG, W Perry M, et al. IL-10 and TGF-beta genotype in irritable bowel syndrome: evidence to support an inflammatory component? Gastroenterology 2000; 118(suppl 1).

101. Simone DA et al. Neurogenic hyperalgesia: central neural correlates in responses of spinothalamic tract neurons. J Neurophysiol 1991; 66(1):228–246.

102. Dougherty PM, Willis WD. Enhanced responses of spinothalamic tract neurons to excitatory amino acids accompany capsaicin-induced sensitization in the monkey. J Neurosci 1992; 12(3):883–894.

103. Kenshalo DR Jr et al. Facilitation of the response of primate spinothalamic cells to cold and to tactile stimuli by noxious heating of the skin. Pain 1982; 12(2):141–152.

104. Hylden JL et al. Expansion of receptive fields of spinal lamina I projection neurons in rats with unilateral adjuvant-induced inflammation: the contribution of dorsal horn mechanisms. Pain 1989; 37(2):229–243.

105. Verne GN, Robinson ME, Price DD. Hypersensitivity to visceral and cutaneous pain in the irritable bowel syndrome. Pain 2001; 93(1):7–14.
106. Munakata J et al. Repetitive sigmoid stimulation induces rectal hyperalgesia in patients with irritable bowel syndrome. Gastroenterology 1997; 112(1):55–63.
107. Coffin B et al. Alteration of the spinal modulation of nociceptive processing in patients with irritable bowel syndrome. Gut 2004; 53(10):1465–1470.
108. Mayer EA. Spinal and supraspinal modulation of visceral sensation. Gut 2000; 47(suppl 4):iv69–72; discussion iv76.
109. Whitehead WE et al. Effects of stressful life events on bowel symptoms: subjects with irritable bowel syndrome compared with subjects without bowel dysfunction. Gut 1992; 33(6):825–830.
110. Gwee KA et al. The role of psychological and biological factors in postinfective gut dysfunction. Gut 1999; 44(3):400–406.
111. Garrett VD et al. The relation between daily stress and Crohn's disease. J Behav Med 1991; 14(1):87–96.
112. Gwee KA et al. Psychometric scores and persistence of irritable bowel after infectious diarrhoea. Lancet 1996; 347(8995):150–153.
113. Stam R, Akkermans LM, Wiegant VM. Trauma and the gut: interactions between stressful experience and intestinal function. Gut 1997; 40(6):704–709.
114. Drossman DA et al. Sexual and physical abuse and gastrointestinal illness. Review and recommendations. Ann Intern Med 1995; 123(10):782–794.
115. Arntz A, Dreessen L, Merckelbach H. Attention, not anxiety, influences pain. Behav Res Ther 1991; 29(1):41–50.
116. Mertz H et al. Regional cerebral activation in irritable bowel syndrome and control subjects with painful and nonpainful rectal distention. Gastroenterology 2000; 118(5):842–848.
117. Naliboff BD et al. Cerebral activation in patients with irritable bowel syndrome and control subjects during rectosigmoid stimulation. Psychosom Med 2001; 63(3):365–375.
118. Berman S et al. Gender differences in regional brain response to visceral pressure in IBS patients. Eur J Pain 2000; 4(2):157–172.
119. Silverman DH et al. Regional cerebral activity in normal and pathological perception of visceral pain. Gastroenterology 1997; 112(1):64–72.
120. Bonaz B et al. Central processing of rectal pain in patients with irritable bowel syndrome: an fMRI study. Am J Gastroenterol 2002; 97(3):654–661.
121. Chen CL, Orr WC. Autonomic responses to heartburn induced by esophageal acid infusion. J Gastroenterol Hepatol 2004; 19(8):922–926.
122. Heitkemper M et al. Increased urine catecholamines and cortisol in women with irritable bowel syndrome. Am J Gastroenterol 1996; 91(5):906–913.
123. Heitkemper M et al. Autonomic nervous system function in women with irritable bowel syndrome. Dig Dis Sci 2001; 46(6):1276–1284.
124. Piccirillo G et al. Abnormal passive head-up tilt test in subjects with symptoms of anxiety power spectral analysis study of heart rate and blood pressure. Int J Cardiol 1997; 60(2):121–131.
125. Thayer JF, Friedman BH, Borkovec TD. Autonomic characteristics of generalized anxiety disorder and worry. Biol Psychiatry 1996; 39(4):255–266.
126. Berntson GG et al. Heart rate variability: origins, methods, and interpretive caveats. Psychophysiology 1997; 34(6):623–648.
127. Koizumi K, Kollai M. Multiple modes of operation of cardiac autonomic control: development of the ideas from Cannon and Brooks to the present. J Auton Nerv Syst 1992; 41(1–2):19–29.
128. Fukudo S, Nomura T, Hongo M. Impact of corticotropin-releasing hormone on gastrointestinal motility and adrenocorticotropic hormone in normal controls and patients with irritable bowel syndrome. Gut 1998; 42:845–849.
129. Stefanini GF et al. Oral disodium cromoglycate treatment on irritable bowel syndrome: an open study on 101 subjects with diarrheic type. Am J Gastroenterol 1992; 87(1):55–57.
130. Posserud I et al. Altered visceral perceptual and neuroendocrine response in patients with irritable bowel syndrome during mental stress. Gut 2004; 53(8):1102–1108.
131. Patacchioli FR, et al. Actual stress, psychopathology and salivary cortisol levels in the irritable bowel syndrome (IBS). J Endocrinol Invest 2001; 24(3):173–177.
132. Elsenbruch S, Orr WC. Diarrhea- and constipation-predominant IBS patients differ in postprandial autonomic and cortisol responses. Am J Gastroenterol 2001; 96(2):460–466.
133. Morris-Yates A et al. Evidence of a genetic contribution to functional bowel disorder. Am J Gastroenterol 1998; 93(8):1311–1317.
134. Levy RL et al. Irritable bowel syndrome in twins: heredity and social learning both contribute to etiology. Gastroenterology 2001; 121(4):799–804.
135. Kim DY, Camilleri M. Serotonin: a mediator of the brain-gut connection. Am J Gastroenterol 2000; 95(10):2698–2709.
136. Yeo A et al. Association between a functional polymorphism in the serotonin transporter gene and diarrhoea predominant irritable bowel syndrome in women. Gut 2004; 53(10):1452–1458.
137. Lesch KP et al. Association of anxiety-related traits with a polymorphism in the serotonin transporter gene regulatory region. Science 1996; 274(5292):1527–1531.

138. McCaffery JM et al. Allelic variation in the serotonin transporter gene-linked polymorphic region (5-HTTLPR) and cardiovascular reactivity in young adult male and female twins of European-American descent. Psychosom Med 2003; 65(5):721–728.

139. Bharucha AE et al. Adrenergic modulation of human colonic motor and sensory function. Am J Physiol 1997; 273(5 Pt 1):997–1006.

140. Kobilka BK et al. Cloning, sequencing, and expression of the gene coding for the human platelet alpha 2-adrenergic receptor. Science 1987; 238(4827):650–656.

141. Kim HJ et al. Association of distinct alpha(2) adrenoceptor and serotonin transporter polymorphisms with constipation and somatic symptoms in functional gastrointestinal disorders. Gut 2004; 53(6):829–837.

142. Holtmann G et al. G-protein beta 3 subunit 825 CC genotype is associated with unexplained (functional) dyspepsia. Gastroenterology 2004; 126(4):971–979.

143. Kleuss C et al. Different beta-subunits determine G-protein interaction with transmembrane receptors. Nature 1992; 358(6385):424–426.

144. Baumgart D et al. G protein beta3 subunit 825T allele and enhanced coronary vasoconstriction on alpha(2)-adrenoceptor activation. Circ Res 1999; 85(10):965–969.

145. Zill P et al. Evidence for an association between a G-protein beta3-gene variant with depression and response to antidepressant treatment. Neuroreport 2000; 11(9):1893–1897.

146. Lindemann M et al. The G protein beta3 subunit 825T allele is a genetic marker for enhanced T cell response. FEBS Lett 2001; 495(1–2):82–86.

11 Visceral Pain: Lessons from Functional Brain Imaging

Emeran A. Mayer
Center for Neurovisceral Sciences and Women's Health, David Geffen School of Medicine at UCLA, Los Angeles, California, U.S.A.

Bruce Naliboff
VA Greater Los Angeles Healthcare System, Los Angeles, California, U.S.A.

INTRODUCTION

A variety of brain regions identified as central pain-processing circuitry ("central pain matrix"), previously described in somatic pain studies (1,2) and well supported by neuroanatomical data (3) [in particular, the insula, the dorsal aspects of the anterior cingulate cortex (dACC), and the thalamus], have also been found to be activated consistently in response to visceral stimuli (4). However, other brain areas including somatosensory, limbic, paralimbic, and pontine regions have also been reported as activated by visceral stimulation though less consistently (4). Due to the lack of rigorous study designs able to isolate specific networks involved in various aspects of visceral stimulus processing [e.g., cognitive/affective influences on pain modulation, attention, anticipation, arousal, and autonomic responses to visceral stimuli (4)], functional brain imaging studies of functional disorders such as irritable bowel syndrome (IBS) to date have not clearly identified reproducible alterations in brain–gut interactions necessary to explain satisfactorily explain the phenomena of enhanced visceral perception, altered autonomic responses, or the frequently co-occurring nongastrointestinal symptoms such as fatigue, loss of energy, and other symptoms of physical discomfort. For example, it is not clear if the primary central abnormality in IBS is related to (i) enhanced selective attentional processes toward symptom-related cues (hypervigilance) and associated endogenous facilitation of visceral perception, (ii) a compromised endogenous pain inhibition system, or (iii) normal processing of pathological visceral input from the periphery.

Visceral pain and discomfort is a subjective, conscious experience, which results from an interpretation of the visceral afferent input influenced by memories and emotional, motivational, and cognitive factors. In principle, altered perception of visceral stimuli could result from activity changes in visceral afferent signal-processing areas alone (reflecting increased visceral afferent input to the brain from the gut), alterations in pain modulation circuits alone ("central pain amplification"), or variable combinations of these two overlapping circuitries (5–7). In the following, we will first briefly review published findings of brain activation by visceral stimuli in healthy control subjects and patient populations up to 2002, followed by a more detailed review of more recent studies in patient populations primarily done in IBS patients. In this latter discussion, we will highlight studies focusing on five aspects of altered visceral pain perception: (i) alterations in visceral afferent ascending pathways, (ii) altered central modulation of afferent signals, (iii) alterations in descending modulation, (iv) sex-related differences, and (v) pharmacological modulation of brain responses.

REVIEW OF PUBLISHED STUDIES ON BRAIN RESPONSES TO VISCERAL STIMULI
Review of Studies up to 2002

Following the initial publication in 1997 (8), there has been a series of studies describing the brain areas activated during brief, experimental, visceral stimulation. The majority of these studies has used phasic balloon distension in the rectum as the primary stimulus but there are also significant data on esophageal distension and a few studies of gastric distension and chemical-induced discomfort in the esophagus. Consistent with the focus on responses to phasic stimuli, these studies have used either $H_2{}^{15}O$-positron-emission tomography ($H_2{}^{15}O$-PET) or functional magnetic resonance imaging (fMRI) brain imaging technologies. Derbyshire published a comprehensive review of neuroimaging studies using visceral stimulation up to May of 2002 (4). The review had several aims: (i) to summarize studies using functional brain imaging to investigate brain responses during stimulation of the upper and lower gastrointestinal (GI) tract, (ii) to identify key regions in which activation has been consistently reported during distension, and (iii) to identify potential differences in processing between stimuli and groups. Based on a Medline search, he found 15 relevant articles with 21 independent study samples (8–22). The studies included PET and fMRI assessments of an active sensation condition (usually balloon distension of a hollow viscus) compared to a nondistension or reduced sensation baseline condition. Fourteen of the 15 studies involved brain responses to controlled distension of the upper (esophagus and stomach) (9–12,16) or lower GI tract (anus, rectum, and sigmoid) (8,14,15,17–22), and one study involved drug-induced cardiac pain (13). Overall, the regions reported as being activated by the experimental visceral stimuli were comparable to those reported in studies of noxious somatic stimulation (23,24) or cognition (25). The single most consistently activated brain region in all reports was the insular cortex, a multifunctional brain region that has been referred to as the interoceptive cortex (26) and is involved in the integration of somatic and visceral information, as well as affect. Through its connections with the amygdala and subregions of the ACC, the insular cortex is part of a limbic/paralimbic circuitry involved in regulation of emotion and autonomic responses.

Consistent with the neurophysiological model for somatic pain processing, Derbyshire found that a majority of studies also reported activation of cortical regions including the prefrontal cortex (PFC), the ACC, and primary sensory cortex. Although activation of these areas were found for both upper and lower GI stimulation, it appears as if lower GI stimulation (primarily rectal distension) was associated more consistently with activation in prefrontal regions and anterior portions of the ACC that have direct connections with limbic and brain stem structures (including the amygdala). In contrast, upper GI stimulation (primarily of the esophagus) was more consistently associated with activation of areas involved in sensory and motor processing including more posterior aspects of the cingulate cortex, posterior insula, S1, and motor cortex. One may speculate that this reflects, at least in part, a difference in the central representation of visceral afferents from a foregut structure (in particular, the proximal portion of the esophagus) and of hindgut structures.

Several of the initial descriptive imaging studies also examined the differences between patients with IBS and healthy controls during visceral stimulation (8,14,15) and anticipation of visceral stimulation (15). The findings suggested that patients showed similar areas of activation to controls (4) but evidenced greater activation in some regions, especially in the dACC and perhaps in limbic areas including the hypothalamus, infragenual cingulate cortex, and amygdala (15). Decreased activation in the dorsal pons [in the region of the periaqueductal gray (PAG)] was also reported in IBS patients (15), and these results gave rise to an initial hypothesis that patients might have increased affective and attentional responses to actual or anticipated visceral stimuli (hypervigilance), as well as potentially decreased descending pain inhibition (15). Another interesting early study compared subliminal rectal distension to perceived and uncomfortable stimulation in healthy controls and found similar areas of response, but smaller global activation measures during subliminal stimuli, suggesting similar brain responses across a wide range of stimulus intensities (27).

It should be emphasized that the great majority of the studies published up to 2002 (as summarized above) were descriptive, not hypothesis driven, and did not control for various important factors such as expectation, response requirements, previous exposure to the stimulus, affective comorbidity, symptom-related anxiety, or sex of the subjects. Thus, one may speculate that the most consistently reported regions in these studies (such as insula and dACC), which also are consistently activated in somatic pain studies and across patient and healthy populations, may be those that are less dependent on non–stimulus-related variables. This may be particularly true about the anterior insula which has been referred to as the interoceptive cortex, and activation of which has been found to covary with stimulus intensity (18). Other areas that are found to be significantly activated in some studies, but not others (in particular, limbic and prefrontal regions, as well as thalamus), may be more influenced by factors not directly related to visceral afferent stimulation.

Review of More Recent Studies (2002–2005)
Differences in Brain Responses to Visceral and Somatic Pain Stimuli

Extensive visceral (esophageal balloon distension) and somatic (contact heat on the midline chest) animal and human experimental studies have demonstrated that the perceptual, autonomic, and behavioral responses to noxious stimulation of somatic structures differ from those of the viscera (28,29). These differences have been explained based on the functional neuroanatomic differences between visceral and somatic pain processing. Experimentally induced aversive visceral sensations in humans are generally described as more unpleasant than somatic sensations (30,31). A series of studies from Bushnell's laboratory evaluated perceptual and central nervous system responses to visceral and cutaneous painful stimuli to the chest. In these studies, the authors used controlled balloon distension of the esophagus as a visceral stimulus and contact heat exposure of the chest as a corresponding somatic stimulus, matched in terms of perceived intensity within the same dermatome (30,32,33). In an initial psychophysical study in healthy volunteers, they found that the visceral, mechanical stimulus was experienced as more unpleasant, diffuse, and variable than cutaneous thermal pain of similar intensity, independent of the duration of the stimulus (30). Using the same stimulation paradigm, Strigo et al. studied regional brain responses and associated behavioral responses in seven healthy subjects with fMRI during visceral and somatic stimulation (32). A similar set of regions, including secondary somatosensory and parietal cortices, thalamus, basal ganglia, and cerebellum was activated by both stimuli. However, preferential activation of certain regions by visceral versus somatic stimuli was observed. For example, cutaneous heat pain evoked higher activations in the bilateral anterior insular cortex and ventrolateral PFC. On the other hand, visceral mechanical pain evoked in the same dermatome was associated with activation of bilateral inferior primary somatosensory cortex, bilateral primary motor cortex, and a more rostral region within the dACC. As in previous psychophysiological studies, subjects rated esophageal pain with higher affective scores than cutaneous pain. In a follow-up study, the authors provided evidence for a segregation of nociceptive inputs from the cutaneous trunk and distal esophagus with the parasylvian cortex in the parietal opercula (33). Visceral stimulation of the esophagus resulted in the activation of a more lateral region in the parasylvian cortex than cutaneous stimulation of the trunk. Evaluating differential brain responses to visceral and somatic stimuli of the lower body, Hobday et al. found similar brain activation to visceral (rectal) and somatic (anal) distension, even though a greater activation of motor cortex by the somatic stimulus was observed (17). Tracey's group used fMRI scanning of the brain to evaluate the cortical processing of visceral (rectal) and somatic stimuli in 10 healthy control subjects (34). Each subject received noxious somatic stimulation (in the form of cutaneous contact heat) to the left foot and midline lower back and noxious visceral stimulation (controlled balloon distension of the rectum). Stimulus unpleasantness was matched for visceral and somatic stimuli, resulting in different stimulus intensities: Somatic stimuli were rated as mild to moderately painful, while visceral stimuli did not reach the pain threshold. Thus, similar to the findings in the chest, the relative unpleasantness of the subjective experience of the visceral mechanical stimuli was higher than that of the somatic thermal stimuli. Visceral stimuli were associated with deactivation of the perigenual anterior cingulate cortex (pACC; a finding also reported in somatic pain studies) (35), with a relatively greater activation of the right anterior insula. Somatic (but not visceral) pain was associated with left dorsolateral PFC, a region concerned with cognitive processes. In a follow-up study (36), the authors compared brain stem responses to the same two stimuli. Ten healthy subjects (five females) were studied twice with 3T fMRI, during which they received matched, moderately painful, electrical stimuli to either the midline lower abdomen or the rectum. Significant activation associated with both stimuli was observed in several brain stem regions including the PAG, the parabrachial nucleus, the locus coeruleus complex (LCC), and the nucleus cuneiformis (NCF). Marked spatial similarities in activation were observed for the visceral and somatic pain conditions. However, two regions showed greater responses during the visceral pain condition: A significantly greater activation of a region identified as the NCF and a significant correlation of the right PAG with anxiety ratings. The authors concluded from these findings that the observed differences may represent a greater nocifensive response and a greater emotive salience of visceral pain. It needs to be kept in mind that in all of the studies comparing brain and subjective responses to visceral and somatic pain stimuli, these stimuli also differed in the pain modality used (mechanical vs. thermal), and that placement of a stimulus device into the upper or lower GI tract by itself is an uncomfortable procedure, regardless of the actual stimulus delivered.

Two studies have looked at differences in central processing of somatic and visceral experimental stimuli in patients with IBS. These studies follow from a series of psychophysiological studies showing increased perception of visceral stimulation in IBS, but less consistent findings regarding IBS sensitivity to noxious somatic stimuli. However, depending on the somatic pain stimulus used, different investigators have reported normal (37–40), reduced (41), and enhanced (31) perceptual responses to somatic pain stimuli. One of the two imaging studies done to date comparing visceral and somatic stimuli in IBS used thermal pain (31) and the other cutaneous pressure (41). Verne et al. studied brain responses with fMRI to rectal distension (35–55 mmHg) and to cutaneous heat (foot immersion in 45°C and 47°C water bath) in nine IBS patients (six females) and in a group of healthy age- and sex-matched controls (31). They report that both noxious stimuli evoked greater neural activity in brain regions of patients compared to controls. These regions included both those related to somatosensory processing (thalamus, somatosensory, and insular cortices) and those more related to cognitive and emotional modulation (anterior and posterior cingulate and prefrontal cortices). Enhanced brain responses to both types of stimuli were observed within the same brain structures. The authors interpreted these findings as supporting their original hypothesis that visceral and cutaneous hypersensitivity in IBS patients is related to increased afferent processing in ascending pathways, rather than to altered cognitive and/or emotional modulation at higher brain levels. Chang et al. reached a somewhat different conclusion based on findings in female patients with IBS with ($n = 10$) and without ($n = 10$) a comorbid diagnosis of fibromyalgia (42). Brain responses to somatic pressure (administered with a dolorimeter) and rectal distension (via barostat) were evaluated with $H_2{}^{15}O$-PET; subjective stimulus ratings were quantified by rating scales. The somatic stimulus was perceived as less aversive than the visceral stimulus by the IBS patients, while IBS + fibromyalgia patients rated both stimuli as equally aversive. Group differences in regional brain activation were only observed within the dACC, where IBS patients showed a greater response to visceral stimuli and IBS + fibromyalgia patients showed a greater response to somatic stimuli. The authors concluded from their findings that chronic stimulus-specific enhancement of dACC responses to sensory stimuli in both syndromes may be associated with cognitive enhancement of either visceral (IBS) or somatic (IBS + fibromyalgia) sensory input. The fact that no group differences were observed in primary sensory areas (thalamus, somatosensory cortex, and insula) is consistent with the concept that afferent input that reaches the brain is not different between the two patient populations, while arousal and attentional mechanisms may differ.

In summary, a growing number of brain imaging studies have addressed the question of how brain responses to somatic and visceral pain stimuli may differ, in both healthy control subjects and patients with IBS. The literature on differences in the greater subjective affective rating of visceral pain stimuli (in terms of unpleasantness) has been fairly consistent. This perceptual difference may be related in part to the difference in response options for the two stimuli (inescapable for visceral pain; requirement for motor response for somatic pain) and to the greater unpleasantness related to the placement of the visceral stimulus device. In contrast, a consistent difference in brain processing of visceral and somatic stimuli has not emerged from published studies. For example, consistent evidence for an expected greater activation of limbic and paralimbic brain regions for visceral stimuli (correlating with the greater affective responses) or differences in arousal and antinociceptive mechanisms between visceral and somatic stimuli have not been reported. This lack of consistency may be due, in large part, to differences in study design (imaging modality, study paradigms, nature of stimuli used, previous exposure of subjects to similar stimuli, sex of participants, etc.) and the relatively small number of studies reported for upper and lower GI tract so far.

Evidence for Sensitization of Visceral Afferent Pathways

One important question in the pathophysiology of functional GI disorders is related to the nature and pathophysiology of the enhanced perceptual responses observed in a large number of experimental pain studies (43). While acute gut inflammation in both human and animal experimental models is typically associated with peripheral and central sensitization (as well as important, time-dependent modulatory influences from the brain in the form of both facilitatory and inhibitory modulation), chronic visceral pain is likely to involve additional sensitization at supraspinal levels, as well as cognitive and emotional modulation of the chronic visceral pain experience related to coping mechanisms and symptom-related anxiety (28). Brain imaging in human subjects is one modality, which may allow us to differentiate between these different pain modulation mechanisms.

Addressing the brain's response to acute visceral sensitization, Aziz's group has provided convincing evidence for the alteration of visceral afferent pathways, consistent with central sensitization (44). Sarkar et al. used cortex-evoked potentials to study the effect of a 30-minute perfusion of 0.15 M HCl acid into the distal esophagus of healthy control subjects on esophageal pain thresholds and associated latencies (44). They found a reduction of the pain threshold to electrical stimulation of the proximal, non–acid-exposed esophagus and an associated reduction in the latency of the N1 and P2 components of the esophagus-evoked potential. The authors interpreted their findings as an indication for hyperexcitability within the central visceral pain pathway contributing to the secondary hyperalgesia/allodynia within the proximal esophagus. It will be of great interest to evaluate the effect of this intervention on brain responses assessed with fMRI, and to compare them with findings in patients with functional esophageal pain.

Although they have not measured sensitization directly, several imaging studies have interpreted their results as suggestive of upregulated afferent activity in IBS. As outlined above, Verne et al. studied patients with IBS and healthy control subjects using fixed intensities of visceral stimulation (35 and 55 mmHg) and concluded from their findings of enhanced responses in both somatosensory and paralimbic and prefrontal regions that IBS patients primarily show evidence for increased afferent processing in ascending pathways, rather than evidence for altered cognitive and/or emotional modulation of the visceral pain signal at higher brain levels (45,46).

In a recent study, Kwan et al. used a different paradigm to evaluate possible differences of brain responses between healthy controls ($n = 11$; seven females) and IBS patients ($n = 9$; six females) associated with either the stimulus or the time series of continuous subjective rating of the stimulus (percept-related brain responses) (47). Brain responses were assessed in response to previously determined individual stimulus intensities required to induce a sensation of urge or pain. On the day of the fMRI study, distension pressures were adjusted to a level that evoked moderate intensities (50/100 on a verbal rating scale) of urge or pain. Using a similar psychophysical technique, the authors had previously reported that the perceptual responses to rectal stimuli are time locked to the stimulus period in healthy subjects, but are dissociated from the duration and intensity of rectal stimuli in IBS patients (48,49). Percept-related activations were more extensive than stimulus-related activations in control subjects, a finding the authors explained with a better temporal fit with the percept compared with the stimulus pressure curve. In addition, the authors reported abnormal brain responses of the IBS patients associated with the rectal distension–evoked sensations in several brain regions: IBS patients, but not controls, showed urge-related activation in primary somatosensory cortex and pain-related activations in medial thalamus and hippocampus. Controls, but not IBS patients, showed pronounced urge- and pain-related activations in the right anterior insula and right ACC. The authors interpreted their surprising findings as consistent with IBS visceral hypersensitivity (increased activation in primary sensory cortex), but with possible deficits in interoceptive processing (lack of anterior insular activation) and decreased attentional engagement in IBS patients. The design, findings, and conclusions of this study are clearly different from those reported by other investigators (14,15,45).

Another unorthodox approach to dissect different aspects of visceral pain processing and modulation was taken by Kern and Shaker. In order to minimize cognitive/emotional modulation of the visceral afferent signal, they used a technique of "subliminal" visceral stimulation, whereby a rectal balloon is inflated to pressures below conscious perception, and associated brain responses are recorded with fMRI (27). They recently reported their studies of brain responses in 10 female diarrhea-predominant IBS patients and 10 age-matched healthy control subjects during three levels of subliminal distension pressures (10, 15, and 20 mmHg). By using a nonconventional way of quantifying fMRI brain responses in terms of activity volumes, they reported that IBS patients showed a larger response to all three distension pressures than the control group. The authors interpreted their findings as evidence for an increased sensitivity of visceral afferent pathways, regardless of the stimulus-related cognitive processes (50). As pointed out by an accompanying editorial (51), there are alternative explanations for these findings, in particular, as they relate to aversive stimulus expectation.

In summary, published evidence supports the feasibility of studying the effect of acute central sensitization using evoked potential recordings. Unfortunately, the small number of published studies in patients with chronic functional visceral pain do not provide conclusive evidence for a selective sensitization of afferent pathways in IBS patients. Differences in experimental design (percept- vs. stimulus-related activation, subliminal vs. supraliminal stimulus intensities, and individualized stimulus intensities to produce discomfort vs. fixed pressure stimuli) and analysis may be largely responsible for the widely different findings of published studies. Even though several authors interpreted their findings as being consistent with sensitization of ascending pathways, rather than with alterations in central pain modulation, such interpretations are open to alternative explanations. For example, it may be assumed that, other than in fully anesthetized subjects, cognitive and emotional modulation of the afferent signal will always occur and influence the subjective experience of the stimulus. Such modulation is likely to occur at the level of the brain, for example via locally released opioids (52), or by activation of descending pain-inhibitory and -facilitatory pathways modulating excitability of the spinal cord (53,54).

Evidence for Central Pain Amplification

The brain has multiple ways to modulate the perception of afferent information, and this modulation is influenced by cognitive factors (e.g., attention), the emotional state of the individual (e.g., fear, anxiety, or anger), or memories of previous sensory events. Considerable progress has been made on both preclinical and, more recently, clinical levels to identify brain regions, circuits, and mechanisms that play a role in the facilitation and inhibition of the subjective pain experience (53,55).

Phillips et al. used a study paradigm involving viewing of emotional faces and nonpainful esophageal distension to evaluate the neural mechanisms underlying the effect of emotional context on visceral perception (56). In a first paradigm, they studied brain responses of eight healthy subjects (seven males) to nonpainful esophageal distension using a 1.5T fMRI. Brain responses to the esophageal stimulation during either neutral or negative emotional context were evaluated. Activation within the right anterior insular cortex and bilateral dACC by the visceral stimulus was significantly greater while viewing fearful faces compared to neutral faces. In a second paradigm, they studied anxiety, discomfort, and brain responses in another eight healthy male subjects during the same esophageal stimulus while viewing faces with low, moderate, or high intensity of fear expression. During the high-intensity fearful visual stimulus, significantly greater discomfort, anxiety, and brain activation were observed, compared to the low-intensity fearful stimulus. Greater brain activation was seen predominantly in the left dACC and bilateral anterior insular cortex. These findings clearly demonstrated the powerful effect of emotional context on the perceptual, emotional, and brain response to an innocuous visceral stimulus.

A second study from the same group looked at the modulatory role of attention on the brain responses to visceral (esophageal) distension in seven healthy volunteers (six males) (57). Brain responses to phasic visual and esophageal (nonpainful balloon distension) stimuli were presented simultaneously while subjects were asked to focus their attention on either the esophageal or the visual stimulus (selective attention). During another manipulation, subjects were asked to focus on a change in frequency of both stimuli (divided attention). Selective attention on the esophageal stimulus was associated with activation of sensory (somatosensory cortex) and cognitive (dACC) networks, while selective attention on the visual stimulus activated the visual cortex. During the divided attention task, more brain regions in the sensory and cognitive domains were activated to process esophageal stimuli, in comparison to those processing visual stimuli. These findings emphasize the importance of attentional processes in the modulation of sensory information from the body and the relative biological importance placed on visceral sensation, compared to other sensory modalities.

Yaguez et al. studied brain responses during different phases of visceral aversive conditioning in eight healthy volunteers (five males) using 1.5T fMRI (58). The authors used a classical conditioning paradigm in which different colored circles were used as conditioned stimuli and were paired with painful esophageal distension (learning phase), airpuff to the wrist, or nothing. Brain responses associated with the learning phase, expectation phase, and extinction were acquired. Brain responses during the learning phase (delivery of aversive esophageal distension) were seen in regions of the pain matrix (including dACC, insula, and somatosensory cortex). During the anticipation and extinction phase of the paradigm, brain activity resembled that seen during actual esophageal distension. These findings are similar to earlier published studies using somatic pain stimuli and emphasize the importance of central influences, such as expectation and memory recall, on brain activation seen in visceral pain paradigms.

Recent brain imaging studies in patient populations provide support for alterations in corticolimbic pontine pain modulation networks in IBS patients, leading to visceral hyper-sensitivity. Mayer et al. (59) examined three groups ($n = 9$ in each group) of male subjects, ulcerative colitis patients with quiescent disease, patients with IBS, and healthy male controls, during actual and anticipated but undelivered rectal distensions using $H_2^{15}O$-PET. This study found similar responses in all three groups in anterior insula and dACC, the viscerosensory input regions most strongly activated in association with the experience of pain (4). However, IBS patients compared to both the ulcerative colitis and control groups showed consistently greater activation of limbic/paralimbic brain regions (amygdala, hypothalamus, ventral/rostral ACC, and dorsomedial PFC) suggestive of increased activation of pain-facilitatory pathways. In addition, the results showed activation in the ulcerative colitis and control subjects, but not in IBS patients, in the lateral frontal regions and a brain region including the PAG. A connectivity analysis using structural equation modeling supported these regions acting as part of a pain inhibition network that involves lateral and medial frontal influences on the PAG.

Several lines of evidence indicate that patients with IBS and other functional disorders have hypervigilance for symptom relevant sensations (60). Repeated exposure to experimental visceral stimuli can lead to decreased hypervigilance and, therefore, discomfort. In a longitudinal study of IBS patients exposed to six sessions of rectal inflations over a 12-month period, we examined regional cerebral blood flow to the inflations and anticipation of inflations using PET at the first and last session (61). Subjective ratings of the rectal inflations normalized over the 12 months of the study, while IBS symptom severity did not, indicating decreased vigilance independent of changes in disease activity. In response to rectal distension, stable activation of the central pain matrix (including thalamus and insula) was observed over the 12-month period, while activity in limbic, paralimbic, and pontine regions decreased. During the anticipation condition, there were significant decreases in amygdala, dACC, and dorsal brain stem (perhaps involving the LCC) activation at 12 months. An analysis examining the covariation of these brain regions supported the hypothesis of changes in an arousal network including limbic, pontine, and cortical areas underlying the decreased perception seen over the multiple stimulation studies. These two examples show preliminary support for IBS-related alterations in corticolimbic pontine networks involved in affective and cognitive modulation of pain and discomfort.

In summary, the studies reviewed in this section clearly demonstrate the power of using functional brain imaging approaches to test specific hypothesis related to central pain modulation. Both studies in healthy control subjects and two-patient studies illustrate an important influence of cognitive and affective modulation on brain responses to experimental visceral stimuli. In contrast to the highly variable results seen in studies looking at group differences between IBS patients and healthy control subjects using simple distension paradigms, these hypothesis-driven studies are consistent with each other as well as with an extensive literature on the powerful role of cognitive and emotional factors in the modulation of pain perception (5,6).

Evidence for Alterations in Descending Pain Modulation

Since the beginning of the 20th century it has been known that the brain can tonically inhibit spinal cord excitability, thereby regulating the amount of peripheral sensory information reaching the central nervous system. More recent evidence has demonstrated the activity of both pain-inhibitory and -facilitatory mechanisms that can tonically and phasically regulate spinal cord excitability (55,62,63). While top-down tonic pain-inhibitory modulation appears to predominate in healthy individuals, an upregulation of descending pain-facilitatory systems has been demonstrated in the maintenance of hyperalgesia in animal models of peripheral nerve injury (64). An alteration in the balance between inhibitory and facilitatory pain-modulatory systems has been proposed as a possible mechanism underlying chronic pain syndromes such as fibromyalgia (65) and IBS (66,67). Zambreanu et al. were the first to demonstrate the activation of brain stem regions in the context of central sensitization in healthy human volunteers (68). Using 3T fMRI, they compared whole brain responses, including the brain stem, to punctuate mechanical stimulation in an area of secondary hyperalgesia (induced by heat/capsaicin sensitization model) or in a control area. They found greater activation during stimulation of the hyperalgesic region in several cortical regions, including posterior insula and anterior and posterior cingulate cortex, as well as the thalamus and pons. The brain stem activation was localized to the NCF and the PAG, two regions that receive inputs from corticolimbic networks (including the rostral ACC), send projections to the rostroventral medulla, and are part of a corticolimbic pontine pain modulation circuit (69,70). These intriguing findings correlate nicely with recent findings in rodents demonstrating the upregulation of spino bulbo spinal loops, which play a role in the maintenance of hyperalgesia following peripheral injury (64). There is preliminary evidence to suggest that patients with IBS may also show abnormal activation of brain stem regions involved in pain modulation, in particular a reduced activation of endogenous pain inhibition systems. Mayer et al. demonstrated that while healthy control subjects and asymptomatic patients with longstanding, quiescent ulcerative colitis showed normal activation of corticolimbic pontine pain modulation circuits, IBS patients showed significantly less activation of the pontine region (59). The limited spatial resolution of PET imaging used in this study did not allow identification of the specific brain stem nucleus involved. Wilder-Smith et al. performed an fMRI study in 10 female patients with IBS (5 constipated- and 5 diarrhea-predominant bowel habit) and 10 female healthy control subjects to test the hypothesis that IBS patients show abnormal activation of diffuse noxious inhibitory controls (DNICs) systems in response to a noxious stimulus (71). DNIC activation can be quantified by the perceptual modulation of a painful stimulus (in this case noxious rectal balloon distension) by a secondary heterotypically applied nociceptive stimulus (in this case ice water immersion of the foot). They found that subjective pain ratings of rectal volume distension by the heterotypic cold pain stimulus was reduced in healthy controls but not in the IBS patient group, suggesting an inadequate activation of DNICs in the patients. Interestingly, prior to the heterotypic pain stimulus, patients showed less activation in the ACC, pACC, and PFC during painful distension compared with baseline. This decreased activation is interpreted as possibly relating to a preexisting saturation of the entire pain/anxiety system or ceiling effect. Following the heterotypic cold stimulus, a complex set of differences in response to rectal pain were found among the controls and the two IBS subgroups (constipation and diarrhea). These included a decreased insular, thalamus, and PAG activation in the controls (perhaps reflecting the DNIC process) that was absent in the IBS subjects.

While intriguing, several methodological issues make this study more difficult to interpret and suggest further replication. First, the rectal stimuli were balloon volumes done manually using a syringe. Computer-controlled phasic pressure pulses using a barostat are known to give more accurate stimuli for sensory measurement. Pain thresholds determined in terms of distension volume do not allow differentiation of perceptual differences from differences in rectal compliance. Second, the small sample size and the subgrouping of IBS patients into even smaller samples further increase the potential unreliability of the pairwise group differences.

Sex Differences in Brain Responses to Visceral Stimuli

A series of observations demonstrates that women are more likely to suffer from IBS, develop the so-called postinfectious IBS, and develop comorbidities such as fibromyalgia or interstitial cystitis (72). A variety of mechanisms have been proposed to explain these sex differences, including differences in the response of the central nervous system to pelvic visceral stimuli. Several investigators have addressed this question using functional brain imaging.

Berman et al. reported the first study of brain responses in two samples of a total of 30 IBS patients (13 females; 6 with constipation-predominant bowel habit) with $H_2{}^{15}O$-PET in response to rectal distension (18). Despite similar subjective stimulus ratings by male and female patients, regional brain activations were stronger in males. In males, but not females, rectal distension was associated with activation of regions within the central pain matrix (including anterior insula and dACC). Insula activation correlated most strongly with the objective intensity of the stimulus (rectal pressure), whereas ACC activation correlated most strongly with the subjective discomfort rating of the stimulus. The authors interpreted their findings in IBS patients as possibly being related to the greater sympathetic nervous system responses to rectal distension seen in male patients (73).

Naliboff et al. studied brain responses in 42 (23 females) nonconstipated IBS patients to a visceral (rectal) stimulus of moderate intensity and during expectation of such distension using $H_2^{15}O$-PET (74). In response to the visceral stimulus, both male and female patients showed activation of the expected pain regions (dACC and anterior insula), in addition to prefrontal and brain stem regions. Female patients showed greater activation in limbic (amygdala) and paralimbic regions (ventromedial PFC, infragenual cingulate cortex, and dACC), whereas male patients showed greater activation of the midposterior insula, dorsolateral PFC, and dorsal pons. Similar sex-related differences were observed during the expectation condition. This study replicated the finding from the earlier study showing greater activation by male patients of the insular cortex. The findings also suggested that female patients in response to a pelvic aversive stimulus show greater responses of limbic and paralimbic regions, while male patients show greater activation of regions belonging to a corticolimbic pain inhibition system.

Kern et al. studied brain responses in 28 healthy control subjects (age 20–44; 15 females) to barostat-controlled rectal distension using a 1.5T fMRI (22). Individual stimulus intensities were set at the perception threshold, as well as 10 mmHg above (supraliminal) and 10 mmHg below (subliminal) that threshold. Increase in maximum percent signal change and total volume of cortical activity was used to quantify brain responses to the stimuli. The average distension pressure at the perception threshold (which was neither associated with pain nor discomfort) was similar in male (32 mmHg) and female (28 mmHg) subjects. Interestingly, these threshold values are similar to thresholds reported from several laboratories as discomfort thresholds in healthy control subjects. Male subjects showed localized clusters of fMRI activity primarily in the sensory motor cortex and parieto occipital regions, whereas female subjects also showed activity in the dACC and prefrontal regions and insular cortex. In both sexes, increasing stimulus intensity was associated with increases in brain activation as assessed by the two measures. Volume of cortical activity during distension was significantly greater in females than that for males at all distension levels. For example, when the clustering criterion was eliminated, and all voxels were included in the regional activity volume calculation, female subjects showed a progressive increase in the activation volume in the insular and ACC/prefrontal region with progressive stimulus intensity (while males showed virtually no response at any distension pressures).

In summary, the published literature on sex difference in brain activation by visceral stimuli is sparse and contradictory. Studies with different results are difficult to compare in terms of methodology, study population (controls vs. patients), and data analysis. Future studies will need to establish group differences in brain activation to standardized stimuli between healthy males and females, and between female and male patients with IBS.

Modulation of Brain Responses by Pharmacological Treatments

Despite the lack of consensus regarding brain responses to rectal stimuli in healthy controls and group differences between IBS patients and control subjects, several studies have been reported using functional brain imaging to identify changes in cerebral activation associated with various treatment modalities, including pharmacological treatments (75–77) and non-pharmacological treatments (78,79). Only a few of the reported studies were of sufficient quality (statistical power, blinding, and homogeneous study populations) to allow any conclusions from the results.

Morgan et al. studied 22 females with pain-predominant IBS (Rome II positive, 11 with diarrhea, 7 with constipation, and 4 with alternating bowel habit) (75). No patients had significantly elevated symptoms for depression, anxiety, and general psychological distress on the Symptom Check List-90 (SCL-90) instrument. The study was designed as a randomized, placebo-controlled, double-blind crossover trial. Patients initially took 25 mg (one week), and later 50 mg, of amitriptyline at bedtime for three weeks, followed by a three-week washout before switching over to the alternate treatment. Cerebral activation during controlled rectal distension (15, 30, and 50 mmHg distension pressure) was compared between placebo and amitriptyline groups by fMRI. Distensions were performed alternately during auditory stress (babies crying) and relaxing music (stress reduction tape), and a total number of nine distensions in random order were given during each condition. Subjective ratings of rectal pain were associated with significant activation of the pACC, right insula, and right PFC. Amitriptyline treatment was not associated with either a significant subjective symptom improvement or changes in brain activation during the relaxing music condition. However, decreased activation in the pACC and the left posterior parietal cortex was observed during distension when associated with the auditory stressor. Even though adequately powered, this study had several shortcomings that may have affected the outcome. Patients had significant psychological comorbidities, making it difficult to determine if the effect of the drug was on IBS symptoms or anxiety. Given the well-known side effects of amitriptyline, it would seem that the study was inadequately blinded, and that exposure to drug during the initial session significantly affected the placebo response during the second session. Finally, the finding of pACC during the relaxation condition is different from generally observed activation of dACC during rectal distension. Since brain images during the relaxation and stress conditions (without rectal distension) were not obtained, it is difficult to determine if the drug effect was primarily on the brain response to the auditory stressor or to the visceral stimulus.

Berman et al. reported a double-blind, randomized, placebo-controlled study in 49 Rome I positive, nonconstipated IBS patients (26 females) who underwent $H_2^{15}O$-PET scanning before and after a three-week course of the 5-HT$_3$ receptor antagonist alosetron (75). The study aimed to evaluate the mechanisms underlying the therapeutic effects of alosetron on IBS symptoms. It was hypothesized that a viscero analgesic effect would primarily be seen as a reduction of distension-induced regional cerebral blood flow increases in regions of the central pain matrix, in particular, the anterior insula cortex. This interoceptive region had previously been shown to correlate with subjective intensity ratings of rectal distension (18). Alternatively, if the compound acted on limbic brain regions, which have known 5-HT$_3$ receptor localization (such as the amygdala), an effect would be expected on such limbic brain regions and arousal circuits (including amygdala, paralimbic cortex, and pons), and this effect would be seen primarily during the nondistension conditions. Thirty-seven patients completed the entire study. Brain responses at baseline, during 45-mmHg rectal distension, and during announced but undelivered aversive distension (expectation condition) were given twice, the second time following a train of repeated noxious sigmoid distensions (60 mmHg). Alosetron treatment was associated with reduced blood flow in limbic regions, including the amygdala and the ventral striatum, ventromedial PFC, and a pontine region, but not with significant changes in areas of the pain matrix (insula, dACC, and thalamus). Significant reductions were seen only at baseline and during the expectation condition, but not during the rectal distension. IBS symptom improvement was correlated with regional cerebral blood flow in the amygdala, ventral striatum, and pons. The alosetron-mediated reduction in regional cerebral blood flow in ventromedial PFC and infragenual cingulate was reversed following the train of repeated noxious sigmoid distensions. These findings are most consistent with an effect of alosetron treatment on limbic brain regions, by either a direct effect on 5-HT$_3$ receptors in these areas or an indirect effect mediated by vagal afferent input to the brain; 5-HT$_3$ receptors have been demonstrated on peripheral and central terminals of vagal afferents.

Drossman et al. reported a case study of a severe female IBS patient with significant psychological distress, a history of sexual abuse, and severe functional GI symptoms (80). Evaluation during symptom flare showed high subjective ratings of GI and psychological symptoms, a low rectal discomfort threshold, and distension-induced activation of multiple brain regions, including the dACC. Following symptom improvement, the studies were repeated. Symptom improvement was associated with normalization of the perceptual hypersensitivity to rectal balloon distension and with a significant decrease in distension-induced activation of the dACC, the somatosensory cortex, and a prefrontal region. Unfortunately, since the authors did not rule out that repeated exposure to rectal distension by itself may be associated with decreased brain responses, in particular of the dACC, it cannot be differentiated from the results if the observed brain changes were secondary to symptom improvement, or to habituation to the rectal stimulus. Preliminary evidence for such a decrease in brain and perceptual responses to repeated rectal sensitivity testing has been reported (81).

Lackner et al. studied six severe female Rome II positive IBS patients using $H_2^{15}O$-PET before and after a brief course of cognitive behavioral therapy (82). Comparing pretreatment resting scans (without rectal distension) with posttreatment scans, a reduction in regional cerebral blood flow was found in the parahippocampal gyrus and the ventral portion of the ACC.

These brain changes were associated with significant improvement in GI symptoms and psychological functioning. Reduced blood flow in the left pons was correlated with post-treatment anxiety ratings.

In summary, the information gained from a small number of published neuroimaging studies of brain activity associated with treatment responses in IBS patients has to be considered as preliminary. The finding of selective effects of alosetron treatment on limbic, but not primary pain regions, and the correlation of these limbic effects with IBS symptom ratings demonstrate the potential strength of this technique to understanding the action of new IBS treatments. Well-designed treatment studies, with adequate sample size, homogeneous study populations, and reproducible study paradigms are needed to confirm the validity of this approach to monitor treatment effects and predict possible clinical outcomes.

CONCLUSIONS AND FUTURE DIRECTIONS

In summary, the literature in the area of brain imaging of visceral perception published since 2002 clearly indicates significant progress in study design, methodology, and analyses techniques. While consensus is evolving in some areas (including the cognitive and emotional modulation of pain perception), considerable differences in reported results remain in other areas, from the comparison of brain responses to somatic and visceral pain stimuli to differences between control subjects and IBS patients to sex differences in brain activation. However, given the rapid advances that are being made in the such diverse fields as somatic pain modulation, emotion regulation, and imaging genomics, it is likely that the application of neuroimaging techniques to the study of brain–gut interactions in health and disease will lead to breakthroughs in the understanding of pathophysiology of chronic visceral pain conditions, including functional GI disorders and in the prediction of treatment responses in the near future.

Figure 1 summarizes an evolutionary process in brain imaging. The vast majority of studies described in this review have involved detecting and determining the extent of regional brain activation across levels of an independent variable such as stimulus intensity or group. This is essentially a univariate analysis in that each brain volume or *a priori*–chosen region is examined separately and the statistical threshold is adjusted for the large number of individual comparisons made. While important for generating hypotheses about what parts of the brain might be involved in visceral sensation and the response to these sensations, this descriptive approach to imaging clearly does not capture the critical interrelationships among structures that form the foundation of brain function. The brain operates as functional networks and activations in specific brain areas may have very different interpretations based on the coactivation of other regions that are connected via a network of inputs and projections (83). The first step toward understanding networks involves detection of regional

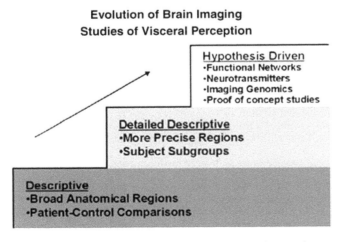

Figure 1 Evolution of brain imaging studies of visceral perception.

pairwise associations. This bivariate correlational technique can be labeled functional connectivity analysis and can show important relationships between separate regions, but does not allow for directly testing the nature of these associations over time or across conditions, provides no information on how these associations may come about, and permits only rudimentary inferences regarding the characterization of neural networks. Effective connectivity analyses, on the other hand, employ sophisticated multivariate techniques such as partial least squares (84,85), principal components analysis (86), and structural equation modeling (86). These covariance-based methods permit examination of integrated neural systems (86), as well as the identification of spatial and temporal clustering of neuroimaging data. Thus, unlike its functional counterpart, effective connectivity analysis incorporates anatomical connections and considers neural interactions simultaneously to quantify explicitly the effect brain structures exert on one another in a network and provides a means to test theories regarding neural networks (87). A very simplified example of connectivity analysis is the structural equation model testing corticolimbic pontine interactions operating during noxious visceral stimulation discussed above (59). In this example, three brain regions were simultaneously examined for direct and indirect connections leading to increased activity in the dorsal brain stem and potentially increased descending pain-inhibitory action.

Shown is a schematic illustrating the evolution from the earlier, purely descriptive studies to hypothesis-driven designs and toward novel application of imaging technology and analysis.

Much more sophisticated connectivity analyses that include a much larger set of highly specific brain regions are now becoming possible and they go hand-in-hand with other advances in brain imaging, including increased spatial and temporal scanner resolution (36), use of radioligand tracers specific to molecules of interest (52), and the application of genetic analyses related to the development of specific brain circuitry (88). These new analytical tools should yield important breakthroughs in our understanding of central processes related to the pathophysiology of visceral pain disorders.

REFERENCES

1. Jones AK, Kulkarni B, Derbyshire SW. Functional imaging of pain perception. Curr Rheumatol Rep 2002; 4:329–333.
2. Casey KL. Concepts of pain mechanisms: the contribution of functional imaging of the human brain. Prog Brain Res 2000; 129:277–287.
3. Craig AD. How do you feel? Interoception: the sense of the physiological condition of the body. Nat Rev Neurosci 2002; 3:655–666.
4. Derbyshire SW. A systematic review of neuroimaging data during visceral stimulation. Am J Gastroenterol 2003; 98:12–20.
5. Petrovic P, Ingvar M. Imaging cognitive modulation of pain processing. Pain 2002; 95:1–5.
6. Villemure C, Bushnell MC. Cognitive modulation of pain: how do attention and emotion influence pain processing? Pain 2002; 95:195–199.
7. Price DD. Psychological and neural mechanisms of the affective dimension of pain. Science 2000; 288:1769–1772.
8. Silverman DH, Munakata JA, Ennes H, et al. Regional cerebral activity in normal and pathological perception of visceral pain. Gastroenterology 1997; 112:64–72.
9. Binkofski F, Schnitzler A, Enck P, et al. Somatic and limbic cortex activation in esophageal distension: a functional magnetic resonance imaging study. Ann Neurol 1998; 44:811–815.
10. Kern MK, Birn RM, Jaradeh S, et al. Identification and characterization of cerebral cortical response to esophageal mucosal acid exposure and distension. Gastroenterology 1998; 115:1353–1362.
11. Aziz Q, Andersson JL, Valind S, et al. Identification of human brain loci processing esophageal sensation using positron emission tomography. Gastroenterology 1997; 113:50–59.
12. Aziz Q, Thompson DG, Ng VWK, et al. Cortical processing of human somatic and visceral sensation. J Neurosci 2000; 20:2657–2663.
13. Rosen SD, Paulesu E, Frith CD, et al. Central nervous pathways mediating angina pectoris. Lancet 1994; 344:147–150.
14. Mertz H, Morgan V, Tanner G, et al. Regional cerebral activation in irritable bowel syndrome and control subjects with painful and nonpainful rectal distension. Gastroenterology 2000; 118:842–848.
15. Naliboff BD, Derbyshire SWG, Munakata J, et al. Cerebral activation in irritable bowel syndrome patients and control subjects during rectosigmoid stimulation. Psychosom Med 2001; 63:365–375.
16. Ladabaum U, Minoshima S, Hasler WL, et al. Gastric distention correlates with activation of multiple cortical and subcortical regions. Gastroenterology 2001; 120:369–376.

17. Hobday DI, Aziz Q, Thacker N, et al. A study of the cortical processing of ano-rectal sensation using functional MRI. Brain 2001; 124:361–368.

18. Berman S, Munakata J, Naliboff B, et al. Gender differences in regional brain response to visceral pressure in IBS patients. Eur J Pain 2000; 4:157–172.

19. Baciu MV, Bonaz BL, Papillon E, et al. Central processing of rectal pain: a functional MR imaging study. Am J Neuroradiol 1999; 20:1920–1924.

20. Lotze M, Wietek B, Birbaumer N, et al. Cerebral activation during anal and rectal stimulation. Neuroimage 2001; 14:1027–1034.

21. Bernstein CN, Frankenstein UN, Rawsthorne P, et al. Cortical mapping of visceral pain in patients with GI disorders using functional magnetic resonance imaging. Am J Gastroenterol 2002; 97:319–327.

22. Kern MK, Jaradeh S, Arndorfer RC, et al. Gender differences in cortical representation of rectal distension in healthy humans. Am J Physiol Gastrointest Liver Physiol 2001; 281:G1512–G1523.

23. Peyron R, Laurent B, García-Larrea L. Functional imaging of brain responses to pain. A review and meta-analysis. Neurophysiol Clin 2000; 30:263–288.

24. Derbyshire SWG. Metareview of functional imaging studies with noxious stimuli reveals reproducible patterns of central activation [abstr]. J Pain 2001; 2:655.

25. Bush G, Luu P, Posner MI. Cognitive and emotional influences in anterior cingulate cortex. Trends Cogn Sci 2000; 4:215–222.

26. Craig AD. Interoception: the sense of the physiological condition of the body. Curr Opin Neurobiol 2003; 13:500–505.

27. Kern MK, Shaker R. Cerebral cortical registration of subliminal visceral stimulation. Gastroenterology 2002; 122:290–298.

28. Mayer EA, Gebhart GF. Basic and clinical aspects of visceral hyperalgesia. Gastroenterology 1994; 107:271–293.

29. Mayer EA, Raybould HE. Role of visceral afferent mechanisms in functional bowel disorders. Gastroenterology 1990; 99:1688–1704.

30. Strigo IA, Bushnell MC, Boivin M, et al. Psychosocial analysis of visceral and cutaneous pain in human subjects. Pain 2002; 97:235–246.

31. Verne GN, Robinson ME, Price DD. Hypersensitivity to visceral and cutaneous pain in the irritable bowel syndrome. Pain 2001; 93:7–14.

32. Strigo IA, Duncan GH, Boivin M, et al. Differentiation of visceral and cutaneous pain in the human brain. J Neurophysiol 2003; 89:3294–3303.

33. Strigo IA, Albanese MC, Bushnell MC, et al. Visceral and cutaneous pain representation in parasylvian cortex. Neurosci Lett 2005; 384:54–59.

34. Dunckley P, Wise RG, Aziz Q, et al. Cortical processing of visceral and somatic stimulation: differentiating pain intensity from unpleasantness. Neuroscience 2005; 133:533–542.

35. Porro CA, Cettolo V, Francescato MP, et al. Functional activity mapping of the mesial hemispheric wall during anticipation of pain. Neuroimage 2003; 19:1738–1747.

36. Dunckley P, Wise RG, Fairhurst M, et al. A comparison of visceral and somatic pain processing in the human brainstem using functional magnetic resonance imaging. J Neurosci 2005; 25:7333–7341.

37. Cook IJ, Van Eeden A, Collins SM. Patients with irritable bowel syndrome have greater pain tolerance than normal subjects. Gastroenterology 1987; 93:727–733.

38. Whitehead WE, Holtkotter B, Enck P, et al. Tolerance for rectosigmoid distention in irritable bowel syndrome. Gastroenterology 1990; 98:1187–1192.

39. Accarino AM, Azpiroz F, Malagelada JR. Selective dysfunction of mechanosensitive intestinal afferents in irritable bowel syndrome. Gastroenterology 1995; 108:636–643.

40. Zighelboim J, Talley NJ, Phillips SF, et al. Visceral perception in irritable bowel syndrome. Dig Dis Sci 1995; 40:819–827.

41. Chang L, Mayer EA, Johnson T, et al. Differences in somatic perception in female patients with irritable bowel syndrome with and without fibromyalgia. Pain 2000; 84:297–307.

42. Chang L, Berman S, Mayer EA, et al. Brain responses to visceral and somatic stimuli in patients with irritable bowel syndrome with and without fibromyalgia. Am J Gastroenterol 2003; 98:1354–1361.

43. Mertz H. Review article: visceral hypersensitivity. Aliment Pharmacol Ther 2003; 17:623–633.

44. Sarkar S, Hobson AR, Furlong PL, et al. Central neural mechanisms mediating human visceral hypersensitivity. Am J Physiol Gastrointest Liver Physiol 2001; 281:G1196–G1202.

45. Verne GN, Himes NC, Robinson ME, et al. Central representation of visceral and cutaneous hypersensitivity in the irritable bowel syndrome. Pain 2003; 103:99–110.

46. Verne GN, Price DD. Irritable bowel syndrome as a common precipitant of central sensitization. Curr Rheumatol Rep 2002; 4:322–328.

47. Kwan CL, Diamant NE, Pope G, et al. Abnormal forebrain activity in functional bowel disorder patients with chronic pain. Neurology 2005; 65:1268–1277.

48. Kwan CL, Diamant NE, Mikula K, et al. Characteristics of rectal perception are altered in irritable bowel syndrome. Pain 2005; 113:160–171.

49. Kwan CL, Mikula K, Diamant NE, et al. The relationship between rectal pain, unpleasantness, and urge to defecate in normal subjects. Pain 2002; 97:53–63.

50. Lawal A, Kern M, Sidhu H, et al. Novel evidence for hypersensitivity of visceral sensory neural circuitry in IBS patients. Gastroenterology 2006; 130:26–33.

51. Naliboff BD, Mayer EA. Brain imaging in IBS: drawing the line between cognitive and non-cognitive processes. Gastroenterology 2006; 130:267–270.
52. Zubieta JK, Smith YR, Bueller JA, et al. Mu-opioid receptor-mediated antinociceptive responses differ in men and women. J Neurosci 2002; 22:5100–5107.
53. Tracey I. Nociceptive processing in the human brain. Curr Opin Neurobiol 2005; 15:478–487.
54. Tracey I. Functional connectivity and pain: how effectively connected is your brain? Pain 2005; 116:173–174.
55. Tracey I, Dunckley P. Importance of anti- and pro-nociceptive mechanisms in human disease. Gut 2004; 53:1553–1555.
56. Phillips ML, Gregory LJ, Cullen S, et al. The effect of negative emotional context on neural and behavioural responses to oesophageal stimulation. Brain 2003; 126:669–684.
57. Gregory LJ, Yaguez L, Williams SC, et al. Cognitive modulation of the cerebral processing of human oesophageal sensation using functional magnetic resonance imaging. Gut 2003; 52:1671–1677.
58. Yaguez L, Coen S, Gregory LJ, et al. Brain response to visceral aversive conditioning: a functional magnetic resonance imaging study. Gastroenterology 2005; 128:1819–1829.
59. Mayer EA, Berman S, Suyenobu B, et al. Differences in brain responses to visceral pain between patients with irritable bowel syndrome and ulcerative colitis. Pain 2005; 115:398–409.
60. Mayer EA, Craske MG, Naliboff BD. Depression, anxiety and the gastrointestinal system. J Clin Psychiatry 2001; 62:28–36.
61. Naliboff BD, Berman S, Suyenobu B, Labus JS, Chang L, Stians J, Mandelkerh MA, Mayer EA. Longitudinal change in perceptual and brain activation response to visceral stimuli in irritable bowel syndrome patients. Gastroenterology 2006; 131:352–365.
62. Gebhart GF. Descending modulation of pain. Neurosci Biobehav Rev 2004; 27:729–737.
63. Porreca F, Ossipov MH, Gebhart GF. Chronic pain and medullary descending facilitation. Trends Neurosci 2002; 25:319–325.
64. Suzuki R, Morcuende S, Webber M, et al. Superficial NK1-expressing neurons control spinal excitability through activation of descending pathways. Nat Neurosci 2002; 5:1319–1326.
65. Clauw DJ, Crofford LJ. Chronic widespread pain and fibromyalgia: what we know, and what we need to know. Best Pract Res Clin Rheumatol 2003; 17:685–701.
66. Munakata J, Naliboff B, Harraf F, et al. Repetitive sigmoid stimulation induces rectal hyperalgesia in patients with irritable bowel syndrome. Gastroenterology 1997; 112:55–63.
67. Chang L, Naliboff BD, Labus JS, et al. Effect of sex on perception of rectosigmoid stimuli in irritable bowel syndrome. Am J Physiol Regul Integr Comp Physiol 2006; 291:R277–R284.
68. Zambreanu L, Wise RG, Brooks JC, et al. A role for the brainstem in central sensitisation in humans. Evidence from functional magnetic resonance imaging. Pain 2005; 114:397–407.
69. Petrovic P, Petersson KM, Hansson P, et al. Brainstem involvement in the initial response to pain. Neuroimage 2004; 22:995–1005.
70. Petrovic P, Dietrich T, Fransson P, et al. Placebo in emotional processing—induced expectations of anxiety relief activate a generalized modulatory network. Neuron 2005; 46:957–969.
71. Wilder-Smith CH, Schindler D, Lovblad K, et al. Brain functional magnetic resonance imaging of rectal pain and activation of endogenous inhibitory mechanisms in irritable bowel syndrome patient subgroups and healthy controls. Gut 2004; 53:1595–1601.
72. Mayer EA, Berman S, Chang L, et al. Sex-based differences in gastrointestinal pain. Eur J Pain 2004; 8:451–463.
73. Tillisch K, Labus JS, Naliboff BD, et al. Characterization of the alternating bowel habit subtype in patients with irritable bowel syndrome. Am J Gastroenterol 2005; 100:896–904.
74. Naliboff BD, Berman S, Chang L, et al. Sex-related differences in IBS patients: central processing of visceral stimuli. Gastroenterology 2003; 124:1738–1747.
75. Morgan V, Pickens D, Gautam S, et al. Amitriptyline reduces rectal pain related activation of the anterior cingulate cortex in patients with irritable bowel syndrome. Gut 2005; 54:601–607.
76. Berman SM, Chang L, Suyenobu B, et al. Condition-specific deactivation of brain regions by 5-HT$_3$ receptor antagonist alosetron. Gastroenterology 2002; 123:969–977.
77. Drossman DA, Toner BB, Whitehead WE, et al. Cognitive-behavioral therapy versus education and desipramine versus placebo for moderate to severe functional bowel disorders. Gastroenterology 2003; 125:19–31.
78. Lackner JM, Mesmer C, Morley S, et al. Psychological treatments for irritable bowel syndrome: a systematic review and meta-analysis. J Consult Clin Psychol 2004; 72:1100–1113.
79. Lieberman MD, Jarcho JM, Berman S, et al. The neural correlates of placebo effects: a disruption account. Neuroimage 2004; 22:447–455.
80. Drossman DA, Ringel Y, Vogt BA, et al. Alterations of brain activity associated with resolution of emotional distress and pain in a case of severe irritable bowel syndrome. Gastroenterology 2003; 124:754–761.
81. Naliboff BD, Derbyshire SWG, Munakata J, et al. Evidence for decreased activation of central fear circuits by expected aversive visceral stimuli in IBS patients [abstr]. Gastroenterology 2000; 118:A137.
82. Lackner JM, Lou Coad M, Mertz HR, et al. Cognitive therapy for irritable bowel syndrome is associated with reduced limbic activity, GI symptoms, and anxiety. Behav Res Ther 2006; 44:621–638.

83. McIntosh AR. Mapping cognition to the brain through neural interactions. Memory 1999; 7:523–548.
84. McIntosh AR, Bookstein FL, Haxby JV, et al. Spatial pattern analysis of functional brain images using partial least squares. Neuroimage 1996; 3:143–157.
85. McIntosh AR, Lobaugh NJ. Partial least squares analysis of neuroimaging data: applications and advances. Neuroimage 2004; 23:S250–S263.
86. McIntosh AR, Grady CL, Ungerleider LG, et al. Network analysis of cortical visual pathways mapped with PET. J Neurosci 1994; 14:655–666.
87. Friston KJ. Functional and effective connectivity in neuroimaging: a synthesis. Hum Brain Mapp 1994; 2:56–78.
88. Hariri AR, Weinberger DR. Imaging genomics. Br Med Bull 2003; 65:259–270.

12 | The Neural Basis of Referred Visceral Pain

Maria Adele Giamberardino
Department of Medicine and Science of Aging, "G. d'Annunzio" University of Chieti, Chieti, Italy

Fernando Cervero
Anesthesia Research Unit (Faculty of Medicine), Faculty of Dentistry and McGill Center for Pain Research, McGill University, Montreal, Quebec, Canada

INTRODUCTION

There are many clinical features of visceral pain but the one that makes it more distinctive is the frequent referral of the painful sensation to areas of the body away from the diseased organ. This is what Henry Head called "referred pain," a painful sensation reported in a region of the body remote from the originating lesion (1). Referred pain is a useful diagnostic tool in the clinic because the patterns of referral produced by a lesion in a given internal organ are constant across subjects (2). It is also a phenomenon of considerable neurobiological interest, which implies that the brain can attribute a painful sensation to the wrong location and generate a mismatch between the real and the perceived sites of injury.

Pain is usually regarded as a protective sensation, the "psychical adjunct of a protective reflex" (3) and a reasonably accurate location of the sensation would be necessary to produce an effective protection of the injured site. However, visceral pain shows a number of clinical and neurobiological properties that question a purely defensive role for the organism (4). Many internal organs are insensitive to pain and there is often no relation between the extent of damage to internal organs and the intensity of the resulting pain (5). The sensory innervation of the viscera is sparse and the functional characteristics of the sensory receptors that innervate internal organs also differ from those of cutaneous or muscle nociceptors (4) (Chapter 5) Visceral pain is often dull and persistent in its early phases and, although it is subsequently projected to more superficial areas of the body, it follows temporal and spatial patterns that cannot be confounded with the kinds of superficial pain felt by somatic injuries (6,7). In this way, pain from internal organs often forces the patient to take rest or seek help and in doing so can contribute to the defense of the organism.

In this chapter, we review the phenomenon of referred visceral pain from a variety of perspectives. We describe its clinical features and properties, the experimental models—both in animals and in humans—that are being used in its study and the neurobiological and molecular mechanisms that may be involved in its generation. In this way, we hope to present the reader with a multidisciplinary approach to this unique feature of visceral pain, combining clinical observations with potential neurological mechanisms.

REFERRED PAIN PHENOMENA IN THE CLINICAL CONTEXT
Referred Pain/Hyperalgesia

Referral of pain to distant structures is a typical feature of visceral nociception (2,8). It is only in the very first episode, or early phases of the first episode, in fact, that pain symptoms from internal organs are perceived in a common site for all viscera (i.e., usually along the midline, in the thorax or abdomen, anteriorly, or posteriorly). At this stage, the symptom is a vague and poorly defined sensation, accompanied by marked neurovegetative signs and emotional reactions (the so-called "true visceral pain"). Soon after this phase (minutes or, at most, hours), visceral pain is "transferred" (and called übertragener Schmertz, i.e., transferred pain, by German authors) to somatic areas of the body wall, which differ according to the specific viscus and which are generally located within the related metameric field (2). Secondary hyperalgesia (increased sensitivity to painful stimuli/decreased pain threshold) most often takes place in the referred areas, starting in the skeletal muscle layer, to also extend upwards to the overlying subcutis and skin, especially in the case of recurrent and/or prolonged visceral stimuli (*referred pain without and with hyperalgesia*) (7,9).

In the clinical context, myocardial infarction is one of the most paradigmatic forms of the progression of pain in internal organs from the phase of "true visceral pain" to the phase of pain referral with secondary hyperalgesia. The early stages are characterized by a vague sensation of malaise and oppression in the lowest sternal area and/or epigastrium, or aching in the interscapular region, with accompanying neurovegetative symptoms such as nausea, vomiting, pallor, sweating, alvus disturbances, and strong emotional alarm reactions (e.g., anguish or feeling of impending death). Subsequent phases, occurring after a few minutes to a few hours, are instead featured by a sharper and better defined pain sensation, which is perceived at the level of the thoracic wall, either anteriorly or posteriorly, and very often in the upper limbs, most commonly the left one (ulnar side of the arm and forearm) (referred pain). Hyperalgesia is typically found in muscles of the referred area, mostly the pectoralis major and muscles of the interscapular region and forearm, sometimes also the trapezius and deltoid muscles. In a low percentage of cases, the hypersensitivity also extends upwards to the subcutis and skin of the referred area, within dermatomes C8-T1 on the ulnar side of the upper limb (10).

Urinary colics from calculosis, among the most intense forms of pain that a human being can experience, are other typical examples of referred pain from internal organs. The symptom is normally felt at lumbar level on the affected side, with radiation to the ipsilateral flank and anteriorly to the groin. Deep hyperalgesia is detectable in muscles of the lumbar and flank area (quadratus lumborum and oblique muscles) (11). In symptomatic biliary calculosis, pain is referred to the upper right quadrant of the abdomen with radiation toward the back. Hyperalgesia typically affects the rectus abdominis at the cystic point, i.e., level of junction of the 10th rib with the outer margin of the same muscle (12). In pelvic pain conditions, e.g., dysmenorrhea, pain is referred to the lower abdomen, perineum, and sacral region, with radiation toward the groin and upper part of the thighs. Tenderness typically affects the lowest part of the rectus abdominis and muscles of the pelvic region (13). In all the previous examples, hyperalgesia may also possibly involve the subcutis and skin overlying the tender muscles, in cases of repeated and/or prolonged painful episodes (10).

The referred sensory changes (hyperalgesia) can be detected by clinical means and precisely quantified instrumentally. The clinical maneuvers reveal the hypersensitivity in an "on–off" manner, i.e., vigorous pain reaction by the subject upon firm manual compression of the muscle tissue, pinch palpation of the subcutis, and scratching of the point of a needle over an area of altered dermographic reactivity of the skin (14). The instrumental procedures mostly involve evaluation of the pain threshold, i.e., the minimum intensity of a stimulus corresponding to the first report of pain by the subject (15), with a threshold decrease indicating hyperalgesia. For the muscle and subcutis, mechanical (myometer for muscle and pinch algometer for subcutis), electrical (impulses delivered through needle electrodes), and chemical (injections of algogenic substances of progressively increasing concentrations) stimuli are usually employed. For the skin, thermal stimulation (thermal algometer) is also used in addition to mechanical (von Frey hairs) and electrical (impulses delivered through surface electrodes) stimuli (7,6,13,16).

These various procedures have been used to assess the profile of the referred sensory changes in different algogenic conditions from internal organs, e.g., the digestive system [gallbladder pathologies, irritable bowel syndrome (IBS)], urinary tract (calculosis), and female reproductive organs (dysmenorrhea and endometriosis) (6,7,9,13,17–20). The global outcome of these studies indicates that referred visceral hyperalgesia, mostly involving the skeletal muscle layer of the affected body wall area, is an early phenomenon, in that it is detected soon after the first visceral pain episodes. It is accentuated in extent by the repetition of the episodes (e.g., colics and painful menstruations), that is, the more numerous the episodes, the lower the threshold, and outlasts the spontaneous pain, being detectable in the pain-free intervals and sometimes remaining even after recovery from the primary visceral disease. An example is provided by the profile of muscle hyperalgesia in urinary calculosis, where hypersensitivity of the oblique musculature at L1 appears soon after the first one to two colics, increases in extent with their repetition, and is detectable in between the painful episodes (Fig. 1).

In about 90% of the cases, it also persists (for months and even years) after the urinary stone has been eliminated (6,7,9,17). As a general rule, it has been found that a minimum pain

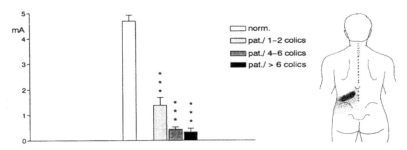

Figure 1 Referred sensory changes at muscle level in urinary colics from calculosis. Pain thresholds to electrical stimulation of the obliquus externus muscle ipsilateral to the affected urinary tract in different groups of patients who had experienced a progressively higher number of colics (recordings performed in the pain-free interval) as compared to thresholds measured in normal subjects at the same level. Note the progressively significant decrease in threshold with respect to normal. Asterisks refer to comparison between patients and normal subjects. *Source*: From Ref. 22.

perception is required for the secondary sensory changes to take place. Asymptomatic diseases of internal organs, in fact, are not able to trigger referred hyperalgesia, as shown by the sensory normality of body wall tissues in the areas of projection of the gallbladder or the kidney/ureter in the case of silent calculosis (i.e., calculosis without colics). In contrast, painful nonorganic visceral diseases do provoke referred sensory changes, as happens in biliary diskinesia (19) or in IBS. Regarding the latter, in fact, recent studies have shown somatic hyperalgesia in the abdominal referred pain area, which was particularly accentuated in the muscle layer (20).

In acute inflammatory visceral pain, the referred hyperalgesia tends to also involve the superficial somatic tissues. Patients with acute appendicitis show increased ratings to pinprick (von Frey hairs) and thermal stimuli (warm and cold metal rollers), together with a reduction of cutaneous pain thresholds to electrical stimuli and of pain thresholds to pressure stimuli, in the referred abdominal pain area (McBurney's point) versus the contralateral control area. The pain thresholds to electrical and pressure stimuli are lower in the referred pain area in patients compared with the same area in healthy control subjects (21). In acute cholecystitis, there is hypersensitivity to pinprick, heat, cold, pressure, and single and repeated cutaneous electrical stimulation in the referred pain area and in the contralateral control area of the abdomen. However, the hypersensitivity appears normalized after cholecystectomy (21–23). This latter finding is different from the above-reported results on the persistence of some degree of hyperalgesia even after removal of the primary visceral focus. It probably indicates that repeated algogenic inputs from viscera (e.g., recurrent conditions such as colics or painful menstruations) rather than isolated acute episodes, are required to leave persistent hyperalgesic traces in the referred area.

Referred Pain/Hyperalgesia and "Viscero–Visceral" Interactions

In the clinical context, it is common to observe that algogenic conditions may affect simultaneously more than one internal organ in the same patient. Especially when two viscera are involved, which share at least part of their central sensory projection, this circumstance gives rise to the so-called phenomenon of "viscero-visceral hyperalgesia," due to which the patient experiences an enhancement of both spontaneous referred pain and referred hyperalgesia (22). The concomitant presence of coronary heart disease and gallbladder calculosis, for instance, tends to produce more numerous anginal attacks and biliary colics in the patients than does one condition only (common sensory projection between heart and gallbladder: T5) (24). The association of dysmenorrhea with IBS (common projection between uterus and colon: T10-L1) (25) frequently produces more menstrual pain, intestinal pain, and somatic abdominal/pelvic hyperalgesia (in the areas of referral from the uterus and from the intestine) than dysmenorrhea or IBS only (unpublished observation). Dysmenorrhea/endometriosis combined with urinary calculosis in the same patient (common projection between uterus and upper urinary tract: T10-L1) (25) has been shown to produce increased menstrual pain,

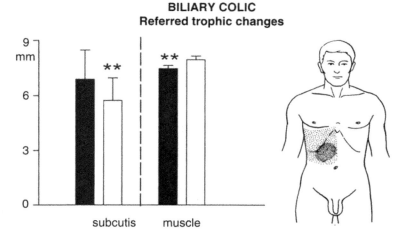

Figure 2 Referred trophic changes in subcutis (*increased thickness*) and muscle (*decreased thickness*) measured via ultrasounds at the cystic point (*black column*) and contralateral side (*white column*) in patients with symptomatic gallbladder calculosis. Asterisks refer to comparison between the two sides. *Source*: From Ref. 19.

urinary colic pain, and somatic abdomino-pelvic/lumbar hyperalgesia (in the areas of referred pain from the uterus and from the urinary tract), with respect to one condition only (18). The phenomenon of "viscero-visceral hyperalgesia" has important therapeutic implications. Effective treatment of one condition, in fact, may significantly improve typical symptoms from the other, e.g., decrease in urinary pain and referred hyperalgesia at lumbar level after hormonal treatment of dysmenorrhea or decrease in menstrual pain and referred abdomino-pelvic hyperalgesia after urinary stone elimination following lithotripsy (18,22).

Referred Trophic Changes

Referred pain with hyperalgesia is frequently accompanied by changes in trophism of the deep layers of the body wall, namely an increased thickness of the subcutis and a decreased thickness of the muscle (tendency to muscle atrophy) (2,10). These changes are easily detectable clinically by pinch palpation. Instrumental quantification via ultrasounds has also been performed. In symptomatic urinary and biliary calculosis, as well as in symptomatic gallbladder shape abnormality, in fact, subcutis thickness was found to be significantly higher and muscle thickness significantly lower on the side ipsilateral to the affected organ than on the contralateral side (Fig. 2).

No changes were observed, in contrast, in patients with asymptomatic gallbladder, urinary stones, or asymptomatic gallbladder shape abnormality (9,19). Thus, similarly to the hyperalgesia, also the referred trophic changes from viscera appear only in the case of painful visceral conditions. It has recently been shown, however, that while the hyperalgesia tends to decrease with the progressive fading of the painful manifestations from the visceral focus (though remaining still significant), the trophic changes do not. Patients with symptomatic gallbladder calculosis presenting both hyperalgesia and trophic changes in the cystic point area in basal conditions were reevaluated after a period of six months, during which a subgroup of them had not complained of further colics while another subgroup had continued to present with colics. In the symptomatic subgroup, the hyperalgesia was accentuated while in the asymptomatic subgroup it was diminished; in contrast, trophic changes remained unaltered in both (19). Thus, while referred hyperalgesia appears strictly modulated by the algogenic input from the viscera, the referred trophic changes would rather seem an on–off phenomenon.

REFERRED PAIN PHENOMENA IN THE EXPERIMENTAL CONTEXT

Referred pain phenomena from internal organs have been the subject of increasing experimental studies in recent decades. This exponential rise reflects the need to assess, and consequently interpret, visceral pain in standardized, controllable conditions, which are rarely found in the clinical context. A number of studies have been performed both in humans and in animals.

Human Studies

Most experimental studies have applied controlled stimuli of different nature—mechanical, thermal, electrical, and chemical—to various internal organs in healthy volunteers (16,26–29).

These studies have characterized the different areas of distribution of the evoked pain and have also shown the phenomenon of enlargement of these areas after "sensitization" of the viscera due to repeated visceral stimulation or experimental inflammation of the organs ("visceral hyperalgesia") (22). For example, a first mechanical distension of a 25 cm tract of the sigmoid colon in healthy volunteers for 30 seconds at a pressure of 60 mm Hg was not painful, but only induced nonalgogenic sensations in the lower abdomen, perineum, and upper part of the lumbar region (30). With repeated distension, the referral areas increased progressively and the sensation became frankly painful at the 10th distension. IBS represents the clinical counterpart of this experiment. IBS is regarded as a paradigmatic form of visceral hyperalgesia, because a lowered pain threshold has been demonstrated at different levels of the gastrointestinal (GI) tract, with exaggerated responses to distensions of various GI portions and significantly larger areas of referral compared to normal subjects (31). IBS patients typically experience pain even to physiologic stimuli, such as the intestinal transit, and also naturally report a progressive enlargement of the areas of pain referral with the progression of their disease (32).

Enlargement of referred pain areas as a consequence of visceral hyperalgesia has also been demonstrated experimentally in the urinary bladder (33). Repeated filling of the organ in female volunteers progressively increased the physiological and perceptual responses to pain and the extent of the referred somatic areas.

Similar results were obtained with stimuli other than mechanical applied to internal organs. Continuous electrical stimulation of the gut provoked a progressive enlargement of the referred pain area as the duration of the stimulation was increased from 30 to 120 seconds (16). Thermal stimulation of the esophagus after sensitization with acid resulted in a significant increase in the referred pain area in human volunteers (34). Multimodal stimulation of the same organ (electrical, mechanical, cold, and warmth stimuli) showed a precise relationship between stimulus intensity and pain intensity. The referred pain area increased with increasing intensity of the electrical and mechanical stimuli (26), with women showing significantly larger areas than men, a result interpreted as a reflection of sex differences in central pain processing (which may explain why gut functional disorders prevail in women) (35).

Chemical stimulation of the ileum (increasing volumes of chemical activators) in subjects with an ileostoma induced referred pain around the stomal opening with a correlation between the pain area and pain intensity (29).

Experimental stimulation of the internal organs has also been successfully used to study secondary sensory somatic changes. Sensitization of the esophagus with acid increased by 100% the amplitude of the nociceptive withdrawal reflex to electrical stimuli at the ankle (used to assess the interaction between visceral and somatic pathways) (28), indicating the presence of central hyperexcitability. The experimenters interpreted this result as an indication of the fact that even short-lasting visceral hyperalgesia can generate central sensitization.

Though most experimental visceral studies in humans have concerned the GI organs or the urinary tract, other districts have also been investigated. Experimental noxious stimulation (repeated dilatations) of the uterine cervix of healthy females evoked pain in all subjects, with referral to the hypogastric and low back regions (36). The word descriptors and the areas of referred sensations were similar to those seen clinically in abortion, labor, and menstrual pain.

Animal Studies

A number of animal models of visceral nociception have been set up, mostly in the course of recent decades (37,38). However, only a percentage of them have been specifically designed to assess referred phenomena. The parameter monitored has mostly been referred deep and/or superficial hyperalgesia, assessed in various ways in somatic tissues, e.g., by recording withdrawal reactions to application of mechanical and thermal stimuli or by measuring vocalization thresholds to different stimuli (mechanical and electrical), because vocalization is a highly integrated test, regarded as a reliable index of perceived pain in animals (38). Some examples are provided below.

Prolonged noxious electrical stimulation of the ureter in the awake rat produces not only behavioral signs indicative of direct visceral pain (abdominal stretching/contractions) but also referred hypersensitivity of the ipsilateral oblique musculature (L1), as shown by a significant reduction of vocalization thresholds to electrical muscle stimulation for 30 to 40 minutes after the end of ureter stimulation (39). Formation of an artificial stone in one ureter (through injection of dental cement into the upper third of the lumen) produces more long-lasting direct and referred phenomena in rats. The animals display not only spontaneous visceral pain behavior (multiple "ureteral crises") over a period of four days postoperatively, but also referred hypersensitivity of the oblique musculature ipsilateral to the affected ureter, as testified by a significant decrease in the vocalization threshold to muscle electrical and mechanical stimulation, which lasts over a week. The extent of the referred muscle hyperalgesia is proportional to the amount of spontaneous pain behavior (number and duration of ureteral crises) and is dose-dependently reduced by treatment with morphine, tramadol, metamizol, nonsteroidal anti-inflammatory drugs (NSAIDs), or spasmolytics (40–42).

The combination of an artificial ureteric stone with experimental endometriosis in female rats produces particularly pronounced algogenic effects. In this model, mimicking the "viscero-visceral hyperalgesia" observed in women with urinary calculosis and endometriosis, an enhancement is, in fact, observed not only of the spontaneous pain behavior (both "ureteral" and "uterine") but also of the referred lumbar muscle hyperalgesia, with a post-stone decrease in vocalization thresholds to electrical muscle stimulation significantly more pronounced than in rats with a stone only or rats with sham-endometriosis plus stone. Similarly to what is observed in humans, treatment of only one condition in this model relieves symptoms from the other, i.e., treatment of endometriosis before stone formation (with NSAIDs or tramadol) prevents the enhancement of pain symptoms from the ureter (ureteral crises and referred lumbar muscle hyperalgesia) (43).

Experimental noxious stimulation of the bladder also produces referred hyperalgesia. For instance, application to the rat bladder of irritants such as 25% turpentine, 2.5% mustard oil, or 2% croton oil (44) produces hypersensitivity to noxious stimuli applied to the tail or caudal abdomen. Bladder inflammation with 50% turpentine oil also produces referred somatic hyperalgesia to thermal stimuli (45) and punctate mechanical stimuli of the hind limb (testified by a decrease in the limb withdrawal thresholds to these stimuli), which is observable two hours after turpentine instillation and persists for at least 24 hours (46). The referred thermal hyperalgesia is mimicked by intravesical instillation of nerve growth factor (NGF) (in place of turpentine) and attenuated, in the turpentine model, by prior administration of an NGF sequestering molecule, trkA-IgG (45); it is also dose-dependently reduced by endocannabinoids (anandamide and palmitoylethanolamide) (47). The referred mechanical hyperalgesia is attenuated by the capsaicin analogue SDZ249–665, administered systemically (46).

Intravesical instillation of xylene (a well-known C-fiber irritant) through a chronically implanted catheter in rats provokes behavioral reactions indicative of visceral pain, that is, hind paw hyperextension and licking and biting of the lower abdomen and perineum in an area corresponding to dermatomes innervated by the same spinal segments that receive afferents from the bladder. The behavioral responses directed toward these somatic structures may well represent the equivalent of the referred pain from the bladder experienced by patients (48).

Cyclophosphamide-induced cystitis in mice, in addition to behavioral signs of direct visceral pain (49), also produces referred hyperalgesia of the tail base, which is inhibited dose dependently by morphine (50).

Injection of mustard oil into the right horn of the uterus in female rats elicits not only spontaneous pain behavior (major episodes of movements/postures indicative of pelvic pain) over four days postoperatively but also referred hyperalgesia in the ipsilateral flank muscles, as testified by a significant decrease in vocalization thresholds to electrical muscle stimulation over the same period. In this model, mimicking women's pelvic inflammatory pain, the areas of referred muscle hyperalgesia are also the sites of neurogenic plasma extravasation in the skin, the first experimental evidence of trophic changes in sites of referred pain from viscera (51,52).

Neurogenic plasma extravasation in L5 to S2 dermatomes (primarily in L6 and S1) has also been documented in male rats after experimental prostatitis (chemical irritation of the prostate) and in rats receiving bladder irritation (53).

In the mouse, chemical stimulation of the colon (e.g., mustard oil or capsaicin) evokes dose-dependent visceral pain behaviors (licking of abdomen, stretching, contractions of abdomen, etc.) and referred abdominal hyperalgesia, as shown by a significant increase in withdrawal responses to application of von Frey hairs to the abdomen. All these nociceptive behavioral responses are dose-dependently reversed by morphine (54).

The murine models of visceral pain/referred hyperalgesia from both the GI tract and the urinary tract are being increasingly used to investigate referred phenomena from viscera in genetic studies. As will be discussed in more detail in the sections devoted to pathophysiological mechanisms, transgenic mice that lack the receptor for substance P (NK1), for instance, fail to develop both primary hyperalgesia after visceral inflammation (intracolonic capsaicin or acetic acid, and cyclophosphamide cystitis) and referred hyperalgesia or tissue edema (55), while mice lacking the tetrodotoxin-resistant sodium channel alpha subunit Nav1.8 (which is expressed exclusively in primary sensory neurons) show weak pain and no referred hyperalgesia to intracolonic capsaicin, a model in which behavior is sustained by ongoing activity in nociceptors sensitized by the initial application (56).

Genetic studies, as well as electrophysiological, pharmacological, anatomical, or immunohistochemical investigations performed on the described animal models of visceral nociception, have allowed several hypotheses on the pathophysiology of referred phenomena to be tested in standardized experimental contexts (57–59).

NEUROPHYSIOLOGICAL BASIS OF REFERRED PAIN

While the sparse innervation of internal organs (60) and the widespread divergence of visceral afferents in the central nervous system (CNS) explain the dull, vague, and not well-localized nature of the first phase of a visceral pain sensation (5), the referral of visceral sensations to areas of the body away from the injured organ has always been interpreted as the consequence of convergence of somatic and visceral afferent information onto the same sensory neurons. The rationale for this interpretation is that the brain receives information from both internal organs and somatic areas through the same sensory channel and attributes the origin of the sensation to the somatic domain.

There are two major assumptions in this interpretation. The first one is that the brain locates the origin of a sensory stimulus through a direct sensory channel—a string is pulled at one end and a bell rings at the other telling the brain where the string has been pulled. We now know that things are not so simple and that parallel processing through various specific and nonspecific sensory channels is more likely to mediate a complex painful experience. The second assumption is that the brain will always attribute the origin of a stimulus to a somatic location even when the point stimulated is in the viscera. In other words, regardless of how a convergent sensory pathway is activated—by its somatic or visceral inputs—the final result is always a sensation felt in the somatic region. This assumption implies that somatic locations have a priority over visceral ones when it comes to the assessment by the brain of the origin of a given stimulus. This interpretation of the neural mechanisms of referred pain is based on the principle that sensory perceptions are shaped by a learning process. When a viscerosomatic convergent pathway is activated, the brain attributes the origin of the stimulus to the region, which is the most frequent source of sensory experiences, that is, the somatic area.

Two models of viscerosomatic convergence have been put forward to explain referred visceral pain: a peripheral model of dichotomizing primary afferent fibers and a central model of viscerosomatic convergence onto second-order neurons in the CNS. Both are supported by experimental evidence, although the CNS model is by far the most popular and the one that has received the greatest experimental support.

The peripheral model of viscerosomatic convergence is based on the existence of primary afferent neurons with cell bodies in the dorsal root ganglia (DRG) and whose peripheral projections have several branches with separate endings in internal organs and in somatic structures. In this way, the same primary sensory neuron will have receptive endings in somatic and visceral tissues. Such DRG neurons have been described in several species using anatomical and electrophysiological methods (51,61–64), suggesting that dichotomizing afferent fibers could mediate referred sensations from a variety of viscera including the heart, the GI tract, and the reproductive organs. On the other hand, these reports have also met with some skepticism from alternative studies of dichotomizing afferents showing that, although such afferents can sometimes be observed anatomically or electrophysiologically, their very low numbers (less than 1% of the total number of afferents) make them unlikely candidates as mediators of referred visceral pain (65–67). It is also not known if the sensory endings of such dichotomizing afferents are functionally active in all their various locations and if so, whether all the endings have similar receptive properties (mechanical, thermal, chemical, etc.).

The second model of viscerosomatic convergence is based on the existence of second order neurons in the spinal cord and of other CNS neurons in sensory pathways that receive convergent inputs from somatic and visceral tissues. This interpretation forms the basis of the Convergence-Projection theory of referred visceral pain put forward by Ruch in 1946. The rationale of the theory is that viscerosomatic convergent neurons, when activated by afferent impulses from the viscera, send information to the brain that is interpreted as coming from the somatic areas. The pattern of referral will be determined by the pattern of viscerosomatic convergence so that, for example, if neurons with inputs from cardiac nociceptors have receptive fields in the left thorax and left arm, the pain will be felt in these regions of the body rather than in the heart.

There is considerable experimental evidence in support of this interpretation. Numerous studies have described viscerosomatic convergent neurons in the spinal cord and other regions of the CNS (68–73). The patterns of viscerosomatic convergence from a given organ coincide with the zones of referred visceral pain from the same organ in humans (Fig. 3) and with the somatic areas in experimental animals, which generate behavioral nociceptive patterns (41). Moreover, the fact that viscerosomatic convergence occurs on CNS sensory neurons offers the possibility of substantial integration and modulation at each synaptic relay and therefore a likely substrate for more complex sensory experiences than those mediated exclusively by primary afferents.

Referred Hyperalgesia

As already discussed above, most forms of visceral pain produce an increased tenderness of remote and superficial areas of the body known as referred visceral hyperalgesia (22). The fact that referred hyperalgesia appears to originate from otherwise healthy tissues strongly suggests that their locus of origin is in the CNS rather than in the periphery. The conceptual framework underpinning the central organization of visceral hyperalgesia originates from James MacKenzie, who in his classical 1909 publication, proposed that signals from a diseased viscus arriving in the spinal cord would converge onto somatic pathways and set up an "irritable focus" in the cord responsible for the enhanced pain sensitivity referred to the somatic area and for the increased motor and autonomic activity characteristic of visceral pain states. This "irritable focus" in the CNS was the predecessor of what is known today as "central sensitization."

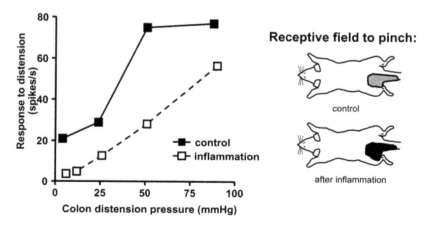

Figure 3 Viscerosomatic convergence in the spinal cord. The figure shows the responses of a viscerosomatic convergent neuron in the spinal cord of the rat to controlled distension of the colon (*graph on the left*) and the cutaneous receptive field of the neuron (*figurines on the right*). The responses of the neuron before (control) and after the induction of a colonic inflammation are shown. Note that the inflammation enhances the responses of the neuron to colonic distension and enlarges its cutaneous receptive field. *Source*: From Ref. 74.

The properties of the "irritable focus" (central sensitization) have been extensively studied, providing plenty of evidence in support of an enhanced excitability of spinal cord neurons as the mechanism responsible for the manifestation of visceral hyperalgesic states (69,75,76). An injury or inflammation applied to a given viscus will not only result in an enhancement of the responses of the neurons to stimulation of the viscus, but also in an increase in the excitability of the responses mediated by the somatic afferent drives (Fig. 3). This general increase in the excitability of viscerosomatic convergent neurons to all their inputs has been interpreted as the substrate for the generation of referred hyperalgesic states.

A similar mechanism can be hypothesized for referred hyperalgesia in the case of concurrent algogenic conditions from two internal organs sharing at least part of their central sensory projection (viscero-visceral hyperalgesia). Along with viscerosomatic convergence, in fact, experimental evidence exists for viscero-visceral convergence in the CNS, e.g., between the gallbladder and the heart, and between colon and rectum, bladder, vagina and uterine cervix (24,77,78). Thus, increases in the excitability of viscero-viscero-somatic convergent neurons, triggered by the afferent barrage from one visceral organ, could mediate the increased reactivity to impulses from the second visceral organ and the somatic area of referral (43).

As already reported in the section on animal models, referred visceral hyperalgesia can also be detected in animals. For instance, instillation of capsaicin or mustard oil into the colon in the rat evokes not only an immediate, and short-lived, pain reaction of the animal but also leaves an area of referred mechanical hyperalgesia in the abdomen that lasts for more than 24 hours after the initial insult (54) (Fig. 4A). This model has been extensively used to examine the cellular and molecular mechanisms of referred visceral pain and hyperalgesia.

Molecular Mechanisms of Referred Visceral Hyperalgesia

The neurobiological mechanisms of referred visceral pain and hyperalgesia include a peripheral component of enhanced activity from nociceptors and a central component of alteration

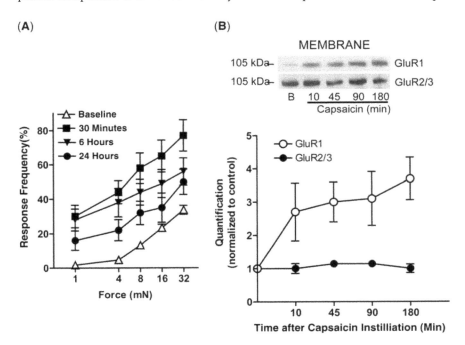

Figure 4 Trafficking of AMPA receptors in spinal cord neurons induced by a visceral hyperalgesic state. (**A**) Model of referred visceral hyperalgesia in the mouse. The animals received an intracolonic instillation of capsaicin and the mechanical sensitivity of the abdomen was measured 30 minutes to 24 hours later. Note the rapid enhancement of the responses (mechanical hyperalgesia) at the 30-minute interval, which are still present 24 hours later. *Source*: From Ref. 54. (**B**) Time course of subcellular distribution of GluR1 and GluR2/3 in the plasma membrane fraction of spinal cord tissue before and after intracolonic instillation of capsaicin. Lane marked "B" in the immunoblot contain control (basal) tissue. The graph below shows quantification of GluR1 and GluR2/3 normalized to levels detected in control spinal tissue. *Source*: From Ref. 79.

in the central processing of low threshold inputs (59). The peripheral component mediates spontaneous pain and primary hyperalgesia and the central component underlies secondary (or referred) hyperalgesia. In the case of visceral pain, secondary referred hyperalgesia appears in a somatic region away from the diseased organ and is mediated through CNS viscerosomatic convergence on neurons with inputs from both the injured viscus and the somatic referral area. In the following paragraphs, several potential targets involved in the generation of visceral hyperalgesic states and that have been the object of recent research are discussed.

Role of Neurokinins in Referred Visceral Pain and Hyperalgesia

The tachykinin family of peptide neurotransmitters are involved both in the control of intestinal motility and secretion, and in the pain and hyperalgesia (80). One of the most ubiquitous tachykinins, substance P, is present in a very high proportion of visceral afferent neurons (>80%) (81) and is thought to play a very significant role in visceral pain and hyperalgesia. For instance, mice with a deletion of the substance P receptor (NK1) show profound alterations in the visceral pain and hyperalgesia normally evoked by sensitizing noxious stimuli like those applied to the viscera (55).

The role of tachykinin NK1 receptors in the responses of spinal neurons to the stimulation of colon afferents after the induction of acute colonic inflammation in rats has been studied using selective tachykinin NK1 receptor antagonists (58). It was shown that NK1 receptors are involved in the enhanced responses of viscerosomatic neurons following colonic inflammation (82), implicating central NK1 receptors in the expression of referred hyperalgesia. The role of tachykinin NK2 receptors in the responses of spinal neurons to the stimulation of colon afferents in normal rats, and after the induction of acute colonic inflammation has also been examined (74). The effect of cumulative doses of a selective NK2 receptor antagonist on responses to these stimuli was tested in control conditions and 45 minutes after intracolonic instillation of acetic acid. After colonic inflammation, neuronal responses to colorectal distension and pelvic nerve stimulation were significantly greater and the NK2 antagonist dose-dependently inhibited the enhanced responses to colorectal distension after inflammation (74). These observations are consistent with previous behavioral and reflex studies in rats showing that NK2 receptor antagonists inhibit the enhanced responses to gut distension evoked by inflammation induced by trinitrobenzenesulphonic acid or nematode infestation (83,84).

Role of Intracellular Signaling Kinases in Referred Visceral Pain and Hyperalgesia

Mitogen-activated protein (MAP) kinases, also known as extracellular signal-regulated kinases (ERKs), are members of a family of serine/threonine protein kinases that mediate intracellular signal transduction in response to a variety of stimuli. Upon activation by upstream MAP kinases, ERKs translocate into the nucleus, phosphorylate transcription factors, and regulate the transcription of related genes. In the nervous system, ERKs play an established role in learning, memory, and synaptic plasticity.

Recent evidence suggests a role for ERKs in spinal processing of visceral pain, and particularly in the development of referred visceral hyperalgesia (85). ERK1/2 activation was detected in the spinal cord of mice that had previously received an intracolonic injection of capsaicin, a procedure known to evoke referred visceral hyperalgesia (54). ERK activation was detected in the lumbosacral spinal cord, but not in the thoracic region, extracted 30 minutes after the noxious visceral stimulus (85).

ERK activation correlates well with the expression of hyperalgesia and is specifically localized to the lumbosacral spinal region where colonic afferents have been shown to terminate in the mouse. However, intracolonic mustard oil and capsaicin instillation induce an accumulation of phosphorylated ERK1/2 in the nucleus of the neurons at 90 minutes poststimulus, which is still significantly greater than basal levels at 180 minutes posttreatment. This time course and subcellular localization of the effects observed suggest that ERK is involved in transcriptional events underlying the maintenance of secondary hyperalgesia. Therefore ERK activation seems to play an important and specific role in maintaining prolonged referred hyperalgesia, but does not seem to participate in other features of the pain behavior such as acute pain and primary hyperalgesia.

AMPA Receptor Trafficking and Referred Visceral Hyperalgesia

Hyperalgesia is the result of plasticity in the pain pathway. A well-known example of synaptic plasticity is long-term potentiation, whereby brief, conditioning stimuli evoke enhancement of responses to subsequent stimuli by a mechanism that involves trafficking of the alpha-amino-3-hydroxy-5-methyl-4-isoxazolepropionic acid (AMPA) subclass of glutamate receptors from the cytosol to the membrane (86). Glutamate is the main fast excitatory neurotransmitter in the spinal dorsal horn and it has been suggested that synaptic potentiation of spinal neurons is associated with the insertion of AMPA-R subunits into synapses (87). Recently it has been shown, using a model of referred visceral hyperalgesia in the mouse, that glutamate receptor trafficking mediates the synaptic plasticity in the spinal cord that leads to pain hypersensitivity (79).

Induction of visceral pain and hyperalgesia by intracolonic application of capsaicin was associated with a pronounced increase in the abundance of the AMPA-R subunit GluR1 in the membrane fraction with a peak 3.7-fold increase 180 minutes after treatment and a corresponding decrease in the levels in the cytosolic fraction. In contrast to the pronounced effects of the painful visceral stimulus on GluR1 distribution, capsaicin treatment had no effect on the intracellular distribution of GluR2/3 in spinal tissue (Fig. 4B). This is consistent with observations in other brain areas and with the proposal that GluR1 insertion into the membrane is an inducible and tightly regulated process, whereas GluR2/3 subunits are constitutively cycled in and out of the membrane to maintain normal transmission (86). The trafficking of GluR1 to the membrane of spinal neurons induced by the painful visceral stimulus was also shown to be dependent on the activation of calcium-calmodulin kinase II (CaMKII) showing that the process shared cellular properties with other forms of synaptic plasticity such as long-term potentiation. Interestingly, inhibition of the functional exocytotic machinery of the neurons prevented the GluR1 accumulation in the neuronal membrane and inhibited the referred visceral hyperalgesia induced by intracolonic capsaicin (79). These results suggest that synaptic incorporation of GluR1 plays an important role in the development and expression of visceral hyperalgesia.

These observations show that natural activation of the visceral pain pathway in intact adult animals in vivo provokes trafficking of GluR1 subunits in the spinal cord and reveals an association between GluR1 trafficking and the development of hyperalgesia in a model of visceral pain. They also confirm that the molecular mechanisms of synaptic plasticity that mediate process such as learning or memory is shared by the visceral pain pathway.

Phosphorylation and Membrane Recruitment of the NKCC1 Cotransporter and Referred Visceral Hyperalgesia

The $Na+-K+-2Cl^-$ cotransporter isoform 1 (NKCC1) is a member of the cation-dependent Cl^- transporter family whose main function is to move chloride ions into the cell using the energy of the sodium gradient created by the Na-K-ATPase pump (88). The function of the NKCC1 cotransporter is tightly regulated by phosphorylation of Thr184 and Thr189 in the intracellular N-terminal domain and this has been demonstrated to be a mechanism for the enhancement of the cotransporter's activity (89). The activity of the NKCC1 cotransporter is a key contributor to the postsynaptic actions of gamma-aminobutyric acid (GABA) (90).

Recently, several studies have suggested a role for the NKCC1 cotransporter in nociceptive processing and in the generation and maintenance of hyperalgesic states. Disruption of the gene encoding NKCC1 causes an impaired behavioral response to the hot plate test (91) and a reduction in stroking hyperalgesia (touch-evoked pain or allodynia) evoked by capsaicin injections (92). NKCC1 is expressed in primary afferent neurons and in sensory neurons in the spinal cord and the induction of an experimental arthritis alters the expression of NKCC1 in these neurons (93). The process by which NKCC1 may be involved in pain processing involves the role of the cotransporter in the generation of presynaptic inhibition in the spinal cord (94), a mechanism proposed in the gate control theory of pain (95) to explain interactions between low- and high-threshold afferents in spinal nociceptive processing.

The upregulation of NKCC1 during the generation of a visceral hyperalgesic state has been studied recently (96). Using a murine model of visceral hyperalgesia (54), it was found that the noxious visceral stimulus induces a delivery of the NKCC1 cotransporter to the plasma membrane of neurons in the spinal cord. Additionally, the noxious visceral stimulation evokes a rapid and transient phosphorylation of the NKCC1 cotransporter in the membrane fraction of the lumbosacral spinal cord (Fig. 5) (96).

(A)

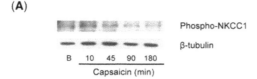

(B)

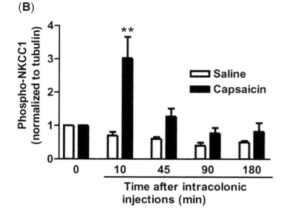

Figure 5 Intracolonic capsaicin induces Na$^+$-K$^+$-2Cl$^-$ cotransporter isoform 1 cotransporter phosphorylation. (**A**) Western blot from membrane protein extracts showing the time course of NKCC1 phosphorylation. Lane marked "B" in the immunoblot contains control (basal) tissue. (**B**) Quantification of phospho-NKCC1 normalized to β-tubulin values after intracolonic capsaicin. Asterisks indicate a significant difference from control levels ($p < 0.01$). *Source*: From Ref. 96.

If the membrane mobilization of NKCC1 occurred in the spinal cord terminals of primary afferents, this would produce an increase in the intracellular concentration of chloride and an enhanced GABA-mediated primary afferent depolarization (PAD). It has been proposed that such an enhancement of PAD can lead to touch-evoked pain (97,98); it has been demonstrated that PAD can be increased by inflammatory stimuli to levels that will evoke spike activity (99).

Manipulation of anion gradients in primary afferent neurons, particularly those involved in nociceptive signalling, represents an entirely novel approach to the development of new therapeutic strategies for the treatment and prevention of persistent pain. Traditional pharmacological approaches are usually based on targeting neurotransmitters and their receptors or the enzymes responsible for their metabolism. The results described above offer a new avenue in pain control by approaching the ionic basis of the actions of some neurotransmitters particularly those, such as GABA, that can change from inhibitory under normal conditions to excitatory in certain pain states.

Mechanisms of Referred Trophic Changes

The areas of referred pain/hyperalgesia are frequently the sites of referred trophic changes, as already reported above. If the hyperalgesic state can be explained by central mechanisms, it is difficult to postulate a similar mechanism for the occurrence of objective changes in the periphery. Thus alternative mechanisms need to be hypothesized. Regarding changes in muscle, one hypothesis is a reflex arc activation involving sensory fibers from the internal organ, as the afferent branch of the reflex, and somatic efferents to the skeletal muscle, as the efferent branch of the reflex. This mechanism has been postulated based on the clinical observation that the area of pain referral from viscera is often the site of sustained muscle contraction (2,22); the activation of somatic efferents would thus produce sustained contraction in the skeletal muscle, the first possible step toward a dystrophic reaction of the tissue. The muscle contraction could also contribute to the hypersensitivity via sensitization of nociceptors locally. A recent study in the rat model of referred muscle hyperalgesia from artificial ureteric calculosis has indeed provided some experimental support for this so far hypothetical mechanism. Positivity was found for a number of ultrastructural indices of contraction in the hyperalgesic muscle ipsilateral to the affected ureter at the lumbar level but not in the contralateral, nonhyperalgesic muscle, and the extent of these indices was proportional to the degree of visceral pain behavior and referred hyperalgesia recorded in the animals. In the same model, c-Fos activation was found in the spinal cord not only in sensory neurons but also in motoneurons, significantly more on the affected side (100,101).

Reflex arc activations have been indicated as contributing mechanisms also to the skin/subcutis referred changes (102). In this case, the efferent branch of the reflex would be represented by sympathetic efferents toward the superficial somatic tissues. This hypothesis, based on the clinical observation of the reduction of referred superficial changes in patients after blocking of the sympathetic efferents toward the referred area, still needs to be confirmed experimentally in standardized conditions (103–105).

CONCLUSION

The referral of visceral sensations to superficial somatic tissues, a constant feature in visceral nociception, has been known for a long time clinically, but the pathophysiological bases of the phenomenon have been the subject of research investigation only in relatively recent times. The execution of studies in patients in standardized conditions involving quantitative measurement of referred phenomena and the setting up of a number of animal models of visceral nociception (with clear behavioral indicators of referred changes) reproducing the clinical conditions are important advances of the last decades. Basic research studies on these models, often using sophisticated technical approaches, have represented a fundamental step toward identification of neurophysiological and molecular mechanisms underlying referred phenomena, especially the hyperalgesia. Though some interpretative questions still remain open—like the nature of referred dystrophic changes accompanying secondary hyperalgesia—the results so far obtained cast a new light on the generation and the mediators of the referred component of nociception from internal organs. This opens new avenues for treatment strategies, not merely symptomatic, of one of the most prominent forms of pain that a human being can experience in the medical context.

REFERENCES

1. Head H. On disturbances of sensation with special reference to the pain of visceral disease. Brain 1893; 16:1–133.
2. Procacci P, Zoppi M, Maresca M. Clinical approach to visceral sensation. In: Cervero F, Morrison JFB, eds. Visceral Sensation, Progress in Brain Research. Amsterdam: Elsevier, 1986:21–28.
3. Sherrington CS. Cutaneous sensations. In: Schäffer EA, ed. Textbook of Physiology. Edinburgh: Y.J. Pentland, 1900:920–1001.
4. Cervero F. Sensory innervation of the viscera: Peripheral basis of visceral pain. Physiol Rev 1994; 74:95–138.
5. Cervero F, Laird JMA. Visceral pain. Lancet 1999; 353:2145–2148.
6. Giamberardino MA, de Bigontina P, Martegiani C, Vecchiet L. Effects of extracorporeal shock-wave lithotripsy on referred hyperalgesia from renal/ureteral calculosis. Pain 1994; 56:77–83.
7. Vecchiet L, Giamberardino MA, Dragani L, Albe-Fessard D. Pain from renal/ureteral calculosis: evaluation of sensory thresholds in the lumbar area. Pain 1989; 36:289–295.
8. Cervero F. Visceral pain—central sensitisation. Gut 2000; 47:56–57.
9. Vecchiet L, Giamberardino MA, Dragani L, Galletti R, Albe-Fessard D. Referred muscular hyperalgesia from viscera: clinical approach. Adv Pain Res Ther 1990; 13:175–182.
10. Vecchiet L, Vecchiet J, Giamberardino MA. Referred muscle pain: clinical and pathophysiological aspects. Curr Rev Pain 1999; 3:489–498.
11. Vasavada SP, Comiter CV, Raz S. Painful diseases of the kidney and ureter. In: Loeser JD, ed. Bonica's Management of Pain. Philadelphia: Lippincott, Williams & Wilkins, 2001:1309–1325.
12. Graham DD, Bonica JJ. Painful diseases of the liver, biliary system and pancreas. In: Loeser JD, ed. Bonica's Management of Pain. Philadelphia: Lippincott, Williams & Wilkins, 2001:1293–1308.
13. Giamberardino MA, Berkley KJ, Iezzi S, de Bigontina P, Vecchiet L. Pain threshold variations in somatic wall tissues as a function of menstrual cycle, segmental site and tissue depth in non-dysmenorrheic women, dysmenorrheic women and men. Pain 1997; 71:187–197.
14. Vecchiet L, Pizzigallo E, Iezzi S, Affaitati G, Vecchiet J, Giamberardino MA. Differentiation of sensitivity in different tissues and its clinical significance. J Musculoske Pain 1998; 6:33–45.
15. Merskley H, Bogduk N. Classification of Chronic Pain: Descriptions of Chronic Pain Syndromes and Definitions of Pain Terms. 2nd ed. Seattle: IASP Press, 1994.
16. Arendt-Nielsen L. Induction and assessment of experimental pain from human skin, muscle and viscera. In: Jensen TS, Turner JA, Wiesenfeld-Hallin Z, eds. Proc 8th World Congress on Pain, Progress in Pain Research and Management. Vol. 8. Seattle: IASP Press, 1997:393–425.
17. Vecchiet L, Giamberardino MA, de Bigontina P. Referred pain from viscera: when the symptom persists despite the extinction of the visceral focus. Adv Pain Res Ther 1992; 20:101–110.

18. Giamberardino MA, De Laurentis S, Affaitati G, Lerza R, Lapenna D, Vecchiet L. Modulation of pain and hyperalgesia from the urinary tract by algogenic conditions of the reproductive organs in women. Neurosci Lett 2001; 304:61–64.

19. Giamberardino MA, Affaitati G, Lerza R, Lapenna D, Costantini R, Vecchiet L. Relationship between pain symptoms and referred sensory and trophic changes in patients with gallbladder pathology. Pain 2005; 114:239–249.

20. Caldarella MP, Giamberardino MA, Laterza F, et al. Visceral and somatic hypersensitivity in patients with the irritable bowel syndrome (IBS). Gastroenterology 2002; 122(4):448.

21. Stawowy M, Bluhme C, Arendt-Nielsen L, Drewes AM, Funch-Jensen P. Somatosensory changes in the referred pain area in patients with acute cholecystitis before and after treatment with laparoscopic or open cholecystectomy. Scand J Gastroenterol 2004; 39:988–993.

22. Giamberardino MA. Visceral Hyperalgesia. In: Devor M, Rowbotham MC, Wiesenfeld-Hallin Z, eds. Progress in Pain Research and Management. Vol. 16. Seattle: IASP Press, 2000:523–550.

23. Stawowy M, Rossel P, Bluhme C, Funch-Jensen P, Arendt-Nielsen L, Drewes AM. Somatosensory changes in the referred pain area following acute inflammation of the appendix. Eur J Gastroenterol Hepatol 2002; 14:1079–1084.

24. Foreman RD. Integration of viscerosomatic sensory input at the spinal level. In: Mayer EA, Saper CB, eds. Progress in Brain Research. Vol. 122. Amsterdam: Elsevier, 2000:209–221.

25. Bonica JJ. The Management of Pain. 2nd ed. Philadelphia, London: Lea & Febiger, 1990.

26. Drewes AM, Schipper KP, Dimcevski G, et al. Multimodal assessment of pain in the esophagus: a new experimental model. Am J Physiol Gastrointest Liver Physiol 2002; 283:95–103.

27. Drewes AM, Babenko L, Birket-Smith L, Funch-Jensen P, Arendt-Nielsen L. Induction of non-painful and painful intestinal sensations by hypertonic saline: a new human experimental model. Eur J Pain 2003a; 7:81–91.

28. Drewes AM, Schipper KP, Dimcevski G, et al. Multi-modal induction and assessment of allodynia and hyperalgesia in the human oesophagus. Eur J Pain 2003; 7:539–549.

29. Drewes AM, Schipper KP, Dimcevski G, et al. Gut pain and hyperalgesia induced by capsaicin: a human experimental model. Pain 2003c; 104:333–341.

30. Ness TJ, Metcalf AM, Gebhart GF. A psychophysical study in humans using phasic colonic distension as a noxious visceral stimulus. Pain 1990; 43:377–386.

31. Aspirotz F. Dimensions of gut dysfunction in irritable bowel syndrome: altered sensory function. Can J Gatroenterol 1999; 13:12–14.

32. Naliboff B, Lembo A, Mayer EA. Abdominal pain in irritable bowel syndrome. Curr Rev Pain 1999; 3:144–152.

33. Ness TJ, Richter HE, Varner RE, Fillingim RB. A psychophysical study of discomfort produced by repeated filling of the urinary bladder. Pain 1998; 7:661–669.

34. Pedersen J, Reddy H, Funch-Jensen P, Arendt-Nielsen L, Gregersen H, Drewes AM. Cold and heat pain assessment of the human oesophagus after experimental sensitisation with acid. Pain 2004b; 110:393–399.

35. Pedersen J, Reddy H, Funch-Jensen P, Arendt-Nielsen L, Gregersen H, Drewes AM. Differences between male and female responses to painful thermal and mechanical stimulation of the human esophagus. Dig Dis Sci 2004a; 49:1065–1074.

36. Bajaj P, Drewes AM, Gregersen H, Petersen P, Madsen H, Arendt-Nielsen L. Controlled dilatation of the uterine cervix—an experimental visceral pain model. Pain 2002; 99:433–442.

37. Joshi SK, Gebhart GF. Visceral Pain. Curr Rev Pain 2000; 4:499–506.

38. Le Bars D, Gozariu M, Caaden SW. Animal models of nociception. Pharmacol Rev 2001; 53:597–652.

39. Giamberardino MA, Rampin O, Laplace JP, Vecchiet L, Albe-Fessard D. Muscular hyperalgesia and hypoalgesia after stimulation of the ureter in rats. Neurosci Lett 1988; 87:29–34.

40. Giamberardino MA, Valente R, de Bigontina P, Iezzi S, Vecchiet L. Effects of spasmolytics and/or non-steroidal anti-inflammatories on muscle hyperalgesia of ureteral origin in rats. Eur J Pharmacol 1995a; 278:97–101.

41. Giamberardino MA, Valente R, de Bigontina P, Vecchiet L. Artificial ureteral calculosis in rats: behavioural characterization of visceral pain episodes and their relationship with referred lumbar muscle hyperalgesia. Pain 1995b; 61:459–469.

42. Laird JM, Roza C, Olivar T. Antinociceptive activity of metamizol in rats with experimental ureteric calculosis: central and peripheral components. Inflamm Res 1998; 47:389–395.

43. Giamberardino MA, Berkley KJ, Affaitati G, et al. Influence of endometriosis on pain behaviors and muscle hyperalgesia induced by a ureteral calculosis in female rats. Pain 2002; 95:247–257.

44. McMahon SB, Abel C. A model for the study of visceral pain states: chronic inflammation of the chronic decerebrate rat urinary bladder by irritant chemicals. Pain 1987; 28:109–127.

45. Jaggar SI, Scott HC, Rice AS. Inflammation of the rat urinary bladder is associated with a referred thermal hyperalgesia, which is nerve growth factor dependent. Br J Anaesth 1999; 83:442–448.

46. Jaggar SI, Scott HC, James IF, Rice AS. The capsaicin analogue SDZ249–665 attenuates the hyperreflexia and referred hyperalgesia associated with inflammation of the rat urinary bladder. Pain 2001; 89:229–235.

47. Farquhar-Smith WP, Rice AS. Administration of endocannabinoids prevents a referred hyperalgesia associated with inflammation of the urinary bladder. Anesthesiology 2001; 94:507–513.

48. Abelli L, Conte B, Somma V, Maggi CA, Giuliani S, Meli A. A method for studying pain arising from the urinary bladder in conscious, freely moving rats. J Urol 1989; 141:148–151.

49. Olivar T, Laird JM. Cyclophosphamide cystitis in mice: behavioural characterisation and correlation with bladder inflammation. Eur J Pain 1999; 3:141–149.

50. Bon K, Lichtensteiger CA, Wilson SG, Mogil JS. Characterization of cyclophosphamide cystitis, a model of visceral and referred pain, in the mouse: species and strain differences. J Urol 2003; 170:1008–1012.

51. Wesselmann U, Lai J. Mechanisms of referred visceral pain: uterine inflammation in the adult virgin rat results in neurogenic plasma extravasation in the skin. Pain 1997; 73:309–317.

52. Wesselmann U, Czakanki PP, Affaitati G, Giamberardino MA. Uterine inflammation as a noxious visceral stimulus: behavioral characterization in the rat. Neurosci Lett 1998; 246:73–76.

53. Ishigooka M, Zermann DH, Doggweiler R, Schmidt RA. Similarity of distributions of spinal c-Fos and plasma extravasation after acute chemical irritation of the bladder and the prostate. J Urol 2000; 164:1751–1756.

54. Laird JMA, Martinez-Caro L, Garcia-Nicas E, Cervero F. A new model of visceral pain and referred hyperalgesia in the mouse. Pain 2001a; 92:335–342.

55. Laird JMA, Olivar T, Roza C, De Felipe C, Hunt SP, Cervero F. Deficits in visceral pain and hyperalgesia of mice with a disruption of the tachykinin NK1 receptor gene. Neuroscience 2000; 98:345–352.

56. Laird JM, Souslova V, Wood JN, Cervero F. Deficits in visceral pain and referred hyperalgesia in Nav1.8 (SNS/PN3)-null mice. J Neurosci 2002; 22:8352–8356.

57. Gebhart GF. Pathobiology of visceral pain: molecular mechanisms and therapeutic implications. Am J Physiol Gastrointest Liver Physiol 2000; 278:834–838.

58. Cervero F, Laird JMA. Referred visceral hyperalgesia: from sensations to molecular mechanisms. In: Brune K, Handwerker HO, eds. Hyperalgesia: molecular mechanisms and clinical implications. Seattle: IASP Press, 2004a:229–250.

59. Cervero F, Laird JMA. Understanding the signalling and transmission of visceral nociceptive events. J Neurobiol 2004b; 61:45–54.

60. Cervero F, Connell LA, Lawson SN. Somatic and visceral primary afferents in the lower thoracic dorsal root ganglia of the cat. J Comp Neurol 1984; 228:422–431.

61. Pierau FK, Taylor DC, Abel W, Friedrich B. Dichotomizing peripheral fibres revealed by intracellular recording from rat sensory neurones. Neurosci Lett 1982; 31:123–128.

62. Pierau FK, Fellmer G, Taylor DC. Somato-visceral convergence in cat dorsal root ganglion neurones demonstrated by double-labelling with fluorescence tracers. Brain Res 1984; 321:63–70.

63. Alles A, Dom RM. Peripheral sensory nerve fibers that dichotomize to supply the brachium and the pericardium in the rat: a possible morphological explanation for referred cardiac pain? Brain Res 1985; 342:382–385.

64. Dawson NJ, Schmid H, Pierau F-K. Pre-spinal convergence between thoracic and visceral nerves of the rat. Neurosci Lett 1992; 138:149–152.

65. Bahr R, Blumberg H, Janig W. Do dichotomizing afferent fibers exist which supply visceral organs as well as somatic structures? A contribution to the problem or referred pain. Neurosci Lett 1981; 24:25–28.

66. Devor M, Wall PD, McMahon SB. Dichotomizing somatic nerve fibers exist in rats but they are rare. Neurosci Lett 1984; 49:187–192.

67. Habler HJ, Janig W, Koltzenburg M. Dichotomizing unmyelinated afferents supplying pelvic viscera and perineum are rare in the sacral segments of the cat. Neurosci Lett 1988; 94:119–124.

68. Cervero F, Tattersall JEH. Somatic and visceral sensory integration in the thoracic spinal cord. In: Cervero F, Morrison JFB, eds. Visceral Sensation. Progress in Brain Research. Vol. 67. Amsterdam: Elsevier, 1986:189–205.

69. Garrison DW, Chandler MJ, Foreman RD. Viscerosomatic convergence onto feline spinal neurons from esophagus, heart and somatic fields: Effects of inflammation. Pain 1992; 49:373–382.

70. Euchner-Wamser I, Sengupta JN, Gebhart GF, Meller ST. Characterization of responses of T2-T4 spinal cord neurons to esophageal distension in the rat. J Neurophysiol 1993; 69:868–883.

71. Keay KA, Clement CI, Owler B, Depaulis A, Bandler R. Convergence of deep somatic and visceral nociceptive information onto a discrete ventrolateral midbrain periaqueductal gray region. Neuroscience 1994; 61:727–732.

72. Brüggemann J, Shi T, Apkarian AV. Squirrel monkey lateral thalamus. II. Viscerosomatic convergent representation of urinary bladder, colon, and esophagus. J Neurosci 1994; 14:6796–6814.

73. Brüggemann J, Shi T, Apkarian AV. Viscero-somatic neurons in the primary somatosensory cortex (SI) of the squirrel monkey. Brain Res 1997; 756:297–300.

74. Laird JMA, Olivar T, Lopez-Garcia JA, Maggi CA, Cervero F. Responses of rat spinal neurons to distension of inflamed colon: role of tachykinin NK2 receptors. Neuropharmacology 2001b; 40: 696–701.

75. Hummel T, Sengupta JN, Meller ST, Gebhart GF. Responses of T2–4 spinal cord neurons to irritation of the lower airways in the rat. Am J Physiol Regul Integr Comp Physiol 1997; 273:R1147–R1157.

76. Roza C, Laird JMA, Cervero F. Spinal mechanisms underlying persistent pain and referred hyperalgesia in rats with an experimental ureteric stone. J Neurophysiol 1998; 79:1603–1612.

77. Berkley KJ, Guilbaud G, Benoist JM, Gautron M. Responses of neurons in and near the thalamic ventrobasal complex of the rat to stimulation of uterus, cervix, vagina, colon, and skin. J Neurophysiol 1993; 69:557–568.

78. Berkley KJ, Hubscher CH, Wall PD. Neuronal responses to stimulation of the cervix, uterus, colon and skin in the rat spinal cord. J Neurophysiol 1993; 69:533–544.

79. Galan A, Laird JMA, Cervero F. In vivo recruitment by painful stimuli of AMPA receptor subunits to the plasma membrane of spinal cord neurons. Pain 2004; 112:315–323.

80. Holzer P, Holzer-Petsche U. Tachykinins in the gut. Part I. Expression, release and motor function. Pharmacol Ther 1997; 73:173–217.

81. Perry MJ, Lawson SN. Differences in expression of oligosaccharides, neuropeptides, carbonic anhydrase and neurofilament in rat primary afferent neurons retrogradely labelled via skin, muscle or visceral nerves. Neuroscience 1998; 85:293–310.

82. Olivar T, Cervero F, Laird JMA. Responses of rat spinal neurones to natural and electrical stimulation of colonic afferents: effect of inflammation. Brain Res 2000; 866:168–177.

83. McLean PG, Picard C, Garcia-Villar R, Moré J, Fioramonti J, Buéno L. Effects of nematode infection on sensitivity to intestinal distension: Role of tachykinin NK2 receptors. Eur J Pharmacol 1997; 337:279–282.

84. Toulouse M, Coelho AM, Fioramonti J, Lecci A, Maggi C, Buéno L. Role of tachykinin NK2 receptors in normal and altered rectal sensitivity in rats. Br J Pharmacol 2000; 129:193–199.

85. Galan A, Cervero F, Laird JM. Extracellular signalling-regulated kinase-1 and -2 (ERK 1/2) mediate referred hyperalgesia in a murine model of visceral pain. Brain Res Mol Brain Res 2003; 116: 126–134.

86. Malinow R, Malenka RC. AMPA receptor trafficking and synaptic plasticity. Annu Rev Neurosci 2002; 25:103–126.

87. Woolf CJ, Salter MW. Neuronal plasticity: increasing the gain in pain. Science 2000; 288:1765–1769.

88. Alvarez-Leefmans FJ, Nani A, Marquez S. Chloride transport, osmotic balance and presynaptic inhibition. In: Rudomin P, Romo R, Mendell LM, eds. Presynaptic Inhibition and Neural Control. New York: Oxford University Press, 1998:50–79.

89. Darman RB, Forbush B. A regulatory locus of phosphorylation in the N terminus of the Na-K-Cl cotransporter, NKCC1. J Biol Chem 2002; 277:37542–37550.

90. Price TJ, Cervero F, de KY. Role of cation-chloride-cotransporters (CCC) in pain and hyperalgesia. Curr Top Med Chem 2005; 5:547–555.

91. Sung KW, Kirby M, McDonald MP, Lovinger DM, Delpire E. Abnormal GABAA receptor-mediated currents in dorsal root ganglion neurons isolated from Na-K-2Cl cotransporter null mice. J Neurosci 2000; 20:7531–7538.

92. Laird JMA, García-Nicas E, Delpire EJ, Cervero F. Presynaptic inhibition and spinal pain processing in mice: a possible role of the NKCC1 cation-chloride co-transporter in hyperalgesia. Neurosci Lett 2004; 361:200–203.

93. Morales-Aza BM, Chillingworth NL, Payne JA, Donaldson LF. Inflammation alters cation chloride cotransporter expression in sensory neurons. Neurobiol Dis 2004; 17:62–69.

94. Rudomin P, Schmidt RF. Presynaptic inhibition in the vertebrate spinal cord revisited. Exp Brain Res 1999; 129:1–37.

95. Melzack R, Wall PD. Pain mechanisms: A new theory. Science 1965; 150:971–979.

96. Galan A, Cervero F. Painful stimuli induce in vivo phosphorylation and membrane mobilization of mouse spinal cord NKCC1 co-transporter. Neuroscience 2005; 133:245–252.

97. Cervero F, Laird JMA. Mechanisms of touch-evoked pain (allodynia): a new model. Pain 1996; 68:13–23.

98. Cervero F, Laird JM, Garcia-Nicas E. Secondary hyperalgesia and presynaptic inhibition: an update. Eur J Pain 2003; 7:345–351.

99. Willis WD Jr. Dorsal root potentials and dorsal root reflexes: a double-edged sword. Exp Brain Res 1999; 124:395–421.

100. Giamberardino MA, Affaitati G, Lerza R, et al. Evaluation of indices of skeletal muscle contraction in areas of referred hyperalgesia from an artificial ureteric stone in rats. Neurosci Lett 2003; 338:213–216.

101. Aloisi A, Ceccarelli I, Affaitati G, et al. c-Fos expression in the spinal cord of female rats with artificial ureteric calculosis. Neurosci Lett 2004; 361:212–215.

102. Davis L, Pollock LJ. The peripheral pathway for painful sensations. Arch Neurol Psychiatr 1930; 24:883–898.

103. Galletti R, Procacci P. The role of the sympathetic system in the control of somatic pain and of some associated phenomena. Acta Neuroveg (Wien) 1966; 28:495–500.

104. Procacci P, Francini F, Zoppi M, Maresca M. Cutaneous pain threshold changes after sympathetic block in reflex dystrophies. Pain 1975; 1:167–175.

105. Jänig W, Häbler H-J. Visceral-autonomic integration. In: Gebhart GF, ed. Visceral Pain. Progress in Pain Research and Management. Seattle: IASP Press, 1995:311–348.

13 | From Sensation to Perception: The Gut–Brain Connection

Fernando Azpiroz

Digestive System Research Unit, University Hospital Vall d'Hebron, Autonomous University of Barcelona, Barcelona, Spain

GENERAL OVERVIEW

The digestive system is controlled by a complex net of feedback mechanisms, by which the gut is able to sense and react to a variety of stimuli. Feedback control of gut function is operated via reflex pathways distributed within the enteric nervous system and both the sympathetic and parasympathetic nervous systems. This organization allows the digestive system a high degree of versatility and adaptation to a wide range of situations. Nevertheless, under some circumstances gut stimuli may activate perception pathways and induce conscious sensations. The peripheral neurons of this viscerosensory system are located in the posterior root ganglia with a visceral projection along sympathetic-splanchnic pathways and central projection into the spinal cord (1–3). Hence, while the operation of the digestive system is assured by a complex wiring of reflex arcs, there is also a sensory alarm system that may be activated to signal dysfunction, translated into symptoms, that is, abnormal conscious sensations. To some extent, the sensory system may be also involved in pleasant gut sensations, that may contribute to gastrointestinal comfort and well-being, but this aspect is still virtually unexplored.

GASTROINTESTINAL WELL-BEING

The concept of unspecific gastrointestinal well-being has been proposed, but supporting experimental evidence in still scarce. Uncontrolled observations suggest that specific pleasant sensations may originate from the gastrointestinal tract. Such sensations are primarily related with the intake of meals and the evacuation of feces, in particular, gratifying sensations, such as satiation and complete rectal evacuation, and conceivably also preparatory sensations, such as appetite or call for stools. Other physiological events, such as eructation and farting, and nonspecific sensation, such as "easy digestion," may also contribute to gastrointestinal well-being. In contrast to perception of symptoms (ill-being), very little is known about gastrointestinal "well-being" and perception of pleasant sensations originating in the gut. The conceptual and methodological developments derived from pathophysiological studies could be applied to investigate this area that may become very important in the future.

Abdominal pain is one of the sensations that may arise from abdominal viscera, but it is relatively infrequent as compared to other abdominal symptoms, such as pressure, fullness, bloating, borborygmi among others. In fact, there is some debate as to whether pain is a distinctive sensation or just an intensity qualifier of perception. This chapter will primarily deal with abdominal symptoms in general, not strictly with abdominal pain, and will review the mechanisms of visceral sensation both in physiological conditions and in the pathophysiology of abdominal symptoms, particularly in patients without no detectable cause, i.e., patients with functional gut disorders. Furthermore, this chapter will basically refer to the digestive system, but the general schema and the concepts discussed also apply, at least in part, to other abdominal systems.

FUNCTIONAL GUT DISORDERS

More than half of the patients in a gastroenterological clinic complain of abdominal symptoms, without demonstrable cause by conventional diagnostic tests. In the absence of positive findings, unexplained abdominal symptoms have been categorized as functional gastrointestinal disorders, and several syndromes, such as noncardiac chest pain, functional dyspepsia, and the irritable bowel syndrome (IBS), have been defined. Noncardiac chest pain refers to patients with thoracic symptoms without cardiac, pulmonary, or esophageal disorders. Functional dyspepsia applies to symptoms such as epigastric pain, pressure, fullness, and bloating that presumably originate from the upper gastrointestinal tract, and that are frequently precipitated by meals. The IBS is attributable to the distal gut, and is characterized by abdominal pain or discomfort associated to disordered bowel habit. The diagnosis of those syndromes is solely based on clinical criteria, because their underlying pathophysiology has not yet been unestablished. It is noteworthy that similar types of functional syndromes have also been described in urology (interstitial cystitis), gynecology (some forms of chronic pelvic pain), and the musculoskeletal system (fibromyalgia). Some data suggest that patients with different visceral functional disorders could have a sensory dysfunction, so that physiological stimuli that are normally unperceived, activate perception pathways and produce their symptoms. This concept has attracted much attention in the field of visceral sensitivity.

EVALUATION OF VISCERAL SENSITIVITY IN HUMANS

Evaluation of visceral sensitivity can be performed by means of provocative tests, measuring the responses to standard stimuli.

What Are the Effective Stimuli that Activate Perception Pathways?

Since physiological stimuli are normally not perceived, evaluation of visceral sensitivity requires probing stimuli that activate perception pathways and induce conscious sensations. However, visceral sensitivity seems different than somatic sensitivity, particularly the skin, in terms of effective stimuli. Abdominal surgeries performed under local anesthesia have demonstrated that cutting or crushing the gut is not perceived, while traction and distension induce conscious sensations (4).

Distension of Hollow Viscera

Gut distension has been widely used to test sensitivity, both in experimental animals and in conscious man. Gastrointestinal distension in healthy subjects induces sensations such as abdominal pressure and fullness, referred to the epigastrium and the paraumbilical region. The type of sensations induced by distension is rather homogeneous from the stomach down to the mid small bowel (5–8), which indicates that the expression of the gut in response to stimuli, and the discriminative value of symptoms in relation to the site of origin in the gut are both relatively poor. A small proportion of distensions in the stomach and proximal duodenum induce nausea, which is rarely induced by jejunal distension. In contrast, jejunal distensions are frequently perceived as colicky or stinging sensation. To note, these sensations induced by experimental stimuli in healthy subjects are similar to the symptoms reported by patients with functional gut disorders in the clinic.

The intensity of perception is stimulus related, small stimuli are unperceived, and the intensity of the conscious sensations increases from the perception threshold up to the threshold for discomfort. Interestingly, the same type of sensations are induced by barely perceptible and by uncomfortable distensions (5). However, perception of gut distension may also depend on the method used.

Several methods to produce distension may be used. Distensions can be produced by manual inflation using a syringe, with automated pumps or with a barostat, which applies fixed intraluminal pressures (9–12). However, these methods do not allow standardization of the distending stimuli when the compliance of the gut varies. For instance, using fixed-volume distension, if the gut contracts, both intraluminal pressure and the intensity of perception increase. Using fixed-pressure distensions, the result is quite different: if the gut contracts, both intraluminal volume and perception decrease (12). Hence, using these methods, perception of gut distension depends on the muscular activity of the gut, and varies upon contraction and relaxation. To overcome these problems, a new methodological approach, the tensostat, has been developed (13). The tensostat is a computerized air pump that applies fixed tension levels on the gut wall. Based on intraluminal pressure and intraluminal volume, the system calculates wall tension, by applying Laplace's law (either for the sphere or for the cylinder) and drives in the pump to maintain the desired tension level on the gut wall. Applying fixed-tension distensions, if the gut contracts, intraluminal volume decreases and intraluminal pressure increases, but perception remains unaffected. These data indicate that perception of gut distension in healthy subjects depends on stimulation of tension receptors, rather than on intraluminal volume or pressure (13). Hence, the tensostat may allow a better standardization of distending stimuli in situations in which the capacity and compliance of the gut is different, for instance, in patients with the IBS who may have either a normal, small, or very large rectum. The tensostat may also be ideally suited to investigate sensory effects of nutrients or drugs that also modify gut motor activity (14). Furthermore, since gut motor activity determines in part the intensity of perception, in the evaluation of gut sensitivity it is good council to control for gut motor activity.

GUT DISTENSION: METHODOLOGICAL ASPECTS

Gut distension can be performed by means of a distending device, a balloon or something similar, mounted over a tube. High-compliance latex balloons made with condoms have relatively low intrinsic pressures, and compliance can be calculated with a reasonably small error. Flaccid bags with negligible intrinsic pressure require no corrections and may be preferable. However, the bag has to be oversized, because when the capacity of the bag is attained during distension, the gut is not being really tested. Most studies use air to produce gut distension, because its resistance to flow through small tubes is relatively low. Furthermore, in contrast to liquids, air does not present the problem of hydrostatic pressure differences along the connecting line. However, air is compressible, and hence, the actual distending volume depends on the pressure within the distending device. In a conventional balloon inflated with a syringe, this compression is negligible. However, using large pumps, air compression within the pump may be considerable, and requires careful corrections before interpreting distension data. Furthermore, the compliance of the pump, specially with bellows pumps that are deformable, may require an additional correction factor.

Nonmechanical Stimuli

As compared to visceral pain, somatic pain is a much more developed area. Indeed, somatic afferents can be precisely investigated using a series of stimulation techniques that allow a selective activation of specific pathways (15,16). Some of these techniques can also be adapted for visceral stimulation.

Electrical Nerve Stimulation

Transmucosal electrical nerve stimulation has been applied in the gut via intraluminal electrodes mounted over a tube (5,6,17–21). Whereas distending stimuli activate sensory pathways and induce perception by specific stimulation of mechanoreceptors on the gut wall, transmucosal nerve stimulation induces similar perception by nonspecific stimulation of afferent pathways, that is, without relying on any specific receptor (5,6).

Thermal Stimulation

Methods for thermal stimulation, involving both cold and warm stimuli, have also been developed to test visceral afferents (22). Thermal stimulation of the gut can be produced via intraluminal bags by recirculating water at adjusted temperatures. It has been shown that the stomach and the intestine exhibit similar stimulus-related thermal sensitivity, but still gastrointestinal thermosensitivity in humans, and specifically the type of afferents activated by warm and cold stimuli, remain poorly explored. Nevertheless, thermal stimuli are potentially applicable in conjunction with mechanical and electrical stimuli for the evaluation of sensory dysfunctions of the gut. These combined techniques may help to identify the specific pathways affected and the level of the dysfunction.

What Kind of Responses Can Be Evaluated?

Basically, three types of responses to gut stimuli can be measured: conscious perception, evoked potentials at various levels of the afferent pathways, and reflex responses. The methodology for the first two has been developed in the area of somatic pain and later applied to viscerosensory testing.

Measurement of Conscious Perception

Perception of probe stimuli applied into the gut can be evaluated in the laboratory by detection of sensory thresholds using various paradigms of stimuli presentation. The intensity and the quality of perception can be measured by means of rating scales, analog, numeric, or descriptive. There is little experience about the affective dimension of visceral sensation, i.e., unpleasantness, which seems independent of the intensity of perception.

Sensory-Evoked Potentials

Visceral sensitivity has also been evaluated using sensory-evoked potentials, the responses evoked by gut stimuli can be recorded at different levels of the afferent pathways using cortical evoked potentials and magnetoencephalography. The problem with these techniques is that it cannot be ascertained as to whether the responses that are recorded relate to perception or to reflex pathways. New imaging techniques, such as positron emission tomography, single-photon emission computer tomography, and functional magnetic resonance imaging use different tracers to detect focal changes in brain blood flow and metabolic activity in response to different stimuli. These techniques provide images of the brain regions activated by visceral stimulation, but their application is limited by their restricted availability. A detailed description of these techniques is provided in Chapter 11.

Reflex Responses

Gut stimuli may also induce reflex motor responses. Reflex responses to gut stimuli in humans can be investigated in the laboratory using different methods to measure gut motor activity. The gut generates both phasic, pulse contractions, and tonic, sustained contractions. Phasic activity can be recorded by measuring pressure changes within the gut using conventional manometry. Tonic contractions do not produce detectable changes in intraluminal pressure, and thus, evaluation of tonic activity requires a more sophisticated methodology. Changes in gut tone can be measured by means of the barostat, as changes in the volume of air within an intraluminal bag, maintained at a fixed pressure level by an electronic air pump (9–11). When the gut relaxes, the barostat injects air into the intraluminal bag to prevent a pressure fall, and when the gut contracts, the barostat withdraws air. Using this isobaric approach, a volume expansion reflects a relaxation, and a volume reduction a contraction. The barostat has proven particularly useful for studying reflex activity, because brief inhibitory reflexes may be missed by recording intermittent phasic activity (7,8).

In contrast to the uniformity of perception, the reflex responses to gut distension are quite heterogeneous, and some data indicate that perception and reflex responses are dissociable and probably mediated by different mechanisms (7,8). From a pathophysiological standpoint this finding may be very important, because it means that perception and reflex responses to gastrointestinal stimuli may be independently altered in some conditions. Indeed, despite that gross motor abnormalities cannot be detected in patients with functional gut disorders using conventional techniques, more refined studies on reflex activity indicate that the dysfunction in these patients involves not only sensory pathways, but also regulatory motor pathways.

Some reflex responses involving central mechanisms may be directly related to conscious perception. For instance, it has been shown that visceral perception produces a parallel inhibition of a somatic flexion reflex, and the latter has been used as an objective equivalent of perception (23).

MODULATION OF VISCERAL PERCEPTION

The sensory signals traveling along the gut–brain connection are modulated by various mechanisms located at multiple levels between sensory nerve terminals in the gut and the brain-cortex. Final perception depends on the interaction of these modulatory mechanisms.

Stimulus-Related Mechanisms

As stated before, perception depends on the intensity of the effective stimulus, so that the level of conscious sensation is related to the magnitude of the stimulus applied. However, the responses to gut stimuli depend also on the number of receptors activated, and specifically, visceral perception in humans is substantially modified by spatial summation phenomena (24,25). The area of stimulation in the intestine, that is, the extension exposed to a distending stimulus, determines the intensity of perception. Moreover, summation effects are similar whether adjacent or distant fields are stimulated, at least over the proximal half of the small bowel (25). These observations suggest that the intestine may tolerate circumscribed activation of sensory terminals without perception, but additional recruitment of afferents at other areas, even at distant sites of the gut, may induce symptoms.

The interaction of different types of stimuli in the gut also modifies conscious perception. For instance, transmucosal electrical nerve stimulation, even at a very low unperceived level, heightens perception of concomitant gut distension, and this sensitizing effect is not explained by changes in intestinal compliance (20,26,27).

Intraluminal Nutrients

Intraluminal nutrients increase gut perception, and this effect depends on the concentration and the type of nutrient. At physiological loads, lipids have a marked effect, but the influence of carbohydrates is much weaker (28). Nutrients modify gut motor activity, but their effects on perception are independent. Indeed, the sensitization induced by lipids seems specifically related to mechanoreceptors, because perception of transmucosal electrical stimulation of the gut, which activates gut afferents without relaying on any specific receptor, is not modified by intraluminal lipids (27). Cholecystokinin (CCK) has been shown to increase the mechanoreceptive response (29), and hence, it could be involved in these effects. Furthermore, in the presence of intestinal lipids, loxiglumide, a CCK-A receptor antagonist, reduces perception of gastric distension (30).

Somatovisceral Interactions

Somatic pain is modulated by a complex neural circuitry that can be activated by somatic stimulation, a phenomenon known as counterirritation or stimulation analgesia. Some data indicate that a neuronal link at the brain stem exerts control over spinal transmission via descending inhibitory pathways, as well as at higher levels of the somatic projection system (31–33). Conceivably, spinal and supraspinal circuits with specific modulatory effects may be activated depending on the type of stimulation (32). This control system of somatic pain perception also modulates visceral sensitivity. It has been shown that transcutaneous electrical nerve stimulation applied on the hand reduces the discomfort produced by gastric or duodenal distensions (34). This viscerosensory modulation by somatic afferents is exerted without alteration of basal gut tone or visceral reflexes (34). Some forms of counterirritation require painful stimulation (31,33,35), but visceral discomfort can be reduced by painless somatic stimuli (34). Furthermore, somatic stimuli may decrease the perception of uncomfortable, but not necessarily painful, visceral sensations. Theoretically, impairment of these modulatory mechanisms could result in visceral hypersensitivity, and conversely, therapeutic techniques to reduce visceral perception via somatic stimulation could potentially benefit patients with abdominal symptoms (33–35).

Role of the Autonomic Nervous System

Experimental data indicate that increased sympathetic activity magnifies perception of gut stimuli, without affecting somatic perception (36). Sympathetic control of visceral perception could be exerted via descending inhibitory pathways of supraspinal origin (37,38). Patients with the IBS display increased sympathetic activity (39), and it is precisely these patients who exhibit a sensory disturbance that is similar to that produced by sympathetic activity—namely, they manifest visceral hypersensitivity, but normal or even increased tolerance to somatic stimuli (6,40). Hence, sympathetic dysregulation of visceral sensitivity may be clinically relevant. The vagus does not seem to be involved in afferent transmission of perception signals, but may exert a central modulatory role (1,41). It remains to be shown whether or not the vagus plays a role in the visceral hypersensitivity of patients with functional gut disorders.

Cognitive Processes

Conscious perception is finally modulated at the highest level of the brain–gut axis. It has been shown that anticipatory knowledge as compared to mental distraction increases perception and the referral area of intestinal stimuli without modifying intestinal reflexes (42). Hence, cognitive processes selectively regulate the sensitivity to gut stimuli, while visceral reflexes operate independently. These data raise the possibility that functional patients are hypervigilant and pay more attention to gut events. It has been further shown that psychological mechanisms also modulate gut perception. Symptoms of colonic distension in healthy subjects are modified by anxiety induced by mental stress and, to a lesser intent, by active relaxation (43). Cognitive-affective modulation of visceral perception may also have therapeutic implications. Hypnosis, which may activate this type of mechanism, has been shown to reduce perception of rectal distension in patients with the IBS, and rectal hypersensitivity and to improve clinical symptoms (44–46).

DYSFUNCTION OF THE SENSORY SYSTEM: FUNCTIONAL GUT DISORDERS

In case of structural diseases or motility disorders of the digestive system, activation of sensory pathways and symptoms are indicative of malfunction. However, some patients exhibit abdominal symptoms without detectable abnormalities, i.e., functional disorders, and in them the alarm system is activated without apparent reason. In some of these patients, malfunction of the alarm system itself may be the cause of the symptoms. Indeed, it has been consistently shown that these patients have a visceral hypersensitivity, so that physiological stimuli that are not perceived by healthy subjects induce their symptoms.

VISCERAL HYPERSENSITIVITY: HISTORICAL BACKGROUND

Some reports in the 1970s described disturbances of gut perception in patients with the irritable bowel and related syndromes, but these studies remained largely ignored. These classic observations were later reconfirmed and expanded, clearly showing a colonic and rectal hypersensitivity in these patients. Further studies tested whether symptoms after meal ingestion in patients with functional dyspepsia were due to a sort of gastric rigidity, that is, to altered compliance and an abnormal response of the stomach to distension. Gastric accommodation to a meal was experimentally reproduced by distending the stomach with an air-filled bag, either with fixed volumes or at fixed pressure levels maintained by a barostat. With both the methods, the results were equivalent. Gastric distension studies showed that the pressure–volume relationship, that is, compliance, was normal. However, the patients developed their customary symptoms at distending levels that were largely unperceived by healthy subjects. It is important to note that these studies were performed in fasted subjects, and hence, did not entirely reproduce the conditions of meal accommodation. Nevertheless, these data suggested that dyspeptic symptoms could be related to gastric hypersensitivity. Similar type of gut hypersensitive responses were also recognized in patients with noncardiac chest pain, and these data altogether suggested that patients with functional gut disorders could have a sensory dysfunction, so that physiological stimuli induced symptoms. Increased sensitivity to mechanical stimuli may arise from reduced compliance of the gut wall, but this hypersensitivity mechanism has been systematically ruled out, because in most studies, gut compliance was shown to be normal. Hence, hypersensitivity seems related to a dysfunction of afferent perception pathways. Over the past decade, the initial observations of visceral hypersensitivity in functional gastrointestinal disorders have been expanded, and the sensory dysfunctions have been further characterized by an extensive series of studies.

Topography of the Sensory Dysfunction

Several lines of evidence indicate that altered sensitivity in patients with functional gut syndromes affects exclusively the visceral territory. Somatic sensitivity, both to the cold pressure test and to transcutaneous electrical nerve stimulation, is normal or even reduced both in dyspeptic and IBS patients (6,40,47,48). This increased tolerance of somatic pain has been related to the pain reporting behavior characteristic of painful conditions. In contrast to these data showing a selective visceral sensory dysfunction, it seems that patients with IBS have an increased incidence of somatic pain disorders, such as fibromyalgia and various myofascial pain syndromes (49–52). The reason for this association is unknown. It remains to be established whether patients with IBS and concomitant fibromyalgia are different than those with irritable bowel alone.

Several studies have attempted to define the regions of the gut and the specific pathways affected in different subsets of patients, and there seems to be a region specificity (6). Increased gastric but normal duodenal sensitivity was shown in a specific subset of patients with motility-like dyspepsia predominantly complaining of postcibal bloating (48). In this study, dyspeptic patients invariably recognized that gastric distension, but not duodenal distension, reproduced their customary symptoms, whereas in healthy subjects both stimuli were perceived alike.

In IBS patients, colonic hypersensitivity to distension has been well documented (22,40, 53–56), and it has been further demonstrated that other regions of the gut, such as the jejunum and even the esophagus also display heightened perception, suggesting a widespread sensory dysfunction (6,57,58). However, the sensory dysfunction in IBS does not affect all types of afferents, but exhibits fiber specificity. Studies using both mechanical stimuli and transmucosal nerve stimulation have shown that patients with IBS have increased perception of mechanical stimuli (distension) with normal perception of electrical stimulation (6). These data suggest that small bowel hypersensitivity in IBS is related to a selective alteration of mechanosensitive pathways. The level of the afferent dysfunction has not been established, but using these techniques, a response bias can be reasonably excluded. It has been postulated that patients with noncardiac chest pain tend to overinterpret esophageal stimuli as painful (59). However, in IBS patients, transmucosal electrical nerve stimulation induces normal perception, even though electrical and mechanical stimuli produce similar, undistinguishable sensations in most tests (6).

Reflex Dysfunctions

The relation between the sensory disturbances detected in the laboratory in patients with functional gut disorders and their clinical complaints is still unclear. Sensitivity tests do not allow a clear discrimination between patients and healthy controls, which indicates that altered perception per se may not entirely explain the symptoms. Conceivably, real life situations involve a larger number of stimuli than the testing conditions, and may recruit a wider pool of altered responses, including both altered perception and reflexes. Indeed, an important question in the pathophysiology of functional gut disorders is whether the neural dysfunction affects exclusively sensory pathways or whether reflex pathways involved in the regulation of motility are also affected.

It has been shown that dyspeptic patients with gastric hypersensitivity also have impaired gastric reflexes (14,48). Physiologically, duodenal distension releases a vagal reflex that induces gastric relaxation. In a group of dyspeptic patients with normal duodenal sensitivity and compliance, duodenal distension induced impaired relaxation of the stomach. It has been suggested that vagal function is impaired in dyspepsia (60), and this could explain the defective duodenogastric reflex. Other studies have shown that IBS patients also display abnormal reflex responses of the gut (40).

Interaction of Sensory and Reflex Dysfunctions

The cause of the concomitant dysfunction of sensory and reflex pathways is not clear, both predisposing and triggering factors may be involved, acting at peripheral and central levels. Potential causes include genetic and early life influences, enteric infection and inflammation, alterations in enteric flora, dietary factors and food intolerance, autonomic dysfunctions, psychosocial stress, and other cognitive factors. In any case, altered reflex activity and altered conscious perception of gut stimuli may combine to different degree in patients with various functional gut syndromes, and their interaction may explain the origin of clinical symptoms. These aspects will be discussed in detail in Section IV, but following are two pathophysiological models in relation to functional dyspepsia and IBS.

Normally, ingestion of a meal induces a relaxation of the proximal stomach to accommodate the meal volume, and the magnitude of the relaxation is regulated by a complex net of reflexes (61,62). Hence, this partial relaxation prevents wall tension increments and symptoms, but still the residual contraction of the proximal stomach gently forces gastric content distally into the antrum and initiates gastric emptying. As the relaxatory input decreases, the proximal stomach regains tone and emptying progresses. A gastric hyporeactivity to relaxatory reflexes would predictably result in a defective volume accommodation of the proximal stomach and antral overload. In patients with functional dyspepsia, gastric tone and compliance are normal during fasting (47,48,63,64). However, the reactivity of the stomach to regulatory reflexes is abnormal, and the proximal stomach does not relax properly in response to reflexes arising from the antrum and the small intestine (14,48,65). Consequently, accommodation of the proximal stomach to a meal is impaired (63,64,66), which results in antral overload (67,68). Antral distension may release symptoms in these patients, because this area is hypersensitive to wall tension increments (14). Furthermore, some experimental data indicate that increased intragastric pressure after a meal, simulating a defective gastric accommodation, produces dyspeptic-type symptoms without disturbing gastric emptying (61), a condition that resembles most patients with functional dyspepsia (69). Hence, the gastric hyporeflexia exacerbates the poor tolerance of dyspeptics to intragastric volumes, and thus, contributes to generation of clinical symptoms in the absence of major motor dysfunctions. Some data further suggest that specific symptoms, such as early satiety and postprandial epigastric pain, may be related to impaired accommodation (62,64).

It has been reported that rectal hypersensitivity in IBS patients is associated with motor hyperactivity in response to gut stimuli (54). Again both hypersensitivity and hyperreactivity could contribute to perception of rectal tenesmus and fecal urgency, which is a common symptom in these patients. Recent studies using a gas challenge test, further substantiate the role of combined sensory-reflex disturbances in IBS. Whereas healthy subjects propel and evacuate as much gas as infused into the jejunum, IBS patients have a poor tolerance to gas loads, and develop gas retention and abdominal symptoms (70,71). Gas transit is normally regulated by gut reflexes (72), and these control mechanisms are altered in IBS patients (73,74). Whether or not intestinal gas is a real problem in IBS remains unclear (75), but the important contribution of the gas challenge studies is the demonstration of abnormal control of gut motility in these patients, which, together with increased gut sensitivity, may produce their symptoms.

SUMMARY AND CONCLUSION

Physiological stimuli in the gut induce regulatory reflexes to accomplish the digestive process, but are normally not perceived. However, under some circumstances, gut stimuli may activate perception pathways and induce conscious sensations. Experimental evidence gathered during the past decade suggests that patients with functional gut disorders and unexplained abdominal symptoms may have a sensory dysfunction of the gut, so that physiological stimuli would induce their symptoms. Assessment of visceral sensitivity is still poorly developed, but in analogy to somatosensory testing, differential stimulation of visceral afferents may be achieved by a combination of stimulation techniques, which may help to characterize sensory dysfunctions. Visceral afferent input is modulated by a series of mechanisms at different levels of the brain–gut axis, and conceivably, a dysfunction of these regulatory mechanisms could cause hypersensitivity. Alteration of visceral perception may result in unexplained symptoms characteristic of functional disorders. Furthermore, these patients also have altered visceral reflexes, and these mixed sensory-reflex dysfunctions may interact to produce the clinical syndrome. Evidence of a gut sensory-reflex dysfunction as a common pathophysiological mechanism in different functional gastrointestinal disorders would suggest that they are different forms of the same process, and that the clinical manifestations depend on the specific pathways affected. This unifying working hypothesis may be also extrapolated to explain the pathophysiology of other extradigestive functional syndromes.

REFERENCES

1. Sengupta JN, Gebhart GF. Gastrointestinal afferents and sensation. In: Johnson, LR, eds. Physiology of the Gastrointestinal Tract. Vol. 1. 3rd ed. New York: Raven, 1994:483–519.
2. Bentley FH, Smithwick RH. Visceral pain produced by balloon distension of the jejunum. Lancet 1940; 2:389.
3. Ray BS, Neill CL. Abdominal visceral sensation in man. Ann Surg 1947; 126:709.
4. Ness TJ, Gebhart GF. Visceral pain: a review of experimental studies. Pain 1990; 41:167.
5. Accarino AM, Azpiroz F, Malagelada J-R. Symptomatic responses to stimulation of sensory pathways in the jejunum. Am J Physiol 1992; 263:G673.
6. Accarino AM, Azpiroz F, Malagelada J-R. Selective dysfunction of mechanosensitive intestinal afferents in the irritable bowel syndrome. Gastroenterology 1995; 108:636.
7. Azpiroz F, Malagelada J-R. Perception and reflex relaxation of the stomach in response to gut distention. Gastroenterology 1990; 98:1193.
8. Rouillon JM, Azpiroz F, Malagelada J-R. Reflex changes in intestinal tone: relationship to perception. Am J Physiol 1991; 261:G280.
9. Azpiroz F, Malagelada J-R. Gastric tone measured by an electronic barostat in health and postsurgical gastroparesis. Gastroenterology 1987; 92:934.
10. Azpiroz F, Malagelada J-R. Physiological variations in canine gastric tone measured by an electronic barostat. Am J Physiol 1985; 248:G229.
11. Azpiroz F, Salvioli B. Barostat measurements. In: Shuster MM, Crowel MD, Koch KL, eds. Schuster Atlas of Gastrointestinal Motility in Health and Disease. 2nd ed. Hamilton, ON: BC Decker, 2002: 151–170.
12. Notivol R, Coffin B, Azpiroz F, Mearin, Serra, Malagelada. Gastric tone determines the sensitivity of the stomach to distension. Gastroenterology 1995; 108:330.
13. Distrutti E, Azpiroz F, Soldevilla, Malagelada J-R, et al. Gastric wall tension determines perception of gastric distension. Gastroenterology 1999; 116:1035.
14. Caldarella MP, Azpiroz F, Malagelada J-R. Antro–fundic dysfunctions in functional dyspepsia. Gastroenterology 2003; 124:1220.
15. Price DD, Long S, Huitt C. Sensory testing of pathophysiological mechanisms of pain in patients with reflex sympathetic dystrophy. Pain 1992; 49:163.
16. Gracely RH. Studies of pain in normal man. In: Wall PD, Melzack R, eds. Textbook of Pain. 3rd ed. Edinburgh: Churchill Livingstone, 1994:315–336.
17. Meunier P, Collet, Duclaux, Chéry-Croze. Endorectal cerebral evoked potentials in human. Int J Neurosci 1987; 37:193.
18. Frieling T, Enck P, Wienbeck M. Cerebral responses evoked by electrical stimulation of the rectosigmoid in normal subjects. Dig Dis Sci 1989; 34:202.
19. Smout AJPM, De Vore, Dalton, Castell. Cerebral potentials evoked by esophageal distension in patients with non-cardiac chest pain. Gut 1992; 33:298.
20. Accarino AM, Azpiroz F, Malagelada J-R. Gut perception in humans is modulated by interacting gut stimuli. Am J Physiol 2002; 282:G220.
21. Kamm MA, Lennard-Jones JE, Nicholls RJ. Evaluation of the intrinsic innervation of the internal anal sphincter using electrical stimulation. Gut 1989; 30:935.
22. Villanova N, Azpiroz F, Malagelada J-R. Perception and gut reflexes induced by stimulation of gastrointestinal thermoreceptors in humans. J Physiol (Lond) 1997; 502:215.
23. Bouhassira D et al. [Authors are Bouhassira, Chollet, Coffin, Lémann, LeBars, Willer, and Jian.] Inhibition of a somatic nociceptive reflex by gastric distension in humans. Gastroenterology 1994; 107:985.
24. Serra J, Azpiroz F, Malagelada J-R. Perception and reflex responses to intestinal distension are modified by simultaneous or previous stimulation. Gastroenterology 1995; 109:1742.
25. Serra J, Azpiroz F, Malagelada J-R. Modulation of gut perception by spatial summation phenomena. J Physiol (Lond.) 1998; 506:579.
26. Feinle C, et al. [Authors are Feinle, Rades, Otto, and Fried.] Fat digestion modulates gastrointestinal sensations induced by gastric distention and duodenal lipid in humans. Gastroenterology 2001; 120:1100.
27. Accarino AM, Azpiroz F, Malagelada J-R. Modification of small bowel mechanosensitivity by intestinal fat. Gut 2001; 48:690.
28. Carrasco M, Azpiroz F, Malagelada J-R. Modulation of gastric accommodation by duodenal nutrients. WJG. 2005; 11:4848–4851.
29. Davison JS, Clarke GD. Mechanical properties and sensitivity to CCK of vagal gastric slowly adapting mechanoreceptors. Am J Physiol 1988; 255:G55.
30. Feinle C, D'Amato M, Read NW. Cholecystokinin-A receptors modulate gastric sensory and motor responses to gastric distension and duodenal lipid. Gastroenterology 1996; 110:1379.
31. De Broucker T. et al. [Authors are De Broucker, Cesaro, Willer, and Le Bars.] Diffuse noxious inhibitory controls in man. Involvement of the spino reticular tract. Brain 1990; 113:1223.
32. Ness TJ, Gebhart GF. Interactions between visceral and cutaneous nociception in the rat. I. Noxious cutaneous stimuli inhibit visceral nociceptive neurons and reflexes. J Neurophysiol 1991; 66:20–28.

33. Melzack R. Folk medicine and the sensory modulation of pain. In: Wall PD, Melzack R, eds. Textbook of Pain. 3rd ed. Edimburgh: Churchill Livingstone, 1994:1209–1217.
34. Coffin B, Azpiroz F, Malagelada J-R. Somatic stimulation reduces perception of gut distension. Gastroenterology 1994; 107:1636.
35. Woolf CJ, Thompson JW. Stimulation fibre-induced analgesia: transcutaneous electrical nerve stimulation (TENS) and vibration. In: Wall PD, Melzack R, eds. Textbook of Pain. 3rd ed. Edinburgh: Churchill Livingstone, 1994:1191–1208.
36. Iovino P, et al. [Authors are Iovino, Azpiroz, Domingo, and Malagelada.] The sympathetic nervous system modulates perception and reflex responses to gut distension in humans. Gastroenterology 1995; 108:680.
37. Tattersall JEH, Cerveró F, Lumb BM. Viscero-somatic neurons in the lower thoracic spinal cord of the cat: excitations and inhibitions evoked by splanchnic and somatic nerve volleys and by stimulation of brain stem nuclei. J Neurophysiol 1986; 56:1411.
38. Cerveró F, Lumb BM. Bilateral inputs and supraspinal control of viscerosomatic neurons in the lower thoracic cord of the cat. J Physiol (Lond.) 1988; 403:221.
39. Aggarwal A, et al. [Authors are Aggarwal, Cutts, Abell, Cardoso, Familoni, Bremer, Karas.] Predominant symptoms in irritable bowel syndrome correlate with specific autonomic nervous system abnormalities. Gastroenterology 1994; 106:945.
40. Whitehead WE, et al. [Authors are Whitehead, Holtkotter, Enck, Hoelzl, Holmes, Anthony, Shabsin, Schuster.] Tolerance for rectosigmoid distension in irritable bowel syndrome, Gastroenterolog 1990; 98:1187.
41. Ren K, Randich A, Gebhart GF. Effects of electrical stimulation of vagal afferents on spinothalamic tract cells in the rat. Pain 1991; 44:311.
42. Accarino AM, Azpiroz F, Malagelada J-R. Attention and distraction: effects on gut perception. Gastroenterology 1997; 113:415.
43. Ford MJ, Camilleri, Zinsmeister, Hanson. Psychosensory modulation of colonic sensation in the human transverse and sigmoid colon. Gastroenterology 1995; 109:1772.
44. Prior A, Colgan JM, Whorwell PJ. Changes in rectal sensitivity after hypnotherapy in patients with irritable bowel syndrome. Gut 1990; 31:896.
45. Whorwell PJ, Prior A, Faragher EB. Controlled trial of hypnotherapy in the treatment of severe refractory irritable bowel syndrome. Lancet 1984; 2:1232.
46. Whorwell PJ, Prior A, Colgan JM. Hypnotherapy in severe irritable bowel syndrome: further experience. Gut 1987; 28:423.
47. Mearin F, Cucala, Azpiroz, Malagelada. The origin of symptoms on the brain gut axis in functional dyspepsia. Gastroenterology 1991; 101:999.
48. Coffin B, Azpiroz, Guarner, Malagelada. Selective gastric hypersensitivity and reflex hyporeactivity in functional dyspepsia. Gastroenterology 1994; 107:1345.
49. Veale D, Kavanagh, Fielding, Fitzgerald O. Primary fibromyalgia and the irritable bowel syndrome different expressions of a common pathogenetic process. Br J Rheumatol 1991; 30:220.
50. Barton A, Whorwell PJ, Marshall D. Increased prevalence of sicca complex and fibromyalgia in patients with irritable bowel syndrome. Am J Gastroenterol 1999; 94:1898.
51. Pace P, Manzionna, Bollani, Sarzi-Puttini, Bianchi-Porro. Visceral sensitivity in patients with fibromyalgia and in normal controls. Gastroenterology 1997; 112:A802.
52. Chang L, Mayer, Johnson, Fitzgerald, Naliboff. Differences in somatic perception in female patients with irritable bowel syndrome with and without fibromyalgia. Pain 2000; 84:297.
53. Ritchie J. Pain from distension of the pelvic colon by inflating a balloon in the irritable bowel syndrome. Gut 1973; 14:123.
54. Whitehead WE, Engel BT, Schuster MM. Irritable bowel syndrome: physiological and psychological differences between diarrhea-predominant and constipation-predominant patients. Dig Dis Sci 1980; 25:404.
55. Distrutti E, Salvioli, Azpiroz, Malagelada. Rectal function and bowel habit in irritable bowel syndrome. Am J Gastroenterol 2004; 99:131.
56. Mertz H, Naliboff, Munakata, Niazi N. Altered rectal perception is a biological marker of patients with irritable bowel syndrome. Gastroenterology 1995; 109:40.
57. Moriarty KJ, Dawson AM. Functional abdominal pain: further evidence that the whole gut is affected. Br Med J 1982; 284:1670.
58. Trimble KC, Farouk, Pryde, Douglas, Heading. Heightened visceral sensations in functional gastrointestinal disease is not site-specific. Evidence for a generalized disorder of gut sensitivity. Dig Dis Sci 1995; 40:1607.
59. Richter JE, Bradley LA. The irritable esophagus. In: Mayer EA, Raybould HE, eds. Pain Research and Clinical Management, Basic and Clinical Aspects of Chronic Abdominal Pain. Vol. 9. Amsterdam: Elsevier, 1993:45–54.
60. Greydanus MP, Vassallo, Camilleri, Nelson, Hanson, Thomforde. Neurohormonal factors in functional dyspepsia: insights on pathophysiological mechanisms. Gastroenterology 1991; 100:1311.
61. Moragas G, Azpiroz, Pavía, Malagelada. Relations among intragastric pressure, postcibal perception and gastric emptying. Am J Physiol 1993; 264:G1112.

62. Mayer EA. The physiology of gastric storage and emptying. In: Johnson LR, ed. Physiology of the Gastrointestinal Tract. Vol. 1. 3rd ed. New York: Raven, 1994:929–976.
63. Tack J, Piessevaux, Coulie, Caenepeel, Janssens. Role of impaired gastric accommodation to a meal in functional dyspepsia. Gastroenterology 1998; 115:1346.
64. Tack J, Caenepeel, Fischler, Piessevaux, Janssens. Symptoms associated with hypersensitivity to gastric distention in functional dyspepsia. Gastroenterology 2001; 121:526.
65. Feinle C, Meier, Otto, D'Amato, Fried. Symptomatic and plasma CCK responses to increasing doses of duodenal lipid in patients with functional dyspepsia (FD) and the role of CCK-A receptors. Gut 2001; 48:347.
66. Salet GAM, Samsom, Roelofs, et al. Responses to gastric distension in functional dyspepsia. Gut 1998; 42:823.
67. Hausken T, Thune, Matre, Gilja, Odegaard, Berstad. Volume estimation of the gastric antrum and the gallbladder in patients with non-ulcer dyspepsia and erosive prepyloric, changes, using three-dimensional ultrasonography. Neurogastroenterol Mot 1994; 6:263.
68. Troncon LEA, Bennett, Akhluwalia, Thompson. Abnormal intragastric distribution of food during gastric emptying in functional dyspepsia patients. Gut 1994; 35:327.
69. Tucci A, Corinaldesi, Stanghellini, et al. Helicobacter pylori infection and gastric function in patients with chronic idiopathic dyspepsia. Gastroenterology 1992; 103:768.
70. Serra J, Azpiroz F, Malagelada J-R. Intestinal gas dynamics and tolerance in humans. Gastroenterology 1998; 115:542.
71. Caldarella MP, Serra, Azpiroz, Malagelada. Prokinetic effects of neostigmine in patients with intestinal gas retention. Gastroenterology 2002; 122:1748.
72. Harder H, Serra, Azpiroz, Malagelada. Reflex control of intestinal gas dynamics and tolerance in humans. Am J Physiol 2004; 286:G89.
73. Serra J, Salvioli, Azpiroz, Malagelada. Lipid-induced intestinal gas retention in the irritable bowel syndrome. Gastroenterology 2002; 123:700.
74. Passos MC, Tremolaterra, Serra, Azpiroz, Malagelada. Impaired reflex control of intestinal gas transit in patients with abdominal bloating. Gut 2005; 54:344.
75. Maxton DG, Martin, Whorwell, Godfrey. Abdominal distension in female patients with irritable bowel syndrome: exploration of possible mechanisms. Gut 1991; 32:662.

14 | Stress, Visceral Pain, and the Brain–Gut Connections

Yvette Taché and Mulugeta Million
CURE/Digestive Diseases Research Center, and Center for Neurovisceral Sciences and Women's Health, Division of Digestive Diseases, Department of Medicine, University of California Los Angeles, and VA Greater Los Angeles Healthcare System, Los Angeles, California, U.S.A.

INTRODUCTION

The first clinical observation of brain–gut interactions dates back to Beaumont's classical monograph published in 1833 that detailed alterations of gastric mucosa in relation with the mental state of his fistulous subject, Alexis St. Martin (1). Seminal reports by Cannon at the beginning of the last century brought experimental proof of the impact of emotion (fear, rage, and hunger) on gastric secretory and motor function in cats (2). However, Selye deserves much of the credit for introducing the term "stress" which he defined as " the adaptive bodily changes to any demands" (3). In his 1936 landmark publication, he identified the gut, immune systems, and endocrine systems as primary targets altered by various physical and chemical challenges (4). Since then, over 200,000 articles are listed in PubMed related to stress and cell or body responses. However, the impact of stress on visceral pain has emerged only recently, largely driven by the early clinical recognition that stressful events exacerbate or even trigger abdominal pain episodes in nearly half of patients with irritable bowel syndrome (IBS) (5) and increase pain response to colorectal distension (CRD) (6,7). Now growing clinical reports document that the manifestations of IBS symptoms, including visceral pain, are modulated by stress (8–10) and that disorders of the brain-gut axis are part of the underlying mechanisms involved in visceral hypersensitivity in IBS patients (11–13). Recently, several laboratories have developed experimental models of visceral pain that recapture some features of IBS symptoms to gain insight into the pathophysiology of this functional bowel disorder.

This chapter will focus on the modulatory effects of stress on visceral pain induced by CRD in experimental animals and aspects of sex differences. Mechanisms of stress-related visceral hyperalgesia will be mainly addressed in the context of activation of brain corticotropin-releasing factor (CRF) and CRF receptors. This brain-signaling pathway has emerged to intimately connect the stress responses (14), including alterations of lower gut function (15) and the development of diseases (16).

STRESS-INDUCED VISCERAL HYPERALGESIA

The body could be subjected to a variety of stressors that have been commonly subdivided into two categories: exteroceptive (psychological or neurogenic) and interoceptive (physical or systemic). Exteroceptive stressors become stressful only after being processed in the context of previous experiences and are, therefore, limbic sensitive. Brain circuits mediating the endocrine and autonomic response to exteroceptive stressors encompass the limbic-sensitive neural network, namely, the cortex (lateral, medial prefrontal, ventromedial, perigenual, and infragenual cingulate), bed nucleus of the stria terminalis, lateral septum, hippocampus, amygdala, hypothalamus (mainly paraventricular nucleus, PVN), and periaqueductal gray (PAG) (Fig. 1A) (17–20). The impacts of exteroceptive stressors on cortical structures are conveyed to these forebrain and hindbrain nuclei which themselves have projections to pontomedullary nuclei (Fig. 1A) (21,22). With regard to interoceptive or limbic-insensitive stressors that represent a threat to the homeostasis (such as immune stress), the cognitive processing is bypassed and brainstem/pontine nuclei such as the lateral parabrachial nucleus, nucleus tractus solitarius, brainstem/pontine catecholaminergic neurons in the ventrolateral medulla and the locus

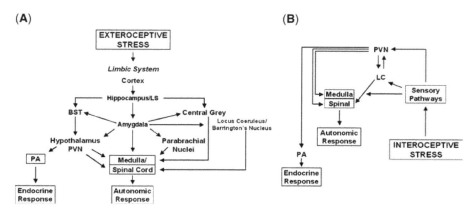

Figure 1 Schematic drawing of the neural circuits by which exteroceptive (**A**) and interoceptive (**B**) stressors induce endocrine and autonomic responses that impact on peripheral organs. *Abbreviations*: BST, bed nucleus of the stria terminalis; LC, locus coeruleus; LS, lateral septum; PA, pituitary adrenal axis; PVN, paraventricular nucleus.

coeruleus (LC), respectively, receive sensory visceral input (Fig. 2) (17–20). In both exteroceptive and interoceptive types of stressors, the PVN serve as the principal gateway conveying actions on the pituitary-adrenal axis (endocrine) and autonomic nervous system which are the two main effector arms of the stress response (Fig. 1) (23–25).

Modulation of Visceral Pain by Stress

Stress influences the manifestations or the development of visceral pain in IBS patients (Table 1) (5,8,9). For instance, IBS patients exposed to an acute psychological or physical stressor exhibit increased visceral sensitivity to rectal electrostimulation (10). Convergent clinical reports established that stressful life events before or after an acute enteric infection are strong predictors of acquiring postinfectious IBS (26). Childhood trauma by biopsychosocial stressful factors (neglect, abuse, loss of caregiver, or life threatening situation) impact the susceptibility to subsequently develop visceral pain and comorbidity with anxiety, depression, and emotional distress (34–36).

Experimental models have been produced to recapture clinical features of IBS symptoms, of which lowered pain threshold and hyperalgesia to repeated sigmoid distensions are hallmarks in IBS patients (32,37). Therefore, the influence of exposure to various stressors, including early life stress (8,9), on visceral pain has been investigated by performing repeated CRD in rodents and monitoring related changes in abdominal contractions, a validated measure of visceral pain (38).

Gué et al. provided the first experimental evidence that stress enhanced visceral pain of colonic origin in rats (39). This and subsequent studies showed that partial restraint, applied for two hours followed 30 minutes later by graded *tonic* rectal distensions, induced hypersensitivity compared with nonstressed groups in male (39) and female Wistar rats (40,41). In contrast, water avoidance stress (WAS) or restraint did not alter abdominal contractions in response to graded intensity of *phasic* CRD performed *immediately* after the stress in Long-Evans, Sprague-Dawley, or Wistar rats (42–45). However, a delayed hyperalgesia to repeated phasic CRD (40 and 60 mmHg) occurred 24 hours after WAS exposure in male Wistar and Long-Evans rats (44,45).

Intermittent maternal separation (MS180) of pups from the dam was developed by Plotsky and Meaney (46) originally as an experimental approach to establish the impact of early adverse experience on stress susceptibility in adulthood. MS180 adult rats showed enduring changes in stress responsiveness and emotionality (47) and responded to CRD by developing visceral hyperalgesia (42,45,48,49). In particular, 64% of male Long-Evans rats, maternally separated for a 180-minute period daily from days 2 to 14 postnatally (MS180) and subjected at 12 weeks of age to phasic CRD immediately after WAS, displayed an immediate visceral hyperalgesia (42,45,49). In addition, at 24 hours after WAS, the hyperalgesic response was further enhanced (45). In another experimental model of genetically prone to

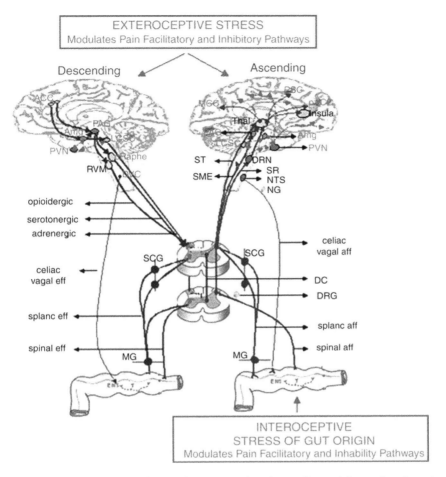

Figure 2 (*See color insert*) Schematic representation of ascending and descending visceral pain pathways and the stress-related neuronal circuitry that potentially modulates these pain pathways. Classical ascending pain pathways are shown in solid blue lines and descending pathways in solid dark brown lines. Thinner blue and dark brown lines represent vagal afferent and efferent pathways, respectively, where some evidence has been shown for their role in the visceral pain circuitry. Brain regions that are activated by both stress and pain stimuli or that are activated by stress and have the potential to modulate the pain pathways are labeled in red. Similarly, brain circuits that are activated by stress and have the potential to modulate the pain pathway are indicated by dashed red lines. The diagram is not intended to represent the exact anatomic localization of the different structures and is not exhaustive. *Abbreviations*: ACC, anterior cingulate cortex; Aff, afferent; Amg, amygdala; cRaphe, caudal raphe nucleus; DC, dorsal column; DRG, dorsal root ganglia; DRN, dorsal reticular nucleus; DVC, dorsal vagal complex; Eff, efferent; ENS, enteric nervous system; MCC, mid cingulate cortex; MG, mesenteric ganglia; NG, nodose ganglia; NTS, solitary tract nucleus; pACC, perigenual anterior cingulate cortex; PAG, periaqueductal gray; PSC, primary somatosensory cortex; PVN, paraventricular nucleus of the hypothalamus; RVM, rostroventral medulla; SCG, sympathetic chain ganglia; SME, spinomesencephalon; Splanc, splanchnic; SR, spinoreticular; ST, spinothalamic; Thal, thalamus.

anxiety male Wistar Kyoto rats, an increased sensitivity to CRD, compared to less anxiety prone rat strains, was observed (50). These studies indicate that early adverse events and genetically anxiety predisposed rats are susceptible to developing persistent visceral sensitization to interoceptive and exteroceptive stressors.

Sex Difference in Stress-Related Visceral Hyperalgesia

Clinical reports have well documented that IBS symptoms including the perception of abdominal pain are three to four times more prevalent in women than in men (51–53). However, experimental studies characterizing sex difference in stress-related visceral pain models are relatively limited (54). In contrast, in the somatic pain field, gonadal hormones

Table 1 Stress-Related Visceral Pain or Hyperalgesia in Humans

Type of Stress	Subjects	Visceral Response	References
Psychosocial + chronic psychosocial stress	IBS	Correlated with ↑ symptoms	(5,26–29)
Acute auditory	IBS	↑ Pain rating	(30)
Cold stress	Ulcerative colitis	↑ Esophageal hyperalgesia	(31)
Repeated sigmoid distension	IBS	↑ Rectal hyperalgesia	(32,33)

Abbreviation: IBS, irritable bowel syndrome.

have received increasing attention in relation to their modulatory influence on the perception and responsiveness to stressful stimuli (55,56), and studies have unraveled alterations of neural processing of pain and pain inhibitory pathways by estrogens (55,56).

Experimental studies to explore sex differences in the visceral pain field indicate that the pressure at which CRD triggers visceromotor response is lower in female than in male Wistar anesthetized rats (57). Likewise, in a rat model of maternal separation involving the removal of the litter from the mother for a few hours from days 1 to 14 postnatally, acute restraint resulted in hypersensitivity to incremental intensity of tonic CRD performed at 12 weeks of age only in female, but not in male Wistar rats (48). Further investigations to assess the role of sex hormones in the sex difference established that ovariectomy abolished restraint stress-induced hypersensitivity that developed with incremental tonic CRD in conscious cycling female rats, while not affecting the nociceptive response proper to CRD (41). Conversely, estrogen replacement in ovariectomized rats, at levels similar to those of normal cycling rats, restored restraint-induced hypersensitivity to incremental tonic CRD, while progesterone had no effect (41). Moreover, estrogen administration in ovariectomized rats induced sensitization to repeated innocuous phasic CRD (58). Lastly, rats in proestrus exhibited the lowest pain threshold of sensitivity to CRD, compared with other estrus cycle phases or male rats (57,59). These observations combined with the immediate and persistent increase in estradiol levels in the proestrus stage or in response to stress in female rats (60) support the notion that fluctuation of estrogens may have a bearing on sex difference in visceral pain of colonic origin.

The facilitation of estrogen-related hypersensitivity can take place at many neuronal sites. Estrogen receptors (ERs) are distributed throughout the central nervous system including the brain (61) and the spinal cord (62), along with the peripheral sensory processing pathway such as the dorsal root ganglia neurons (63). In the lumbosacral spinal cord, ERα immunoreactive neurons have been identified in the superficial laminae where visceral afferents terminate (64). Electrophysiological studies established that estrogen increase spinal cord processing of sensory information activated by CRD (58).

STRESS-INDUCED SOMATIC AND VISCERAL HYPOALGESIA

In contrast to visceral pain exacerbated by wrap restraint in Wistar rats or WAS in MS180 Long-Evans rats, the same study provided evidence that there was somatic hyposensitivity to noxious cutaneous stimuli indicative of analgesia in rats (39,42). Stress initiated by low-intensity–induced somatic analgesia involves a naloxone-sensitive opioid pathway as part of the descending antinociceptive circuits from the amygdala, the PAG, and rostroventral medulla (Fig. 2) (42,65,66). Therefore, the hypersensitivity to CRD induced by stress seems to be restricted to the visceral compartment in these studies. This is in keeping with differences between acute stress-related somatic hypoalgesia and visceral hyperalgesia in IBS patients (7,10,67,68), although there is also a report of cutaneous hypersensitivity in IBS patients (69).

However, recent reports indicate that the activation of descending opioid inhibitory pathways also modulates stress-related visceral responses, because naloxone unmasked WAS-induced hyperalgesia to repeated phasic CRD in normal rats and exacerbated the pain response to CRD in MS180 rats (42). In a different study, WAS attenuated the visceral pain response to graded phasic CRD performed six hours after the stress in wild-type mice or in Sprague-Dawley male rats (43). In contrast, WAS or restraint induced hyperalgesia to repeated phasic CRD in neurotensin knockout mice or in rats pretreated intraperitoneally with the neurotensin receptor antagonist, SR 48692 (43), suggesting a role of neurotensin in WAS-induced visceral hypoalgesia. Interestingly, the study also showed that WAS-induced visceral analgesia to CRD was higher in male than in female rats, while the hyperalgesic response after blockade of neurotensin receptors was increased in female compared to male rats (43). These data suggest that neurotensin may as well contribute to the sex difference in visceral pain sensitivity (43). In another experimental model, the brief (15 minutes) rough handling of rat pups during postnatal days 2 to 14 decreased the visceromotor response to phasic CRD performed immediately after WAS and prevented the development of hyperalgesia at 24 hours after WAS in adult rats (45). This points to the modulation of the susceptibility to develop hyper- or hypoalgesia by postnatal events that impact the plasticity of stress circuitry within a sensitive period of postnatal development (70).

Taken together, these experimental data indicate that rats with an anxiety-like behavior phenotype induced by either early life events such as maternal separation MS180 rats or genetically prone rats (Wistar Kyoto or Fischer rats) display a stress-related visceral hyperalgesia to CRD. In contrast, other strains do not develop immediate but delayed hyperalgesia (42,45,48). The lack of induction of stress-related hypersensitivity under the above specific conditions has been related to the parallel recruitment of pain inhibitory pathways involving opioid and/or neurotensin mechanisms (42,43). It is to note that detailed investigations of hyperalgesic and analgesic pathways recruited by stress under conditions of CRD are still lacking and difference in time interval between stress and CRD and different type of stressors may influence their prevalence.

CRF/CRF$_1$ RECEPTORS AND THE BIOCHEMICAL CODING OF STRESS
Brain CRF

CRF (also known as corticotropin-releasing hormone) was characterized by Vale et al. in 1981 as a novel 41-amino acid hypothalamic-releasing peptide that stimulates the synthesis and release of adrenocorticotropy hormone (ACTH) and β-endorphin from the pituitary (71). With the early recognition that various internal or external cues disrupting homeostasis result in the release of ACTH and glucocorticoids into the circulation, the stimulation of the hypothalamic-pituitary-adrenal (HPA) axis became one of the major neuroendocrine hallmarks of the adaptive response to stress (3). Now, CRF is well established as the prime hypothalamic hormone involved in the stimulation of the HPA axis during stress (71,72). The population of CRF-synthesizing neurons is predominantly expressed in the parvocellular part of the PVN and projects via the external zone of the median eminence to the anterior pituitary (73). During stress, CRF is delivered into the hypophyseal portal blood vessels and stimulates ACTH release from the pituitary corticotropes. Once into the circulation, ACTH increases the secretion of glucocorticoid hormones from the adrenal cortex (73).

Aside from its role as a hypothalamic hypophysiotropic hormone, CRF acts as a neurotransmitter in several brain areas (74). In particular, CRF directly administered into the brain reproduces the overall endocrine, behavioral, autonomic, and visceral changes induced by stress in experimental animals, including monkeys (14,24,75,76). Consistent with these observations, immunohistochemical localization of brain CRF established that the peptide is largely distributed throughout the neocortex (prefrontal and cingulate), which mediates behavioral and cognitive components of stress (77). The central nucleus of the amygdala, which is involved in processing the emotional cues, also contains a high density of CRF neurons (78). These neurons project to the LC and increase their firing rate resulting in the stimulation of the ascending noradrenergic system (79). CRF is also located in the subdivision of the hypothalamic (PVN dorsal cap) and pontine nucleus (Barrington's nucleus/LC) that receive stimulatory input from the colon as well as sends direct projections to the intermediolateral column involved in the regulation of autonomic (preganglionic sympathetic and sacral parasympathetic) outflow to the colon (21,80). Consequently, CRF in the PVN and Barrington's nucleus/LC is well positioned to participate in the reciprocal brain–gut interactions, as it pertains to sensory information from the colon and reflex behavioral and autonomic responses of the viscera.

CRF Receptors

CRF signaling is mediated by CRF receptors, subtype 1 (CRF$_1$) and/or subtype 2 (CRF$_2$), cloned from two distinct genes (14,81). Both receptors belong to the class of seven-transmembrane receptors that signal by coupling to Gs proteins (82,83). One important feature of CRF receptor subtypes is their distinct affinity for mammalian CRF family ligands including CRF and urocortin 1 (also known as urocortin), and the recently discovered urocortin 2 and urocortin 3 (83,84). CRF displays 10- to 40-fold higher affinity for the CRF_1 than CRF_2 receptor. Urocortin 1 binds with equal affinity to CRF_1 and CRF_2 receptors and, compared with CRF, displays approximately 100-fold higher affinity to CRF_2 and roughly a 6-fold higher affinity for CRF_1 (85–87). Both urocortin 2 and urocortin 3 exhibit high selectivity for the CRF_2 receptor (85,86). These binding characteristics have positioned CRF and urocortin 1 as the preferential endogenous ligands for CRF_1 receptors, whereas urocortins; 2 and 3 are likely the natural ligands for CRF_2.

CRF Antagonists

In addition to the mimicry in the responses triggered by stress and central injection of CRF, the evidence for a role of brain CRF-signaling pathways in the stress response came from studies using CRF receptor antagonists injected into the cerebrospinal fluid. Among the specific nonselective CRF_1/CRF_2 antagonists are α-helical CRF_{9-41} (88), D-Phe^{12}CRF$_{12-41}$ (89), and the recently developed, more potent and long acting peptides, astressin (90,91) and astressin B (92).

The potential therapeutic application of CRF_1 receptor antagonists for the treatment of neuropsychiatric disorders, such as anxiety and depression (93–95), led to synthetic nonpeptide selective CRF_1 antagonists that cross the blood–brain barrier (96,97). These include CP-154,526 (97), antalarmin (98), NBI-30775 (formerly R-121919) (99), and the water-soluble compound, NBI-35965 (49,99), and several others (96,100). These CRF_1 antagonists have high brain penetrance upon peripheral, including oral, administration (49,99).

The wealth of evidence based on pharmacologic and genetic approaches clearly indicates that the activation of the brain CRF_1 receptor subtype plays a predominant role in stress-related endocrine (activation of the HPA axis with the release of ACTH and glucocorticoids) (14), behavioral (anxiety and depression) (95), and autonomic (activation of sympathetic and sacral parasympathetic outflow) (101,102) responses as well as gut motor alterations (stimulation of colonic motor function and diarrhea) (15). Recently, selective peptide CRF_2 receptor antagonists, namely, antisauvagine-30, K41498, [D-Phe^{11},His^{12},Nle^{17}]sauvagine$_{11-40}$, and the more potent, long acting analog, astressin$_2$-B, have been developed (103,104). Although the role of CRF_2 receptors in the stress response still needs to be further defined, existing reports indicate that the activation of peripheral CRF_2 receptors diminishes brain CRF_1-mediated endocrine, cardiovascular, and visceral responses (14,105–108).

BRAIN CRF/CRF$_1$-SIGNALING PATHWAYS IN STRESS-RELATED VISCERAL HYPERALGESIA
Biological Evidence

Various stressors activate the brain CRF-signaling pathways in experimental animals. For instance, WAS, largely used to induce stress-related visceral hyperalgesia (42–45,49), induces CRF gene transcription in the PVN within 15 minutes and activates the HPA axis and neurons in the PVN, LC, and lumbosacral parasympathetic nuclei (102,109,110). Changes in postnatal maternal handling also impacts the central CRF system and thereby, the responsiveness to stress (70). The profound and persistent consequences of early maternal separation in adult rats relate to the facilitation of circuitries that underlie stress response (47), which encompasses an exaggerated activation of the HPA axis (47). In addition, there is a heightened basal tone of CRF gene expression and CRF release in the PVN and limbic system (central amygdala and cortex), enhanced levels of CRF in the LC, and upregulation of CRF_1 signal transduction in the PVN, LC, and raphe nuclei leading to anxiety-prone behavior and reactivity to stress in adult rats (36,47,70,111). In contrast, short daily handling (15 minutes) postnatally dampens stress reactivity in adulthood by reducing the activity in the central amygdala-LC CRF system (70). Painful CRD is an interoceptive stressor that activates HPA axis as shown by the increase in ACTH release and corticosterone, and activation of PVN and LC neurons that are prevented by CRF_1 antagonists (112–114).

In humans, early life traumatic events are associated with hyperresponsiveness to stress in adulthood and predisposition to the development of comorbidity with anxiety disorders and IBS (36,115). There is also evidence that alterations in brain neurotransmitters, including brain CRF-signaling pathways, do play a role (36,116). This is supported by the elevation of CRF levels in cerebrospinal fluid of depressed patients (117,118) and the dampening of anxiety and depression by CRF_1 antagonists in rodents, primates, and in a first open-labeled clinical trial (75,119,120).

Pharmacological Evidence

Within the last few years, burgeoning experimental data based on pharmacologic approaches support a role of brain CRF/CRF_1 receptors in stress-related visceral hyperalgesia (15). First, exogenous injection of CRF into the brain mimics the effect of stress-induced visceral hyperalgesia. Studies in Wistar and Fischer rats showed that intracerebroventricular (ICV) injection of CRF enhanced the number of abdominal contractions in response to graded tonic CRD, and CRF action was prevented by the CRF_1 antagonist, antalarmin (39,121). Second, the blockade of CRF receptors impaired the development of stress-related visceral hyperalgesia (Table 2). The initial report by Gué et al. established that the CRF_1/CRF_2 antagonist, α-helical CRF_{9-41}, injected ICV blocked wrap restraint-induced hyperalgesic response to tonic rectal distension (39). Other data showed that the CRF_1/CRF_2 antagonist, astressin B, injected into the cisterna magna, abolished WAS-induced immediate and delayed hypersensitivity to phasic CRD in MS180 Long-Evans rats (45). Moreover, several selective CRF_1 receptor antagonists dampened visceral hyperalgesia (15). For instance, NBI-35965 injected peripherally prevented WAS-induced hyperalgesia to graded phasic CRD (20–80 mmHg) in MS180 Long-Evans male rats (49). CP-154,526 injected before WAS completely antagonized the hypersensitivity to graded intensities of phasic CRD (40–60 mmHg), occurring 24 hours after WAS exposure in Wistar rats as well as the acute and delayed WAS-induced hyperalgesia in MS180 Long-Evans rats (44,45). In contrast, neurokinin 1 antagonist under the same conditions had no effect (44). Antalarmin also prevented the visceral hypersensitivity to tonic CRD induced by pretreatment with an intracolonic noxious stimuli (tonic CRD or acetic acid) in anxiety prone strains of rats (105,121). The intrahippocampal injection of α-helical CRF_{9-41} and peripheral injection of the selective CRF_1 antagonist, JTC-017, also reduced the frequency of abdominal contractions induced by tonic CRD at 80 mmHg in restrained rats (112). Collectively, these data support that activation of CRF_1 receptors is the primary CRF signaling involved in the visceral hyperalgesia induced by various exteroceptive or interoceptive stressors (Table 1).

Role of Barrington's Nucleus/LC

Key to our understanding of brain CRF_1-signaling pathways that may contribute to visceral susceptibility to stress is the neuroanatomical link between the Barrington's nucleus and the LC. The LC encompasses noradrenergic ascending projections to a vast terminal field in the limbic system and cortex along with descending spinal projections and reciprocal inputs from

Table 2 Extero- and Interoceptive Stress-Induced Visceral Hyperalgesia: Blockade by CRF Receptor Antagonists in Rats

Stressors	CRF Antagonists	Administration	Effects	References
Restraint + tonic CRD	α-helical CRF_{9-41}	ICV	↓ SICH	(39)
Restraint + tonic CRD	α-helical CRF_{9-41}	IH	↓ Abdominal contraction	(112)
MS180 + WAS + phasic CRD	Astressin B	IC	↓ SICH (acute + delayed)	(45)
MS180 + WAS + phasic CRD	CP-154,526	SC	↓ SICH (acute + delayed)	(45)
Tonic CRD (2 sets)	Antalarmin	SC	↓ SICH	(105)
WAS + phasic CRD	CP-154,526	SC	↓ Delayed SICH	(44)
MS180 + WAS + phasic CRD	NBI-35965	SC	↓ SICH	(49)
High anxiety rats + tonic CRD	Antalarmin	SC	↓ SICH	(121)

Abbreviations: CRD, colorectal distension; CRF, corticotropin-releasing factor; IC, intracisternal; ICV, intracerebroventricular; IH, intrahippocampal; MS180, maternal separation for 180 min from postnatal day 2–14; SICH, stress-induced colonic hypersensitivity to CRD; SC, subcutaneous; WAS, water avoidance stress.

and to the Barrington's nucleus (Fig. 2) (21,80,122–124). CRF neurons in the Barrington's nucleus innervating the spinal parasympathetic neurons also project to the LC, where CRF exerts an excitatory action resulting in norepinephrine release in the brain cortex (21,80,125,126). Stress upregulates CRF gene expression in the Barrington's nucleus (127,128) and elevates CRF concentration and tyrosine hydroxylase activity in the LC (129,130). Collectively, the ascending and spinal projections from Barrington's nucleus/LC nuclei and the stress-related modulation of CRF expression at these pontine sites positioned them well to coordinate brain–gut interaction with visceral information from the gut impacting on cortical and limbic activities under stress conditions.

Bringing support to this view, recent electrophysiological studies established that tonic or phasic CRD at 40 to 45 mmHg activates LC neurons and forebrain electroencephalogram (EEG) through brain CRF/CRF_1 receptor–dependent mechanisms in rats (114,131,132). The Barrington's nucleus was identified to be the source of CRF that induces CRF receptor–dependent activation of LC neurons in response to a tonic CRD (132,133). In addition, CRD evokes a burst firing pattern of neurons in the LC that is blocked by peripheral injection of CRF_1 antagonist or intracisternal injection of astressin (114). Such a firing pattern is known to facilitate norepinephrine release in the rat prefrontal cortex and hippocampus (134,135) and leads to arousal and anxiogenic behavioral responses in rats (136–138). Recent reports further established that CRD applied during restraint stress increased by twofold the hippocampal noradrenaline levels compared with those induced by restraint alone (112,139). Therefore, there is direct experimental evidence of an interaction between stress and visceral pain in the brain release of the angiogenic amine noradrenaline (140). Pharmacological blockade of CRF receptors within the LC by CRF antagonists attenuates stress-induced angiogenic behaviors such as freezing and withdrawal in rats (141,142). Moreover, CRF_1 antagonists prevented a somatosensory stress-induced increase in cortical norepinephrine release and CRD-evoked rise in noradrenaline levels in the hippocampus along with anxiety- and depression-related responses in several stress models (95,112,143).

These experimental findings may have important clinical relevance and provide insight to some underlying mechanisms of stress modulation of pain sensitivity in IBS. Several reports indicate the presence of perceptual alterations in patients with IBS, as it relates to hypersensitivity to CRD and hypervigilance to rectal phasic stimuli (37,144–146). IBS patients are hyperreactive to auditory stress stimuli as monitored in the activation of frontal brain regions and rate significantly higher levels of anxiety and intensity and unpleasantness of CRD at 45 mmHg during auditory stress (30,147). Based on experimental findings reviewed above (21,114), it is tempting to speculate that the altered threshold of visceral pain to CRD is may be caused by a more pronounced, sustained and/or frequent CRF/CRF_1-mediated activation of LC noradrenergic neurons as reported in experimental animals (114,118). The overstimulation of the CRF/CRF_1 system may play a role in the genesis of increased vigilance and anxiety that may have a bearing on the high incidence of comorbid anxiety/mood disorders in IBS patients (149,150).

Role of Gut Mast Cells

Biopsy specimens of descending colon from patients with IBS showed an increase in mast cells displaying features of degranulation and increased tryptase compared with healthy subjects (151). The study also showed a correlation between the vicinity of mast cells to nerves and the severity and frequency of perceived abdominal pain sensations (151). These data support a possible role of mast cells as effector cells in the visceral nociception in IBS patients. In experimental animals, the mast cell stabilizer, doxantraxoze, which has no effect by itself on the visceral response to rectal distension, suppressed stress-induced hyperalgesia in rats (39). Other reports demonstrate that acute restraint stress degranulates colonic mucosal mast cells through autonomic-dependent pathways, as shown by the increased release of mucosal protease II and histamine in the rat colon (39,40,151–153). In addition, visceral hyperalgesia can be reproduced by peripheral injection of mast cell degradulator, BrX-537 (154). Anatomical support for neurally mediated activation of colonic mucosal mast cells by restraint stress in rats (155) came from anatomical investigation showing that one-half to two-thirds of mast cells are closely apposed to nerves in the intestinal mucosa (156). Mast cell mediators such as tryptase, through activation of protease-activated receptor-2 receptors located on enteric nerves and visceral afferents (157), can induce a delayed hyperalgesia in response to CRD (157,158). Other mediators released from rat mast cells, namely, prostaglandins and serotonin, unlike histamine, may also contribute to the alteration of visceral sensory information (40,154,159,160).

Stress-induced activation of colonic mast cells is consistent with the involvement of brain CRF/CRF receptor–signaling pathways. First, CRF injected ICV mimicked the effects of acute stress by inducing mast cell degranulation and increasing histamine content in the rat colon (153,155). Second, ICV injection of CRF antagonist, α-helical CRF_{9-41}, blocked restraint-induced mucosal mast cell activation and increased histamine content in the colon (153,155). Lastly, central injection of CRF induced a CRF_1-mediated alteration of autonomic regulation of colonic secretory and motor function (15). These data support a brain CRF receptor-mediated intestinal mucosal mast cell degranulation induced by restraint stress.

CONCLUSIONS

Clinical investigations support the notion that stress contributes to visceral hypersensitivity of the gut, and experimental models have been developed that recapture some of the features observed in IBS patients with regard to stress-related hyperalgesia, sex differences, and comorbidity with anxiety/depression. Tremendous progress in our understanding of the biochemical coding of stress, in particular, as it relates to the characterization and brain distribution of CRF ligands, and CRF receptor subtypes and the development of selective CRF antagonists, have allowed us to gain insight into the underlying mechanisms of stress-related gut responses including visceral pain. Converging experimental data using pharmacologic approaches in various models support the notion that the activation of brain CRF_1-signaling pathways contributes to the development of visceral hyperalgesia induced by various exteroceptive or interoceptive stressors, as well as in models of genetically anxiety prone strains. However, there is a glaring lack of knowledge of how dysregulation of the CRF-signaling pathways impact brain circuitry regulating visceral pain at the level of facilitatory and/or inhibitory mechanisms (Fig. 2). In light of the promising functional preclinical reports that CRF_1 receptors alleviate acute and chronic stress-induced visceral hyperalgesia to CRD, CRF_1 antagonists may provide an additional option for future therapeutic interventions by dampening the behavioral, sacral parasympathetic and gut enteric/mast cell response to stress (161).

ACKNOWLEDGMENTS

The authors' work was supported by the National Institute of Arthritis, Metabolism and Digestive Diseases, Grants R01 DK-33061, R01 DK-57238, Center grant DK-41301 (Animal Core), R21 DK-068155, P50 AR-049550, and VA Merit and Senior Scientist Awards. The authors thank Drs. J. Rivier (Salk Institute, La Jolla, CA), D. Grigoriadis (Neurocrine Biosciences Inc., La Jolla, CA), and E.D. Pagani (Center Research Division, Pfizer Inc., Croton, CT) for the generous supply of different CRF agonists and antagonists used in our studies. Miss Teresa Olivas' help in the preparation of the manuscript is gratefully acknowledged.

REFERENCES

1. Beaumont W. In: Osler W, ed. Experiments and Observations on the Gastric Juice and the Physiology of Digestion. New York: Dover Publications Inc., 1833:1–280.
2. Cannon WB. Bodily Changes in Pain, Hunger, Fear and Rage. Boston: Branford, CT, 1953.
3. Selye H. Theories Stress in Health and Disease. Boston-London: Butterworths, 1976:928–1148.
4. Selye H. Syndrome produced by diverse nocuous agents. Nature 1936; 138:32.
5. Whitehead WE, Crowell MD, Robinson JC, et al. Effect of stressful life events on bowel symptoms: subjects with irritable bowel syndrome compared with subjects without bowel dysfunction. Gut 1992; 33:825–830.
6. Ritchie J. Pain from distension of the pelvic colon by inflating a balloon in the irritable colon syndrome. Gut 1973; 14:125–132.
7. Ford MJ, Camilleri M, Zinsmeister AR, et al. Psychosensory modulation of colonic sensation in the human transverse and sigmoid colon. Gastroenterology 1995; 109:1772–1780.

8. Mönnikes H, Tebbe JJ, Hildebrandt M, et al. Role of stress in functional gastrointestinal disorders. Evidence for stress-induced alterations in gastrointestinal motility and sensitivity. Dig Dis 2001; 19:201–211.

9. Mayer EA, Naliboff BD, Chang L, et al. Stress and the gastrointestinal tract. V. Stress and irritable bowel syndrome. Am J Physiol Gastrointest Liver Physiol 2001; 280:G519–G524.

10. Murray CD, Flynn J, Ratcliffe L, et al. Effect of acute physical and psychological stress on gut autonomic innervation in irritable bowel syndrome. Gastroenterology 2004; 127:1695–1703.

11. Mulak A, Bonaz B. Irritable bowel syndrome: a model of the brain-gut interactions. Med Sci Monit 2004; 10:RA52–RA62.

12. Mach T. The brain-gut axis in irritable bowel syndrome—clinical aspects. Med Sci Monit 2004; 10:RA125–RA131.

13. Harris ML, Aziz Q. Brain-gut interaction in irritable bowel syndrome. Hosp Med 2003; 64:264–269.

14. Bale TL, Vale WW. CRF and CRF receptor: role in stress responsivity and other behaviors. Annu Rev Pharmacol Toxicol 2004; 44:525–557.

15. Taché Y, Martinez V, Wang L, et al. CRF_1 receptor signaling pathways are involved in stress-related alterations of colonic function and viscerosensitivity: implications for irritable bowel syndrome. Br J Pharmacol 2004; 141:1321–1330.

16. Bale TL. Sensitivity to stress: dysregulation of CRF pathways and disease development. Horm Behav 2005; 48:1–10.

17. Sawchenko PE, Li HY, Ericsson A. Circuits and mechanisms governing hypothalamic responses to stress: a tale of two paradigms. Prog Brain Res 2000; 122:61–78.

18. Saper CB. The central autonomic nervous system: conscious visceral perception and autonomic pattern generation. Annu Rev Neurosci 2002; 25:433–469.

19. Price JL. Prefrontal cortical networks related to visceral function and mood. Ann N Y Acad Sci 1999; 877:383–396.

20. Vogt BA, Sikes RW. The medial pain system, cingulate cortex, and parallel processing of nociceptive information. Prog Brain Res 2000; 122:223–235.

21. Valentino RJ, Miselis RR, Pavcovich LA. Pontine regulation of pelvic viscera: pharmacological target for pelvic visceral dysfunctions. Trends Pharmacol Sci 1999; 20:253–260.

22. Herman JP, Cullinan WE. Neurocircuitry of stress: central control of the hypothalamo-pituitary-adrenocortical axis. Trends Neurosci 1997; 20:78–84.

23. Sawchenko PE, Brown ER, Chan RK, et al. The paraventricular nucleus of the hypothalamus and the functional neuroanatomy of visceromotor responses to stress. Prog Brain Res 1996; 107:201–222.

24. Tache Y, Martinez V, Million M, et al. Stress and the gastrointestinal tract III. Stress-related alterations of gut motor function: role of brain corticotropin-releasing factor receptors. Am J Physiol 2001; 280:G173–G177.

25. Pothoulakis C, Castagliuolo I, Leeman SE. Neuroimmune mechanisms of intestinal responses to stress. Role of corticotropin-releasing factor and neurotensin. Ann N Y Acad Sci 1998; 840:635–648.

26. Gwee KA, Leong YL, Graham C, et al. The role of psychological and biological factors in postinfective gut dysfunction. Gut 1999; 44:400–406.

27. Bennett EJ, Piesse C, Palmer K, et al. Functional gastrointestinal disorders: psychological, social, and somatic features. Gut 1998; 42:414–420.

28. Gwee KA, Graham JC, McKendrick MW, et al. Psychometric scores and persistence of irritable bowel after infectious diarrhoea. Lancet 1996; 347:150–153.

29. Neal KR, Hebden J, Spiller R. Prevalence of gastrointestinal symptoms six months after bacterial gastroenteritis and risk factors for development of the irritable bowel syndrome: postal survey of patients. BMJ 1997; 314:779–782.

30. Dickhaus B, Mayer EA, Firooz N, et al. Irritable bowel syndrome patients show enhanced modulation of visceral perception by auditory stress. Am J Gastroenterol 2003; 98:135–143.

31. Galeazzi F, Luca MG, Lanaro D, et al. Esophageal hyperalgesia in patients with ulcerative colitis: role of experimental stress. Am J Gastroenterol 2001; 96:2590–2595.

32. Munakata J, Naliboff B, Harraf F, et al. Repetitive sigmoid stimulation induces rectal hyperalgesia in patients with irritable bowel syndrome. Gastroenterology 1997; 112:55–63.

33. Fukudo S, Kanazawa M, Kano M, et al. Exaggerated motility of the descending colon with repetitive distention of the sigmoid colon in patients with irritable bowel syndrome. J Gastroenterol 2002; 37(suppl 14):145–150.

34. Halpert A, Drossman D. Biopsychosocial issues in irritable bowel syndrome. J Clin Gastroenterol 2005; 39:665–669.

35. Kamm MA. The role of psychosocial factors in functional gut disease. Eur J Surg Suppl 1998; 583:37–40.

36. Nemeroff CB. Neurobiological consequences of childhood trauma. J Clin Psychiatry 2004; 65(suppl 1): 18–28.

37. Bouin M, Plourde V, Boivin M, et al. Rectal distention testing in patients with irritable bowel syndrome: sensitivity, specificity, and predictive values of pain sensory thresholds. Gastroenterology 2002; 122:1771–1777.

38. Ness TJ, Gebhart GF. Colorectal distension as a noxious visceral stimulus: physiologic and pharmacologic characterization of pseudoaffective reflexes in the rat. Brain Res 1988; 450:153–169.

39. Gué M, Del Rio-Lacheze C, Eutamene H, et al. Stress-induced visceral hypersensitivity to rectal distension in rats: role of CRF and mast cells. Neurogastroenterol Motil 1997; 9:271–279.
40. Bradesi S, Eutamene H, Garcia-Villar R, et al. Acute and chronic stress differently affect visceral sensitivity to rectal distension in female rats. Neurogastroenterol Motil 2002; 14:75–82.
41. Bradesi S, Eutamene H, Garcia-Villar R, et al. Stress-induced visceral hypersensitivity in female rats is estrogen-dependent and involves tachykinin NK1 receptors. Pain 2003; 102:227–234.
42. Coutinho SV, Plotsky PM, Sablad M, et al. Neonatal maternal separation alters stress-induced responses to viscerosomatic nociceptive stimuli in rat. Am J Physiol Gastrointest Liver Physiol 2002; 282:G307–G316.
43. Gui X, Carraway RE, Dobner PR. Endogenous neurotensin facilitates visceral nociception and is required for stress-induced antinociception in mice and rats. Neuroscience 2004; 126:1023–1032.
44. Schwetz I, Bradesi S, McRoberts JA, et al. Delayed stress-induced colonic hypersensitivity in male Wistar rats: role of neurokinin-1 and corticotropin releasing factor-1 receptors. Am J Physiol Gastrointest Liver Physiol 2003; 286:G683–G691.
45. Schwetz I, McRoberts JA, Coutinho SV, et al. Corticotropin-releasing factor receptor 1 mediates acute and delayed stress-induced visceral hyperalgesia in maternally separated Long-Evans rats. Am J Physiol Gastrointest Liver Physiol 2005; 289:G704–G712.
46. Plotsky PM, Meaney MJ. Early, postnatal experience alters hypothalamic corticotropin-releasing factor (CRF) mRNA, median eminence CRF content and stress-induced release in adult rats. Brain Res Mol Brain Res 1993; 18:195–200.
47. Ladd CO, Thrivikraman KV, Huot RL, et al. Differential neuroendocrine responses to chronic variable stress in adult Long Evans rats exposed to handling-maternal separation as neonates. Psychoneuroendocrinology 2005; 30:520–533.
48. Rosztoczy A, Fioramonti J, Jarmay K, et al. Influence of sex and experimental protocol on the effect of maternal deprivation on rectal sensitivity to distension in the adult rat. Neurogastroenterol Motil 2003; 15:679–686.
49. Million M, Grigoriadis DE, Sullivan S, et al. A novel water-soluble selective CRF$_1$ receptor antagonist, NBI 35965, blunts stress-induced visceral hyperalgesia and colonic motor function in rats. Brain Res 2003; 985:32–42.
50. Gunter WD, Shepard JD, Foreman RD, et al. Evidence for visceral hypersensitivity in high-anxiety rats. Physiol Behav 2000; 69:379–382.
51. Heitkemper M, Jarrett M, Bond EF, et al. Impact of sex and gender on irritable bowel syndrome. Biol Res Nurs 2003; 5:56–65.
52. Naliboff BD, Berman S, Chang L, et al. Sex-related differences in IBS patients: central processing of visceral stimuli. Gastroenterology 2003; 124:1738–1747.
53. Arendt-Nielsen L, Bajaj P, Drewes AM. Visceral pain: gender differences in response to experimental and clinical pain. Eur J Pain 2004; 8:465–472.
54. Tache Y, Million M, Nelson AG, et al. Role of corticotropin-releasing factor pathways in stress-related alterations of colonic motor function and viscerosensibility in female rodents. Gend Med 2005; 2:146–154.
55. Craft RM, Mogil JS, Aloisi AM. Sex differences in pain and analgesia: the role of gonadal hormones. Eur J Pain 2004; 8:397–411.
56. Fillingim RB, Hastie BA, Ness TJ, et al. Sex-related psychological predictors of baseline pain perception and analgesic responses to pentazocine. Biol Psychol 2005; 69:97–112.
57. Holdcroft A, Sapsed-Byrne S, Ma D, et al. Sex and oestrous cycle differences in visceromotor responses and vasopressin release in response to colonic distension in male and female rats anaesthetized with halothane. Br J Anaesth 2000; 85:907–910.
58. Ji Y, Murphy AZ, Traub RJ. Estrogen modulates the visceromotor reflex and responses of spinal dorsal horn neurons to colorectal stimulation in the rat. J Neurosci 2003; 23:3908–3915.
59. Sapsed-Byrne S, Ma D, Ridout D, et al. Estrous cycle phase variations in visceromotor and cardiovascular responses to colonic distension in the anesthetized rat. Brain Res 1996; 742:10–16.
60. Shors TJ, Pickett J, Wood G, et al. Acute stress persistently enhances estrogen levels in the female rat. Stress 1999; 3:163–171.
61. Laflamme N, Nappi RE, Drolet G, et al. Expression and neuropeptidergic characterization of estrogen receptors (ERalpha and ERbeta) throughout the rat brain: anatomical evidence of distinct roles of each subtype. J Neurobiol 1998; 36:357–378.
62. Williams SJ, Papka RE. Estrogen receptor-immunoreactive neurons are present in the female rat lumbosacral spinal cord. J Neurosci Res 1996; 46:492–501.
63. Papka RE, Storey-Workley M, Shughrue PJ, et al. Estrogen receptor-alpha and beta- immunoreactivity and mRNA in neurons of sensory and autonomic ganglia and spinal cord. Cell Tissue Res 2001; 304:193–214.
64. Vanderhorst VG, Gustafsson JA, Ulfhake B. Estrogen receptor-alpha and -beta immunoreactive neurons in the brainstem and spinal cord of male and female mice: relationships to monoaminergic, cholinergic, and spinal projection systems. J Comp Neurol 2005; 488:152–179.
65. Shane R, Acosta J, Rossi GC, et al. Reciprocal interactions between the amygdala and ventrolateral periaqueductal gray in mediating of Q/N(1–17)-induced analgesia in the rat. Brain Res 2003; 980:57–70.

66. Foo H, Helmstetter FJ. Activation of kappa opioid receptors in the rostral ventromedial medulla blocks stress-induced antinociception. Neuroreport 2000; 11:3349–3352.
67. Chang L, Mayer EA, Johnson T, et al. Differences in somatic perception in female patients with irritable bowel syndrome with and without fibromyalgia. Pain 2000; 84:297–307.
68. Posserud I, Agerforz P, Ekman R, et al. Altered visceral perceptual and neuroendocrine response in patients with irritable bowel syndrome during mental stress. Gut 2004; 53:1102–1108.
69. Verne GN, Himes NC, Robinson ME, et al. Central representation of visceral and cutaneous hypersensitivity in the irritable bowel syndrome. Pain 2003; 103:99–110.
70. Francis DD, Caldji C, Champagne F, et al. The role of corticotropin-releasing factor—norepinephrine systems in mediating the effects of early experience on the development of behavioral and endocrine responses to stress. Biol Psychiatry 1999; 46:1153–1166.
71. Vale W, Spiess J, Rivier C, et al. Characterization of a 41-residue ovine hypothalamic peptide that stimulates secretion of corticotropin and b-endorphin. Science 1981; 213:1394–1397.
72. Turnbull AV, Rivier C. Corticotropin-releasing factor (CRF) and endocrine response to stress: CRF receptors, binding protein, and related peptides. Proc Soc Exp Biol Med 1997; 215:1–10.
73. Herman JP, Figueiredo H, Mueller NK, et al. Central mechanisms of stress integration: hierarchical circuitry controlling hypothalamo-pituitary-adrenocortical responsiveness. Front Neuroendocrinol 2003; 24:151–180.
74. Owens MJ, Nemeroff CB. Physiology and pharmacology of corticotropin-releasing factor. Pharmacol Rev 1991; 43:425–473.
75. Habib KE, Weld KP, Rice KC, et al. Oral administration of a corticotropin-releasing hormone receptor antagonist significantly attenuates behavioral, neuroendocrine, and autonomic responses to stress in primates. Proc Natl Acad Sci U S A 2000; 97:6079–6084.
76. Jeong KH, Jacobson L, Pacak K, et al. Impaired basal and restraint-induced epinephrine secretion in corticotropin-releasing hormone-deficient mice. Endocrinology 2000; 141:1142–1150.
77. De Souza EB. Corticotropin-releasing factor receptors: physiology, pharmacology, biochemistry and role in central nervous system and immune disorders. Psychoneuroendocrinology 1995; 20: 789–819.
78. Phelps EA, LeDoux JE. Contributions of the amygdala to emotion processing: from animal models to human behavior. Neuron 2005; 48:175–187.
79. Gray TS, Bingaman EW. The amygdala: corticotropin-releasing factor, steroids, and stress. Crit Rev Neurobiol 1996; 10:155–168.
80. Valentino RJ, Page ME, Luppi PH, et al. Evidence for widespread afferents to Barrington's nucleus, a brainstem region rich in corticotropin-releasing hormone neurons. Neuroscience 1994; 62:125–143.
81. Perrin MH, Vale WW. Corticotropin releasing factor receptors and their ligand family. Ann N Y Acad Sci 1999; 885:312–328.
82. Dautzenberg FM, Hauger RL. The CRF peptide family and their receptors: yet more partners discovered. Trends Pharmacol Sci 2002; 23:71–77.
83. Hauger RL, Grigoriadis DE, Dallman MF, et al. International Union of Pharmacology. XXXVI. Current status of the nomenclature for receptors for corticotropin-releasing factor and their ligands. Pharmacol Rev 2003; 55:21–26.
84. Li C, Vaughan J, Sawchenko PE, et al. Urocortin III-immunoreactive projections in rat brain: partial overlap with sites of type 2 corticotrophin-releasing factor receptor expression. J Neurosci 2002; 22:991–1001.
85. Reyes TM, Lewis K, Perrin MH, et al. Urocortin II: a member of the corticotropin-releasing factor (CRF) neuropeptide family that is selectively bound by type 2 CRF receptors. Proc Natl Acad Sci USA 2001; 98:2843–2848.
86. Lewis K, Li C, Perrin MH, et al. Identification of urocortin III, an additional member of the corticotropin-releasing factor (CRF) family with high affinity for the CRF2 receptor. Proc Natl Acad Sci USA 2001; 98:7570–7575.
87. Vaughan J, Donaldson C, Bittencourt J, et al. Urocortin, a mammalian neuropeptide related to fish urotensin I and to corticotropin-releasing factor. Nature 1995; 378:287–292.
88. Rivier J, Rivier C, Vale W. Synthetic competitive antagonists of corticotropin-releasing factor: effect on ACTH secretion in the rat. Science 1984; 224:889–891.
89. Hernandez JF, Kornreich W, Rivier C, et al. Synthesis and relative potency of new constrained CRF antagonists. J Med Chem 1993; 36:2860–2867.
90. Miranda A, Lahrichi SL, Gulyas J, et al. Constrained corticotropin-releasing factor antagonists with i-(i + 3) Glu-Lys bridges. J Med Chem 1997; 40:3651–3658.
91. Gulyas J, Rivier C, Perrin M, et al. Potent, structurally constrained agonists and competitive antagonists of corticotropin-releasing factor. Proc Natl Acad Sci U S A 1995; 92:10575–10579.
92. Rivier JE, Kirby DA, Lahrichi SL, et al. Constrained corticotropin releasing factor antagonists (astressin analogues) with long duration of action in the rat. J Med Chem 1999; 42:3175–3182.
93. Grammatopoulos DK, Chrousos GP. Functional characteristics of CRH receptors and potential clinical applications of CRH-receptor antagonists. Trends Endocrinol Metab 2002; 13:436–444.
94. Holsboer F. The rationale for corticotropin-releasing hormone receptor (CRH-R) antagonists to treat depression and anxiety. J Psychiatr Res 1999; 33:181–214.

95. Kehne J, De Lombaert S. Non-peptidic CRF1 receptor antagonists for the treatment of anxiety, depression and stress disorders. Curr Drug Target CNS Neurol Disord 2002; 1:467–493.
96. McCarthy JR, Heinrichs SC, Grigoriadis DE. Recent advances with the CRF1 receptor: design of small molecule inhibitors, receptor subtypes and clinical indications. Curr Pharm Des 1999; 5:289–315.
97. Keller C, Bruelisauer A, Lemaire M, et al. Brain pharmacokinetics of a nonpeptidic corticotropin-releasing factor receptor antagonist. Drug Metab Dispos 2002; 30:173–176.
98. Webster EL, Lewis DB, Torpy DJ, et al. In vivo and in vitro characterization of antalarmin, a non-peptide corticotropin-releasing hormone (CRH) receptor antagonist: suppression of pituitary ACTH release and peripheral inflammation. Endocrinology 1996; 137:5747–5750.
99. Heinrichs SC, De Souza EB, Schulteis G, et al. Brain penetrance, receptor occupancy and antistress in vivo efficacy of a small molecule corticotropin releasing factor type I receptor selective antagonist. Neuropsychopharmacology 2002; 27:194–202.
100. Gilligan PJ, Robertson DW, Zaczek R. Corticotropin releasing factor (CRF) receptor modulators: progress and opportunities for new therapeutic agents. J Med Chem 2000; 43:1641–1660.
101. Yokotani K, Murakami Y, Okada S, et al. Role of brain arachidonic acid cascade on central CRF1 receptor-mediated activation of sympatho-adrenomedullary outflow in rats. Eur J Pharmacol 2001; 419:183–189.
102. Million M, Wang L, Martinez V, et al. Differential Fos expression in the paraventricular nucleus of the hypothalamus, sacral parasympathetic nucleus and colonic motor response to water avoidance stress in Fischer and Lewis rats. Brain Res 2000; 877:345–353.
103. Rivier J, Gulyas J, Kirby D, et al. Potent and long-acting corticotropin releasing factor (CRF) receptor 2 selective peptide competitive antagonists. J Med Chem 2002; 45:4737–4747.
104. Ruhmann A, Bonk I, Lin CR, et al. Structural requirements for peptidic antagonists of the corticotropin-releasing factor receptor (CRFR): development of CRFR2b-selective antisauvagine-30. Proc Natl Acad Sci U S A 1998; 95:15264–15269.
105. Million M, Maillot C, Adelson DW, et al. Peripheral injection of sauvagine prevents repeated colorectal distention-induced visceral pain in female rats. Peptides 2005; 26:1188–1195.
106. Million M, Wang L, Wang Y, et al. CRF2 receptor activation prevents colorectal distension-induced visceral pain and spinal ERK1/2 phosphorylation in rats. Gut 2006; 55:172–181.
107. Martinez V, Wang L, Million M, et al. Urocortins and the regulation of gastrointestinal motor function and visceral pain. Peptides 2004; 25:1733–1744.
108. Coste SC, Quintos RF, Stenzel-Poore MP. Corticotropin-releasing hormone-related peptides and receptors: emergent regulators of cardiovascular adaptations to stress. Trends Cardiovasc Med 2002; 12:176–182.
109. Kresse AE, Million M, Saperas E, et al. Colitis induces CRF expression in hypothalamic magnocellular neurons and blunts CRF gene response to stress in rats. Am J Physiol 2001; 281:G1203–G1213.
110. Bonaz B, Tache Y. Water-avoidance stress-induced c-fos expression in the rat brain and stimulation of fecal output: role of corticotropin-releasing factor. Brain Res 1994; 641:21–28.
111. Kalinichev M, Easterling KW, Plotsky PM, et al. Long-lasting changes in stress-induced corticosterone response and anxiety-like behaviors as a consequence of neonatal maternal separation in Long-Evans rats. Pharmacol Biochem Behav 2002; 73:131–140.
112. Saito K, Kasai T, Nagura Y, et al. Corticotropin-releasing hormone receptor 1 antagonist blocks brain-gut activation induced by colonic distention in rats. Gastroenterology 2005; 129:1533–1543.
113. Elsenbruch S, Wang L, Hollerbach S, et al. Pseudo-affective visceromotor responses and HPA axis activation following colorectal distension in rats with increased cholinergic sensitivity. Neurogastroenterol Motil 2004; 16:801–809.
114. Kosoyan H, Grigoriadis D, Tache Y. The CRF$_1$ antagonist, NBI-35965 abolished the activation of locus coeruleus by colorectal distention and intracisternal CRF in rats. Brain Res 2004; 1056:85–96.
115. Francis DD, Champagne FA, Liu D, et al. Maternal care, gene expression, and the development of individual differences in stress reactivity. Ann N Y Acad Sci 1999; 896:66–84.
116. Keck ME, Holsboer F. Hyperactivity of CRH neuronal circuits as a target for therapeutic interventions in affective disorders. Peptides 2001; 22:835–844.
117. Nemeroff CB, Widerlov E, Bissette G, et al. Elevated concentrations of CSF corticotropin-releasing factor-like immunoreactivity in depressed patients. Science 1984; 226:1342–1344.
118. Wong ML, Kling MA, Munson PJ, et al. Pronounced and sustained central hypernoradrenergic function in major depression with melancholic features: relation to hypercortisolism and corticotropin-releasing hormone. Proc Natl Acad Sci U S A 2000; 97:325–330.
119. Keck ME, Ohl F, Holsboer F, et al. Listening to mutant mice: a spotlight on the role of CRF/CRF receptor systems in affective disorders. Neurosci Biobehav Rev 2005; 29:867–889.
120. Zobel AW, Nickel T, Kunzel HE, et al. Effects of the high-affinity corticotropin-releasing hormone receptor 1 antagonist R121919 in major depression: the first 20 patients treated. J Psychiatr Res 2000; 34:171–181.
121. Greenwood-Van Meerveld B, Johnson AC, Cochrane S, et al. Corticotropin-releasing factor 1 receptor-mediated mechanisms inhibit colonic hypersensitivity in rats. Neurogastroenterol Motil 2005; 17:415–422.

122. Valentino RJ, Kosboth M, Colflesh M, et al. Transneuronal labeling from the rat distal colon: anatomic evidence for regulation of distal colon function by a pontine corticotropin-releasing factor system. J Comp Neurol 2000; 417:399–414.
123. Nuding SC, Nadelhaft I. Bilateral projections of the pontine micturition center to the sacral parasympathetic nucleus in the rat. Brain Res 1998; 785:185–194.
124. Pavcovich LA, Yang M, Miselis RR, et al. Novel role for the pontine micturition center, Barrington's nucleus: evidence for coordination of colonic and forebrain activity. Brain Res 1998; 784:355–361.
125. Valentino RJ, Chen S, Zhu Y, et al. Evidence for divergent projections to the brain noradrenergic system and the spinal parasympathetic system from Barrington's nucleus. Brain Res 1996; 732:1–15.
126. Curtis AL, Lechner SM, Pavcovich LA, et al. Activation of the locus coeruleus noradrenergic system by intracoerulear microinfusion of corticotropin-releasing factor: effects on discharge rate, cortical norepinephrine levels and cortical electroencephalographic activity. J Pharmacol Exp Ther 1997; 281:163–172.
127. Imaki T, Nahan J-L, Rivier C, et al. Differential regulation of corticotropin-releasing factor mRNA in rat brain regions by glucocorticoids and stress. J Neurosci 1991; 11:585–599.
128. Imaki T, Vale W, Sawchenko PE. Regulation of corticotropin-releasing factor mRNA in neuroendocrine and autonomic neurons by osmotic stimulation and volume loading. Neuroendocrinology 1992; 56:633–640.
129. Chappell PB, Smith MA, Kilts CD, et al. Alterations in corticotropin-releasing factor-like immunoreactivity in discrete rat brain regions after acute and chronic stress. J Neurosci 1986; 6:2908–2914.
130. Melia KR, Duman RS. Involvement of corticotropin-releasing factor in chronic stress regulation of brain noradrenergic system. Proc Natl Acad Sci U S A 1991; 88:8382–8386.
131. Elam M, Thoren P, Svensson TH. Locus coeruleus neurons and sympathetic nerves: activation by visceral afferents. Brain Res 1986; 375:117–125.
132. Lechner SM, Curtis AL, Brons R, et al. Locus coeruleus activation by colon distention: role of corticotropin-releasing factor and excitatory amino acids. Brain Res 1997; 756:114–124.
133. Rouzade-Dominguez ML, Curtis AL, Valentino RJ. Role of Barrington's nucleus in the activation of rat locus coeruleus neurons by colonic distension. Brain Res 2001; 917:206–218.
134. Florin-Lechner SM, Druhan JP, Aston-Jones G, et al. Enhanced norepinephrine release in prefrontal cortex with burst stimulation of the locus coeruleus. Brain Res 1996; 742:89–97.
135. Palamarchouk VS, Swiergiel AH, Dunn AJ. Hippocampal noradrenergic responses to CRF injected into the locus coeruleus of unanesthetized rats. Brain Res 2002; 950:31–38.
136. Butler PD, Weiss JM, Stout JC, et al. Corticotropin-releasing factor produces fear-enhancing and behavioral activating effects following infusion into the locus coeruleus. J Neurosci 1990; 10:176–183.
137. Aston-Jones G, Rajkowski J, Cohen J. Role of locus coeruleus in attention and behavioral flexibility. Biol Psychiatry 1999; 46:1309–1320.
138. Koob GF. Corticotropin-releasing factor, norepinephrine, and stress. Biol Psychiatry 1999; 46:1167–1180.
139. Saito K, Kanazawa M, Fukudo S. Colorectal distention induces hippocampal noradrenaline release in rats: an in vivo microdialysis study. Brain Res 2002; 947:146–149.
140. Sullivan GM, Coplan JD, Kent JM, et al. The noradrenergic system in pathological anxiety: a focus on panic with relevance to generalized anxiety and phobias. Biol Psychiatry 1999; 46:1205–1218.
141. Smagin GN, Harris RB, Ryan DH. Corticotropin-releasing factor receptor antagonist infused into the locus coeruleus attenuates immobilization stress-induced defensive withdrawal in rats. Neurosci Lett 1996; 220:167–170.
142. Swiergiel AH, Takahashi LK, Rubin WW, et al. Antagonism of corticotropin-releasing factor receptors in the locus coeruleus attenuates shock-induced freezing in rats. Brain Res 1992; 587:263–268.
143. Griebel G, Simiand J, Steinberg R, et al. 4-(2-Chloro-4-methoxy-5-methylphenyl)-N-[(1S)-2-cyclo-propyl-1-(3-fluoro-4- methylphenyl)ethyl]5-methyl-N-(2-propynyl)-1:3-thiazol-2-amine hydrochloride (SSR125543A), a potent and selective corticotrophin-releasing factor(1) receptor antagonist. II. Characterization in rodent models of stress-related disorders. J Pharmacol Exp Ther 2002; 301:333–345.
144. Naliboff BD, Munakata J, Fullerton S, et al. Evidence for two distinct perceptual alterations in irritable bowel syndrome. Gut 1997; 41:505–512.
145. Mertz H, Naliboff B, Munakata J, et al. Altered rectal perception is a biological marker of patients with irritable bowel syndrome. Gastroenterology 1995; 109:40–52.
146. Rey E, Alvarez SA, Diaz-Rubio M. Which is the best distension protocol to study rectal sensitivity in the irritable bowel syndrome? Rev Esp Enferm Dig 2002; 94:211–220.
147. Blomhoff S, Jacobsen MB, Spetalen S, et al. Perceptual hyperreactivity to auditory stimuli in patients with irritable bowel syndrome. Scand J Gastroenterol 2000; 35:583–589.
148. Lejeune F, Millan MJ. The CRF1 receptor antagonist, DMP695, abolishes activation of locus coeruleus noradrenergic neurones by CRF in anesthetized rats. Eur J Pharmacol 2003; 464:127–133.
149. Folks DG. The interface of psychiatry and irritable bowel syndrome. Curr Psychiatry Rep 2004; 6:210–215.
150. Lydiard RB. Irritable bowel syndrome, anxiety, and depression: what are the links? J Clin Psychiatry 2001; 62(suppl 8):38–45.

151. Barbara G, Stanghellini V, De Giorgio R, et al. Activated mast cells in proximity to colonic nerves correlate with abdominal pain in irritable bowel syndrome. Gastroenterology 2004; 126:693–702.
152. Castagliuolo I, Wershil BK, Karalis K, Pasha A, Nikulasson ST, Pothoulakis C. Colonic mucin release in response to immobilization stress is mast cell dependent. Am J Physiol 1998; 274:G1094–1100.
153. Eutamene H, Theodorou V, Fioramonti J, et al. Acute stress modulates the histamine content of mast cells in the gastrointestinal tract through interleukin-1 and corticotropin-releasing factor release in rats. J Physiol 2003; 553:959–966.
154. Coelho AM, Fioramonti J, Bueno L. Mast cell degranulation induces delayed rectal allodynia in rats: role of histamine and 5-HT. Dig Dis Sci 1998; 43:727–737.
155. Castagliuolo I, Lamont JT, Qiu B, et al. Acute stress causes mucin release from rat colon: role of corticotropin releasing factor and mast cells. Am J Physiol 1996; 271:G884–G892.
156. Stead RH. Innervation of mucosal immune cells in the gastrointestinal tract. Reg Immunol 1992; 4:91–99.
157. Vergnolle N. Clinical relevance of proteinase activated receptors (pars) in the gut. Gut 2005; 54: 867–874.
158. Coelho AM, Vergnolle N, Guiard B, et al. Proteinases and proteinase-activated receptor 2: a possible role to promote visceral hyperalgesia in rats. Gastroenterology 2002; 122:1035–1047.
159. Su X, Gebhart GF. Mechanosensitive pelvic nerve afferent fibers innervating the colon of the rat are polymodal in character. J Neurophysiol 1998; 80:2632–2644.
160. Kirkup AJ, Brunsden AM, Grundy D. Receptors and transmission in the brain-gut axis: potential for novel therapies. I. Receptors on visceral afferents. Am J Physiol Gastrointest Liver Physiol 2001; 280:G787–G794.
161. Tache Y. Corticotropin releasing factor receptor antagonists: potential future therapy in gastroenterology? Gut 2004; 53:919–921.

15 | The Biopsychosocial Continuum in Visceral Pain in Chronic Abdominal and Visceral Pain: Theory and Practice

Douglas A. Drossman
UNC Center for Functional GI and Psychiatry, Division of Gastroenterology and Hepatology, University of North Carolina at Chapel Hill, Chapel Hill, North Carolina, U.S.A.

INTRODUCTION

A biopsychosocial understanding of chronic abdominal pain requires integrating the biological processes affecting the pain, both peripheral and central, with knowledge of the contributing psychosocial factors (1). In effect, it is the brain–gut modulation of both enteroceptive (i.e., gut related) and extrinsic (i.e., environmental and stress related) influences on sensation that are unique to the individual. Although nociceptive signals increase with heightened motor reactivity and visceral hypersensitivity, these are not experienced as pain until they reach the brain, where central factors modulate the degree of conscious perception, even independent of gut activity. For example, pain disappears during sleep and pain can be produced in healthy individuals through hypnosis. For the clinician, an understanding of both central and peripheral processes eliciting the pain experience must be understood. This chapter will review how chronic abdominal pain exists on a continuum of severity as modulated through the brain–gut axis. For the clinician, an understanding of the degree of contribution from peripheral (i.e., visceral hypersensitivity and increased motor reactivity) and central (i.e., alteration of descending inhibitory pathways and psychosocial influences) sources will determine the diagnostic options and ultimately the plan of care.

Let us consider the following two case examples:

Case 1

> Ms. L.R., a 38-year-old woman presents with a three month history of lower abdominal pain associated with and relieved by defecation of loose watery stools. There is no prior medical history except for occasional episodes of "gastroenteritis" as a child that resolved in adulthood. Her gastrointestinal (GI) symptoms recurred three months ago after a camping trip in South America with her husband. They both developed acute dysentery that was untreated. Her husband's symptoms resolved within a week; yet hers continued unabated. The camping trip was scheduled just prior to Ms. L.R.'s plans to return to teaching after 10 years; she had taken a leave to raise her three children. She acknowledged that she did not enjoy the camping trip because of considerable anticipatory anxiety about returning to her job. After so many years, she feared she would be inadequate to meet the tasks required.
>
> The medical evaluation, which included complete blood count (CBC), serum electrolytes, sigmoidoscopy, stool for ova and parasites, and bacterial culture, was normal. She was placed on hyoscyamine sublingual tabs and scheduled to return in six weeks. At the follow-up visit, she volunteered that soon after returning to work, her anxiety dissipated as she regained her confidence as a teacher. Concurrently, her GI symptoms had nearly resolved.

This case illustrates a patient who developed postinfectious irritable bowel syndrome (IBS). As will be discussed, its pathogenesis relates in part to the combination of increased visceral sensitivity and motor reactivity probably due to infection-induced alterations in mucosal immune function that occurs concurrent with psychological distress (2). For this patient, with the absence of a lifelong history of bowel difficulties and psychosocial comorbidities, recovery would be expected.

Case 2

> Ms. L.J., a 54-year-old woman was referred for chronic generalized abdominal pain of over 10 years duration that has been refractory to usual treatments. She entered the office, walking slowly and

holding her abdomen. She described the pain with a sense of urgency as "the worst ever" also "sickening" and "tormenting." The pain is constant and disabling, and is unrelated to physical activity, eating, or defecation. Other painful conditions include headache, back pain, fibromyalgia, and, earlier in life, dysmenorrhea diagnosed as endometriosis. The history of painful episodes also led to a cholecystectomy, appendectomy, and three laparoscopies for lysis of adhesions.

Ms. L.J. alluded to having been victimized as a child, and from this, she learned the importance of being independent and stoical. In fact, until this pain began, she had never missed work and was always the "strong one" at times of hardship, such as when her father died (the time when her severe pain began). Notably, while others observe that symptoms flare during times of stress, she strongly denies this association and states that she knows the problem is "real and not in my head." Over time, she has felt unable to control the symptoms, and this has led to dependence on others with a sense of helplessness and reduced self-esteem. Family and friends have taken over many of her activities, and she frequently visits the emergency room for pain shots. Her family doctor is worried about her use of narcotics. Mrs. L.J. says she is willing to accept any method for pain control, but other treatments have not been helpful or she has rejected them because of side effects. Because she can cope no longer with the pain, she now requests inpatient evaluation and is willing (if you agree) to go on disability.

Recent evaluations included upper and lower endoscopy, endoscopic retrograde cholangiopancreatography (ERCP), barium contrast studies, computed tomography (CT), and magnetic resonance (MR) scans. A trial of antidepressants was begun, and cognitive-behavioral counseling was recommended. Two weeks later, the patient phoned requesting pain medication. The antidepressants were discontinued after three days because of side effects, and psychological referral was not initiated, the patient stating she "is not crazy."

This case report is more complex than the first one with regard to the severity of the disorder, its pathophysiology, and treatment options: (i) there is little evidence for bowel dysfunction contributing to the pain; her diagnosis is consistent with functional abdominal pain syndrome (3), (ii) the repeated surgeries and procedures may have contributed to the development of visceral hypersensitivity, and (iii) there is evidence for a strong central contribution to the pain as supported by the following: (a) the constancy and wide distribution of pain over several organs and regions, (b) history of abuse, (c) denial of stress, (d) maladaptive cognitions with catastrophic thoughts, feelings of helplessness, dependency, and lack of control, and (e) chronic pain behaviors with high health-care utilization, possible narcotic seeking, and family reinforcement of the illness state. It is unlikely that this patient would have rapid or full recovery. Therefore, her care must be directed toward the following: (i) establishing an effective physician–patient relationship built on trust, a shared understanding of the illness and mutual agreement on treatment goals, (ii) providing proper education about the pathophysiology and treatment options, and (iii) helping the patient develop adaptive coping strategies and regaining a sense of personal control over a chronic pain disorder. Only when this is achieved, can the patient benefit from a long-term clinical relationship, the effective use of antidepressants for pain control, and possibly ancillary psychological intervention with cognitive-behavioral treatment (4).

THE BIOPSYCHOSOCIAL CONTINUUM

The biopsychosocial model (5) proposes that illness and disease result not from a single (biological) etiology, but from simultaneously interacting systems at the cellular, tissue, organism, interpersonal, and environmental level. Furthermore, psychosocial factors have direct physiological and pathological consequences and vice versa. Finally, it is the unique contributions of both psychosocial and pathophysiological factors that determine the nature of the illness or disease and its severity for every individual (1,5). Given this assumption, we can conceptualize chronic abdominal or visceral pain as existing on a continuum from gut to brain and from mild-to-severe as shown in Figure 1, where there are differing contributions of psychosocial and biological factors that determine the nature and severity of the condition.

Figure 1 conceptualizes chronic abdominal pain as the product of contributions from peripheral (i.e., gut) and central sources that then affect the severity of the condition and determine the types of treatments. For the majority of individuals with mild-to-moderate chronic abdominal pain, a combination of factors affecting gut function (e.g., dietary, motility, infection, bowel injury, and hormonal changes) can lead to increased afferent excitation and upregulation of afferent neuronal activity. However, for the smaller group of patients with more severe and disabling pain (shown to the right of Fig. 1), there is a greater contribution from the central nervous system, and peripheral influences (e.g., motility and visceral

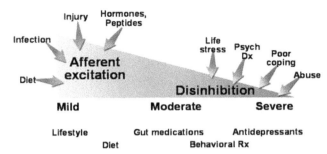

Figure 1 Chronic abdominal pain: the bio-psychosocial continuum. This figure displays the continuum from primarily peripheral (more common) to primarily central (less common) influences on the pain process. In general, the more severe and disabling the pain, the greater the contribution of central processes. See text for details.

hypersensitivity) become less prominent (6). In these cases, pain is amplified due to the impaired central modulation of pain, leading to decreased central inhibitory effects on afferent signals at the level of the spinal cord (disinhibition). Factors contributing to this effect can include life stresses and abuse, comorbid psychiatric diagnoses, and poor coping. Knowing the severity of the disorder and the purported site of action (i.e., gut, brain, or both) can help in the treatment approach, as will be discussed later in this chapter.

PATHOPHYSIOLOGY

What is the physiological basis to justify this conceptual model? Chronic pain is a multidimensional (sensory, emotional, and cognitive) experience, best explained by abnormalities in the neurophysiological functioning at the afferent, spinal, and central nervous system (CNS) levels (7). Chronic pain is distinct from acute pain arising from peripheral/visceral injury or disease, because structural abnormalities, motility disturbances, and tissue damage leading to increased afferent visceral stimuli are not prominent and may not even be present. As pain becomes more chronic, the CNS becomes the primary modulator of the pain experience and can even amplify incoming regulatory (i.e., non-nociceptive) visceral afferent signals to the point of conscious awareness and distress. The discussion below provides a plausible explanation for amplification of chronic pain from both peripheral and central sources (3).

Visceral Pain Transmission to the CNS

Figure 2 shows ascending afferent pathways from the colon, which can occur from inflammation or, as shown here, balloon distension. The first order neuron projects to the spinal cord where it synapses with a secondly order neuron and then ascends to the thalamus and midbrain. Several supraspinal projecting pathways have been identified, which include the spinothalamic, spinoreticular, and spinomesencephalic tracts (8,9). The spinothalamic tract shown on the right terminates in the medial thalamus containing the parafascicular nucleus, and also terminates in the posterior thalamus containing ventral posterior lateral/ventral posterior medial (VPL/VPM) nuclei (nuclei not labeled). Thalamocortical fibers then project to the primary somatosensory cortex (SI). This spinothalamic pathway is important for somatotopic sensory discrimination and localization of visceral and somatic stimuli. The spinoreticular tract (middle pathway) conducts sensory information from the spinal cord to the reticular formation in the brain stem. Unlike the SI, the reticular formation has almost no information about where on the body surface noxious stimulation occurs and it is involved mainly in the reflexive, affective, and motivational properties of such stimulation. The reticulothalamic tract projects from the dorsal and caudal medullary reticular formation [dorsal reticular nucleus (DRN)] to the medial thalamus on the left. The spinomesencephalic tract (pathway on left) ascends the spinal cord with fibers to various regions in the brain stem, including the periaqueductal gray (PAG), locus coeruleus, and DRN in the medulla (three arrows in midbrain). Thalamocortical projections from the medial thalamus transmit sensory input to different areas of the brain, such as the cingulate cortex and insula, that are involved with the processing of noxious visceral and somatic information (three arrows more rostral in brain). The brain regions innervated by these pathways that are activated in response to painful

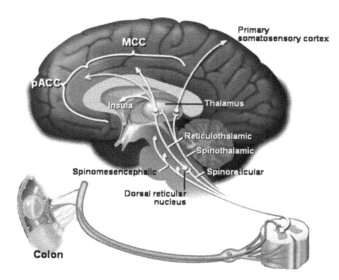

Figure 2 Visceral pain transmission to the central nervous system. This figure shows the ascending pathways from gut to somatosensory and limbic structures in the brain via spinal and midbrain pathways. See text for details. *Abbreviations*: MCC, midcingulate cortex; pACC, perigenual anterior cingulate cortex. *Source*: From Ref. 3.

colorectal stimuli include the thalamus, anterior insula, amygdala, and anterior cingulate cortex (ACC). The latter region comprises two components, perigenual ACC (pACC) and midcingulate cortex (MCC), with the former involved in affect and the latter in behavioral response modification. Other pathways for transmission of noxious visceral stimuli (such as the dorsal column pathway) exist (10), but are not shown in this figure. This multicomponent integration of nociceptive information, dispersed to the somatotopic and intensity area (to the lateral sensory cortex as well as the emotional or motivational-affective area of the medial cortex), explains the variability in the experience and reporting of pain (11).

This conceptual scheme of pain modulation through both sensory- and motivational-affective components has been supported through positron emission tomography (PET) imaging using O^{15}-radiolabeled imaging (12) Among healthy subjects who immersed their hands in hot (47°C.) water, half were hypnotized to experience the immersion as painful and the other half as not painful or even pleasant. Comparison of changes in cortical activation between these two groups found no difference in activity in the SI. However, for those subjects hypnotized to experience the hand immersion as painful, there was significantly greater activation of the ACC of the limbic system. Thus, the hypnotic suggestion differentiated the functioning of these two pain systems; the suggestion of unpleasantness was specifically encoded by the anterior midcingulate portion of the ACC, an area involved with negative perceptions of fear and unpleasantness.

Amplification of Visceral Afferent Signals

There is growing evidence that visceral inflammation and injury can amplify activity in visceral pathways, as has been reported for postinfectious IBS (2) and other painful functional GI disorders (13). Possibly, either an increase in peripheral receptor sensitivity or an increase in the excitability of spinal or higher CNS pain regulatory systems may be responsible for producing a state of hyperalgesia (increased pain response to a noxious signal), allodynia (increased pain response to non-noxious or regulatory signals), and/or chronic pain (14,15).

It is commonly observed that patients with chronic abdominal pain can have prior episodes of frequent or recurrent pain events or procedures that later become generalized to a chronic and persistent symptom presentation. Patients with IBS undergo more abdominal and gynecological operations for painful conditions than control groups (16). Although the surgeries have been attributed to increased health-care seeking and illness behaviors, an alternative explanation is that the surgical insult triggered the painful functional GI disorder and manifested clinically in patients physiologically and psychologically predisposed. Symptoms suggestive of IBS arise de novo in about 10% of women undergoing hysterectomy (17), and preoperative treatment with local or regional anesthesia or nonsteroidal anti-inflammatory medications reduces the severity of postoperative pain (14). These observations suggest that the CNS response to peripheral injury can be modified by prior reduction of afferent input to the spinal cord and CNS. Finally, surgery causes postoperative pain that is inflammatory in nature and associated with reduced stimulus threshold and pain enhancement. Factors predicting the pain response depend upon the site and duration of the surgery and the individual's psychological vulnerability to pain (18). Therefore, recurrent peripheral injury such as repeated abdominal operations in the psychologically predisposed host may sensitize intestinal receptors, making perception of even baseline (regulatory) afferent activity more painful.

These observations are consistent with newer data relating to the development of visceral hypersensitivity and postinfectious IBS. Inflammation and injury to nerve fibers in immature (i.e., neonate) animals can alter the function and structure of peripheral neurons (19) that later yield a greater pain response to visceral distension when they become adults (20). In humans, repetitive balloon inflations in the colon lead to a progressive, though transient increase in pain intensity (21), occurring to a greater degree and for a longer period in patients with IBS (22). There is also a subset of IBS patients with increased mucosal inflammatory cells and cytokine activation (23), which may predispose to the development of visceral hypersensitivity. In one study (24), degranulated mast cells found close to the enteric nerves were associated with clinical reports of greater pain. Thus, in at least a subset of patients with functional GI symptoms, inflammation may play a role in visceral sensitization.

Perhaps the best clinical model for the effects of inflammation on visceral hypersensitivity is the postinfectious IBS model (PI-IBS). This was the diagnosis in the first case report, with Ms. L.R. Recent evidence suggests that PI-IBS actually results from a combination of an inflammation-induced altered mucosal immune system that sensitizes visceral afferent nerves (2), in addition to some degree of central emotional distress. The stress further amplifies the afferent signal to a point of conscious awareness (13,25). In the first prospective study to address this issue, 94 patients hospitalized with acute gastroenteritis and no prior history of bowel complaints were followed up three months later (26). Although most ($n = 72$) of the patients recovered clinically, 22 continued with abdominal pain and bowel dysfunction. Notably, both the symptomatic and the recovered postinfectious groups had similar levels of gut hypermotility and visceral sensitivity. However, greater psychological distress at the time of the infectious episode, and a greater number of mucosal inflammatory cells during the three-month follow-up period, characterized the group with continued pain. It was proposed (25) in this study that while the similar levels of abnormal motility and visceral hypersensitivity relative to the controls were permissive factors, it was the CNS amplification of these peripheral signals occurring in the psychologically distressed group that raised the signals to conscious awareness, thereby perpetuating the symptoms. The increased pain may have also been mediated via CNS influences on peripheral inflammatory/cytokine activity. Further specification for these findings occurred in a more recent more well-powered study (27), which found that PI-IBS patients had significantly higher enterochromaffin cell counts and lamina propria T-lymphocytes, as well as greater anxiety and depression, relative to those with acute gastroenteritis who recovered or control groups. In fact, multivariate analysis showed that both enterochromaffin (EC) cell counts and depression were equally important predictors of developing PI-IBS (relative risk (RR) 3.8 and 3.2, respectively). These data support the contention that for postinfectious IBS to become clinically expressed, there must be evidence for brain–gut dysfunction with both visceral sensitization and high levels of psychological distress.

Descending Modulation of Pain
Figure 3 shows the principal components of the descending pain modulatory system activated in response to the noxious balloon distension of the colon, as postulated in the gate control theory of pain (11). It is believed that the central descending inhibitory system originates in the ACC, an area rich in opioids, (28) as well as from other cortical regions. Activation of this region from peripheral/visceral afferent activity (Fig. 2) may downregulate afferent signals via descending corticofugal inhibitory pathways, as illustrated. Descending connections from the ACC and the amygdala to pontomedullary networks, including the PAG, rostral ventral medulla, and the raphe nuclei, activate inhibitory pathways via opioidergic, serotonergic, and noradrenergic systems (8,29) to the dorsal horn of the spinal cord, which acts like a "gate," to increase or decrease the transmission of afferent impulses arising from peripheral nociceptive sites to the CNS.

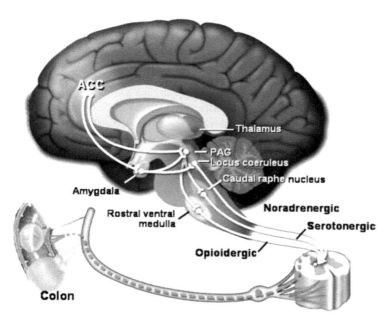

Figure 3 Descending modulation of pain. This figure demonstrates the corticofugal descending inhibitory pathways from the central nervous system to the spinal cord. The descending pathway is consistent with the gate control theory of pain modulation (11). *Abbreviations*: ACC, anterior cingulate cortex; PAG, periaqueductal gray. *Source*: From Ref. 3.

Psychological Distress and its Possible Role in Central Amplification of Pain

As noted, psychological disturbances are associated with greater pain severity and disability, and thus may serve as an amplifying factor to the pain experience, i.e., a CNS type of sensitization. So, while peripheral sensitization may influence the onset and short-term continuation of the pain, the CNS appears involved in the predisposition and perpetuation of pain, leading to the more severe chronic pain condition. As with case #2, L.J., this was evident by the lack of gut dysfunction associated with the pain and by the strong association of psychosocial disturbances and chronic pain behaviors. Empiric data support the idea that comorbid psychiatric diagnosis, major life stress, a history of sexual or physical abuse, poor social support, and maladaptive coping are associated with more severe and chronic abdominal pain and poorer health outcome (6,30–32).

The relationship between psychosocial disturbances, emotional distress, and chronic pain may be mediated through impairment in the limbic system's modulation of visceral signals. The ACC, involved in the motivational and affective components of the limbic or medial pain system, is reported to be dysfunctional in patients with IBS and other chronic painful conditions such as fibromyalgia (33–35). There are different degrees of activation of the pACC, an area rich in opioids associated with emotional encoding, and the posterior ACC, also called the rostral or anterior MCC in response to painful stimuli. The latter region, MCC, is associated with unpleasantness, fear (along with the amygdala), and motor pain behavior (36). When using PET and functional magnetic resonance imaging to evaluate the ACC response to rectal distension or the anticipation of distension, IBS patients preferentially activate the MCC and have less activation of the pACC relative to controls (33,34,37,38). Possibly in IBS, activation of the descending inhibitory pain pathway that originates in the opioid-rich pACC is supplanted by the activation of the MCC, the area associated with fear and unpleasantness. Similar findings occur in patients with somatization (39) and post-traumatic stress disorder (40).

There is preliminary evidence to support an association between psychosocial distress, in particular abuse, and dysfunction of central regulation of pain via the ACC. There may be a synergistic effect of abuse history and IBS leading to greater ACC activation and pain reporting than either condition alone (41,42), and this supports the clinical evidence that patients with functional GI disorders with abuse report more pain and have poorer health behaviors than patients with IBS alone (32) In addition, a strong correlation between life stress

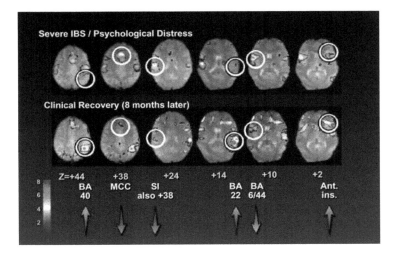

Figure 4 (*See color insert.*) Cingulate activation in irritable bowel syndrome (IBS) before and after clinical recovery. Functional magnetic resonance imaging images show pairs of horizontal sections in a patient with severe IBS and after clinical recovery (eight months later). Each pre- and postsymptomatic pair of sections was selected to show a single cortical area difference. The *Z* level scores are shown with standard color coding (red for highest to blue for lowest). Cortical areas with high initial activation during the severe IBS state on top are circled in white and include midcingulate cortex, primary somatosensory cortex, and prefrontal areas 6/44. Areas with initially low levels of activation that were significantly elevated at clinical recovery (eight months later) are highlighted with black-stroked circles and included the anterior insula among other areas. *Source*: From Ref. 44.

and maladaptive coping with ACC activation has been reported by our group (43). Furthermore, in the case report of a patient with severe chronic IBS pain and abuse history (as shown in the top of Fig. 4), there was marked activation of the MCC and SI. However, after antidepressant treatment and brief psychotherapy, there was marked clinical recovery with a return to a more normal CNS state—reduced MCC and SI activation and increased insular activation (bottom of Fig. 4)(44). Other studies support that there is a reduction of cingulate activity in patients with IBS receiving antidepressants (45), and that among patients with depression cingulate activity can predict a response to antidepressants (46,47).

These data suggest that emotional disturbances may aggravate the dysfunctional central pain regulatory pathways seen in functional GI pain. Although further confirmatory data are needed, the findings are compelling and provide a mechanistic basis for psychological and antidepressant treatments in more severe forms of chronic pain where central contributions are thought to be pre-eminent.

CLINICAL PRESENTATION BASED ON SEVERITY OF PAIN AND IMPLICATIONS FOR TREATMENT

Patients with chronic abdominal and visceral pain can fall under a variety of diagnostic syndromes and categories. This may include longstanding structural diagnoses such as chronic pancreatitis, a variety of functional GI diagnoses (e.g., IBS, functional chest pain or dyspepsia, functional biliary pain, levator syndrome, etc.), or combinations (e.g., inflammatory bowel disease (IBD) with IBS). In this chapter, the proposition is that, independent of diagnosis, the nature and severity of the pain as well as clinical decisions regarding treatment will depend on integrating the relative contributions of the peripheral and central determinants that affect the nature and severity of the pain and its psychosocial concomitants.

Table 1 is a further elaboration of Figure 1 providing the continuum of chronic abdominal pain or other functional GI painful conditions that are broken into specific clinical features based on severity.

Mild Symptoms

The most frequently seen group with abdominal pain has intermittent episodes of mild pain. These patients are usually treated in primary care practices. They maintain normal daily

Table 1 Spectrum of Clinical Features Among Patients with Functional Gastrointestinal Pain

Clinical Feature	Mild	Moderate	Severe
Estimated prevalence	70%	25%	5%
Practice type	Primary	Specialty	Referral
Visceral contribution-altered gut physiology	+ + +	+ +	+
Symptoms constant	0	+	+ + +
Psychosocial difficulties	0	+	+ + +
Healthcare use	+	+ +	+ + +
Chronic pain behavior	0	+	+ + +
Psychiatric diagnoses	0	+	+ + +

Note: 0, generally absent; +, mild; + +, moderate; + + +, marked. *Source*: From Refs. 13, 48.

activities, have little or no psychosocial difficulties (although they may experience symptom exacerbation with stress) or chronic pain behaviors, and are not high health-care utilizers. Like case #1, they commonly have IBS, dyspepsia, or other functional GI disorders where the pain is associated with altered GI motility or sensitivity indicating a greater peripheral (i.e., gut related) contribution to the condition. Treatment involves education, reassurance, and dietary/ lifestyle changes (Fig. 1) or possibly pharmacological treatments (e.g., antidiarrheals and anti-cholinergics) targeted to gut function.

Moderate Symptoms

Patients with moderately painful symptoms have more frequent or severe pain that is at times disabling. There may be symptom-related psychological distress, associated with greater physiological gut reactivity (e.g., worse with eating or stress, relieved by defecation or vomiting) and a greater number of health-care visits. Treatments involve gut-acting pharmacological agents (e.g., anticholinergics, antidiarrheals, or the newer 5-HT receptor–acting agents, etc.), and the psychosocial distress tends to improve concurrent with relief of the GI symptoms. If the symptoms are more persistent, low-dose tricyclic antidepressants and/or psychological treatments can be considered.

Severe Symptoms

Ms. J.L. (case #2) represents the small proportion of patients with severe and refractory symptoms. They are most frequently seen in referral centers. The pain may be constant or frequently recurrent, and is not associated with GI dysfunction. There is usually marked impairment of function (disability is not uncommon), chronic pain behaviors, comorbid psychiatric diagnoses (e.g., depression, anxiety disorders, somatization, or Axis II diagnoses), associated psychosocial difficulties (e.g., major losses or deprivation and sexual/physical abuse), maladaptive coping (e.g., catastrophizing), and high health-care use. Here, antidepressant medication and possibly mental health or pain center referral are needed along with an ongoing relationship with the primary care physician to provide psychosocial support through brief, regular visits (49).

CONCLUSION

The care of patients with chronic abdominal or visceral pain involves an understanding of the mechanisms explaining the pain, i.e., sensitization of peripheral activity or dysfunction of central pain regulatory systems, an appreciation of the clinical and psychosocial features that characterize and amplify the symptoms and behaviors, the establishment of an effective physician–patient relationship, and the implementation of a variety of treatment options tailored to the needs of the patient, often based on the severity of the pain. In most cases, the rationale for the treatments requires that the physician provide adequate information; so the patient sees them as relevant to personal needs. This integrated biopsychosocial treatment approach is intuitively logical. When this approach is properly implemented, the short-term outcome appears improved, and importantly, the process becomes mutually gratifying for the patient and physician (50).

REFERENCES

1. Drossman DA. Presidential address: gastrointestinal illness and biopsychosocial model. Psychosom Med 1998; 60(3):258–267.
2. Spiller RC. Post infectious irritable bowel syndrome. Gastroenterol 2003; 124(5):1662–1671.
3. Drossman DA. Functional abdominal pain syndrome. Clin Gastroenterol Hepatol 2004; 2(5): 353–365.
4. Drossman DA, Toner BB, Whitehead WE, et al. Cognitive-behavioral therapy vs. education and desipramine vs. placebo for moderate to severe functional bowel disorders. Gastroenterol 2003; 125(1):19–31.
5. Engel GL. The need for a new medical model: a challenge for biomedicine. Science 1977; 196: 129–136.
6. Drossman DA, Whitehead WE, Toner BB, et al. What determines severity among patients with painful functional bowel disorders. Am J Gastroenterol 2000; 95(4):974–980.
7. Casey KL. Match and mismatch: Identifying the neuronal determinants of pain. Ann Intern Med 1996; 124(11):995–998.
8. Vogt BA, Sikes RW. The medial pain system, cingulate cortex, and parallel processing of nociceptive information. In: Mayer EA, Saper CB, eds. The Biological Basis for Mind Body Interactions. 1st. Los Angeles: Elsevier Science BV, 2000:223–235.
9. Heimer L. Ascending sensory pathways. In: Heimer L, ed. The Human Brain and Spinal Cord: Functional Neuroanatomy and Dissection Guide. 2nd. New York: Springer-Verlag, 1995:201–216.
10. Willis WD, Al Chaer ED, Quast MJ, Westlund KNA. Visceral pain pathway in the dorsal column of the spinal cord. Proc Natl Acad Sci USA 1999; 96(14):7675–7679.
11. Melzack R, Wall P. Gate-control and other mechanisms. In: Melzack R, Wall P, eds. The Challenge of Pain. 2. London: Pelican Books, 1988:165–193.
12. Rainville P, Duncan GH, Price DD, Carrier B, Bushnell MC. Pain affect encoded in human anterior cingulate but not somatosensory cortex. Science 1997; 277:968–971.
13. Drossman DA, Camilleri M, Mayer EA, Whitehead WE. AGA Technical review on irritable bowel syndrome. Gastroenterol 2002; 123(6):2108–2131.
14. Coderre TJ, Katz J, Vaccarino AL, Melzack R. Contribution of central neuroplasticity to pathological pain: review of clinical and experimental evidence. Pain 1993; 52:259–285.
15. Mayer EA, Gebhart GF. Basic and clinical aspects of visceral hyperalgesia. Gastroenterol 1994; 107(1):271–293.
16. Longstreth GF, Yao JF. Irritable bowel syndrome and surgery: a multivariable analysis. Gastroenterol 2004; 126(7):1665–1673.
17. Prior A, Stanley KM, Smith AR, Read NW. Relation between hysterectomy and the irritable bowel: a prospective study. Gut 1992; 33(6):814–817.
18. Jess P, Jess T, Beck H, Bech P. Neuroticism in relation to recovery and persisting pain after laparoscopic cholecystectomy. Scand J Gastroenterol 1998; 33(5):550–553.
19. Ruda MA, Ling QD, Hohmann AG, Peng YB, Tachibana T. Altered nociceptive neuronal circuits after neonatal peripheral inflammation. Science 2000; 289:628–630.
20. Al-Chaer ED, Kawasaki M, Pasricha PJ. A new model of chronic visceral hypersensitivity in adult rats induced by colon irritation during postnatal development. Gastroenterol 2000; 119(4):1277–1285.
21. Ness TJ, Metcalf AM, Gebhart GF. A psychophysiological study in humans using phasic colonic distension as a noxious visceral stimulus. Pain 1990; 43:377–386.
22. Munakata J, Naliboff B, Harraf F, et al. Repetitive sigmoid stimulation induces rectal hyperalgesia in patients with irritable bowel syndrome. Gastroenterol 1997; 112(1):55–63.
23. Chadwick VS, Chen W, Shu D, et al. Activation of the mucosal immune system in irritable bowel syndrome. Gastroenterol 2002; 122(7):1778–1783.
24. Barbara G, Stanghellini V, DeGiorgio R, et al. Activated mast cells in proximity to colonic nerves correlate with abdominal pain in irritable bowel syndrome. Gastroenterol 2004; 126(3):693–702.
25. Drossman DA. Mind over matter in the postinfective irritable bowel. Gut 1999; 44(3):306–307.
26. Gwee KA, Leong YL, Graham C, et al. The role of psychological and biological factors in post-infective gut dysfunction. Gut 1999; 44:400–406.
27. Dunlop SP, Jenkins D, Neal KR, Spiller RC. Relative importance of enterochromaffin cell hyperplasia, anxiety, and depression in postinfections IBS. Gastroenterology 2003; 125(6):1651–1659.
28. Vogt BA, Watanabe H, Grootoonk S, Jones AKP. Topography of diprenorphine binding in human cingulate gyrus and adjacent cortex derived from coregistered PET and MR images. Hum Brain Mapp 1995; 3:1–12.
29. Heimer L. Brain stem, monoaminergic pathways, and reticular formation. In: Heimer L, ed. The Human Brain and Spinal Cord: Functional Neuroanatomy and Dissection Guide. 2nd ed. New York: Springer-Verlag, 1995:219–238.
30. Creed F, Levy RL, Bradley LA, Francisconi C, Drossman DA, Naliboff BD, Olden KW. Psychosocial aspects of functional gastrointestinal disorders. In: Drossman DA, Corazziari E, Delvaux M, Spiller R, Talley NJ, Thompson WG, Whitehead WE, eds. Rome III: The Functional Gastrointestinal Disorders. 3rd ed. McLean, VA: Degnon Associates, 2006:295–368.

31. Longstreth GF, Thompson WG, Chevy WD, Houghton LA, Mearin F, Spiller R. Functional bowel disorders. In: Drossman DA, Corazziari E, Delvaux M, Spiller R, Talley NJ, Thompson WG, Whitehead WE, eds. Rome III: The Functional Gastrointestinal Disorders. 3rd ed. McLean, VA: Degnon Associates, 2006:487–555.

32. Drossman DA, Li Z, Leserman J, Toomey TC, Hu Y. Health status by gastrointestinal diagnosis and abuse history. Gastroenterol 1996; 110(4):999–1007.

33. Mertz H, Morgan V, Tanner G, et al. Regional cerebral activation in irritable bowel syndrome and control subjects with painful and nonpainful rectal distention. Gastroenterology 2000; 118:842–848.

34. Naliboff BD, Derbyshire SWG, Munakata J, et al. Cerebral activation in irritable bowel syndrome patients and control subjects during rectosigmoid stimulation. Psychosom Med 2001; 63(3):365–375.

35. Chang L, Berman S, Mayer EA, et al. Brain responses to visceral and somatic stimuli in patients with irritable bowel syndrome with and without fibromyalgia. Am J Gastroenterol 2003; 98(6):1354–1361.

36. Vogt BA, Hof PR, Vogt LJ. Cingulate gyrus. In: Paxinos G, Mai JK, eds. The Human Nervous System. 2nd. San Diego and New York: American Press, 2002.

37. Ringel Y, Drossman DA, Turkington TG, et al. Regional brain activation in response to rectal distention in patients with irritable bowel syndrome and the effect of a history of abuse. Dig Dis Sci 2003; 48(9):1774–1781.

38. Silverman DHS, Ennes H, Munakata JA, et al. Differences in thalamic activity associated with anticipation of rectal pain between IBS patients and normal subjects. Gastroenterol 1995; 108:1006.

39. Silverman DHS, Brody AL, Saxena S, Munakata JA, Naliboff BD. Somatization in clinical depression is associated with abnormal function of a brain region active in visceral pain perception. Gastroenterology 1998; 114(4):A839.

40. Shin LM, McNally RJ, Kosslyn SM, et al. Regional cerebral blood flow during script-driven imagery in childhood sexual abuse-related PTSD: a PET investigation. Am J Psychiatry 1999; 156(4):575–584.

41. Ringel Y, Drossman DA, Liu H, et al. fMRI of cingulate activation to painful rectal distension in IBS and sexual/physical abuse. Gastroenterology 2002; 122(4):A311.

42. Ringel Y, Drossman DA, Leserman J, et al. IBS diagnosis and a history of abuse have synergistic effect on the perigenual cingulate activation in response to rectal distention. Gastroenterology 2003; 124(4):A-531.

43. Ringel Y, Drossman DA, Leserman J, et al. Association of anterior cingulate cortex (ACC) activation with psychosocial distress and pain reports. Gastroenterology 2003; 124(4):A-97.

44. Drossman DA, Ringel Y, Vogt B, et al. Alterations of brain activity associated with resolution of emotional distress and pain in a case of severe IBS. Gastroenterol 2003; 124(3):754–761.

45. Mertz H, Pickens D, Morgan V. Amitriptyline reduces activation of the anterior cingulate cortex in irritable bowel syndrome patients during rectal pain. Gastroenterology 2003; 124(4):A-47.

46. Mayberg HS, Liotti M, Brannan SK, et al. Reciprocal limbic-cortical function and negative mood: converging PET findings in depression and normal sadness. Am J Psychiatry 1999; 156(5):675–682.

47. Mayberg HS, Brannan SK, Mahurin RK, et al. Cingulate function in depression: A potential predictor of treatment response. Neuroreport 1997; 8(4):1057–1061.

48. Drossman DA. Review Article: An Integrated Approach to the Irritable Bowel Syndrome. Aliment Pharmacol Ther 1999; 13(Suppl 2)(4):3–14.

49. Drossman DA. Diagnosing and treating patients with refractory functional gastrointestinal disorders. Ann Intern Med 1995; 123(9):688–697.

50. Drossman DA. Challenges in the physician-patient relationship: feeling "drained". Gastroenterol 2001; 121(5):1037–1038.

16 | Chronic Pain and Addiction

Howard Heit
Georgetown University School of Medicine, Washington, D.C., U.S.A.

Douglas Gourlay
The Wasser Pain Management Center, Mount Sinai Hospital, Toronto, Ontario, Canada

INTRODUCTION

Pain is the most common complaint presenting to the clinician's office (1). Approximately 50 to 70 million people in the United States suffer pain that is undertreated or not treated at all (2). Three to 16% of the American population has the disease of addiction (3). Therefore, four to six million Americans with a history of addiction may have pain. Opioids may be indicated in a small percentage of these patients with moderate to severe pain. However, this population may be at higher risk for relapse if opioids are used as part of the treatment plan.

Sickle cell disease and HIV/AIDS often result in chronic and severe pain, requiring potent medications for treatment. A preponderance of patients with these conditions are members of ethnic/racial groups who are known to be undertreated for these painful conditions because of a concurrent addictive disorder and/or prejudice arising from racism, homophobia, and/or opiophobia (4).

The goal of this chapter is to address the often-complex issues associated with the treatment of pain in those persons suffering from concurrent substance-use disorders.

BINARY CONCEPT OF PAIN AND ADDICTION

For many years, pain conditions and addictive disorders were treated as binary phenomena. If there was a legitimate pain diagnosis, which usually meant that the condition made sense to the assessing clinician, the likelihood of there being an addictive disorder was thought to be so small as to not even merit investigation. Unfortunately, if the patient had an obvious substance-use disorder, very real and treatable pain conditions were often ignored. With time, this thinking was tempered somewhat to suggest that, in the absence of a current, past, or family history of an addictive disorder, the aberrant use of the prescribed controlled substance was very low indeed (5). This dichotomous approach to pain and addiction has served neither patients nor clinicians well.

In reality, there is nothing about a real pain condition that is protective against having a concurrent substance-use disorder. Likewise, we now know that persons suffering from addictive disorders who are in methadone maintenance treatment (MMT) programs list severe chronic pain as a major problem (6). While there is no evidence in the literature to suggest that those patients without past histories or increased risk of substance-use disorders become addicted as a result of rational pharmacotherapy for the treatment of any condition, including pain, there is no credible evidence to the contrary ("iatrogenic addiction"). Perhaps, a more relevant question to ask is whether rational pharmacotherapeutic management of acute or chronic pain can reactivate a previously dormant addictive disorder or express an as yet unidentified predisposition toward substance misuse or addiction. The answers to these questions clearly must be, "Yes."

Addiction is not an uncommon occurrence in the general population. The prevalence of addiction has been stated variously at 3% to 16%, but is often quoted at 10% (3). It is hard to imagine that the rates of substance-use disorders in the chronic pain population should be less. Some authors believe that this rate may very much underestimate the prevalence of addiction within the pain management patient population. Regardless of what the real risk is, it is clear that no one specific marker can reliably identify the at-risk pain patient; so careful boundary setting for all patients is strongly recommended. Not all aberrant behavior reflects drug misuse or addiction. Some individuals who do not meet the diagnostic criteria for addiction may also use medications and other drugs problematically. This group is sometimes referred to as "chemical copers" (7). These individuals lack coping skills commonly acquired during childhood and adolescence and tend to turn to external sources for support in dealing with life's problems.

For example, stress can increase pain (8). A pain patient who takes inappropriate additional doses of his or her opioid medication after stressful situations to treat anxiety must be educated that this is not the correct response to the situation. Behavior therapy to improve coping skills is indicated. Specific pharmacotherapy with medications that are less likely to be misused, such as the Selective Serotonin Reuptate Inhibitor (SSRI) antidepressants or tiagabine hydrochloride (Gabitril®) also may be indicated to treat the anxiety. This is an appropriate biopsychosocial approach to the problem that can lead to a sustainable solution to the patient's problem.

In fact, aberrant behavior may also be a function of inadequate pain management. "Pseudoaddiction" as defined by Weissman and Haddox (9) is a term used to describe a pattern of maladaptive behavior that is due to inadequate treatment of pain. When the pain is treated appropriately, inappropriate behavior ceases.

It is only by aggressive investigation and rational pharmacotherapeutic management of the pain that this diagnosis can be confirmed. While it may be said that the diagnosis of addiction is made prospectively, over time, the diagnosis of pseudoaddiction is made retrospectively (10). When reasonable limits and boundaries are placed on a patient, and yet the patient continues to step out beyond these limits, addiction and pseudoaddiction should be in the differential diagnosis. When the patient explains aberrant behavior in terms of inadequate analgesia, it is reasonable to consider a careful review of the treatment plan and, when appropriate, to adjust the prescribed medications upward to achieve the desired functional goals. This increase in medication dose should be tied to a tightening of the dispensing interval/boundaries in order to test safely the possibilities of drug misuse, pseudoaddiction, or addiction. As an example, a patient who continually runs out of medication early that is dispensed on a monthly basis should have the dispensing interval reduced (i.e., to weekly) when the decision to increase the dose is made. If the patient continues to run out of medication early, despite the dose being increased, the diagnosis of pseudoaddiction becomes less plausible.

PAIN AND OPIOID ADDICTION—A CONTINUUM APPROACH

While pain and addiction can and sometimes do exist as comorbid conditions, they may also present as part of a dynamic continuum with pain at one end of the spectrum and addiction at the other extreme. In cases when the identified substance of misuse is one in which there can be no doubt about the medical inappropriateness of ongoing use, such as with alcohol or cocaine use, a comorbid pain and substance-use disorder should be considered. When the drug in question can arguably be both the problem and the solution, depending on clinician training and perspective, a continuum model may better apply. This can be the

Pain and Addiction Continuum

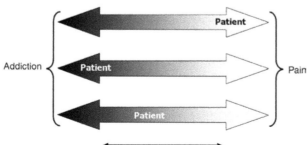

Figure 1 Pain and addiction continuum.

case with opioids used for the treatment of chronic pain. Figure 1 shows diagrammatically this relationship.

With chronic pain, appropriateness of ongoing opioid use may come into question, especially when there is little or no objective improvement in pain relief or function. In this case, the application of the *Diagnostic and Statistical Manual of Mental Disorders* (DSM-IV) criteria for diagnosis of opioid dependence may lead to inappropriate diagnosis of addiction, potentially compromising patient care.

BASIC SCIENCE OF ADDICTION

Drugs of misuse act at local cellular and membrane sites that are within a neurochemical system that is called the Reward and Withdrawal Pathway (11). This pathway is in the meso-limbic dopamine system, and it involves, among other structures, the ventral tegmental area, nucleus accumbens, amygdala, and prefrontal cortex of the primitive brain. Addiction is a neurobiological disease that causes disruption of this pathway. This disruption is mediated via receptor sites and neurotransmitters. Central to this reward and withdrawal pathway is the neurotransmitter dopamine, which has been shown to be relevant not only to drug reward, but also to food, drink, sex, and social reward (12,13). Disruption of this neurochemical pathway by drugs of abuse may lead to addiction. Drug withdrawal can intensify with repeated drug use and can persist during prolonged periods of drug abstinence, a symptom complex known as the protracted abstinence syndrome (14). This sensitization of a neural process related to drug cravings, or to environmental stimuli associated with drugs (referred to as cues), leads, in the at risk individual, to the progressive increase in drug-seeking behavior that characterizes addiction. Such sensitization appears to increase the attractiveness of the drug taking and that of the drug-associated stimuli (15). Addiction is a treatable brain disease; it is a distinct medical condition that may or may not be associated with the patient's pain syndrome (16,17).

Physical dependence, conversely, is a natural expected physiologic response that can occur with opioids, alcohol, benzodiazepines, corticosteroids, antidepressants, diabetic agents, certain cardiac medications, and many other medications used in clinical medicine. Abrupt cessation or rapid dose reduction resulting in decreasing blood level of the substance and/or administration of an antagonist to the substance can produce a withdrawal syndrome that can include, but is not limited to, nausea, vomiting, diaphoresis, diarrhea, abdominal cramps, seizures, or even death (15).

Opioids cause physical dependence and, upon abrupt discontinuation, withdrawal as a result of upregulation of the cyclic aminophosphorase pathway at the locus coeruleus (14). This is a normal physiologic response to this class of medications. It should be noted that most of the medications mentioned above are capable of producing physical dependence, but are not associated with the disease of addiction. A heroin addict may be both addicted and physically dependent on the narcotic, while the pain patient taking opioids is physically dependent, but not addicted. Both will experience withdrawal if the drug is abruptly stopped.

Tolerance is also a natural, expected physiologic response that can occur with exposure to certain classes of drugs, especially alcohol and opioids. Pharmacodynamic tolerance involves adaptations that occur at both the site of the drug action; e.g., receptor, ion channel, and in related systems more distal to the site of the drug action. For example, pharmacodynamic tolerance to opioids is evident at both the level of the opioid receptor in the locus coeruleus (primary) and in the dopaminergic reward pathways afferent to the site of this discrete drug action (secondary) (15). Both persons addicted to heroin and chronic pain patients taking opioids can exhibit tolerance to certain effects of the drug.

The terms "pseudotolerance" and "pseudoaddiction" are very important in pain management. Pseudotolerance, as defined by Pappagallo, is the need to increase medication such as opioids for pain, when other factor(s) are present but unappreciated as disease progression, new disease, increased physical activity, lack of compliance, change in medication, drug interaction, addiction, and/or deviant behavior (18).

The American Academy of Pain Medicine, the American Pain Society, and the American Society of Addiction Medicine [Liaison Committee on Pain and Addiction (LCPA) approved the following definitions in 2001] (19).

ADDICTION

Addiction is a primary, chronic, neurobiologic disease, with genetic, psychosocial, and environmental factors influencing its development and manifestations. It is characterized by behaviors that include one or more of the following: impaired control over drug use, compulsive use, continued use despite harm, and craving.

PHYSICAL DEPENDENCE

Physical dependence is a state of adaptation that is manifested by a drug-class–specific withdrawal syndrome that can be produced by abrupt cessation, rapid dose reduction, decreasing blood level of the drug, and/or administration of an antagonist.

TOLERANCE

Tolerance is a state of adaptation in which exposure to a drug induces changes that result in a diminution of one or more of the drug's effects over time.

Health-care professionals with an improved understanding of the definitions of addiction, physical dependence, tolerance, pseudotolerance, and pseudoaddiction will be able to evaluate and treat chronic pain patients with or without the disease of addiction more effectively.

Diagnostic and Statistical Manual of Mental Disorders-IV

An improved understanding of definitions of addiction, physical dependence, and tolerance would also allow clinicians to more effectively interpret the terminology of the *Diagnostic and Statistical Manual of Mental Disorders-IV* (21).

If one understands the correct definition of physical dependence, it is clear that the DSM-IV misuses the term dependence. By doing so, this has the effect of confusing a pain patient with one with the disease of addiction. Under the section "Criteria for Substance Dependence," DSM-IV defines substance dependence as "a maladaptive pattern of substance use, leading to clinically significant impairment or distress, as manifested by three (or more) of the following during the same 12-month period." It then lists seven criteria for determining if this disorder exists (Table 1) (21). Without differentiating between dependence and addiction, five of the seven criteria for substance-use disorder could apply either to a person with the disease of addiction or a chronic pain patient on opioids. (Table 2) Consequently, a pain patient on opioids may be misdiagnosed with the disease of addiction when he or she is physically dependent, which, as the definitions make clear, is a normal physiological consequence of using opioids. A heroin addict could be both physically dependent and addicted as per the definitions.

Table 1 Criteria for Diagnosis of Substance Dependence

A maladaptive pattern of substance use, leading to clinically significant impairment or distress, as manifested by the occurrence of three (or more) of the following during the same 12-month period:
(1) Tolerance, as defined by either of the following:
   (a) A need for markedly increased amounts of a substance to achieve intoxication or a desired effect
   (b) Markedly diminished effect with continued use of the same amount of a substance
(2) Withdrawal, as manifested by either of the following:
   (a) Symptoms characteristic of withdrawal from a substance,
   (b) The ability to take a substance or one closely related to it, to relieve or avoid withdrawal symptoms
(3) A need to take a substance in larger amounts or over a longer period than intended.
(4) A persistent desire or unsuccessful efforts to cut down or control substance use
(5) A great deal of time spent in activities necessary to obtain a substance (e.g., visits to multiple doctors or driving long distances), to use a substance (e.g., chain smoking), or to recover from its effects.
(6) Abandonment of or absence from important social, occupational, or recreational activities because of substance use
(7) Continued substance use despite knowledge of having a persistent or recurrent physical or psychological problem that is likely to have been caused or exacerbated by the substance (e.g., continued cocaine use despite recognition of cocaine-induced depression, or continued drinking despite recognition that an ulcer is made worse by alcohol consumption)

Table 2 Five Out of Seven of the DSM-IV Criteria for Substance Misuse Could Be for a Pain Patient Appropriately on Opioids or Patient with the Disease of Addiction

1. Tolerance does not equal addiction
2. Withdrawal does not equal addiction
3. Length of use of opioids does not equal addiction
4. Desire to cut down the use of opioids does not equal addiction
5. Time and activity to obtain opioid does not always equal addiction

Source: From Ref. 22.

It is instructive to look at the seven criteria DSM-IV uses to make the diagnosis of substance dependence and apply them to a patient on opioids for chronic pain, taking into account the LCPA's definitions of addiction, physical dependence, and tolerance (23).

1. Tolerance can be present either in an addicted patient or in a pain patient on opioids. Tolerance, as the need to increase the dose of an opioid to achieve intoxication, is consistent with addiction. However, tolerance is also a natural and expected physiologic response to opioids. The opioid dose should be maintained just above the Mean Effective Analgesic Concentration (MEAC) that relieves pain but does not produce impairment and is associated with improved function (24). In clinical pain practice, if the health-care professional or the patient feels that an increase of opioid medication is indicated to reach the goal of decreasing pain and increasing function, this is not tolerance but dose titration.

2. Withdrawal can be present in both addiction and in the pain patient on opioids. Withdrawal is a manifestation of physical dependence that can be part of the disease of addiction. A heroin addict abruptly stops the drug and therefore goes into withdrawal, or the same person enters a narcotic treatment program (NTP), and the opioid substitution relieves the withdrawal syndrome and cravings for heroin. A chronic pain patient enters the hospital on opioids for surgery for a failed back syndrome and the order for his opioid medication is mistakenly not conveyed to his surgeon from his prescribing outpatient physician. The pain patient may go into withdrawal, resulting in increased pain, until his daily opioid requirements have been met. By failing to maintain adequate opioid levels in the physically dependent opioid user, an "opioid debt" may result. "Opioid debt" may be defined as that condition which results from failure to adequately maintain serum levels of chronically used opioids in those patients who have become physically dependent upon these drugs. This is not addiction but rather a normal physiologic response consistent with the definition of physical dependence (25–27).

3. Both an addict and a pain patient may often take a substance/opioid in larger amounts or over a longer period than was intended. Certainly, the heroin addict takes the drug in larger amounts secondary to tolerance and longer than intended to prevent withdrawal, cravings, or as a result of poor coping skills. The chronic pain patient may have to increase the opioid dose due to tolerance, but also to decrease pain and increase function. The chronic pain patient under proper evaluation desires to decrease the opioid dose, if the source of the pain is decreasing or the pathology is corrected. Although both of these patients would appropriately be classified as substance dependent using the improved definitions, only the heroin addict would appropriately be diagnosed with a substance-use disorder.

4. Both an addict and a pain patient can have a persistent desire or unsuccessful effort to cut down or control substance use. The heroin addict desires to cut down or control his/her drug use for a variety of reasons, not the least of which is cost. The pain patient on opioids typically desires to decrease his/her medication if the physical condition improves or is corrected. In addition, the pain patient is always under control with all the medications and takes them as prescribed (28). Would both of these patients be considered to have substance-use disorders? The heroin user suffering from the disease of addiction would; the pain patient should not.

5. An addicted patient spends a great deal of time in activities necessary to obtain the substance/opioid. Very seldom does one evaluate a "happy" person with the disease of addiction, because most of their waking hours are spent either trying to get their drug of choice or using it once obtained. However, a chronic pain patient who is not treated or inadequately treated for pain may also spend a great deal of time trying to obtain medication, which fits the definition of pseudoaddiction (9). Would both of these patients

be considered to have a substance-use disorder? The heroin user suffering from the disease of addiction should; the pain patient should not.

6. Only the addicted patient gives up or reduces important social, occupational, or recreational activities because of substance use. The drug causes a decrease in one's quality of life. This person would correctly be diagnosed as having a substance-use disorder. The goal of opioid therapy for pain, as with any pharmacotherapy, is that the medication increases the quality of life (28).

7. Only the addicted patient continues to use the substance despite knowledge of having a persistent or recurrent physical or psychological problem that is likely to have been caused or exacerbated by the substance. Again, the drug causes a decrease in one's quality of life and the diagnosis of substance-use disorder is correct (Fig. 2).

Broad adoption of standard definitions of addiction, physical dependence, and tolerance would improve the clinical practice of both pain and addiction medicine. The LCPA definitions should be incorporated into the future Substance-Use Disorder section of DSM-V. Until that occurs, clinicians should understand and apply the definitions that reflect accurate and current knowledge in basic science and clinical medicine. Health-care professionals who understand these definitions will be better able to evaluate and treat their patients if opioids are being prescribed for pain and to diagnose the disease of addiction if present (Table 2).

BASIC CONCEPTS IN THE USE OF OPIOIDS

Knowledge of pharmacokinetics and pharmacodynamics of medications such as opioids is essential in prescribing "rational pharmacotherapy." Pharmacokinetics is the absorption, distribution, binding (or distribution) in tissue, biotransformation, and excretion of the drug. It is "what the body does to the drug." Pharmacodynamics is the mechanism by which drugs produce their effect. It is "what the drug does to the body" (29).

Differences Between a Pain Patient and an Addicted Patient

Pain Patient	Addicted Patient
Not out of control with medications	Out of control with medications
Medications improve quality of life	Medications cause decreased quality of life
Will want to decrease medication if side effects are present	Medication continues or increases despite side effects
Concern about the physical problem	Unaware or in denial about any problems
Follows the agreement for the use of the opioids	Does not follow the agreement for use of the opioids
Frequently has medicines left over	Does not have medicines left over, loses prescriptions, and always has a "story"

Figure 2 Differences between a pain patient and an addicted patient. *Source*: From Ref. 28.

The terms "modified release" and "long acting" are often used interchangeably when referring to the opioid class of drugs. This has caused some confusion, especially when considering the pharmacologic characteristics of these medications. In fact, there are relatively few truly long-acting opioids available for clinical use, such as methadone and buprenorphine.

Opioids may be divided into short-acting and long-acting agents. The short-acting group may be further divided into immediate release and modified release. It is important to note that at the receptor level, the drug remains the same in both preparations. The primary effect of the modified-release system is to reach and maintain steady levels of the parent molecule. This becomes extremely important when comparing risk of misuse of various forms of the same drug. These comparisons rely on the delivery system used to modify the rate of release of drug remaining intact. Given that with sufficient time and determination, all clever delivery systems can be defeated, some more easily than others, it is important not to lose sight of the intrinsic abuse liability of the parent molecule.

MODIFIED-RELEASE DELIVERY SYSTEMS

In the case of morphine sulfate, this drug is available in both the immediate- and modified-release forms. As a first-generation modified-release system, the active ingredient is suspended in a wax-like matrix from which it is slowly delivered to the patient. The drug is leeched out of the matrix in a monophasic fashion. The drug has slow onset, which is thought to lower the abuse liability of the active ingredient, morphine (30). However, when the drug is crushed, this slow-release system is compromised, allowing for much more rapid absorption and delivery of the morphine sulfate. In fact, first-generation modified-release forms of morphine have been used as a source of injectable morphine by crushing the tablets up and heating the powder in water. When the resultant solution cools, the waxy matrix residue may be peeled off the surface leaving a potent aqueous morphine solution.

In the case of the second-generation modified-release preparations, a portion of the active ingredient is immediately available to help reach satisfactory blood levels, while the remainder of the drug is released slowly, over time. OxyContin®, a modified-release version of oxycodone, is an example of this system.

In OxyContin, approximately 38% of the dose is released rapidly, whereas the remainder of the drug is delivered over the 12 hours, twice-daily dosing schedule (31). For most patients, this results in rapid onset of analgesic effect and stable blood levels of oxycodone over the 24-hour period. This benefit becomes a liability in those patients who have used oxycodone as a drug of misuse, because by simply crushing the tablet, the clever delivery system is compromised, and the OxyContin becomes essentially an immediate-release product.

Opioid level instability, in the physically dependent patient, may also lead to a situation in which the need to continue opioid analgesics is driven not by dramatic improvement in pain and/or function, but rather by how badly things seem to go upon discontinuation. This information is sometimes gained incidentally by patients when they run out of medication on a weekend or if their prescriber attempts to taper the drug too quickly. In some cases, such as neuropathic pain, the pain problem may be less opioid responsive, requiring higher doses (32). Opioid withdrawal will lead to a hyperadrenergic state that will exacerbate virtually all types of pain (33). The use of a modified-release opioid may result in a transient improvement in pain relief sometimes referred to as the "honeymoon" period. In these cases, once opioid stability is achieved, it may be useful to revisit some of the adjunctive agents that were previously tried, even if they appeared to be ineffective at the time of their initial trial. In fact, in cases of poorly responsive pain, it may be useful to carefully try to discontinue the use of opioids, once these adjunctive measures are in place.

For sometime now, it has been known that some forms of pain may benefit from preemptive approaches to pain management. In 1995, Suzuki reviewed the relationship between injury response and acute and chronic pain in the context of preemptive analgesia (34). More recently, a randomized double-blind study of the involvement of presurgical pain in preemptive analgesia for orthopedic surgery showed a statistically significant difference in effectiveness of preemptive analgesia at the time of surgery for those cases where there was significant pain present prior to surgery as compared to matched controls who were pain-free at the time of surgery (35). Of course, the taking of opioid medications in advance of pain can, in some patients, lead to dose escalation and problematic use of medication. It may be that, in properly chosen patients, the use of appropriate doses of an immediate-release (IR) opioid prior to engaging in a painful procedure or activity may help to improve control of existing chronic pain syndromes in those who already suffer from these conditions. It remains to be seen if preemptive analgesia will reduce the development of chronic pain in those patients who suffer from acute episodes of pain (36).

IR opioids may be indicated in the treatment of moderate to severe acute pain. IR opioids are also indicated in incident or transitory exacerbations of pain with relatively stable and adequately controlled baseline (cancer or noncancer) pain. Prevalence of incident pain varies between 40% and 86% and usually lasts less than one hour (37,38). This appropriate use of IR opioids saves money secondary to decreased hospitalizations, emergency room (ER) visits, and office visits (39).

LONG-ACTING DRUGS

Our selection of long-acting opioids is practically limited to two agents. The first and most widely used is methadone. The second is sublingual buprenorphine with or without naloxone, which is an agent with "off-label" use in the pain management realm but is gaining popularity as a maintenance drug for use in the treatment of opioid addiction. The Drug Enforcement Administration (DEA) permits off-label use of approved medications. The buprenorphine products Suboxone® and Subutex® are the two Schedule III narcotic medications currently approved for the treatment of opioid dependence under the federal Drug Addiction Treatment Act of 2000 (DATA 2000). The off-label use of the sublingual formulations of buprenorphine (Suboxone/Subutex) for the treatment of pain is not prohibited under current DEA requirements. Therefore, a clinician may prescribe off-label use of buprenorphine (Suboxone/Subutex) for the treatment of pain. In addition, if a clinician uses buprenorphine (Suboxone/Subutex) for the treatment of pain, the prescriber does not need the special waiver that is required to prescribe buprenorphine for addiction (40).

Methadone is extremely effective in once-daily dosing when used in the opioid agonist maintenance treatment paradigm (41). However, methadone's analgesic duration of action is markedly shorter, typically lasting only six to eight hours. While the biphasic nature of this drug (alpha redistribution and beta elimination) may help to explain this apparent discrepancy, the exact mechanism of action remains unclear. Clinically, it appears that the serum level of methadone required to eliminate opioid withdrawal and reduce cravings in the physically dependent opioid user is markedly lower than that which is required to achieve and maintain analgesia (42,43).

Interestingly, the duration of action of buprenorphine when used in opioid agonist substitution therapy is over 24 hours (41). When buprenorphine is used parenterally as an analgesic, the duration of action is only six to eight hours (44). The mechanism for these discrepancies between analgesic duration of action in the management of pain and withdrawal elimination based on once-daily dosing has not yet been clearly elucidated in the literature. Clinical experience has demonstrated better pain control with t.i.d. or q.i.d. dosing of either methadone or buprenorphine sublingual (S/L) (Personal Communication).

OPIOIDS FOR ANALGESIA OR OPIOID STABILIZING EFFECT?

Not all pain syndromes are equally responsive to opioids (45). In cases in which a patient is physically dependent on opioids, as one would expect with prolonged use of this class of drug, it can sometimes be useful to consider the appropriateness of continuation of opioid therapy, especially when treatment goals of improved function and decreased pain remain unmet, despite aggressive opioid therapy.

Most pain is, to some degree, opioid responsive especially when the patient is opioid naive. As well, despite years of experience with opioid therapy, it remains unclear who will achieve a sustained opioid response for the treatment of chronic pain.

We know that chronic opioid therapy can reduce pain tolerance in certain individuals (46). The ability to control acute pain in the opioid-dependent individual as compared to the opioid-naive patient is much reduced. In studies looking at pain tolerance in MMT patients, there is a significant decrease in the ability of the MMT patients to tolerate a cold pressor model of neuropathic pain as compared to a matched control population (47). The continued use of opioids, in the absence of analgesic effect, is not without its cost.

When the patient and practitioner define the need to remain on opioid therapy not by how well the patient is doing but rather by how poorly things go whenever they try to reduce the dose, it may be time to reexamine the therapeutic role of opioids. When opioid levels in a physically dependent pain patient fall below a certain level, early withdrawal may occur. In the context of opioid abstinence induced hyperalgesia, it would be expected that the pain complaint should worsen (26). It is something of a myth that pain patients who no longer need opioids come off them easily.

We often see in MMT patients who present with addiction to short-acting, immediate-release opioids a dramatic 24-hour improvement in their pain relief with only once-daily dosing. This is despite the fact that we understand the duration of action of methadone as an analgesic is only six to eight hours (48). In this case, the dominant role of methadone may be to stabilize widely fluctuating opioid levels thereby reducing opioid withdrawal mediated hyperalgesia rather than acting as a primary analgesic.

UNIVERSAL PRECAUTIONS IN PAIN MEDICINE

As we begin to gain an understanding of the prevalence of substance-use disorders within the chronic pain population, it has become clear that no one behavior is pathognomonic of addiction. With this in mind, the importance of carefully inquiring into drug and alcohol histories in all patients becomes evident. This information is vital to any clinician treating complex medical and psychological problems. Alcoholism, for example, is a disease that intrudes into many aspects of the care of affected patients seeking medical treatment. Unresponsive hypertension, intractable mood disorders, difficult interpersonal relations, and poor sleep are all part of the life of an untreated alcoholic. While the use of potent medications including opioids in such cases is likely to be more complicated than in a similar patient who is not afflicted with this disorder, the need for the treating health-care professional to explore issues related to drugs and alcohol is not because of a choice to prescribe any particular medication. It is simply because an undiagnosed substance-use disorder, when it exists, can make even routine health care difficult.

Surprisingly, some clinicians struggle with the idea of taking a drug and alcohol history in all patients. Even asking about drug and alcohol misuse is seen as minimizing or dismissing the patients' complaints of pain. In no other area of medicine would such an attitude exist. The fact is that alcohol and drug addiction is present in virtually all areas of medicine, without particular respect for socioeconomic status, race, age, or sex. While the nature and distribution of these problems vary, it is unwise to limit one's inquiry into substance use based on classical societal stereotypes.

Since it is difficult to determine in advance, with any degree of certainty, who will become a problematic patient, there should be a uniform and respectful way of assessing all patients within the health-care setting. Of course, for those patients who are at increased risk for substance-use disorders, this basic level of inquiry can be expanded.

While the majority of pain patients who present to family practice offices are unlikely to be complicated by substance-use disorders, it may be useful to triage these patients into three groups, according to risk and recommended management strategies (27).

GROUP I PRIMARY CARE MANAGEMENT

This group of patients lacks personal or significant family history of substance-use disorders. They are not complicated by untreated psychopathology. This group likely represents the majority of patients who present for management of chronic pain. These patients should be considered the mainstay of primary care pain management and generally do not require referral either to tertiary level pain or addiction treatment.

GROUP II PRIMARY CARE WITH CONSULTATIVE SUPPORT

These patients are somewhat more complicated by virtue of either a significant past history of problems with drugs or alcohol or a significant family history. This group might benefit from a single consultation or concurrent management with a clinician knowledgeable in pain and addictive disorders. In some cases, a person who has suffered from a substance-use disorder is understandably anxious about using prescription medications to treat his or her pain. An important point is that the patient does not have an active substance-use disorder at the present time. A careful assessment of risk coupled with recommendations for tight boundary setting will help ensure optimum pain management with a minimum of risk.

GROUP III SPECIALTY REFERRAL

Group III represents the most complex and difficult population of patients to assess and treat. They are actively addicted and may be unable to see beyond their chronic pain condition. In the absence of concurrent assessment and treatment of the active addictive disorder, it is unlikely that even aggressive investigation and management of the pain complaint will lead to resolution of either the pain problem or the substance-use disorder. This group should be very tightly managed until they can be referred on to specialist assessment and care. While it is appropriate that the primary care practitioner manages the overall health of the patient, prescribing medications for pain may be inappropriate until the patient has sufficiently stabilized to qualify in Group II.

Two important points should be remembered. The first is that many patients will only become clearly identified as being at risk when a strong therapeutic alliance between practitioner and patient develops. The diagnosis of addiction is made prospectively, over time. Likewise, the unstable patient in Group III may, with effective treatment, move into Group II and be quite appropriate for primary care management with specialist support.

In this sense, Group II and Group III are dynamic; patients potentially move between these two groups as the relative dominance of the pain or addictive disorder changes.

The pain patient who is in recovery from the brain disease of addiction (16) faces multiple barriers to appropriate pharmacologic pain management. The barriers may be insurmountable if the addictive disease is both active and dominant. The reasons are multifactorial: inadequate education in pain and addiction medicine (49); misunderstanding of common definitions used in pain and addiction medicine (19); fear of misuse/addiction and diversion secondary to prescribing a controlled substance such an opioid; and concerns of sanctions from the regulatory agencies for prescribing a controlled substance (23).

The management of the chemically dependent patient does present some diagnostic and therapeutic challenges to the treatment team. In these patients who are physically dependent, due to either appropriate or inappropriate use of opioid agonist medications, it is important to have a strategy to assess and manage this patient population, thus the value of a "universal precautions" approach in pain management.

CLASSIFICATION OF PAIN

Pain can be divided into two main groups: acute and chronic. Acute pain may be further divided into anticipated and unanticipated pain. The following will outline basic strategies to assist in the safe and effective management of pain in the physically dependent patient.

In general, patients suffering acute pain while on opioid medications are at risk for inadequate pain relief. Some clinicians incorrectly believe that opioids used chronically prior to the acute episode may contribute to an acute analgesic effect. This is not true. The pre-event opioid use does nothing to help manage the acute episode and may in fact lower pain thresholds in some patients. If the daily expected dose of opioid is not given as a base upon which more opioids are added to effect analgesic relief, the patient runs the risk of experiencing an "opioid debt" that will certainly complicate acute pain management.

Take for example the patient who has been maintained on 30 mg t.i.d. of modified-release morphine sulfate for chronic osteoarthritis. The patient is scheduled for a total knee arthroplasty. If in the postoperative period, the patient is not given an equivalent of 90 mg/day of morphine sulfate, some degree of opioid withdrawal can be expected. Opioid withdrawal, which may either be objective (with classic opioid withdrawal symptoms evident) or subjective (which appears early in the withdrawal picture as a dysphoric state largely without outward signs of frank opioid withdrawal), is a hyperadrenergic state that can exacerbate the perceptions of any painful stimuli. Thus the failure to provide opioids beyond the 90 mg morphine sulfate per day previously experienced by the patient is apt to create an "opioid debt". Even elegant regional techniques used to manage postoperative pain may be suboptimal in such cases.

In these cases, it is important for prescribers to communicate with the acute pain team to ensure a smooth transition from chronic agonist therapy to the acute setting. These principles apply equally to patients who are physically dependent on maintenance agonist medications such as methadone. In the case of patients whose clinical picture is complicated by active addictive disorders, acute identification and stabilization are the first steps to successful management. In particular, attempts at weaning problematic drug use should be replaced with efforts to substitute medications with more favorable pharmacokinetic/pharmacodynamic profiles in order to affect pharmacologic stability. Consultation with or referral to a substance-use disorder professional is strongly recommended.

SPECIFIC PAIN CONDITION

The sickle cell anemia patient is a particularly good example of the potential complicating effects of unstable opioid levels in the often physically dependent patient. In this case, chronic, episodic use of opioids can lead to a state of physical dependency. When the opioids used are unable to provide pharmacologic stability, withdrawal symptoms including arthralgia and abdominal pain may be misinterpreted as acute, vaso-occlusive disease.

Not uncommonly, infrequent, discrete vaso-occlusive episodes are treated with parenteral opioids, particularly meperidine. This choice of drug is problematic for several reasons. The first is that meperidine is metabolized to normeperidine, which is a neurotoxic metabolite that at low levels can cause subtle personality changes while at higher levels can lead to frank seizure activity. This becomes particularly problematic in those sickle cell anemia patients who have compromised renal function secondary to vaso-occlusive illness. Unfortunately, sickle cell disease can lead to frequent crises episodes resulting in continuous use of potent opioids. Due to the relatively short duration of action of short-acting opioids such as meperidine, physically dependent patients may cycle through periods of opioid withdrawal that may be indistinguishable from their underlying vaso-occlusive disease.

By stabilizing the physically dependent opioid user with a truly long-acting agent such as methadone, true vaso-occlusive episodes of sickle cell crisis–driven arthralgia and abdominal pain can be identified and appropriately treated.

Patients with sickle cell disease, who have recurrent ER visits, have been called "frequent flyers." These patients usually have been treated in the hospital or ER with opioids. If upon discharge, the now physically dependent patient is sent out without opioid medication, approximately 24 to 48 hours later, the patient may develop abdominal and joint pain. Is this a manifestation of physical dependence with withdrawal or a recurrent crisis? Physical dependence can occur within hours or days with the use of certain medications such as opioids (50,51). By compassionate treatment of the patient with sickle cell anemia, the demeaning term "frequent flyers" can be eliminated from the medical terminology.

FEDERAL REGULATIONS FOR PRESCRIBING A SCHEDULED CONTROLLED SUBSTANCE

It is essential that prescribing clinicians understand the federal regulations that address administering, prescribing, and dispensing scheduled controlled substances whether they treat patients in a medical office, a hospital, a long-term care facility, or a hospice setting. This knowledge is necessary not only to reduce diversion and misuse of controlled substances, but also to protect the clinician's ability to provide care while following state and federal regulations in prescribing a controlled substance. It may be equally important for clinicians to have sufficient comfort with their knowledge that they do not invariably err on the side of caution and thereby provide inadequate care (1,40).

The government's role regarding controlled substances is determined by dual imperatives and the central principle of balance. One mandate is to establish a system of controls to prevent misuse and diversion of controlled substances. The second mandate is to ensure availability of controlled substances for medical and scientific purposes and for these medications to be accessible to all who legitimately need them (52).

The clinician must comply with both federal and state regulations that govern prescribing scheduled controlled substances (53). When federal law or regulations differ from state law or regulation, the more stringent rule would apply. Therefore, if there is a question about prescribing a controlled substances, the clinician should call his or her state medical board.

One regulation governing the prescription of a controlled substance is that a lawful prescription must be issued for a legitimate medical purpose by an individual acting in the usual course of his/her professional practice (21 CFR 1306.04). The clinician may administer, prescribe, or dispense a Schedule II controlled substance to a person with intractable pain, in which no relief or cure is possible or none has been found after a reasonable effort (21 CFR 1306.07). A chronic pain patient certainly falls into this classification.

The clinician may treat acute/chronic pain with a Schedule II controlled substances in a recovering narcotic-addicted patient (21 CFR 1306.07). Federal law or regulations do not restrict the prescribing, dispensing, or administering of a narcotic medication to a narcotic-addicted patient for the purpose of alleviating pain, if such prescribing is medically appropriate within standards set by the medical community

However, one *must* keep good records to document that the clinician is treating a pain syndrome, not the disease of narcotic addiction (opioid maintenance or detoxification). If the clinician is going to administer or dispense directly (but not prescribe), a Schedule II narcotic drug to a narcotic-dependent person for detoxification or maintenance treatment, the clinician *must* have a separate registration with the DEA as a NTP (21 CFR 1306.07).

DEA does not impose any limitations on a physician or authorized hospital staff to administer or dispense but not prescribe narcotic drugs in a hospital to maintain or detoxify a narcotic-dependent person as an incidental adjunct to medical or surgical treatment of conditions other than addiction (21 CFR 1306.07).

The clinician must never postdate a prescription for a Schedule II controlled substances such as an opioid. The prescription must be signed and dated usually in the upper right-hand corner on the day written. The regulation states the prescriptions for controlled substances shall be dated as of, and signed on, the date issued (21 CFR 1306.05) (40).

DATA 2000 for office-based opioid treatment with buprenorphine (Suboxone/Subutex) is a major step forward for more widespread treatment of the disease of opioid addiction. Buprenorphine with or without naloxone (in the form of Subutex® or Suboxone®) can be prescribed by certified and specially trained physicians. The physician must apply for and receive a waiver from the requirement to register as an NTP from the Center for Substance Abuse Treatment of the Substance Abuse and Mental Health Services Administration. However, one can prescribe buprenorphine in any form, off label for pain management without the above waiver (40).

Therefore, federal regulations in the United States are clear that the clinician can prescribe a Schedule II medication such as an opioid to a patient without the disease of addiction, in recovery from the disease of addiction, and even with an active addiction as long as the medical record documents the Schedule II medication such as an opioid is prescribed for pain, not for the disease of addiction.

CONCLUSION

Both health-care professionals and patients must understand their respective responsibilities in the effective management of chronic pain. Through this partnership, a balance between the prevention of diversion and misuse of prescription opioids, and the assurance of the availability of these medications to all who need them for the relief of pain is achieved. This concept of "balance" has been clearly described by the Pain and Policy Studies Group at the University of Wisconsin (51).

The purpose of effective pain management in any patient population, including those suffering from substance-use disorders, is to reduce pain while improving function. When a drug does "more to you than for you, and yet continues to be used," an active addictive disorder must be considered. Failure to identify such a comorbid state will render even the most ardent efforts at pain management ineffective and frustrating. As Marquis de Sade said about pain in "120 Days of Sodom," "No kind of sensation is keener or more active than that of pain; its impressions are unmistakable."

REFERENCES

1. Glajchen M. Chronic pain: treatment barriers and strategies for clinical practice. J Am Board Fam Pract 2001; 14(3):211–218.
2. Krames ES, Olson K. Clinical realities and economic considerations: patient selection in intrathecal therapy. J Pain Symptom Manage 1997; 14(Suppl 3):S3–S13.
3. Savage SR. Long-term opioid therapy: assessment of consequences and risks. J Pain Symptom Manage 1996; 11(5):274–286.
4. Pohl M. Pain in special populations. In: Graham A et al., eds. Principles of Addiction Medicine. 3rd ed. Chevy Chase, MD: American Society of Addiction Medicine, 2003:1417–1419.
5. Portenoy RK, Savage SR. Clinical realities and economic considerations: special therapeutic issues in intrathecal therapy—tolerance and addiction. J Pain Symptom Manage 1997; 14(Suppl 3):S27–S35.
6. Rosenblum A et al. Prevalence and characteristics of chronic pain among chemically dependent patients in methadone maintenance and residential treatment facilities. JAMA 2003; 289(18): 2370–2378.
7. Passik SD, Weinreb HJ. Managing chronic nonmalignant pain: overcoming obstacles to the use of opioids. Adv Ther 2000; 7(2):70–83.
8. Compton P, Gebhart G. The Neurophysiology of pain and interfaces with Addiction. In: Graham A et al., eds. Principles of Addiction Medicine. Chevy Chase, MD: American Society of Addiction Medicine, 2003:1385–1404.
9. Weissman DE, Haddox JD. Opioid pseudoaddiction—an iatrogenic syndrome. Pain 1989; 36(3): 363–366.
10. Gourlay DL, Heit HA, Passik SD. Exploring the Misconceptions: Opioids in Pain Management. 2004, Pharma Com Group, 76 Progress Drive, Stamford, CT 06902.
11. Koob GF, Le Moal M. Drug addiction, dysregulation of reward, and allostasis. Neuropsychopharmacology 2001; 24(2):97–129.
12. Nestler EJ, Landsman D. Learning about addiction from the genome. Nature 2001; 409(6822): 834–835.
13. Nestler EJ. Molecular basis of long-term plasticity underlying addiction. Nat Rev Neurosci 2001; 2(2):119–128.
14. Kasser C et al. Principles of detoxification. In: Graham A, Schultz T, eds. Principles of Addiction Medicine. 2nd ed. Chevy Chase, MD: American Society of Addiction Medicine, 1998.
15. Nestler EJ, Hyman SE, Malenka RC. Reinforcement and addictive disorders. In: In: Molecular Neuropharmacology: A Foundation for Clinical Neuroscience. New York: McGraw-Hill Companies Inc., 2001.
16. Wise RA. Addiction becomes a brain disease. Neuron 2000; 26(1):27–33.
17. Leshner AI. Drug abuse and addiction treatment research. The next generation. Arch Gen Psychiatry 1997; 54(8):691–694.
18. Pappagallo M. The concept of pseudotolerance to opioids. J Pharm Care Pain Symptom Control 1998; 6:95–98.
19. Savage SR et al. Definitions related to the medical use of opioids: evolution towards universal agreement. J Pain Symptom Manage 2003; 26(1):655–667.
20. Oaklander A. The pathology of pain. Neuroscientist 1999; 5(5):302–310.
21. Diagnostic and Statistical Manual of Mental Disorders - TR. 4th ed. Washington, DC: American Psychiatric Association, 2000.
22. Heit HA. Addiction, Physical Dependence, and Tolerance: Precise Definitions to Help Clinicians Evaluate and Treat the Patient with Chronic Pain. J Pain and Palliative Care Pharmacotherapy, March/April 2003.
23. American Academy of Pain Medicine, American Pain Society, and American Society Addiction Medicine. Definitions Related to the Use of Opioids for the Treatment of Pain, Glenview, IL, American Academy of Pain Medicine, 2001.
24. Stimmel B, Kreek MJ. Neurobiology of addictive behaviors and its relationship to methadone maintenance. Mt Sinai J Med 2000; 67(5–6):375–380.
25. Compton P, Charuvastra VC, Ling W. Pain intolerance in opioid-maintained former opiate addicts: effect of long-acting maintenance agent. Drug Alcohol Depend 2001; 63(2):139–146.
26. Li X, Clark JD. Hyperalgesia during opioid abstinence: mediation by glutamate and substance p. Anesth Analg 2002; 95(4):979–984. table of contents.
27. Gourlay D, Heit H, Almarhezi A. Universal precautions in pain medicine: a rational approach to the management of chronic pain. Pain Med 2005; 6(2):107–112.
28. Schnoll SH, Finch J. Medical education for pain and addiction: making progress toward answering a need. J Law Med Ethics 1994; 22(3):252–256.
29. Karan KD, Zajicek A, Pating DR. Pharmacokinetic and Pharmacodynamic Principles. In: Graham A et al, ed. Principles of Addiction Medicine. Chevy Chase, MD: American Society of Addiction Medicine, 2003:83–100.
30. Farre M, Cami J. Pharmacokinetic considerations in abuse liability evaluation. Br J Addict 1991; 86(12):1601–1606.

31. Mandema JW et al. Characterization and validation of a pharmacokinetic model for controlled-release oxycodone. Br J Clin Pharmacol 1996; 42(6):747–756.
32. Scadding JW. Treatment of neuropathic pain: historical aspects. Pain Med 2004; 5(suppl 1):S3–S8.
33. Compton P et al. Pain responses in methadone-maintained opioid abusers. J Pain Symptom Manage 2000; 20(4):237–245.
34. Suzuki H. Recent topics in the management of pain: development of the concept of preemptive analgesia. Cell Transplant 1995; 4(suppl 1):S3–S6.
35. Aida S et al. Involvement of presurgical pain in preemptive analgesia for orthopedic surgery: a randomized double blind study. Pain 2000; 84(2–3):169–173.
36. Van Elstraete AC et al. Are preemptive analgesic effects of ketamine linked to inadequate perioperative analgesia. Anesth Analg 2004; 99(5):1576.
37. Portenoy RK, Hagen NA. Breakthrough pain: definition, prevalence and characteristics. Pain 1990; 41(3):273–281.
38. Zeppetella G, O'Doherty CA, Collins S. Prevalence and characteristics of breakthrough pain in cancer patients admitted to a hospice. J Pain Symptom Manage 2000; 20(2):87–92.
39. Fortner BV, Okon TA, Portenoy RK. A survey of pain-related hospitalizations, emergency department visits, and physician office visits reported by cancer patients with and without history of breakthrough pain. J Pain 2002; 3(1):38–44.
40. Heit HA, Covington E, Good PM, Dear DEA. Pain Medicine 2004; 5(3):303–308.
41. Fiellin DA, O'Connor PG. Clinical practice. Office-based treatment of opioid-dependent patients. N Engl J Med 2002; 347(11):817–823.
42. Inturrisi CE, Verebely K. Disposition of methadone in man after a single oral dose. Clin Pharmacol Ther 1972; 13(6):923–930.
43. Inturrisi CE, Verebely K. The levels of methadone in the plasma in methadone maintenance. Clin Pharmacol Ther 1972; 13(5):633–637.
44. Resnick RB et al. Buprenorphine treatment of heroin dependence (detoxification and maintenance) in a private practice setting. J Addict Dis 2001; 20(2):75–83.
45. Dellemijn P. Are opioids effective in relieving neuropathic pain. Pain 1999; 80(3):453–462.
46. White JM. Pleasure into pain: the consequences of long-term opioid use. Addict Behav 2004; 29(7):1311–1324.
47. Doverty M et al. Hyperalgesic responses in methadone maintenance patients. Pain 2001; 90(1–2):91–96.
48. Wheeler WL, Dickerson ED. Clinical application of methadone. Am J Hospice Palliat Care 17(3): 22–77.
49. Weinstein SM et al. Medical students' attitudes toward pain and the use of opioid analgesics: implications for changing medical school curriculum. South Med J 2000; 93(5):472–478.
50. Krystal JH, Redmond DE Jr. A preliminary description of acute physical dependence on morphine in the vervet monkey. Pharmacol Biochem Behav 1983; 18(2):289–291.
51. Bickel WK et al. Acute physical dependence in man: effects of naloxone after brief morphine exposure. J Pharmacol Exp Ther 1988; 244(1):126–132.
52. Joranson DE et al. Achieving Balance in Federal and State Pain Policy: A Guide to Evaluation. Madison, Wisconsin: University of Wisconsin Comprehensive Cancer Center, 2003.
53. Model Policy for the Use of Controlled Substances for the Treatment of Pain. Federation of State Medical Boards of the United States Inc., 2004:1–9.

17 | Treating Visceral Pain Via Molecular Targets on Afferent Neurons: Current and Future

Peter Holzer

Department of Experimental and Clinical Pharmacology, Medical University of Graz, Graz, Austria

VISCERAL PAIN THERAPY: CURRENT AND FUTURE

The current treatment of visceral pain associated, for instance, with functional bowel disorders (FBDs) such as functional dyspepsia and irritable bowel syndrome (IBS) is unsatisfactory. Therapeutic advances are badly needed in view of the high prevalence of chronic or recurrent visceral pain and its socioeconomic burden as outlined in Chapters I/1 and I/2. This gap in the pharmacologic management of visceral pain reflects the incomplete understanding of the underlying mechanisms, which lags behind the knowledge of somatic pain mechanisms. In addition, the utility of nonsteroidal anti-inflammatory drugs and opiates, which are the mainstay in somatic pain management, is limited by their severe adverse effects on gastrointestinal (GI) mucosal homeostasis and motility, respectively. Although progress in the use of opioid and nonopioid drugs for the treatment of abdominal pain is being made (see Chapters III/18 and III/19), there is clearly a need to identify new targets for visceral pain therapy.

There are multiple mechanisms that contribute to the initiation and maintenance of FBDs at the level of the GI tract, the afferent nervous system and the brain. Novel therapies of FBDs may therefore be targeted (i) at the derangements of digestive functions, (ii) the hypersensitivity of afferent neurons, (iii) the exaggerated processing of afferent information in the brain in the context of a variety of psychosocial factors (gut–brain axis), and (iv) the disturbed control of GI functions by the brain through the autonomic nervous system and endocrine mechanisms (brain–gut axis). Besides neurophysiologic, psychologic, complementary, and integrative treatment strategies (see other chapters of this volume), medicines addressing hypersensitive afferent neurons represent a potentially important strategy (Table 1). In addition, drugs that help normalize the disturbances in GI function seen in FBDs may indirectly reduce visceral pain. This article focuses on sensory neuron–specific receptors (SNSR), ion channels, and messenger molecules that have potential in the therapy of visceral hyperalgesia.

SENSORY NEURONS AND GI HYPERSENSITIVITY

Studies of the possible mechanisms underlying FBDs have shown that abdominal hypersensitivity is an important factor in noncardiac chest pain, functional dyspepsia, and IBS (see Chapters II/3, II/6, II/7, II/9 and II/10). The concept that primary afferents are a relevant target for treating abdominal pain implies that these neurons are sensitized in states of hyperalgesia or undergo other functional changes that are relevant to hypersensitivity. Indeed, most extrinsic afferents innervating the gut have the ability to sensitize in response to a number of proinflammatory mediators and display enhanced excitability following experimentally induced inflammation. The mechanisms whereby hypersensitivity and hyperexcitability of afferent neurons are initiated and maintained are thus of prime pharmacologic interest, if therapeutic options to prevent or reverse sensitization are pursued.

Table 1 Gastrointestinal Hypersensitivity and Primary Afferent Neurons

The pharmacologic treatment of abdominal pain such as that associated with functional bowel disorders (FBDs) is unsatisfactory.

Since the prevalence of FBDs, particularly of functional dyspepsia and irritable bowel syndrome, can be as high as 20%, FBDs represent a significant burden in terms of direct health care and productivity costs.

Emerging evidence indicates that the discomfort and pain in many FBD patients is due to persistent hypersensitivity of primary afferent neurons, which may develop in response to infection, inflammation, or other insults.

This concept identifies sensory neurons as important targets for novel therapies of gastrointestinal hyperalgesia.

Sensory neuron–specific targets can be grouped in three categories: receptors and sensors at the peripheral nerve terminals, ion channels relevant to nerve excitability and conduction, and transmitter receptors.

Particular therapeutic potential is attributed to targets that are selectively expressed by afferent neurons and whose number and function are altered in abdominal hypersensitivity, such as transient receptor potential ion channels of vanilloid type 1 and tetrodotoxin-resistant Na^+ channels.

Permanent increases in the sensory gain may be related to changes in the expression of transmitters, receptors, and ion channels, changes in the subunit composition and biophysical properties of receptors and ion channels, or changes in the phenotype, structure, connectivity, and survival of afferent neurons. From a therapeutic point of view, it would be important to know why sensitization is maintained long after the initiating event has gone, because this would help to design strategies to effectively reverse hypersensitivity. A similar issue relates to the question why some patients affected with infectious gastroenteritis develop FBDs whereas others do not. Although the comorbidity of FBDs with depression, anxiety, and related brain disorders (see Chapter II/15) suggests that GI hyperalgesia involves many disturbances in the gut–brain and brain–gut axis, sensory neurons stage as the first element at which to aim novel therapies to control GI pain. In addition, drugs that target nociceptive afferent neurons can be configured such that they do not enter the brain and hence are free of adverse effects on brain functions (1). Sensory neuron–targeting drugs, though, can also have disadvantages if they interfere with important physiologic functions of primary afferents relevant to digestion and with the regulatory roles of peripheral neurons of the enteric and autonomic nervous system. Furthermore, they will be ineffective if hyperalgesia is solely the result of central sensitization processes.

CRITERIA FOR THE DESIGN OF EFFICACIOUS SENSORY NEURON–TARGETING DRUGS

Ideally, sensory neuron–targeting drugs should block the exaggerated signaling of hypersensitive afferents, which implies that they aim at molecular targets that are altered in disease (1). Without doubt, the complex innervation of the GI tract complicates the search for specific traits on nociceptive afferents supplying the gut. In exploiting such molecular targets, it is important to address several key questions that are crucial to the development of efficacious and safe drugs (Table 2). Among these, it is most important to identify receptors, ion channels, or other molecular traits that are selectively expressed by primary afferents, to elucidate their causal involvement in hypersensitivity, and to establish that their pharmacologic manipulation is efficacious in the treatment of GI hyperalgesia.

Table 2 Key Questions to be Addressed in the Design of Efficacious Sensory Neuron–Targeting Drugs

Which mechanical and chemical stimuli, noxious or innocuous, are relevant to visceral pain?

Which receptors and ion channels on primary afferents are relevant to visceral hyperalgesia?

Which extrinsic afferents (vagal or spinal) do contribute to abdominal discomfort and pain?

Are different stimulus modalities signaled by anatomically and neurochemically distinct populations of visceral afferent neurons?

Do visceral nociceptive neurons express receptors, ion channels, or other molecular traits in a cell-selective manner?

Is the expression of sensory neuron–specific molecular targets altered in states of visceral hypersensitivity?

Is it possible to block or even to reverse the pathologic hypersensitivity of afferent neurons while their physiologic role in regulating visceral functions is maintained?

Is it possible to pharmacologically differentiate between the transduction of noxious vs. innocuous stimuli?

Is drug interference with molecular targets on visceral afferents efficacious and safe in the treatment of abdominal hyperalgesia?

THREE CLASSES OF SENSORY NEURON–TARGETING DRUGS

Sensory neuron–specific targets can be grouped into three categories: (i) receptors and sensors at the peripheral terminals of afferent neurons that are relevant to stimulus transduction, (ii) ion channels that govern the excitability and conduction properties of afferent neurons, and (iii) transmitters and transmitter receptors that mediate communication between primary afferents and second-order neurons in the spinal cord and brain stem. There is a large number of receptors and sensors on afferent nerve terminals as listed in Table 3, although, importantly, not all of them are selectively expressed by sensory neurons. Among the ion channels relevant to nerve excitability and conduction, much attention is put on sensory neuron–specific ion channels such as the tetrodotoxin-resistant $Na_v1.8$ sodium channel. Primary sensory neurons can be differentiated by their chemical coding in terms of transmitter expression, with glutamate, calcitonin gene–related peptide (CGRP), and the tachykinins substance P and neurokinin A being the prevalent messenger molecules (2,3). In assessing the significance of targets on sensory neurons in visceral hyperalgesia, it is important to explore whether number, subunit composition, and biophysical properties of sensory neuron–specific ion channels and receptors are persistently altered in GI disease (1,4). Appropriate experimental models of GI disease (5) and clinical proof-of-concept studies are needed to evaluate critically which quantitative contribution various sensory neuron–specific targets make to the induction and/or maintenance of visceral hyperalgesia and whether modulation of a single target is therapeutically sufficient.

SENSORY NEURON–SPECIFIC RECEPTORS AND SENSORS
Sensory Neuron–Specific Orphan G Protein–Coupled Receptors

The murine genome contains more than 50 Mas-related genes (Mrgs), subdivided into subfamilies termed MrgA, MrgB, MrgC, and MrgD, which encode orphan G protein–coupled receptors that are expressed by specific subsets of nociceptive afferent neurons (6–9). This diversity of Mrgs appears to be an atypical feature of mice (8), since rats and gerbils have

Table 3 Three Classes of Drug Targets on Sensory Neurons and Their Transmission Relays

Receptors and sensors on afferent nerve terminals
   5-Hydroxytryptamine (5-HT$_3$ and 5-HT$_4$) receptors
   Adenosine A$_1$ and A$_2$ receptors
   Ionotropic purinoceptors of type P2X$_2$, P2X$_3$, and P2X$_{2/3}$
   Transient receptor potential ion channels of type TRPV1 and TRPV4
   Acid-sensing ion channels of type ASIC1, ASIC2, ASIC3, and ASIC2b/3
   Bradykinin B$_1$ and B$_2$ receptors
   Prostaglandin EP$_1$, EP$_2$, EP$_3$, EP$_4$ and IP receptors
   Protease–activated receptors of type PAR-1 and PAR-2
   Cholecystokinin CCK$_1$ receptors
   Corticotropin-releasing factor receptors
   Somatostatin sst$_2$ receptors
   Ionotropic and metabotropic glutamate receptors
   μ-, κ- , and δ-opioid receptors
   Cannabinoid CB$_1$ receptors
   Orphan G protein–coupled receptors (Mrgs)
   Neurotrophin receptors
   Mechanosensitive K^+ and Ca^{2+} channels
Ion channels relevant to sensory neuron excitability and conduction
   Voltage-gated Ca^{2+} channels
   Voltage-gated K^+ channels
   Tetrodotoxin-resistant voltage-gated Na^+ channels
Receptors for transmitters relevant to sensory neuron signaling
   Ionotropic and metabotropic glutamate receptors
   Calcitonin gene–related peptide receptors
   Tachykinin NK$_1$, NK$_2$, and NK$_3$ receptors
   α$_2$-Adrenoceptors
   μ-, κ- , and δ-opioid receptors
   Cannabinoid CB$_1$ receptors

Abbreviation: TRPV, transient receptor potential ion channels of the vanilloid type.

considerably fewer Mrg genes, and humans contain a related but nonorthologous family of genes, called MrgXs or SNSR. MrgD encodes an orphan G protein–coupled receptor termed TGR7, which is predominantly expressed in dorsal root ganglia (DRG) of rats and monkeys in which it is found on small diameter neurons bearing $P2X_3$ purinoceptors and transient receptor potential ion channels of vanilloid type 1 (TRPV1) (9). It awaits to be elucidated which stimuli and agonists other than RF-amide-related peptides (6), proenkephalin A gene products (7), and β-alanine (9) can activate these receptors and whether Mrgs are relevant to visceral hypersensitivity.

5-Hydroxytryptamine Receptors

Many efforts to develop drugs for FBDs have been directed at 5-hydroxytryptamine (5-HT) receptors as is discussed in Chapter III/18. Most of the 5-HT present in the body is formed in the GI enterochromaffin cells, wherefrom it is released by a variety of luminal stimuli. Being a paracrine messenger, this indoleamine can activate intrinsic and extrinsic sensory nerve fibers as well as other enteric neurons through activation of multiple 5-HT receptors (10–12). There is emerging evidence that the 5-HT system and the serotonin reuptake transporter (SERT) are modified in IBS and intestinal inflammation, which will alter the availability of 5-HT at 5-HT receptors (13–17). Thus, a strong association between the deletion/deletion polymorphic genotype in the SERT promotor region and the diarrhea-predominant IBS phenotype has been reported (17).

In terms of drug development, $5-HT_3$ and $5-HT_4$ receptors have been in the focus of interest, because their pharmacologic manipulation may correct both the functional disturbances in the gut and the pain associated with FBDs (12). This is particularly true for $5-HT_3$ receptors, which are present on vagal afferent neurons originating in the nodose ganglia, spinal afferents originating in the DRG, enteric neurons, and other cells of the gut. 5-HT–evoked excitation of extrinsic sensory neurons is primarily mediated by $5-HT_3$ receptors (10,12,18). Antagonism of $5-HT_3$ receptor–mediated stimulation of vagal afferents inhibits emesis induced by release of 5-HT from enterochromaffin cells (10), and blockade of $5-HT_3$ receptor–mediated activation of spinal afferents by alosetron depresses the afferent signaling of colorectal distension in the rat (19). Accordingly, alosetron has been found to reduce the discomfort and pain in female patients suffering from functional dyspepsia or diarrhea-predominant IBS to a moderate, but significant extent (12). However, the beneficial effect of alosetron is limited by its propensity to cause constipation and to increase the incidence of ischemic colitis in IBS patients (12). It remains to be seen whether other $5-HT_3$ receptor antagonists such as cilansetron will fare better in this respect.

The partial $5-HT_4$ receptor agonist tegaserod has been approved for the treatment of constipation-predominant IBS. While stimulating colonic transit, tegaserod also seems to reduce pain and other symptoms in female patients with constipation-predominant IBS (12) and to attenuate the pain evoked by rectal distension in healthy subjects (20). This antinociceptive activity of tegaserod is in line with experimental studies in which the drug has been found to inhibit the afferent signaling of colorectal distension in the rat and cat, particularly if there is inflammation in the colon (21,22). The mechanism behind this action of tegaserod is little understood, much as it is unknown whether blockade of $5-HT_{2B}$ receptors (23) contributes to its therapeutic profile. Novel insights into tegaserod's mode of action may come from the finding that 5-HT can sensitize polymodal DRG neurons innervating the mouse colon, this effect being mediated by metabotropic $5-HT_2$ and $5-HT_4$ receptors and TRPV1 (24). $5-HT_{1B/D}$ receptor agonists such as sumatriptan have been reported to relax the stomach, which may indirectly contribute to its discomfort-relieving effect in functional dyspepsia (12). $5-HT_3$ receptor antagonists likewise relax the intestine, an effect that may be a factor in their ability to reduce abdominal pain. It is also conceivable that $5-HT_7$ receptors participate in visceral nociception, because these receptors are present on dorsal root ganglion neurons with a putative role in nociception (25).

Cholecystokinin CCK_1 Receptors

Cholecystokinin (CCK) is both a hormone released from duodenal endocrine cells and an enteric neurotransmitter. CCK excites vagal afferents (26), which express predominantly CCK_1 receptors (27–30). These receptors may be relevant targets for the treatment of functional dyspepsia, since the CCK_1 receptor antagonist dexloxiglumide attenuates the meal-like fullness and nausea associated with intraduodenal lipid administration during gastric distension of normal volunteers and dyspeptic patients (31). Since in IBS patients CCK causes exaggerated intestinal motor responses and abdominal pain (32,33) and intestinal infection and inflammation causes upregulation of the CCK system (34,35), it is thought that CCK_1 receptor antagonists may also be beneficial in IBS (36).

Somatostatin Receptors

Somatostatin in the gut is expressed by both endocrine D cells and neurons. An implication of somatostatin in GI pain has been deduced from the ability of octreotide, a long-acting analog of somatostatin, to reduce the perception of gastric and rectal distension in healthy volunteers and IBS patients (37–43). Since octreotide increases discomfort thresholds in IBS patients, but not controls, at baseline and during experimentally induced hyperalgesia, it has been proposed that octreotide exerts primarily an antihyperalgesic rather than an analgesic effect (43). This effect could take place both at a peripheral and at a central site of action. Thus, somatostatin sst_2 receptor activation by octreotide inhibits the activity of chemo- and mechanosensitive spinal afferent nerve fibers innervating the rat jejunum (44), and the heptapeptide analog of somatostatin, TT-232, inhibits phenylquinone-induced writhing by a peripheral site of action (45). On the other hand, mechanonociception in the rat colon is inhibited by octreotide via a target within the spinal cord (46).

Prostaglandin Receptors

Inflammation induces the synthesis of large quantities of prostaglandins (PGs) through cyclooxygenase-2, and PGs such as PGE_2 and PGI_2 are key mediators of inflammatory hyperalgesia. As suppression of PG production in the gut by cyclooxygenase inhibitors carries the risk of severe GI mucosal damage, blockade of PG receptors expressed by sensory neurons appears to be an alternative way of preventing the proalgesic action of PGs. Primary sensory neurons express PG receptors of the EP_1, EP_2, EP_{3C}, EP_4, and IP type (47–51), and PGE_2 excites mesenteric afferent nerve fibers supplying the rat jejunum by a direct action on neuronal EP_1 receptors (52). In addition, PGs sensitize abdominal afferents to other algesic chemicals such as bradykinin (53). Experiments with isolated or cultured DRG neurons indicate that EP_1, EP_2, EP_{3C}, and EP_4 receptors contribute to the PGE_2-induced sensitization of sensory neurons (48–50). Likewise, EP_3 and IP receptors participate in the endotoxin-evoked sensitization of peritoneal afferents in mice as assessed by the writhing response to intraperitoneal acetic acid (54). The acid-induced sensitization of the human esophagus to electrically induced pain is attenuated by the EP_1 receptor antagonist ZD6416 (55). However, the implication of PG receptors in experimental models of FBDs has not yet been explored.

Bradykinin Receptors

Bradykinin is a proinflammatory and algesic mediator that can act via two types of receptor, B_1 and B_2 (56). While the acute effects of bradykinin are mediated by B_2 receptors, B_1 receptors come into play in chronic inflammatory processes and persistent hyperalgesia. There is experimental evidence that bradykinin contributes to visceral pain, given that intraperitoneal bradykinin gives rise to abdominal constriction responses (57) and to cardiovascular and gastric reflex responses (58). These reactions are brought about by the activation of B_2 receptors and most likely related to the kinin's ability to stimulate serosal afferents from the intestine (53,59). The bradykinin B_2 receptor–mediated excitation of afferent nerve fibers in the mesentery is augmented by PGE_2, adenosine, and histamine (53,60), while, vice versa, bradykinin can enhance the activity of TRPV1 (61,62). The potential of bradykinin receptor blockade in visceral hyperalgesia (63) is borne out by a number of experimental studies. For instance, genetic knockout of neutral endopeptidase, an enzyme that cleaves bradykinin, leads to peritoneal hyperalgesia that is reduced by the B_2 receptor antagonist icatibant (64). Icatibant likewise counteracts the inflammation-induced increase in the abdominal constriction response to colorectal distension and intraperitoneal acetic acid (65). In a model of nematode-induced intestinal infection, it has been shown that both B_1 and B_2 receptor antagonists can attenuate the postinfection hypersensitivity to jejunal distension (66). Interstitial cystitis is associated with enhanced levels of bradykinin in the urine (67), and experimental cystitis leads to upregulation of B_1 and B_2 receptors in the urothelium (68). A role of bradykinin in the pathophysiology of cystitis can be concluded from the findings that the hyperreflexia of the detrusor muscle caused by experimental cystitis is reduced by both B_1 and B_2 receptor antagonists, B_1 receptor antagonists having an effect only after inflammation has set in (68–70).

Protease-Activated Receptors

Protease-activated receptors (PARs) of type PAR-1 and PAR-2 are expressed by DRG neurons containing CGRP and substance P (71–73). However, the role of PAR-1 and PAR-2 in visceral nociception is different, PAR-1 being antinociceptive, whereas PAR-2 is pronociceptive. Thus, PAR-1 agonists inhibit the pain responses elicited by intraperitoneal injection of acetic acid, colorectal distension, or intracolonic administration of capsaicin (73,74). In contrast, PAR-2 agonists excite spinal afferents in rat jejunal mesenteric nerves (75) and release CGRP from DRG neurons in culture (76). Likewise, administration of subinflammatory doses of trypsin or a synthetic PAR-2 agonist into the pancreatic duct or into the colon elicits afferent input to the spinal cord, as visualized by *c-fos* expression, and evokes a behavioral pain response (76–78). In addition, activation of PAR-2 gives rise to delayed and prolonged visceral hyperalgesia. Thus, stimulation of mucosal PAR-2 in the rat colon enhances the visceromotor response to colorectal distension (77), and administration of a PAR-2 agonist into the rat pancreatic duct or mouse colon sensitizes spinal afferents to the excitatory effect of capsaicin (74,76). The hypersensitivity to capsaicin appears to arise from a cross talk between PAR-2 and TRPV1 mediated by protein kinase C (79,80).

From these findings, it would appear that PAR-2 antagonists have potential in the control of visceral pain and hyperalgesia. In addition, they may have anti-inflammatory activity, given that the levels of the PAR-2 agonists trypsin and mast cell tryptase are elevated in the colon of inflammatory bowel disease patients, and administration of PAR-2 agonists into the mouse colon induces inflammation via a mechanism involving sensory neurons (81,82). Furthermore, exposure of the mouse colon to a PAR-2 agonist enhances the expression of PAR-2 mRNA (81) much as the expression of PAR-2 on colonic mast cells is upregulated in ulcerative colitis (83). The available evidence indicates that the proalgesic and proinflammatory effects of PAR-2 activation are not necessarily interrelated, given that pain and hyperalgesia can be evoked by subinflammatory doses of PAR-2 agonists (76–78). PAR-1 antagonists may likewise display anti-inflammatory activity, given that PAR-1 stimulation induces intestinal inflammation, and PAR-1 has been implicated in inflammatory bowel disease (84). It is, at present, difficult to say, however, whether PAR-2 antagonists are useful therapeutics for GI hyperalgesia, given that these receptors are also present on enteric neurons and GI effector cells and play a role in normal digestive functions (71–73,85).

Ionotropic Purinoceptors

P2X purinoceptors are ligand-gated membrane cation channels that open when extracellular adenosine triphosphate (ATP) is bound. They are assembled as homo- or heteromultimers of several subunits, seven of which ($P2X_1$–$P2X_7$) have been identified at the gene and protein level (86,87). The P2X receptors on nodose ganglion neurons and DRG neurons projecting to the urinary bladder via the pelvic nerves comprise predominantly homomultimeric $P2X_2$ and some heteromultimeric $P2X_{2/3}$ receptors, whereas on other DRG neurons homomultimeric $P2X_3$ prevail over heteromultimeric $P2X_{2/3}$ receptors (86,88). ATP is released from a number of cellular sources in response to both physiologic and pathologic stimuli and excites vagal, mesenteric, and pelvic afferent neurons of the rat via the activation of P2X receptors (87,89–93). These receptors are hence potential targets for controlling visceral sensation. For instance, ATP seems to be relevant to mechanosensory transduction in the colorectum, ureter, and urinary bladder where ATP released from epithelial cells by distension activates P2X receptors on pelvic afferents and thereby contributes to the reflex regulation of micturition and colorectal function (90–92,94,95).

An implication of P2X receptors in GI nociception may be inferred from the observations that (i) following pepsin-induced inflammation of the ferret esophagus, ATP sensitizes vagal afferents to mechanical stimuli (96), (ii) $P2X_2$ homo- and heteromultimers are sensitized by acidosis (87,97), and (iii) P2X receptors on sensory neurons are upregulated by experimental inflammation (98). Likewise, interstitial cystitis leads to an increased expression of $P2X_2$ and $P2X_3$ protein in the urothelium (99), and inflammatory bowel disease is associated with an increased number of $P2X_3$ receptors in the colon (100). Pharmacologic evidence points to a role of P2X receptors in abdominal chemonociception, since trinitrophenyl-ATP (a $P2X_1$, $P2X_3$, and $P2X_{2/3}$ receptor blocker) and A-317491 (a non-nucleotide $P2X_3$ and $P2X_{2/3}$ receptor antagonist) suppress the nociceptive behavior provoked by intraperitoneal injection of acetic acid in mice (101,102). In contrast, the visceromotor pain response to colonic distension in the rat and the colitis-induced mechanical hyperalgesia are not attenuated by A-317491 (102). The further evaluation of the therapeutic potential of $P2X_3$ and $P2X_{2/3}$ receptors in acid-related, inflammation-, and ischemia-induced disturbances of gut sensation will need to take account of the presence of P2X receptors on enteric neurons and GI smooth muscle cells (86,93), which may limit their selectivity of action.

Transient Receptor Potential Ion Channels of Vanilloid Type 1

The superfamily of transient receptor potential (TRP) ion channels (103) represents a hot spot in the current research on sensory transduction mechanisms. TRP channels have evolved as an ancient sensory apparatus of the cell, responding to temperature, touch, sound, osmolarity, pH, and various chemical messengers (103). One of the many remarkable properties of TRP channels is that TRPV1, TRPV2, TRPV3, TRPV4, TRPM8, and TRPA1 are thermosensors that cover the full range of temperatures from noxious cold to noxious heat (104). The existence of the "capsaicin receptor" TRPV1, which originally was named VR1 (105), has long been envisaged on the basis of the sensory neuron–selective actions of capsaicin (106,107). Like other TRP channels, functional TRPV1 channels are thought to be homo/heterotetramers that operate as nonselective cation channels with high permeability for Ca^{2+} (103). Importantly, TRPV1 behaves as a polymodal nociceptor that is excited by noxious heat, ligands containing a vanillyl moiety such as capsaicin and resiniferatoxin, H^+ ions, and a variety of arachidonic acid–derived lipid mediators (108–112). Both heat and the chemical ligands appear to activate TRPV1 by shifting its voltage-dependent activation curve (113).

In the urinary tract, TRPV1 is contained both in afferent nerve terminals and in the urothelium (114), whereas in the gut, TRPV1 appears to be exclusively associated with primary afferent neurons (112). This inference has been proved by immunohistochemical studies in the rat, guinea pig, and mouse GI tract in which numerous TRPV1-positive nerve fibers occur in the musculature, enteric nerve plexuses, and mucosa (115–119). Since enteric neurons do not stain for TRPV1, it follows that the TRPV1-positive nerve fibers in the intestine represent processes of spinal afferents and, in the stomach, of some vagal afferents (115–117,119,120). Further analysis has revealed that the majority of nodose ganglion neurons projecting to the stomach and of DRG neurons projecting to the gut and urinary tract of rats express TRPV1 (118,119,121). It remains to be elucidated whether the TRPV1-like immunoreactivity, which some investigators have seen in guinea pig, porcine, and human enteric neurons and rat gastric epithelial cells (122–125), is authentic TRPV1 or represents a nonfunctional protein such as TRPV1-β derived from alternative splicing of the *trpv1* gene (126).

Capsaicin-induced gating of TRPV1 stimulates extrinsic afferents of the gut (53,127–129) and gives rise to GI pain in humans (130,131) and mice (132,133). Genetic deletion of TRPV1 abolishes the sensitivity of jejunal afferent neurons to capsaicin and reduces their responsivity to acid and distension, similar effects being seen with the TRPV1 blocker capsazepine (129). Furthermore, there is evidence that TRPV1 contributes to GI hypersensitivity as shown for DRG neurons innervating the mouse colon. The 5-HT–induced sensitization of these neurons to heat, acid, and capsaicin is absent in TRPV1 knockout mice (24). Further analysis has revealed that the effect of 5-HT to sensitize colonic DRG neurons is mediated by metabotropic $5-HT_2$ and $5-HT_4$ receptors, which appear to enhance TRPV1 activity by downstream phosphorylation pathways (24). This finding is in keeping with the concept that TRPV1 is a key molecule in afferent neuron hypersensitivity, because its activity is regulated by many proalgesic pathways. For instance, activation of PGE_2 or bradykinin B_2 receptors can sensitize TRPV1 through phosphorylation of the channel or other mechanisms and thereby enhance the probability of channel gating by heat and other stimuli (61,62). Mild acidosis (pH 7 to 6) likewise sensitizes TRPV1, whereas a fall of the extracellular pH below 6 directly gates the channel (108). A common result of these sensitization processes is that the temperature threshold for TRPV1 activation (43 °C) is lowered to a level permissive for channel gating at normal body temperature (134). The relevance of TRPV1 to inflammatory hyperalgesia is borne out by the finding that TRPV1 knockout mice do not develop thermal hyperalgesia in response to experimental inflammation (135,136).

As a consequence, suppression of TRPV1 activity is explored as a possible strategy to treat visceral hyperalgesia. Given that TRPV1-like immunoreactivity is upregulated in esophagitis (137), painful inflammatory bowel disease (138), rectal hypersensitivity, fecal urgency (125), and neurogenic bladder overactivity (139), one therapeutic approach is to dampen the activity of TRPV1 as well as of the sensory neurons expressing TRPV1 by overstimulation with TRPV1 agonists. It has long been known that stimulation of TRPV1 by excess capsaicin or resiniferatoxin is followed by a state of sensory refractoriness (106), which is associated with downregulation of TRPV1 (107,139). Such a state of functional desensitization can be achieved by systemic administration of high doses of capsaicin to experimental animals or by repeated topical administration of moderate doses of capsaicin or resiniferatoxin to humans. Capsaicin pretreatment of rats blocks the visceromotor response to gastric acid challenge (140), suppresses the cardiovascular pain response to noxious jejunal distension in the rat (141), and prevents the inflammation-induced hypersensitivity to colonic distension (142,143). Chronic administration of capsaicin or resiniferatoxin is also beneficial in patients with urinary bladder pain, urinary bladder hyperreflexia (139,144,145), or GI hyperalgesia. For instance, intractable idiopathic pruritus ani can be relieved by a four-week treatment course with topical capsaicin (146), and daily intragastric administration of red pepper containing capsaicin for five weeks significantly reduces epigastric pain and other symptoms of functional dyspepsia (147).

A disadvantage of the TRPV1 agonist therapy with capsaicin is its initial pungency, which may involve a transient exacerbation of dyspeptic and IBS symptoms (147,148). Consequently, TRPV1 agonists such as SDZ 249–665, which cause little excitation of sensory neurons but effectively induce sensory neuron refractoriness, have been developed (144). SDZ 249–665 is able to inhibit the visceromotor pain response to intraperitoneal administration of acetic acid (149) and to attenuate the hyperreflexia and referred hyperalgesia associated with experimental inflammation of the rat urinary bladder (150). Another approach that is actively pursued is the development of TRPV1 blockers, which would prevent nociceptive afferents from being activated by stimuli that involve TRPV1 (112,144). Following the discovery of capsazepine more than a decade ago (151), several new TRPV1 blockers have been discovered in the past years (112). Apart from being antihyperalgesic, these drugs may also have anti-inflammatory activity, given that, in rodents, TRPV1 appears to be involved in the ileitis evoked by *Clostridium difficile* toxin A (152) and in the colitis elicited by dextran sulphate sodium (153,154). In developing TRPV1 blockers as drugs, there is one caveat to be considered, however, inasmuch as TRPV1-bearing afferent neurons also subserve a protective role in the GI mucosa (120,155). The challenge, therefore, is to find out whether TRPV1-mediated GI inflammation and hyperalgesia can pharmacologically be differentiated from TRPV1 involved in GI mucosal protection (156).

Acid-Sensing Ion Channels

Acid-sensing ion channels (ASICs) are voltage-insensitive Na^+ channels that are encoded by four different genes: ASIC1, ASIC2, ASIC3, and ASIC4 (97,157–159). ASIC1 and ASIC2 each have alternative splice variants termed "ASIC1a" and "ASIC1b" as well as ASIC2a and ASIC2b. Functional channels are made up of different ASIC subunits, most of which are expressed by primary afferent neurons, although to different degrees (160,161). Importantly, ASIC2b, which is inactive as a homomultimer, can form functional heteromultimers with other ASIC subunits, particularly ASIC3, which is exclusively expressed by small and large DRG cells (157,160–162) and, for this reason, is also termed "DRASIC." As their name implies, ASIC1, ASIC2 and ASIC3 are gated by a drop in the external pH below 6.9 (97,157–159). In addition, ASICs are mechanoreceptors (159,163), and studies involving deletion of the ASIC2 and ASIC3 genes point to a role in the transduction of low- and high-threshold mechanosensation in the skin, respectively (164–166). ASIC1, to the contrary, does not contribute to cutaneous mechanotransduction, but plays a role in visceral mechanoreceptor function, given that ASIC1 gene knockout results in increased mechanosensitivity of gastroesophageal and colonic afferent neurons (167). Although an implication in visceral pain has remained unexplored, ASICs could conceivably participate in GI hypersensitivity to mechanical and chemical noxae (97). A role in GI pathology may also be envisaged from the upregulation of ASIC3, but not ASIC1 and ASIC2, in inflammatory bowel disease (168) and the stimulation of ASIC3 transcription by nerve growth factor and proinflammatory mediators such as 5-HT, interleukin-1, and bradykinin (169).

Acid-Sensitive Background K$^+$ Channels

Besides TRPV1 and ASICs, two-pore (or tandem-pore) domain potassium (KCNK) channels may function as chemo- and mechanosensors of afferent neurons. Thus, many members of this family belonging to the tandem of pore domains in a weak inwardly rectifying K$^+$ channel (TWIK), TWIK-related K$^+$ channel (TREK), TWIK-related acid sensitive K$^+$ channel (TASK), and TWIK-related arachidonic acid-stimulated K$^+$ channel (TRAAK) subfamilies are found in DRG neurons and in the GI tract of humans and rats (97). Their basic function is to operate as background channels that play a role in setting the resting membrane potential and the excitability of neurons (170,171). In addition, several KCNK channels are extremely sensitive to variations in the extracellular or intracellular pH in a narrow physiologic range (97). Some of them, such as TREK, are also mechanosensitive (172,173).

Mechanosensitive Ion Channels

Low- and high-threshold mechanosensitive afferents innervate all regions of the alimentary canal and have the ability to sensitize in response to inflammatory mediators (4,174). Their mechanosensitivity depends on the presence of sensors that detect stretch, contraction, or other mechanical deformations of the gut wall. One of these sensors, a mechanosensitive K$^+$ channel, has been characterized by single-channel recordings from sensory neurons in the rat colon (175). DRG neurons innervating the stomach and colon exhibit stretch-sensitive calcium fluxes that are inhibited by gadolinium, a blocker of mechanosensitive ion channels (176). Other mechanosensitive ion channels comprise ASIC1, ASIC2, ASIC3 (163–166), TRPV4 (177), and members of the KCNK channels such as TREK-2 (172). It is uncertain whether blockade of mechanosensitive ion channels is of therapeutic utility, given that mechanically triggered motor and secretory reflexes regulating digestion may also be impaired.

ION CHANNELS REGULATING SENSORY NERVE EXCITABILITY, CONDUCTION, AND TRANSMISSION
Sensory Neuron-Specific Na$^+$ Channels

Voltage-gated Na$^+$ channels, composed of one pore-forming α-subunit and one or more auxiliary β-subunits, are crucial for neuronal excitability and propagation of action potentials (178,179). Among the 10 known α-subunits are two tetrodotoxin-resistant Na$^+$ channels, Na$_v$1.8 (previously termed SNS/PN3) and Na$_v$1.9 (SNS2/NaN) and one tetrodotoxin-sensitive Na$^+$ channel, Na$_v$1.7 (PN1), that are preferentially expressed by nociceptive DRG neurons (178–182). Tetrodotoxin-resistant Na$^+$ currents are also present in vagal and spinal afferent neurons supplying the rat stomach (183) and in DRG neurons projecting to the rat ileum and colon (127,184–186). There is mounting evidence that tetrodotoxin-resistant Na$^+$ channels play a role in neuropathic and inflammatory hyperalgesia (178,179). Experimental gastritis and trinitrobenzene sulphonic acid (TNBSA)-induced ileitis enhance the excitability of DRG neurons predominantly via an increase of Na$_v$1.8 currents (183,186,187). Similar alterations in vagal afferents are seen in rats with acetic acid–induced gastric ulcers (188). The upregulation of tetrodotoxin-resistant Na$^+$ currents in DRG neurons following GI inflammation and injury involves nerve growth factor and proinflammatory mediators such as PGE$_2$ (184,189,190).

Antisense probe–induced inhibition of Na$_v$1.8 expression in rat spinal afferents prevents the effect of intravesical acetic acid to induce urinary bladder hyperalgesia (191). Null mutation of the Na$_v$1.8 gene does not alter behavioral pain responses to acute noxious stimulation of abdominal viscera, but attenuates the behavioral reactions to colonic sensitization by capsaicin or mustard oil and prevents referred hyperalgesia (192). It would seem, therefore, that tetrodotoxin-resistant Na$^+$ channels, particularly Na$_v$1.8, constitute a new target for the treatment of visceral hyperalgesia due to inflammation. While selective blockers for tetrodotoxin-resistant Na^+ channels have not yet been disclosed, nonselective inhibitors of voltage-gated Na^+ channels such as lidocaine (193,194), mexiletine, and carbamazepine (195) suppress the central signaling of colonic distension by spinal afferents. It has been suggested that the analgesic effect of the antidepressant drug amitryptiline may also arise from a use-dependent block of voltage-dependent Na^+ channels on sensory neurons (196).

Sensory Neuron–Specific K^+ Channels

Pathologic hyperexcitability of sensory neurons can, conceivably, result from downregulation of voltage-gated potassium (K_v) channels whose function is to repolarize the cell membrane (197,198). Some of these channels such as $K_v1.4$ appear to be selectively expressed by nociceptive afferent neurons (199). TNBSA-induced ileitis increases the excitability and conduction velocity in nociceptive DRG neurons, a change that is in part attributed to a decrease in the transient A-type and sustained outward rectifier K^+ currents (185,186). Acetic acid–induced gastric ulceration leads to a similar rise of excitability and fall of A-type K^+ current density in spinal and vagal afferents innervating the rat stomach (200). Pharmacologic enhancement of A-type K^+ currents would hence be expected to counteract hyperalgesia, a mode of action whereby compound KW-7158 depresses the excitability of pelvic afferents and inhibits inflammation-induced bladder overactivity (201).

Sensory Neuron–Specific Ca^{2+} Channels

The contention that certain voltage-gated Ca^{2+} channels on sensory neurons are of relevance to visceral pain is based on the antinociceptive effect of gabapentin and pregabalin, two anticonvulsant drugs with high affinity for the $\alpha2\delta1$ Ca^{2+} channel subunit in DRG neurons (197,202,203). Gabapentin and pregabalin are able to counteract the colonic hyperalgesia elicited by septic shock (204) and inflammation due to TNBSA (205). The writhing response to intraperitoneal injection of acetic acid is also inhibited by gabapentin (206). Since pregabalin does not alter the visceromotor response to distension of the normal colon (205), it is inferred that pregabalin-sensitive Ca^{2+} channels play a specific role in inflammation-evoked sensitization of GI afferents. Another Ca^{2+} channel targeted by analgesic drugs is the high voltage-gated N-type Ca^{2+} channel, which is of paramount importance for transmitter release. Inhibition of this channel by intrathecal administration of ziconotide affords relief from chronic pain by blocking transmitter release from the central terminals of spinal afferent neurons (207). In this way, ziconotide also suppresses the spinal transmission of nociceptive information from mesenteric afferents (208).

RECEPTORS RELEVANT TO AFFERENT NEURON TRANSMISSION
Glutamate Receptors

Glutamate is thought to be the principal transmitter of vagal and spinal afferent neurons (3,209). Glutamatergic transmission between primary afferents and secondary projection neurons in the spinal cord and brain stem is accomplished via ionotropic N-methyl-D-aspartate (NMDA), α-amino-3-hydroxy-5-methyl-4-isoxazolepropionic acid (AMPA) and kainate receptors as well as group I metabotropic receptors of subtype 1 and 5 (3,209). In addition, primary afferent neurons themselves express glutamate receptors that are transported into their peripheral axons. These receptors include ionotropic receptors of the NMDA, AMPA, and kainate type (210,211), group I metabotropic glutamate receptors of subtype 1 and 5 (mGluR5) (212,213), and group II metabotropic receptors of subtype 2 and 3 (214). The NR1 subunit of NMDA receptors has also been localized to spinal afferent nerve fibers in the rat colon (211).

Antagonists of both NMDA and non-NMDA ionotropic glutamate receptors reduce the spinal input evoked by noxious colorectal distension in rats (211,215–217) and counteract the mechanical hyperalgesia induced by colonic inflammation (218). The colorectal hypersensitivity induced by repeated distension (219) and the behavioral pain response to bradykinin in experimental pancreatitis (220) are inhibited by intraspinal administration of an NMDA receptor antagonist. NMDA receptors do not appear to mediate the normal micturition reflex at the spinal cord level but contribute to the hyperreflexia that develops after induction of urinary bladder inflammation (221). A similar enhancement of NMDA receptor function in the spinal cord is seen following repeated colorectal distension, a condition that induces inflammation (215,217). In addition, there is evidence that group I metabotropic glutamate receptors participate in visceral pain, given that mGluR5 antagonists depress the neurochemical and behavioral pain responses to intraperitoneal injection of acetic acid (222–224). Glutamate receptors likewise play a role in vagal afferent transmission within the brain stem (3). Non-NMDA ionotropic glutamate receptors participate in cisplatin-induced emesis in ferrets (225), whereas both NMDA and AMPA/kainate receptors contribute to the activation of brain stem neurons in response to gastric distension or intraduodenal administration of nutrients (226–228). The afferent signaling of an acute gastric mucosal acid insult to the rat brain stem remains unaltered by NMDA and non-NMDA ionotropic glutamate receptor antagonists (229). When, however, the stomach is repeatedly injured by acid, a role of NMDA receptors in the communication from the acid-threatened stomach to the brain stem becomes obvious (229).

The presence of NMDA receptors on spinal afferent nerve fibers innervating the rat colon hints at a new possibility to control visceral pain, which is borne out by the observation that the NMDA receptor antagonist memantine inhibits the excitation of pelvic afferents due to colorectal distension (211). It has been hypothesized, therefore, that the memantine-induced inhibition of the visceromotor response to colorectal distension arises from the blockade of NMDA receptors on the peripheral axons of sensory neurons (211). This inference is corroborated by the finding that intrathecal administration of the NMDA receptor antagonist MK-801 fails to alter the visceromotor pain response to distension of the noninflamed colon (217). It is not clear, however, whether blockade of peripheral NMDA receptors is sufficient to counteract visceral hyperalgesia; the exaggerated visceromotor pain response to distension of the zymosan-inflamed colon is inhibited by intrathecal injection of MK-801 (217).

The utility of brain-penetrable NMDA receptor antagonists in pain therapy has remained limited because of their adverse actions on brain function (230). Consequently, attempts are made to develop NMDA receptor antagonists that prevent the pathologic activation of NMDA receptors but allow their physiologic activation (231). This goal may be approached by designing moderate affinity blockers that selectively target the glycine$_B$ or NR2B site of the NMDA receptors (231). Other developments relate to glutamate receptor antagonists with a peripherally restricted site of action and to antagonists of non-NMDA ionotropic and metabotropic glutamate receptors with a role in pain (211,232,233). In pursuing this approach, it is important to realize, however, that glutamate receptors are expressed by enteric neurons and participate in enteric neurotransmission (211,234) and that hence glutamate receptor antagonists may interfere with normal digestive function.

Calcitonin Gene–Related Peptide Receptors

Almost all DRG neurons supplying the viscera of the rat, mouse, and guinea pig express CGRP (2,118,235,236), and there is experimental evidence that this peptide contributes to visceral pain in two different ways. First, intraperitoneal administration of exogenous CGRP or acetic acid–induced release of endogenous CGRP triggers a visceromotor pain reaction (237–239). These findings suggest that, within the peritoneal cavity, CGRP triggers events that indirectly increase the sensory gain of primary afferent neurons (63). Second, CGRP appears to be a cotransmitter of spinal afferents involved in visceral pain and hyperalgesia. Thus, the visceromotor pain response that rats exhibit following colorectal distension or intraperitoneal injection of acetic acid is attenuated by CGRP receptor blockade (142,238). More importantly, the mechanical hyperalgesia in the rat colon due to acetic acid–induced inflammation or repeated distension is reversed by the CGRP receptor antagonist CGRP$_{8-37}$ (142,240). Since in this respect intrathecal administration of CGRP$_{8-37}$ is more potent than intravenous administration of the CGRP receptor antagonist or a monoclonal CGRP antibody, it has been concluded that the site of CGRP-mediated hyperalgesia is primarily in the spinal cord (240). The available evidence indicates, therefore, that CGRP receptor antagonists have potential in the treatment of visceral hyperalgesia. This conjecture is corroborated by the discovery that the nonpeptide CGRP receptor antagonist BIBN 4096 BS is effective in the treatment of acute migraine attacks (241).

Tachykinin Receptors

Most DRG neurons supplying the visceral organs of rodents contain substance P and neurokinin A, and tachykinin NK$_1$, NK$_2$, and NK$_3$ receptors are expressed at many levels of the gut–brain axis (242–244). A double-blind pilot study has shown that the tachykinin NK$_1$

Table 4 Effects of Tachykinin Receptor Blockade or Deletion in Experimental Models of Visceral Hyperalgesia and Pain

Beneficial effects of NK$_1$ receptor blockade or deletion
  Cardiovascular pain response to peritoneal irritation and jejunal distension in rats
  Visceromotor pain response to colonic distension in rats
  Mechanical hyperalgesia caused by repeated noxious colonic distension in rats
  Stress-induced hypersensitivity to noxious colonic distension in rats
  Cardiovascular pain response to colonic irritation by capsaicin or acetic acid in mice
  Mechanical hyperalgesia in irritated colon of mice
  Inflammation-induced hypersensitivity to noxious colonic distension in rabbits
Beneficial effects of NK$_2$ receptor blockade
  Cardiovascular pain response to peritoneal irritation and jejunal distension in rats
  Visceromotor pain response to gastric and colorectal distension in rats
  Enhanced *c-fos* expression in spinal cord after trinitrobenzene sulphonic acid–induced irritation of rat colon
  Inflammation- and stress-induced hypersensitivity to noxious rectal distension in rats
  Enhanced firing of lumbosacral afferents after distension of inflamed rat colon
  Infection-induced hypersensitivity to noxious jejunal distension in rats
Beneficial effects of NK$_3$ receptor blockade
  Visceromotor pain response to colorectal distension in rats
  Inflammation-induced hypersensitivity to noxious colorectal distension in rats
  Mechanical hyperalgesia caused by repeated noxious colonic distension in rats

receptor antagonist CJ-11,974 reduces IBS symptoms and attenuates the emotional response to rectosigmoid distension (245). These observations are in keeping with preclinical studies that attest to a role of tachykinin receptors in visceral pain and hyperalgesia (Table 4) (242–244). For instance, genetic deletion of NK$_1$ receptors in mice prevents intracolonic acetic acid and capsaicin from inducing primary mechanical hyperalgesia in the colon and referred mechanical hyperalgesia in the abdominal skin (246). In addition, NK$_1$ receptor–deficient mice fail to respond to intracolonic acetic acid and capsaicin with cardiovascular responses indicative of pain, whereas the reaction to distension is normal (246).

Experimental studies with selective tachykinin receptor antagonists indicate that all three tachykinin receptors play a role in visceral nociception and inflammation-induced hyperalgesia (242–244). The visceromotor pain response to gastric and colorectal distension in the rat is inhibited by NK$_2$ and NK$_3$ receptor antagonists but left unaltered by NK$_1$ receptor antagonists (247–252). In contrast, the inflammation- or stress-induced colonic hypersensitivity to colorectal distension in the rabbit, rat, and guinea pig is reduced by NK$_1$ receptor antagonists (253–256). The cardiovascular reaction to jejunal distension in the absence of intestinal infection and the analogous reaction to peritoneal irritation are attenuated by both NK$_1$ and NK$_2$ receptor antagonists (238,257,258). The inflammation- and stress-induced hypersensitivity to rectal distension is largely prevented by an NK$_2$ receptor antagonist (249), and the cardiovascular reaction to jejunal distension, which is exaggerated in rats infected with *Nippostrongylus brasiliensis*, is likewise normalized by an NK$_2$ receptor antagonist (259).

Tachykinin receptor antagonists may target multiple relays in the nociceptive pathways from the periphery to the brain. One site of action is within the spinal cord where tachykininergic transmission from primary afferents is interrupted. This appears to be true for the antihyperalgesic effect of the NK$_1$ receptor antagonist TAK-637 in the rabbit and guinea pig (253,255). One study reports that the visceromotor pain response to colorectal distension in rats and the hypersensitivity caused by repeated distension is blocked by intrathecal administration of an NK$_1$ or NK$_3$, but not NK$_2$, receptor antagonist (260). In another study, it has been found that the inflammation-induced hypersensitivity to noxious colorectal distension in rats is inhibited by the intrathecal administration of an NK$_3$ receptor antagonist or a combination of an NK$_1$ and NK$_2$ receptor antagonist, whereas NK$_1$ and NK$_2$ receptor antagonists given singly are without effect (261). These observations point to a site of action within the spinal cord and, in addition, suggest that the antinociceptive efficacy of multi-/pan-tachykinin receptor antagonists is superior to that of monoreceptor antagonists. Similarly, the afferent signaling of a noxious acid stimulus from the stomach to the rat brain stem is attenuated only by simultaneous administration of an NK$_1$, an NK$_2$, and a ionotropic NMDA-type glutamate receptor antagonist (229). Further consistent with a central site of the antinociceptive action of NK$_1$ receptor antagonists is the finding that experimental colitis or cystitis in the rat leads to an upregulation and de novo expression of NK_1 receptors in the dorsal horn of the spinal cord (262–264).

Apart from blocking tachykininergic transmission in the spinal cord, NK_1 and NK_2 receptor antagonists may be antihyperalgesic by a peripheral site of action on nociceptive afferents. Although the expression of tachykinin receptors by primary afferent nerve fibers remains to be clarified (243), the NK_2 receptor antagonist nepadutant has been observed to inhibit the enhanced firing, which lumbosacral afferent neurons exhibit after distension of the experimentally inflamed rat colon (250). Since the activity in pelvic and somatic afferent neurons is not affected, nepadutant has been proposed to be antihyperalgesic by a peripheral action on hypersensitive afferents supplying the colon (250). In addition, peripheral nepadutant suppresses the effect of acute irritation of the colon with TNBSA, but not non-noxious colorectal distension, to stimulate neurons in the spinal cord as visualized by *c-fos* expression (265). The effect of intraperitoneally injected tachykinin receptor agonists to elicit visceromotor pain reactions (238,266) and to increase vagal afferent nerve acticity via an NK_1 receptor–mediated mechanism (267) also point to an action on peripheral axons of afferent neurons. Part of these pronociceptive actions of tachykinins in the periphery may be indirect and due to their ability to modify GI motility and secretion and to promote inflammatory processes (243,244). This is true for tachykinin actions mediated by NK_1 and NK_2 receptors and, possibly, for those brought about by NK_3 receptors. The available evidence indicates that NK_3 receptor antagonists are antihyperalgesic both by a peripheral and by a central site of action. On the one hand, intrathecal administration of an NK_3 receptor antagonist effectively inhibits the visceromotor response to noxious distension of the inflamed or sensitized rat colon (260,261). On the other hand, systemic administration of the non—brain-penetrant NK_3 receptor antagonist SB-235375 is able to inhibit the visceromotor reaction to painful colorectal distension in rats without affecting colonic motility (252,268). Since mechanonociception in the skin is not affected, it has been proposed that NK_3 receptor antagonists exhibit intestine-specific antinociceptive activity (252).

Taken all experimental findings together, tachykinin receptor antagonists appear to have potential for the treatment of visceral pain and FBDs (Table 4) (242–244). This may, in particular, apply to IBS and other disorders where the tachykinin system is deranged in several ways. By correcting hyper- or hypomotility, hypersecretion and inflammation, tachykinin receptor antagonists may reduce the sensory gain of extrinsic afferents in the GI tract and, in addition, block tachykininergic transmission in the spinal cord. Furthermore, the effects of brain-penetrant NK_1 receptor antagonists at the level of the gut and afferent system may favorably combine with their inhibitory actions on emesis, anxiety, depression, and stress reactions in the brain (269,270). In extrapolating these preclinical observations to the development of effective drugs for visceral pain, it needs to be clarified which types of tachykinin receptors are most relevant in the initiation and/or maintenance of visceral pain syndromes in humans.

Opioid Receptors

Both spinal and vagal sensory neurons express different numbers of μ-, δ-, and κ-opioid receptors (271–274). Opioid receptors on the peripheral axons of nociceptive afferent neurons have attracted considerable interest, because activation of these receptors by drugs that do not enter the brain may afford analgesia without adverse effects on brain function (275). The treatment options provided by peripheral opioid receptors are discussed in Chapter III/19.

α_2-Adrenoceptors

Noradrenaline dampens pain pathways at several levels in the brain (276,277). In the spinal cord, it inhibits the transmission of nociceptive signals, because DRG neurons express α_2-adrenoceptors, which, in humans, are preferentially of the α_{2B} and α_{2C} subtype (278,279). Activation of these presynaptic α_2-adrenoceptors inhibits the release of glutamate and substance P from afferent nerve terminals in the rat spinal cord (280,281). This inhibitory effect appears to be mediated by the $\alpha_{2A/D}$ adrenoceptor subtype (282) and is likely to have a bearing on visceral pain. Thus, intrathecal administration of the α_2-adrenoceptor agonists clonidine, fadolmidine, or dexmedetomidine depresses the activation of spinal neurons by distension of the normal and inflamed colon (277,283). The effect of intrathecal fadolmidine is associated with only minor hypotensive and sedative side effects. Intrathecal clonidine also inhibits the cardiovascular pain responses evoked by noxious stimulation of the rat mesentery, an effect that is augmented by the N-type calcium channel blocker ziconotide (208). This antinociceptive activity is relevant to FBDs, given that clonidine is able to reduce the sensation and discomfort associated with gastric and colorectal distension (284,285). Likewise, antidepressant drugs can ameliorate the pain associated with FBDs (286,287), and there is some evidence that the antinociceptive effect of these drugs is related to the extracellular accumulation of noradrenaline acting mostly through α_2-adrenoceptors (288), although a peripheral action unrelated to inhibition of monoamine reuptake may also contribute (289).

Cannabinoid Receptors

The biological actions of exogenous and endogenous cannabinoids are brought about by the activation of two types of cannabinoid receptors, CB_1 and CB_2 (290,291). The implication of cannabinoids in pain mechanisms is related to the presence of CB_1, but not CB_2, receptors on DRG neurons (292,293). Synthesized in the somata, CB_1 receptors are transported not only to the central terminals of sensory neurons in the spinal cord, where their activation inhibits the release of substance P (294), but also to the peripheral terminals of sensory neurons (295), where their activation interferes with nerve excitation by noxious stimuli (296,297). Although activation of CB_1 receptors on peripheral and central vagal afferent pathways counteracts nausea and emesis, a particular aspect of GI discomfort (291), it is not yet clear whether cannabinoid receptor agonists have beneficial effects in visceral hyperalgesia. Owing to observations on somatic pain, it has been proposed that CB_1 receptor agonists may suppress nociception both at a peripheral and at a central level (298,299). If efficacious, cannabinoid receptor agonists with a peripherally restricted site of action would have the advantage of being devoid of psychotropic effects that follow the recruitment of central CB_1 receptors (291,296). Disadvantages may arise from the ability of CB_1 receptor agonists to interfere with enteric nerve function because CB_1 receptors are expressed by neurons of the myenteric and submucosal plexus (291,300).

It should not go unnoticed that there is some cross talk between cannabinoid receptors and TRPV1. Thus endocannabinoids such as anandamide can enhance TRPV1 activity via stimulation of protein kinase C (61). Vice versa, capsaicin-related compounds such as olvanil and arvanil, which are largely devoid of an excitatory influence on TRPV1, but induce a TRPV1-mediated state of sensory neuron refractoriness, are known to bind to CB_1 receptors (297). The ability of endocannabinoids to enhance TRPV1 activity may be the reason that under conditions of inflammation, endocannabinoids may actually contribute to visceral hyperalgesia. Thus, cyclophosphamide-induced cystitis enhances the anandamide content of the urinary bladder, which goes in parallel with the development of bladder hyperreflexia (301). The effect of anandamide to induce reflex hyperactivity in the bladder is prevented by the TRPV1 blocker capsazepine (301). In another study, it has been found, however, that anandamide prevents and reverses bladder hyperreflexia caused by turpentine-induced inflammation through blockade of CB_1 receptors and that peripheral CB_2 receptors also come into play in the inflamed tissue and mediate part of the antihyperalgesic effects of cannabinoid receptor agonists (302). Croton oil–induced inflammation of the mouse small intestine enhances endocannabinoid turnover, the expression of CB_1 receptors, and the potency of CB_1 receptor agonists to slow intestinal motility (303), but it is not known whether anandamide participates in GI hyperalgesia under these conditions.

CONCLUSIONS

There is now good reason to assume that visceral pain involves persistent sensitization of GI afferent neurons. Although central sensitization processes and a distorted processing and representation of the incoming information in the brain are also involved, the contribution made by sensory neurons should not be underestimated. It is via these afferents that the discomfort and pain localized to abdominal viscera is signaled to the brain. Furthermore, visceral sensory neurons are usually polymodal and all of them seem to have the capacity to sensitize (4). In view of these properties, it can be predicted that sensitization of visceral afferents by inflammatory events may tremendously increase the afferent input to the brain (4). If this state of exaggerated responses to peripheral stimuli persists after inflammation has

Table 5 Unsolved Issues in Visceral Pain Research

There is no animal model equivalent of painful functional bowel disorders, although it is possible to model individual symptoms.

The available animal models of visceral hyperalgesia do not assess the perception of pain but record pseudoaffective responses that are interpreted as being indicative of pain.

Reliable quantitation and analysis of pain perception and emotional-affective alterations in animals will require real-time functional brain imaging.

Most animal models of visceral pain (as well as clinical studies) are modality biased inasmuch as they assess only reactions to mechanical, but not chemical, stimuli.

The study of visceral pain has been focused on the spinal afferent innervation of the gut, while the emerging implication of vagal afferent pathways in foregut nociception has been neglected.

Nausea may be seen as a particular form of gastrointestinal discomfort and pain that is mediated by vagal afferents.

Sensory neuron-directed drugs will be efficacious in visceral pain only if visceral hyperalgesia is to a significant extent due to peripheral sensitization.

It is at present difficult to predict whether or not targeting a single receptor or ion channel on visceral afferents will be sufficient to manage visceral hyperalgesia.

subsided, physiologic processes in the alimentary canal may be interpreted by the brain as inappropriately painful (4). For all these reasons, afferent neurons represent an intriguing target at which to aim novel therapies for visceral discomfort and pain (1,10,304).

Efforts to identify molecular traits that are specific for sensory neurons and therefore hold potential for therapeutic exploitation have been remarkably successful (Table 3). These targets include, among others, TRPV1, ASICs (ASIC2b/3), tetrodotoxin-resistant Na^+ channels ($Na_v1.8$), and ionotropic purinoceptors ($P2X_{2/3}$ and $P2X_3$). Since many of these sensors and ion channels are selectively expressed by subpopulations of afferent neurons thought to subserve a nociceptive function, drugs directed at those targets may be antinociceptive without necessarily interfering with physiologic functions of afferent neurons. Changes in the expression and functional properties of sensory neuron-specific molecules in visceral hyperalgesia may add to the selectivity of drugs directed at these molecules. This concept is borne out by observations that blockade of certain sensory neuron-specific targets reverses experimentally induced visceral hyperalgesia but does not influence acute nociception. In addition, selectivity for targets on nociceptive afferent neurons, and preferentially to visceral but not somatic afferents, will be a considerable asset for drug safety. However, despite the identification of sensory neuron-specific drug targets, there is a number of issues that need to be resolved before these advances in basic research can be translated to the development of efficacious and safe drugs for visceral pain (Table 5).

REFERENCES

1. Holzer P. Gastrointestinal pain in functional bowel disorders: sensory neurons as novel drug targets. Expert Opin Ther Targets 2004; 8:107–123.
2. Perry MJ, Lawson SN. Differences in expression of oligosaccharides, neuropeptides, carbonic anhydrase and neurofilament in rat primary afferent neurons retrogradely labelled via skin, muscle or visceral nerves. Neuroscience 1998; 85:293–310.
3. Hornby PJ. Receptors and transmission in the brain-gut axis. II. Excitatory amino acid receptors in the brain-gut axis. Am J Physiol 2001; 280:G1055–G1060.
4. Gebhart GF. Pathobiology of visceral pain: molecular mechanisms and therapeutic implications. IV. Visceral afferent contributions to the pathobiology of visceral pain. Am J Physiol 2000; 278: G834–G838.
5. Mayer EA, Collins SM. Evolving pathophysiologic models of functional gastrointestinal disorders. Gastroenterology 2002; 122:2032–2048.
6. Han SK, Dong X, Hwang JI, Zylka MJ, Anderson DJ, Simon MI. Orphan G protein-coupled receptors MrgA1 and MrgC11 are distinctively activated by RF-amide-related peptides through the $Galpha_{q/11}$ pathway. Proc Natl Acad Sci USA 2002; 99:14740–14745.
7. Lembo PMC, Grazzini E, Groblewski T, et al. Proenkephalin a gene products activate a new family of sensory neuron-specific GPCRs. Nat Neurosci 2002; 5:201–209.
8. Zylka MJ, Dong X, Southwell AL, Anderson DJ. Atypical expansion in mice of the sensory neuron-specific Mrg G protein-coupled receptor family. Proc Natl Acad Sci USA 2003; 100:10043–10048.
9. Shinohara T, Harada M, Ogi K, et al. Identification of a G protein-coupled receptor specifically responsive to beta-alanine. J Biol Chem 2004; 279:23559–23564.

10. Andrews PL, Sanger GJ. Abdominal vagal afferent neurones: an important target for the treatment of gastrointestinal dysfunction. Curr Opin Pharmacol 2002; 2:650–656.

11. Gershon MD. Plasticity in serotonin control mechanisms in the gut. Curr Opin Pharmacol 2003; 3:600–607.

12. De Ponti F. Pharmacology of serotonin: what a clinician should know. Gut 2004; 53:1520–1535.

13. Miwa J, Echizen H, Matsueda K, Umeda N. Patients with constipation-predominant irritable bowel syndrome (IBS) may have elevated serotonin concentrations in colonic mucosa as compared with diarrhea-predominant patients and subjects with normal bowel habits. Digestion 2001; 63:188–194.

14. Camilleri M, Atanasova E, Carlson PJ, et al. Serotonin-transporter polymorphism pharmacogenetics in diarrhea-predominant irritable bowel syndrome. Gastroenterology 2002; 123:425–432.

15. Linden DR, Chen JX, Gershon MD, Sharkey KA, Mawe GM. Serotonin availability is increased in mucosa of guinea pigs with TNBS-induced colitis. Am J Physiol 2003; 285:G207–G216.

16. Coates MD, Mahoney CR, Linden DR, et al. Molecular defects in mucosal serotonin content and decreased serotonin reuptake transporter in ulcerative colitis and irritable bowel syndrome. Gastroenterology 2004; 126:1657–1664.

17. Yeo A, Boyd P, Lumsden S, et al. Association between a functional polymorphism in the serotonin transporter gene and diarrhoea predominant irritable bowel syndrome in women. Gut 2004; 53:1452–1458.

18. Kirkup AJ, Brunsden AM, Grundy D. Receptors and transmission in the brain-gut axis: potential for novel therapies. I. Receptors on visceral afferents. Am J Physiol 2001; 280:G787–G794.

19. Kozlowski CM, Green A, Grundy D, Boissonade FM, Bountra C. The 5-HT$_3$ receptor antagonist alosetron inhibits the colorectal distention induced depressor response and spinal c-fos expression in the anaesthetised rat. Gut 2000; 46:474–480.

20. Coffin B, Farmachidi JP, Rüegg P, Bastie A, Bouhassira D. Tegaserod, a 5-HT$_4$ receptor partial agonist, decreases sensitivity to rectal distension in healthy subjects. Aliment Pharmacol Ther 2003; 17:577–585.

21. Yu S, Long JM, Mathis C, Nass PH, Lacy BE, Crowell MD. A 5-HT$_4$ receptor partial agonist, tegaserod maleate, inhibits cortical and subcortical c-fos activation following noxious colorectal distension in the mouse. Neurogastroenterol Motil 2001; 13:445.

22. Schikowski A, Thewissen M, Mathis C, Ross HG, Enck P. Serotonin type-4 receptors modulate the sensitivity of intramural mechanoreceptive afferents of the cat rectum. Neurogastroenterol Motil 2002; 14:221–227.

23. Beattie DT, Smith JA, Marquess D, et al. The 5-HT$_4$ receptor agonist, tegaserod, is a potent 5-HT$_{2B}$ receptor antagonist in vitro and in vivo. Br J Pharmacol 2004; 143:549–560.

24. Sugiuar T, Bielefeldt K, Gebhart GF. TRPV1 function in mouse colon sensory neurons is enhanced by metabotropic 5-hydroxytryptamine receptor activation. J Neurosci 2004; 24:9521–9530.

25. Meuser T, Pietruck C, Gabriel A, Xie GX, Lim KJ, Pierce Palmer P. 5-HT$_7$ receptors are involved in mediating 5-HT–induced activation of rat primary afferent neurons. Life Sci 2002; 71:2279–2289.

26. Wei J-Y, Wang YH. Effect of CCK pretreatment on the CCK sensitivity of rat polymodal gastric vagal afferents in vitro. Am J Physiol 2000; 279:E695–E706.

27. Moriarty P, Dimaline R, Thompson DG, Dockray GJ. Characterization of cholecystokinin-A and cholecystokinin-B receptors expressed by vagal afferent neurons. Neuroscience 1997; 79:905–913.

28. Sternini C, Wong H, Pham T, et al. Expression of cholecystokinin A receptors in neurons innervating the rat stomach and intestine. Gastroenterology 1999; 117:1136–1146.

29. Broberger C, Holmberg K, Shi TJ, Dockray G, Hökfelt T. Expression and regulation of cholecystokinin and cholecystokinin receptors in rat nodose and dorsal root ganglia. Brain Res 2001; 903: 128–140.

30. Patterson LM, Zheng H, Berthoud HR. Vagal afferents innervating the gastrointestinal tract and CCKA-receptor immunoreactivity. Anat Rec 2002; 266:10–20.

31. Fried M, Feinle C. The role of fat and cholecystokinin in functional dyspepsia. Gut 2002; 51(suppl 1): i54–i57.

32. Kellow JE, Phillips SF, Miller LJ, Zinsmeister AR. Dysmotility of the small intestine in irritable bowel syndrome. Gut 1988; 29:1236–1243.

33. Roberts-Thomson IC, Fettman MJ, Jonsson JR, Frewin DB. Responses to cholecystokinin octapeptide in patients with functional abdominal pain syndromes. J Gastroenterol Hepatol 1992; 7: 293–297.

34. Gay J, Fioramonti J, Garcia-Villar R, Bueno L. Enhanced intestinal motor response to cholecystokinin in post-Nippostrongylus brasiliensis-infected rats: modulation by CCK receptors and the vagus nerve. Neurogastroenterol Motil 2001; 13:155–162.

35. Leslie FC, Thompson DG, McLaughlin JT, Varro A, Dockray GJ, Mandal BK. Plasma cholecystokinin concentrations are elevated in acute upper gastrointestinal infections. Qart J Med 2003; 96: 870–871.

36. Varga G, Balint A, Burghardt B, D'Amato M. Involvement of endogenous CCK and CCK$_1$ receptors in colonic motor function. Br J Pharmacol 2004; 141:1275–1284.

37. Plourde V, Lembo T, Shui Z, et al. Effects of the somatostatin analogue octreotide on rectal afferent nerves in humans. Am J Physiol 1993; 265:G742–G751.

38. Bradette M, Delvaux M, Staumont G, Fioramonti J, Buéno L, Frexinos J. Octreotide increases thresholds of colonic visceral perception in IBS patients without modifying muscle tone. Dig Dis Sci 1994; 39:1171–1178.

39. Hasler WL, Soudah HC, Owyang C. Somatostatin analog inhibits afferent response to rectal distention in diarrhea-predominant irritable bowel patients. J Pharmacol Exp Ther 1994; 268:1206–1211.

40. Chey WD, Beydoun A, Roberts DJ, Hasler WL, Owyang C. Octreotide reduces perception of rectal electrical stimulation by spinal afferent pathway inhibition. Am J Physiol 1995; 269:G821–G826.

41. Mertz H, Walsh JH, Sytnik B, Mayer EA. The effect of octreotide on human gastric compliance and sensory perception. Neurogastroenterol Motil 1995; 7:175–185.

42. Foxx-Orenstein A, Camilleri M, Stephens D, Burton D. Effect of a somatostatin analogue on gastric motor and sensory functions in healthy humans. Gut 2003; 52:1555–1561.

43. Schwetz I, Naliboff B, Munakata J, et al. Anti-hyperalgesic effect of octreotide in patients with irritable bowel syndrome. Aliment Pharmacol Ther 2004; 19:123–131.

44. Booth CE, Kirkup AJ, Hicks GA, Humphrey PP, Grundy D. Somatostatin sst_2 receptor-mediated inhibition of mesenteric afferent nerves of the jejunum in the anesthetized rat. Gastroenterology 2001; 121:358–369.

45. Szolcsányi J, Bolcskei K, Szabo A, et al. Analgesic effect of TT-232, a heptapeptide somatostatin analogue, in acute pain models of the rat and the mouse and in streptozotocin-induced diabetic mechanical allodynia. Eur J Pharmacol 2004; 498:103–109.

46. Su X, Burton MB, Gebhart GF. Effects of octreotide on responses to colorectal distension in the rat. Gut 2001; 48:676–682.

47. Bley KR, Hunger JC, Eglen RM, Smith JAM. The role of EP receptors in hyperalgesia. Trends Pharmacol Sci 1998; 19:141–147.

48. Minami T, Nakano H, Kobayashi T, et al. Characterization of EP receptor subtypes responsible for prostaglandin E_2-induced pain responses by use of EP_1 and EP_3 receptor knockout mice. Br J Pharmacol 2001; 133:438–444.

49. Southall MD, Vasko MR. Prostaglandin receptor subtypes, EP_{3C} and EP_4, mediate the prostaglandin E_2-induced cAMP production and sensitization of sensory neurons. J Biol Chem 2001; 276: 16083–16091.

50. Bar KJ, Natura G, Telleria-Diaz A, et al. Changes in the effect of spinal prostaglandin E_2 during inflammation: prostaglandin E (EP_1-EP_4) receptors in spinal nociceptive processing of input from the normal or inflamed knee joint. J Neurosci 2004; 24:642–651.

51. Nakayama Y, Omote K, Kawamata T, Namiki A. Role of prostaglandin receptor subtype EP_1 in prostaglandin E_2-induced nociceptive transmission in the rat spinal dorsal horn. Brain Res 2004; 1010:62–68.

52. Haupt W, Jiang W, Kreis ME, Grundy D. Prostaglandin EP receptor subtypes have distinct effects on jejunal afferent sensitivity in the rat. Gastroenterology 2000; 119:1580–1589.

53. Maubach KA, Grundy D. The role of prostaglandins in the bradykinin-induced activation of serosal afferents of the rat jejunum in vitro. J Physiol (London) 1999; 515:277–285.

54. Ueno A, Matsumoto H, Naraba H, et al. Major roles of prostanoid receptors IP and EP_3 in endotoxin-induced enhancement of pain perception. Biochem Pharmacol 2001; 62:157–160.

55. Sarkar S, Hobson AR, Hughes A, et al. The prostaglandin E_2 receptor-1 (EP-1) mediates acid-induced visceral pain hypersensitivity in humans. Gastroenterology 2003; 124:18–25.

56. Marceau F, Regoli D. Bradykinin receptor ligands: therapeutic perspectives. Nat Rev Drug Discov 2004; 3:845–852.

57. Heapy CG, Shaw JS, Farmer SC. Differential sensitivity of antinociceptive assays to the bradykinin antagonist Hoe 140. Br J Pharmacol 1993; 108:209–213.

58. Holzer-Petsche U, Brodacz B. Traction on the mesentery as a model of visceral nociception. Pain 1999; 80:319–328.

59. Guo ZL, Symons JD, Longhurst JC. Activation of visceral afferents by bradykinin and ischemia: independent roles of PKC and prostaglandins. Am J Physiol 1999; 276:H1884–H1891.

60. Brunsden AM, Grundy D. Sensitization of visceral afferents to bradykinin in rat jejunum in vitro. J Physiol (London) 1999; 521:517–527.

61. Premkumar LS, Ahern GP. Induction of vanilloid receptor channel activity by protein kinase C. Nature 2000; 408:985–990.

62. Prescott ED, Julius D. A modular PIP_2 binding site as a determinant of capsaicin receptor sensitivity. Science 2003; 300:1284–1288.

63. Bueno L, Fioramonti J, Delvaux M, Frexinos J. Mediators and pharmacology of visceral sensitivity: from basic to clinical investigations. Gastroenterology 1997; 112:1714–1743.

64. Fischer HS, Zernig G, Hauser KF, Gerard C, Hersh LB, Saria A. Neutral endopeptidase knockout induces hyperalgesia in a model of visceral pain, an effect related to bradykinin and nitric oxide. J Mol Neurosci 2002; 18:129–134.

65. Julia V, Mezzasalma T, Bueno L. Influence of bradykinin in gastrointestinal disorders and visceral pain induced by acute or chronic inflammation in rats. Dig Dis Sci 1995; 40:1913–1921.

66. McLean PG, Picard C, Garcia-Villar R, et al. Role of kinin B_1 and B_2 receptors and mast cells in post intestinal infection-induced hypersensitivity to distension. Neurogastroenterol Motil 1998; 10:499–508.

67. Rosamilia A, Clements JA, Dwyer PL, Kende M, Campbell DJ. Activation of the kallikrein kinin system in interstitial cystitis. J Urol 1999; 162:129–134.
68. Chopra B, Barrick SR, Meyers S, et al. Expression and function of bradykinin B_1/B_2 receptors in normal and inflamed rat urinary bladder urothelium. J Physiol (London) 2005; 562:859–871.
69. Maggi CA, Santicioli P, Del Bianco E, Lecci A, Guliani S. Evidence for the involvement of bradykinin in chemically-evoked cystitis in anaesthetized rats. Naunyn-Schmiedeberg's Arch Pharmacol 1993; 347:432–437.
70. Jaggar SI, Habib S, Rice AS. The modulatory effects of bradykinin B_1 and B_2 receptor antagonists upon viscero-visceral hyper-reflexia in a rat model of visceral hyperalgesia. Pain 1998; 75:169–176.
71. Kawabata A. Gastrointestinal functions of proteinase-activated receptors. Life Sci 2003; 74:247–254.
72. Ossovskaya VS, Bunnett NW. Protease-activated receptors: contribution to physiology and disease. Physiol Rev 2004; 84:579–621.
73. Vergnolle N. Modulation of visceral pain and inflammation by protease-activated receptors. Br J Pharmacol 2004; 141:1264–1274.
74. Kawao N, Ikeda H, Kitano T, et al. Modulation of capsaicin-evoked visceral pain and referred hyperalgesia by protease-activated receptors 1 and 2. J Pharmacol Sci 2004; 94:277–285.
75. Kirkup AJ, Jiang W, Bunnett NW, Grundy D. Stimulation of proteinase-activated receptor 2 excites jejunal afferent nerves in anaesthetised rats. J Physiol (London) 2003; 552:589–601.
76. Hoogerwerf WA, Zou L, Shenoy M, et al. The proteinase-activated receptor 2 is involved in nociception. J Neurosci 2001; 21:9036–9042.
77. Coelho AM, Vergnolle N, Guiard B, Fioramonti J, Bueno L. Proteinases and proteinase-activated receptor 2: a possible role to promote visceral hyperalgesia in rats. Gastroenterology 2002; 122:1035–1047.
78. Hoogerwerf WA, Shenoy M, Winston JH, Xiao SY, He Z, Pasricha PJ. Trypsin mediates nociception via the proteinase-activated receptor 2: a potentially novel role in pancreatic pain. Gastroenterology 2004; 127:883–891.
79. Amadesi S, Nie J, Vergnolle N, et al. Protease-activated receptor 2 sensitizes the capsaicin receptor transient receptor potential vanilloid receptor 1 to induce hyperalgesia. J Neurosci 2004; 24:4300–4312.
80. Dai Y, Moriyama T, Higashi T, et al. Proteinase-activated receptor 2-mediated potentiation of transient receptor potential vanilloid subfamily 1 activity reveals a mechanism for proteinase-induced inflammatory pain. J Neurosci 2004; 24:4293–4299.
81. Cenac N, Garcia-Villar R, Ferrier L, et al. Proteinase-activated receptor-2-induced colonic inflammation in mice: possible involvement of afferent neurons, nitric oxide, and paracellular permeability. J Immunol 2003; 170:4296–4300.
82. Nguyen C, Coelho AM, Grady E, et al. Colitis induced by proteinase-activated receptor-2 agonists is mediated by a neurogenic mechanism. Can J Physiol Pharmacol 2003; 81:920–927.
83. Kim JA, Choi SC, Yun KJ, et al. Expression of protease-activated receptor 2 in ulcerative colitis. Inflamm Bowel Dis 2003; 9:224–229.
84. Vergnolle N, Cellars L, Mencarelli A, et al. A role for proteinase-activated receptor-1 in inflammatory bowel diseases. J Clin Invest 2004; 114:1444–1456.
85. Gao C, Liu S, Hu HZ, Kim GY, Xia Y, Wood JD. Serine proteases excite myenteric neurons through protease-activated receptors in guinea pig small intestine. Gastroenterology 2002; 123:1554–1564.
86. Dunn PM, Zhong Y, Burnstock G. P2X receptors in peripheral neurons. Prog Neurobiol 2001; 65:107–134.
87. North RA. Molecular physiology of P2X receptors. Physiol Rev 2002; 82:1013–1067.
88. Zhong Y, Banning AS, Cockayne DA, Ford AP, Burnstock G, McMahon SB. Bladder and cutaneous sensory neurons of the rat express different functional P2X receptors. Neuroscience 2003; 120: 667–675.
89. Kirkup AJ, Booth CE, Chessell IP, Humphrey PP, Grundy D. Excitatory effect of P2X receptor activation on mesenteric afferent nerves in the anaesthetised rat. J Physiol (London) 1999; 520:551–563.
90. Burnstock G. Purine-mediated signalling in pain and visceral perception. Trends Pharmacol Sci 2001; 22:182–188.
91. Vlaskovska M, Kasakov L, Rong W, et al. $P2X_3$ knock-out mice reveal a major sensory role for urothelially released ATP. J Neurosci 2001; 21:5670–5677.
92. Wynn G, Rong W, Xiang Z, Burnstock G. Purinergic mechanisms contribute to mechanosensory transduction in the rat colorectum. Gastroenterology 2003; 125:1398–1409.
93. Galligan JJ. Enteric P2X receptors as potential targets for drug treatment of the irritable bowel syndrome. Br J Pharmacol 2004; 141:1294–1302.
94. Cockayne DA, Hamilton SG, Zhu QM, et al. Urinary bladder hyporeflexia and reduced pain-related behaviour in $P2X_3$-deficient mice. Nature 2000; 407:1011–1015.
95. Knight GE, Bodin P, De Groat WC, Burnstock G. ATP is released from guinea pig ureter epithelium on distension. Am J Physiol 2002; 282:F281–F288.
96. Page AJ, O'Donnell TA, Blackshaw LA. P2X purinoceptor–induced sensitization of ferret vagal mechanoreceptors in oesophageal inflammation. J Physiol (London) 2000; 523:403–411.
97. Holzer P. Acid-sensitive ion channels in gastrointestinal function. Curr Opin Pharmacol 2003; 3:618–625.

98. Xu GY, Huang LY. Peripheral inflammation sensitizes P2X receptor-mediated responses in rat dorsal root ganglion neurons. J Neurosci 2002; 22:93–102.
99. Tempest HV, Dixon AK, Turner WH, Elneil S, Sellers LA, Ferguson DR. P2X$_2$ and P2X$_3$ receptor expression in human bladder urothelium and changes in interstitial cystitis. BJU Int 2004; 93:1344–1348.
100. Yiangou Y, Facer P, Baecker PA, et al. ATP-gated ion channel P2X$_3$ is increased in human inflammatory bowel disease. Neurogastroenterol Motil 2001; 13:365–369.
101. Honore P, Mikusa J, Bianchi B, et al. TNP-ATP, a potent P2X$_3$ receptor antagonist, blocks acetic acid-induced abdominal constriction in mice: comparison with reference analgesics. Pain 2002; 96:99–105.
102. Jarvis MF, Burgard EC, McGaraughty S, et al. A-317491, a novel potent and selective non-nucleotide antagonist of P2X$_3$ and P2X$_{2/3}$ receptors, reduces chronic inflammatory and neuropathic pain in the rat. Proc Natl Acad Sci USA 2002; 99:17179–17184.
103. Clapham DE. TRP channels as cellular sensors. Nature 2003; 426:517–524.
104. Patapoutian A, Peier AM, Story GM, Viswanath V. ThermoTRP channels and beyond: mechanisms of temperature sensation. Nat Rev Neurosci 2003; 4:529–539.
105. Caterina MJ, Schumacher MA, Tominaga M, Rosen TA, Levine JD, Julius D. The capsaicin receptor: a heat–activated ion channel in the pain pathway. Nature 1997; 389:816–824.
106. Holzer P. Capsaicin: cellular targets, mechanisms of action, and selectivity for thin sensory neurons. Pharmacol Rev 1991; 43:143–201.
107. Szallasi A, Blumberg PM. Vanilloid (capsaicin) receptors and mechanisms. Pharmacol Rev 1999; 51:159–212.
108. Caterina MJ, Julius D. The vanilloid receptor: a molecular gateway to the pain pathway. Annu Rev Neurosci 2001; 24:487–517.
109. Hwang SW, Oh U. Hot channels in airways: pharmacology of the vanilloid receptor. Curr Opin Pharmacol 2002; 2:235–242.
110. Gunthorpe MJ, Benham CD, Randall A, Davis JB. The diversity in the vanilloid (TRPV) receptor family of ion channels. Trends Pharmacol Sci 2002; 23:183–191.
111. Geppetti P, Trevisani M. Activation and sensitisation of the vanilloid receptor: role in gastrointestinal inflammation and function. Br J Pharmacol 2004; 141:1313–1320.
112. Holzer P. TRPV1 and the gut: from a tasty receptor for a painful vanilloid to a key player in hyperalgesia. Eur J Pharmacol 2004; 500:231–241.
113. Voets T, Droogmans G, Wissenbach U, Janssens A, Flockerzi V, Nilius B. The principle of temperature-dependent gating in cold- and heat-sensitive TRP channels. Nature 2004; 430:748–754.
114. Birder LA, Nakamura Y, Kiss S, et al. Altered urinary bladder function in mice lacking the vanilloid receptor TRPV1. Nat Neurosci 2002; 5:856–860.
115. Patterson LM, Zheng H, Ward SM, Berthoud HR. Vanilloid receptor (VR1) expression in vagal afferent neurons innervating the gastrointestinal tract. Cell Tissue Res 2003; 311:277–287.
116. Ward SM, Bayguinov J, Won KJ, Grundy D, Berthoud HR. Distribution of the vanilloid receptor (VR1) in the gastrointestinal tract. J Comp Neurol 2003; 465:121–135.
117. Kadowaki M, Kuramoto H, Takaki M. Combined determination with functional and morphological studies of origin of nerve fibers expressing transient receptor potential vanilloid 1 in the myenteric plexus of the rat jejunum. Auton Neurosci 2004; 116:11–18.
118. Robinson DR, McNaughton PA, Evans ML, Hicks GA. Characterization of the primary spinal afferent innervation of the mouse colon using retrograde labelling. Neurogastroenterol Motil 2004; 16:113–124.
119. Schicho R, Florian W, Liebmann I, Holzer P, Lippe IT. Increased expression of TRPV1 receptor in dorsal root ganglia by acid insult of the rat gastric mucosa. Eur J Neurosci 2004; 19:1811–1818.
120. Horie S, Yamamoto H, Michael GJ, et al. Protective role of vanilloid receptor type 1 in HCl-induced gastric mucosal lesions in rats. Scand J Gastroenterol 2004; 39:303–312.
121. Avelino A, Cruz C, Nagy I, Cruz F. Vanilloid receptor 1 expression in the rat urinary tract. Neuroscience 2002; 109:787–798.
122. Nozawa Y, Nishihara K, Yamamoto A, Nakano M, Ajioka H, Matsuura N. Distribution and characterization of vanilloid receptors in the rat stomach. Neurosci Lett 2001; 309:33–36.
123. Poonyachoti S, Kulkarni-Narla A, Brown DR. Chemical coding of neurons expressing delta- and kappa-opioid receptor and type I vanilloid receptor immunoreactivities in the porcine ileum. Cell Tissue Res 2002; 307:23–33.
124. Anavi-Goffer S, Coutts AA. Cellular distribution of vanilloid VR1 receptor immunoreactivity in the guinea-pig myenteric plexus. Eur J Pharmacol 2003; 458:61–71.
125. Chan CL, Facer P, Davis JB, et al. Sensory fibres expressing capsaicin receptor TRPV1 in patients with rectal hypersensitivity and faecal urgency. Lancet 2003; 361:385–391.
126. Wang C, Hu HZ, Colton CK, Wood JD, Zhu MX. An alternative splicing product of the murine trpv1 gene dominantly negatively modulates the activity of TRPV1 channels. J Biol Chem 2004; 279:37423–37430.
127. Su X, Wachtel RE, Gebhart GF. Capsaicin sensitivity and voltage–gated sodium currents in colon sensory neurons from rat dorsal root ganglia. Am J Physiol 1999; 277:G1180–G1188.

128. Blackshaw LA, Page AJ, Partosoedarso ER. Acute effects of capsaicin on gastrointestinal vagal afferents. Neuroscience 2000; 96:407–416.
129. Rong W, Hillsley K, Davis JB, Hicks G, Winchester WJ, Grundy D. Jejunal afferent nerve sensitivity in wild-type and TRPV1 knockout mice. J Physiol 2004; 560:867–881.
130. Drewes AM, Schipper KP, Dimcevski G, et al. Gut pain and hyperalgesia induced by capsaicin: a human experimental model. Pain 2003; 104:333–341.
131. Schmidt B, Hammer J, Holzer P, Hammer HF. Chemical nociception in the jejunum induced by capsaicin. Gut 2004; 53:1109–1116.
132. Laird JM, Martinez-Caro L, Garcia-Nicas E, Cervero F. A new model of visceral pain and referred hyperalgesia in the mouse. Pain 2001; 92:335–342.
133. Mansikka H, Lähdesmäki J, Scheinin M, Pertovaara A. Alpha$_{2A}$ adrenoceptors contribute to feedback inhibition of capsaicin-induced hyperalgesia. Anesthesiology 2004; 101:185–190.
134. Reeh PW, Pethö G. Nociceptor excitation by thermal sensitization—a hypothesis. Prog Brain Res 2000; 129:39–50.
135. Caterina MJ, Leffler A, Malmberg AB, et al. Impaired nociception and pain sensation in mice lacking the capsaicin receptor. Science 2000; 288:306–313.
136. Davis JB, Gray J, Gunthorpe MJ, et al. Vanilloid receptor-1 is essential for inflammatory thermal hyperalgesia. Nature 2000; 405:183–187.
137. Matthews PJ, Aziz Q, Facer P, Davis JB, Thompson DG, Anand P. Increased capsaicin receptor TRPV1 nerve fibres in the inflamed human oesophagus. Eur J Gastroenterol Hepatol 2004; 16:897–902.
138. Yiangou Y, Facer P, Dyer NH, et al. Vanilloid receptor 1 immunoreactivity in inflamed human bowel. Lancet 2001; 357:1338–1339.
139. Brady CM, Apostolidis AN, Harper M, et al. Parallel changes in bladder suburothelial vanilloid receptor TRPV1 and pan-neuronal marker PGP9.5 immunoreactivity in patients with neurogenic detrusor overactivity after intravesical resiniferatoxin treatment. BJU Int 2004; 93:770–776.
140. Lamb K, Kang YM, Gebhart GF, Bielefeldt K. Gastric inflammation triggers hypersensitivity to acid in awake rats. Gastroenterology 2003; 125:1410–1418.
141. Lembeck F, Skofitsch G. Visceral pain reflex after pretreatment with capsaicin and morphine. Naunyn-Schmiedeberg's Arch Pharmacol 1982; 321:116–122.
142. Plourde V, St.-Pierre S, Quirion R. Calcitonin gene-related peptide in viscerosensitive response to colorectal distension in rats. Am J Physiol 1997; 273:G191–G196.
143. Delafoy L, Raymond F, Doherty AM, Eschalier A, Diop L. Role of nerve growth factor in the trinitrobenzene sulfonic acid-induced colonic hypersensitivity. Pain 2003; 105:489–497.
144. Bley KR. Recent developments in transient receptor potential vanilloid receptor 1 agonist-based therapies. Expert Opin Investig Drugs 2004; 13:1445–1456.
145. Cruz F. Mechanisms involved in new therapies for overactive bladder. Urology 2004; 63(suppl 1):65–73.
146. Lysy J, Sistiery-Ittah M, Israelit Y, et al. Topical capsaicin - a novel and effective treatment for idiopathic intractable pruritus ani: a randomised, placebo controlled, crossover study. Gut 2003; 52:1323–1326.
147. Bortolotti M, Coccia G, Grossi G, Miglioli M. The treatment of functional dyspepsia with red pepper. Aliment Pharmacol Ther 2002; 16:1075–1082.
148. Schmulson MJ, Valdovinos MA, Milke P. Chili pepper and rectal hyperalgesia in irritable bowel syndrome. Am J Gastroenterol 2003; 98:1214–1215.
149. Urban L, Campbell EA, Panesar M, et al. In vivo pharmacology of SDZ 249–665, a novel, non-pungent capsaicin analogue. Pain 2000; 89:65–74.
150. Jaggar SI, Scott HCF, James IF, Rice ASC. The capsaicin analogue SDZ 249–665 attenuates the hyper-reflexia and referred hyperalgesia associated with inflammation of the rat urinary bladder. Pain 2001; 89:229–235.
151. Bevan S, Hothi S, Hughes G, et al. Capsazepine: a competitive antagonist of the sensory neurone excitant capsaicin. Br J Pharmacol 1992; 107:544–552.
152. McVey DC, Vigna SR. The capsaicin VR1 receptor mediates substance P release in toxin A-induced enteritis in rats. Peptides 2001; 22:1439–1446.
153. Kihara N, De La Fuente SG, Fujino K, Takahashi T, Pappas TN, Mantyh CR. Vanilloid receptor-1 containing primary sensory neurones mediate dextran sulphate sodium induced colitis in rats. Gut 2003; 52:713–719.
154. Kimball ES, Wallace NH, Schneider CR, D'Andrea MR, Hornby PJ. Vanilloid receptor 1 antagonists attenuate disease severity in dextran sulphate sodium-induced colitis in mice. Neurogastroenterol Motil 2004; 16:811–818.
155. Holzer P. Neural emergency system in the stomach. Gastroenterology 1998; 114:823–839.
156. Holzer P. Vanilloid receptor TRPV1: hot on the tongue and inflaming the colon. Neurogastroenterol Motil 2004; 16:697–699.
157. Waldmann R, Lazdunski M. H$^+$-gated cation channels: neuronal acid sensors in the NaC/DEG family of ion channels. Curr Opin Neurobiol 1998; 8:418–424.
158. Kellenberger S, Schild L. Epithelial sodium channel/degenerin family of ion channels: a variety of functions for a shared structure. Physiol Rev 2002; 82:735–767.

159. Krishtal O. The ASICs: signaling molecules?. Modulators?. Trends Neurosci 2003; 26:477–483.
160. Alvarez de la Rosa D, Zhang P, Shao D, White F, Canessa CM. Functional implications of the localization and activity of acid-sensitive channels in rat peripheral nervous system. Proc Natl Acad Sci USA 2002; 99:2326–2331.
161. Benson CJ, Xie J, Wemmie JA, et al. Heteromultimers of DEG/ENaC subunits form H^+-gated channels in mouse sensory neurons. Proc Natl Acad Sci USA 2002; 99:2338–2343.
162. Xie J, Prise MP, Berger AL, Welsh MJ. DRASIC contributes to pH-gated currents in large dorsal root ganglion sensory neurons by forming heteromultimeric channels. J Neurophysiol 2002; 87: 2835–2843.
163. Welsh MJ, Price MP, Xie J. Biochemical basis of touch perception: mechanosensory function of degenerin/epithelial Na^+ channels. J Biol Chem 2002; 277:2369–2372.
164. Price MP, Lewin GR, McIlwrath SL, et al. The mammalian sodium channel BNC1 is required for normal touch sensation. Nature 2000; 407:1007–1011.
165. Price MP, McIlwrath SL, Xie J, et al. The DRASIC cation channel contributes to the detection of cutaneous touch and acid stimuli in mice. Neuron 2001; 32:1071–1083.
166. Chen CC, Zimmer A, Sun WH, Hall J, Brownstein MJ, Zimmer A. A role for ASIC3 in the modulation of high-intensity pain stimuli. Proc Natl Acad Sci USA 2002; 99:8992–8997.
167. Page AJ, Brierley SM, Martin CM, et al. The ion channel ASIC1 contributes to visceral but not cutaneous mechanoreceptor function. Gastroenterology 2004; 127:1739–1747.
168. Yiangou Y, Facer P, Smith JA, et al. Increased acid-sensing ion channel ASIC-3 in inflamed human intestine. Eur J Gastroenterol Hepatol 2001; 13:891–896.
169. Mamet J, Baron A, Lazdunski M, Voilley N. Proinflammatory mediators, stimulators of sensory neuron excitability via the expression of acid-sensing ion channels. J Neurosci 2002; 22:10662–10670.
170. Goldstein SA, Bockenhauer D, O'Kelly I, Zilberberg N. Potassium leak channels and the KCNK family of two-P-domain subunits. Nat Rev Neurosci 2001; 2:175–184.
171. Patel AJ, Honoré E. Properties and modulation of mammalian 2P domain K^+ channels. Trends Neurosci 2001; 24:339–346.
172. Bang H, Kim Y, Kim D. TREK–2, a new member of the mechanosensitive tandem-pore K^+ channel family. J Biol Chem 2000; 275:17412–17419.
173. Honoré E, Maingret F, Lazdunski M, Patel AJ. An intracellular proton sensor commands lipid- and mechano-gating of the K^+ channel TREK-1. EMBO J 2002; 21:2968–2976.
174. Ozaki N, Gebhart GF. Characterization of mechanosensitive splanchnic nerve afferent fibers innervating the rat stomach. Am J Physiol 2001; 281:G1449–G1459.
175. Su X, Wachtel RE, Gebhart GF. Mechanosensitive potassium channels in rat colon sensory neurons. J Neurophysiol 2000; 84:836–843.
176. Raybould HE, Gschossman JM, Ennes H, Lembo T, Mayer EA. Involvement of stretch-sensitive calcium flux in mechanical transduction in visceral afferents. J Auton Nerv Syst 1999; 75:1–6.
177. Suzuki M, Mizuno A, Kodaira K, Imai M. Impaired pressure sensation with mice lacking TRPV4. J Biol Chem 2003; 278:22664–22668.
178. Lai J, Porreca F, Hunter JC, Gold MS. Voltage-gated sodium channels and hyperalgesia. Annu Rev Pharmacol Toxicol 2004; 44:371–397.
179. Wood JN, Boorman JP, Okuse K, Baker MD. Voltage-gated sodium channels and pain pathways. J Neurobiol 2004; 61:55–71.
180. Fang X, Djouhri L, Black JA, Dib-Hajj SD, Waxman SG, Lawson SN. The presence and role of the tetrodotoxin-resistant sodium channel $Na_v1.9$ (NaN) in nociceptive primary afferent neurons. J Neurosci 2002; 22:7425–7433.
181. Djouhri L, Newton R, Levinson SR, Berry CM, Carruthers B, Lawson SN. Sensory and electrophysiological properties of guinea-pig sensory neurones expressing $Na_v1.7$ (PN1) Na^+ channel alpha subunit protein. J Physiol (London) 2003; 546:565–576.
182. Djouhri L, Fang X, Okuse K, Wood JN, Berry CM, Lawson SN. The TTX-resistant sodium channel $Na_v1.8$ (SNS/PN3): expression and correlation with membrane properties in rat nociceptive primary afferent neurons. J Physiol (London) 2003; 550:739–752.
183. Bielefeldt K, Ozaki N, Gebhart GF. Mild gastritis alters voltage-sensitive sodium currents in gastric sensory neurons in rats. Gastroenterology 2002; 122:752–661.
184. Gold MS, Zhang L, Wrigley DL, Traub RJ. Prostaglandin E_2 modulates TTX–R I_{Na} in rat colonic sensory neurons. J Neurophysiol 2002; 88:1512–1522.
185. Moore BA, Stewart TM, Hill C, Vanner SJ. TNBS ileitis evokes hyperexcitability and changes in ionic membrane properties of nociceptive DRG neurons. Am J Physiol 2002; 282:G1045–G1051.
186. Stewart T, Beyak MJ, Vanner S. Ileitis modulates potassium and sodium currents in guinea pig dorsal root ganglia sensory neurons. J Physiol (London) 2003; 552:797–807.
187. Beyak MJ, Ramji N, Krol KM, Kawaja MD, Vanner SJ. Two TTX-resistant Na^+ currents in mouse colonic dorsal root ganglia neurons and their role in colitis-induced hyperexcitability. Am J Physiol 2004; 287:G845–G855.
188. Bielefeldt K, Ozaki N, Gebhart GF. Experimental ulcers alter voltage-sensitive sodium currents in rat gastric sensory neurons. Gastroenterology 2002; 122:394–405.
189. Bielefeldt K, Ozaki N, Gebhart GF. Role of nerve growth factor in modulation of gastric afferent neurons in the rat. Am J Physiol 2003; 284:G499–G507.

190. Rush AM, Waxman SG. PGE$_2$ increases the tetrodotoxin-resistant Na$_v$1.9 sodium current in mouse DRG neurons via G-proteins. Brain Res 2004; 1023:264–271.

191. Yoshimura N, Seki S, Novakovic SD, et al. The involvement of the tetrodotoxin-resistant sodium channel Na$_v$1.8 (PN3/SNS) in a rat model of visceral pain. J Neurosci 2001; 21:8690–8696.

192. Laird JM, Souslova V, Wood JN, Cervero F. Deficits in visceral pain and referred hyperalgesia in Na$_v$1.8 (SNS/PN3)-null mice. J Neurosci 2002; 22:8352–8356.

193. Ness TJ. Intravenous lidocaine inhibits visceral nociceptive reflexes and spinal neurons in the rat. Anesthesiology 2000; 92:1685–1691.

194. Chevrier P, Vijayaragavan K, Chahine M. Differential modulation of Na$_v$1.7 and Na$_v$1.8 peripheral nerve sodium channels by the local anesthetic lidocaine. Br J Pharmacol 2004; 142:576–584.

195. Su X, Joshi SK, Kardos S, Gebhart GF. Sodium channel blocking actions of the kappa-opioid receptor agonist U50,488 contribute to its visceral antinociceptive effects. J Neurophysiol 2002; 87: 1271–1279.

196. Bielefeldt K, Ozaki N, Whiteis C, Gebhart GF. Amitriptyline inhibits voltage-sensitive sodium currents in rat gastric sensory neurons. Dig Dis Sci 2002; 47:959–966.

197. Cervero F, Laird JM. Role of ion channels in mechanisms controlling gastrointestinal pain pathways. Curr Opin Pharmacol 2003; 3:608–612.

198. Ocana M, Cendan CM, Cobos EJ, Entrena JM, Baeyens JM. Potassium channels and pain: present realities and future opportunities. Eur J Pharmacol 2004; 500:203–219.

199. Rasband MN, Park EW, Vanderah TW, Lai J, Porreca F, Trimmer JS. Distinct potassium channels on pain-sensing neurons. Proc Natl Acad Sci USA 2001; 98:13373–13378.

200. Dang K, Bielefeldt K, Gebhart GF. Gastric ulcers reduce A-type potassium currents in rat gastric sensory ganglion neurons. Am J Physiol 2004; 286:G573–G579.

201. Sculptoreanu A, Yoshimura N, de Groat WC. KW-7158 ((2S)-(+)-3,3,3-trifluoro-2-hydroxy-2-methyl-N-(5,5,10-trioxo-4,10-dihydrothieno(3,2-c) (1)benzothiepin-9-yl)propanamide) enhances A-type K$^+$ currents in neurons of the dorsal root ganglion of the adult rat. J Pharmacol Exp Ther 2004; 310:159–168.

202. Newton RA, Bingham S, Case PC, Sanger GJ, Lawson SN. Dorsal root ganglion neurons show increased expression of the calcium channel alpha2delta1 subunit following partial sciatic nerve injury. Mol Brain Res 2001; 95:1–8.

203. Sutton KG, Martin DJ, Pinnock RD, Lee K, Scott RH. Gabapentin inhibits high-threshold calcium channel currents in cultured rat dorsal root ganglion neurones. Br J Pharmacol 2002; 135:257–265.

204. Eutamene H, Coelho AM, Theodorou V, et al. Antinociceptive effect of pregabalin in septic shock-induced rectal hypersensitivity in rats. J Pharmacol Exp Ther 2000; 295:162–167.

205. Diop L, Raymond F, Fargeau H, Petoux F, Chovet M, Doherty AM. Pregabalin (CI-1008) inhibits the trinitrobenzene sulfonic acid-induced chronic colonic allodynia in the rat. J Pharmacol Exp Ther 2002; 302:1013–1022.

206. Feng Y, Cui M, Willis WD. Gabapentin markedly reduces acetic acid-induced visceral nociception. Anesthesiology 2003; 98:729–733.

207. McGivern JG, McDonough SI. Voltage-gated calcium channels as targets for the treatment of chronic pain. Curr Drug Targets CNS Neurol Disord 2004; 3:457–478.

208. Horvath G, Brodacz B, Holzer-Petsche U. Role of calcium channels in the spinal transmission of nociceptive information from the mesentery. Pain 2001; 93:35–41.

209. Fundytus ME. Glutamate receptors and nociception: implications for the drug treatment of pain. CNS Drugs 2001; 15:29–58.

210. Carlton SM, Coggeshall RE. Inflammation-induced changes in peripheral glutamate receptor populations. Brain Res 1999; 820:63–70.

211. McRoberts JA, Coutinho SV, Marvizon JC, et al. Role of peripheral N-methyl-D-aspartate (NMDA) receptors in visceral nociception in rats. Gastroenterology 2001; 120:1737–1748.

212. Bhave G, Karim F, Carlton SM, Gereau RW. Peripheral group I metabotropic glutamate receptors modulate nociception in mice. Nat Neurosci 2001; 4:417–423.

213. Walker K, Reeve A, Bowes M, et al. mGlu5 receptors and nociceptive function. II. mGlu5 receptors functionally expressed on peripheral sensory neurons mediate inflammatory hyperalgesia. Neuropharmacology 2001; 40:10–19.

214. Carlton SM, Hargett GL, Coggeshall RE. Localization of metabotropic glutamate receptors 2/3 on primary afferent axons in the rat. Neuroscience 2001; 105:957–969.

215. Zhai QZ, Traub RJ. The NMDA receptor antagonist MK-801 attenuates c-Fos expression in the lumbosacral spinal cord following repetitive noxious and non-noxious colorectal distention. Pain 1999; 83:321–329.

216. Kozlowski CM, Bountra C, Grundy D. The effect of fentanyl, DNQX and MK-801 on dorsal horn neurones responsive to colorectal distension in the anaesthetized rat. Neurogastroenterol Motil 2000; 12:239–247.

217. Coutinho SV, Urban MO, Gebhart GF. The role of CNS NMDA receptors and nitric oxide in visceral hyperalgesia. Eur J Pharmacol 2001; 429:319–325.

218. Coutinho SV, Meller ST, Gebhart GF. Intracolonic zymosan produces visceral hyperalgesia in the rat that is mediated by spinal NMDA and non-NMDA receptors. Brain Res 1996; 736:7–15.

219. Gaudreau GA, Plourde V. Involvement of N-methyl-D-aspartate (NMDA) receptors in a rat model of visceral hypersensitivity. Behav Brain Res 2004; 150:185–189.
220. Lu Y, Vera-Portocarrero LP, Westlund KN. Intrathecal coadministration of D-APV and morphine is maximally effective in a rat experimental pancreatitis model. Anesthesiology 2003; 98:734–740.
221. Rice AS, McMahon SB. Pre-emptive intrathecal administration of an NMDA receptor antagonist (AP-5) prevents hyper-reflexia in a model of persistent visceral pain. Pain 1994; 57:335–340.
222. Chen Y, Bacon G, Sher E, et al. Evaluation of the activity of a novel metabotropic glutamate receptor antagonist (+/-)-2-amino-2-(3-cis and trans-carboxycyclobutyl-3-(9-thioxanthyl)propionic acid) in the in vitro neonatal spinal cord and in an in vivo pain model. Neuroscience 2000; 95:787–793.
223. Bianchi R, Rezzani R, Borsani E, Rodella L. mGlu5 receptor antagonist decreases Fos expression in spinal neurons after noxious visceral stimulation. Brain Res 2003; 960:263–266.
224. Zhu CZ, Wilson SG, Mikusa JP, et al. Assessing the role of metabotropic glutamate receptor 5 in multiple nociceptive modalities. Eur J Pharmacol 2004; 506:107–118.
225. Fink-Jensen A, Judge ME, Hansen JB, et al. Inhibition of cisplatin-induced emesis in ferrets by the non-NMDA receptor antagonists NBQX and CNQX. Neurosci Lett 1992; 137:173–177.
226. Partosoedarso ER, Blackshaw LA. Roles of central glutamate, acetylcholine and CGRP receptors in gastrointestinal afferent inputs to vagal preganglionic neurones. Auton Neurosci 2000; 83:37–48.
227. Berthoud HR, Earle T, Zheng H, Patterson LM, Phifer C. Food-related gastrointestinal signals activate caudal brainstem neurons expressing both NMDA and AMPA receptors. Brain Res 2001; 915:143–154.
228. Sengupta JN, Petersen J, Peles S, Shaker R. Response properties of antral mechanosensitive afferent fibers and effects of ionotropic glutamate receptor antagonists. Neuroscience 2004; 125:711–723.
229. Jocic M, Schuligoi R, Schöninkle E, Pabst MA, Holzer P. Cooperation of NMDA and tachykinin NK_1 and NK_2 receptors in the medullary transmission of vagal afferent input from the acid-threatened rat stomach. Pain 2001; 89:147–157.
230. Fisher K, Coderre TJ, Hagen NA. Targeting the N-methyl-D-aspartate receptor for chronic pain management. Preclinical animal studies, recent clinical experience and future research directions. J Pain Symptom Management 2000; 20:358–373.
231. Parsons CG. NMDA receptors as targets for drug action in neuropathic pain. Eur J Pharmacol 2001; 429:71–78.
232. Karim F, Bhave G, Gereau RW. Metabotropic glutamate receptors on peripheral sensory neuron terminals as targets for the development of novel analgesics. Mol Psychiatry 2001; 6:615–617.
233. Neugebauer V. Peripheral metabotropic glutamate receptors: fight the pain where it hurts. Trends Neurosci 2001; 24:550–552.
234. Kirchgessner AL. Glutamate in the enteric nervous system. Curr Opin Pharmacol 2001; 1:591–596.
235. Green T, Dockray GJ. Characterization of the peptidergic afferent innervation of the stomach in the rat, mouse, and guinea-pig. Neuroscience 1988; 25:181–193.
236. Sternini C. Enteric and visceral afferent CGRP neurons. Targets of innervation and differential expression patterns. Ann New York Acad Sci 1992; 657:170–186.
237. Friese N, Diop L, Chevalier E, Angel F, Riviere PJM, Dahl SG. Involvement of prostaglandins and CGRP-dependent sensory afferents in peritoneal irritation-induced visceral pain. Regul Pept 1997; 70:1–7.
238. Julia V, Bueno L. Tachykininergic mediation of viscerosensitive responses to acute inflammation in rats: role of CGRP. Am J Physiol 1997; 272:G141–G146.
239. Ghia JE, Crenner F, Metz-Boutigue MH, Aunis D, Angel F. The effect of a chromogranin A-derived peptide (CgA4-16) in the writhing nociceptive response induced by acetic acid in rats. Life Sci 2004; 75:1787–1799.
240. Gschossmann JM, Coutinho SV, Miller JC, et al. Involvement of spinal calcitonin gene-elated peptide in the development of acute visceral hyperalgesia in the rat. Neurogastroenterol Motil 2001; 13:229–236.
241. Olesen J, Diener HC, Husstedt IW, et al. BIBN 4096 BS clinical proof of concept study group. Calcitonin gene-related peptide receptor antagonist BIBN 4096 BS for the acute treatment of migraine. N Engl J Med 2004; 350:1104–1110.
242. Lecci A, Valenti C, Maggi CA. Tachykinin receptor antagonists in irritable bowel syndrome. Curr Opin Investig Drugs 2002; 3:589–601.
243. Holzer P. Role of tachykinins in the gastrointestinal tract. In: Holzer P, ed. Tachykinins. Handbook of Experimental Pharmacology. 164. Vol. 164. Berlin: Springer, 2004:511–558.
244. Sanger GJ. Neurokinin NK_1 and NK_3 receptors as targets for drugs to treat gastrointestinal motility disorders and pain. Br J Pharmacol 2004; 141:1303–1312.
245. Lee O–Y, Munakata J, Naliboff BD, Chang L, Mayer EA. A double blind parallel group pilot study of the effects of CJ-11,974 and placebo on perceptual and emotional responses to rectosigmoid distension in IBS patients. Gastroenterology 2000; 118:A-846.
246. Laird JM, Olivar T, Roza C, De Felipe C, Hunt SP, Cervero F. Deficits in visceral pain and hyperalgesia of mice with a disruption of the tachykinin NK_1 receptor gene. Neuroscience 2000; 98:345–352.
247. Julia V, Morteau O, Bueno L. Involvement of neurokinin 1 and 2 receptors in viscerosensitive response to rectal distension in rats. Gastroenterology 1994; 107:94–102.

248. Julia V, Su X, Bueno L, Gebhart GF. Role of neurokinin 3 receptors on responses to colorectal distention in the rat: electrophysiological and behavioral studies. Gastroenterology 1999; 116:1124–1131.

249. Toulouse M, Coelho AM, Fioramonti J, Lecci A, Maggi CA, Bueno L. Role of tachykinin NK_2 receptors in normal and altered rectal sensitivity in rats. Br J Pharmacol 2000; 129:193–199.

250. Laird JM, Olivar T, Lopez-Garcia JA, Maggi CA, Cervero F. Responses of rat spinal neurons to distension of inflamed colon: role of tachykinin NK_2 receptors. Neuropharmacology 2001; 40:696–701.

251. Toulouse M, Fioramonti J, Maggi C, Bueno L. Role of NK_2 receptors in gastric barosensitivity and in experimental ileus in rats. Neurogastroenterol Motil 2001; 13:45–53.

252. Shafton AD, Bogeski G, Kitchener PD, Lewis VA, Sanger GJ, Furness JB. Effects of the peripherally acting NK_3 receptor antagonist, SB-235375, on intestinal and somatic nociceptive responses and on intestinal motility in anaesthetized rats. Neurogastroenterol Motil 2004; 16:223–231.

253. Okano S, Ikeura Y, Inatomi N. Effects of tachykinin NK_1 receptor antagonists on the viscerosensory response caused by colorectal distention in rabbits. J Pharmacol Exp Ther 2002; 300:925–931.

254. Bradesi S, Eutamene H, Garcia-Villar R, Fioramonti J, Bueno L. Stress-induced visceral hypersensitivity in female rats is estrogen-dependent and involves tachykinin NK_1 receptors. Pain 2003; 102:227–234.

255. Greenwood-Van Meerveld B, Gibson MS, Johnson AC, Venkova K, Sutkowski-Markmann D. NK_1 receptor-mediated mechanisms regulate colonic hypersensitivity in the guinea pig. Pharmacol Biochem Behav 2003; 74:1005–1013.

256. Schwetz I, Bradesi S, McRoberts JA, et al. Delayed stress-induced colonic hypersensitivity in male Wistar rats: role of neurokinin-1 and corticotropin-releasing factor-1 receptors. Am J Physiol 2004; 286:G683–G691.

257. Holzer-Petsche U, Rordorf-Nikolic T. Central versus peripheral site of action of the tachykinin NK_1-antagonist RP 67580 in inhibiting chemonociception. Br J Pharmacol 1995; 115:486–490.

258. McLean PG, Garcia-Villar R, Fioramonti J, Bueno L. Effects of tachykinin receptor antagonists on the rat jejunal distension pain response. Eur J Pharmacol 1998; 345:247–252.

259. McLean PG, Picard C, Garcia-Villar R, More J, Fioramonti J, Bueno L. Effects of nematode infection on sensitivity to intestinal distension: role of tachykinin NK_2 receptors. Eur J Pharmacol 1997; 337:279–282.

260. Gaudreau GA, Plourde V. Role of tachykinin NK_1, NK_2 and NK_3 receptors in the modulation of visceral hypersensitivity in the rat. Neurosci Lett 2003; 351:59–62.

261. Kamp EH, Beck DR, Gebhart GF. Combinations of neurokinin receptor antagonists reduce visceral hyperalgesia. J Pharmacol Exp Ther 2001; 299:105–113.

262. Ishigooka M, Zermann DH, Doggweiler R, Schmidt RA, Hashimoto T, Nakada T. Spinal NK_1 receptor is upregulated after chronic bladder irritation. Pain 2001; 93:43–50.

263. Honore P, Kamp EH, Rogers SD, Gebhart GF, Mantyh PW. Activation of lamina I spinal cord neurons that express the substance P receptor in visceral nociception and hyperalgesia. J Pain 2002; 3:3–11.

264. Palecek J, Paleckova V, Willis WD. Postsynaptic dorsal column neurons express NK_1 receptors following colon inflammation. Neuroscience 2003; 116:565–572.

265. Birder LA, Kiss S, de Groat WC, Lecci A, Maggi CA. Effect of nepadutant, a neurokinin 2 tachykinin receptor antagonist, on immediate-early gene expression after trinitrobenzenesulfonic acid-induced colitis in the rat. J Pharmacol Exp Ther 2003; 304:272–276.

266. Kishimoto S, Kobayashi H, Machino H, Tari A, Kajiyama G, Miyoshi A. High concentrations of substance P as a possible transmission of abdominal pain in rats with chemical induced ulcerative colitis. Biomed Res 1994; 15(suppl 2):133–140.

267. Minami M, Endo T, Yokota H, et al. Effects of CP-99, 994, a tachykinin NK_1 receptor antagonist, on abdominal afferent vagal activity in ferrets: evidence for involvement of NK_1 and 5-HT_3 receptors. Eur J Pharmacol 2001; 428:215–220.

268. Fioramonti J, Gaultier E, Toulouse M, Sanger GJ, Bueno L. Intestinal anti-nociceptive behaviour of NK_3 receptor antagonism in conscious rats: evidence to support a peripheral mechanism of action. Neurogastroenterol Motil 2003; 15:363–369.

269. Rupniak NMJ, Kramer MS. Discovery of the anti-depressant and anti-emetic efficacy of substance P receptor (NK_1) antagonists. Trends Pharmacol Sci 1999; 20:485–490.

270. Andrews PLR, Rudd JA. The role of tachykinins and the tachykinin NK_1 receptor in nausea and emesis. In: Holzer P, ed. Tachykinins. Handbook of Experimental Pharmacology. 164. Vol. 164. Berlin: Springer, 2004:359–440.

271. Ji RR, Zhang Q, Law PY, Low HH, Elde R, Hökfelt T. Expression of mu-, delta-, and kappa-opioid receptor-like immunoreactivities in rat dorsal root ganglia after carrageenan-induced inflammation. J Neurosci 1995; 15:8156–8166.

272. Minami M, Maekawa K, Yabuuchi K, Satoh M. Double in situ hybridization study on coexistence of mu-, delta- and kappa-opioid receptor mRNAs with preprotachykinin A mRNA in the rat dorsal root ganglia. Mol Brain Res 1995; 30:203–210.

273. Ozaki N, Sengupta JN, Gebhart GF. Differential effects of mu-, delta-, and kappa-opioid receptor agonists on mechanosensitive gastric vagal afferent fibers in the rat. J Neurophysiol 2000; 83:2209–2216.

274. Stein C, Schäfer M, Machelska H. Attacking pain at its source: new perspectives on opioids. Nat Med 2003; 9:1003–1008.
275. Riviere PJ. Peripheral kappa-opioid agonists for visceral pain. Br J Pharmacol 2004; 141:1331–1334.
276. Fürst S. Transmitters involved in antinociception in the spinal cord. Brain Res Bull 1999; 48:129–141.
277. Pertovaara A. Antinociceptive properties of fadolmidine (MPV-2426), a novel alpha$_2$-adrenoceptor agonist. CNS Drug Rev 2004; 10:117–126.
278. Birder LA, Perl ER. Expression of alpha$_2$-adrenergic receptors in rat primary afferent neurones after peripheral nerve injury or inflammation. J Physiol (London) 1999; 515:533–542.
279. Ongjoco RRS, Richardson CD, Rudner XL, Stafford-Smith M, Schwinn DA. alpha$_2$-Adrenergic receptors in human dorsal root ganglia. Anesthesiology 2000; 92:968–976.
280. Ono H, Mishima A, Ono S, Fukuda H, Vasko MR. Inhibitory effects of clonidine and tizanidine on release of substance P from slices of rat spinal cord and antagonism by alpha-adrenergic receptor antagonists. Neuropharmacology 1991; 30:585–589.
281. Ueda M, Oyama T, Kuraishi Y, Akaike A, Satoh M. Alpha2-adrenoceptor-mediated inhibition of capsaicin-evoked release of glutamate from rat spinal dorsal horn slices. Neurosci Lett 1995; 188:137–139.
282. Li X, Eisenach JC. Alpha$_{2a}$-adrenoceptor stimulation reduces capsaicin–induced glutamate release from spinal cord synaptosomes. J Pharmacol Exp Ther 2001; 299:939–944.
283. Pertovaara A, Kalmari J. Comparison of the visceral antinociceptive effects of spinally administered MPV-2426 (fadolmidine) and clonidine in the rat. Anesthesiology 2003; 98:189–194.
284. Thumshirn M, Camilleri M, Choi M-G, Zinsmeister AR. Modulation of gastric sensory and motor functions by nitrergic and alpha$_2$-adrenergic agents in humans. Gastroenterology 1999; 116:573–585.
285. Malcolm A, Camilleri M, Kost L, Burton DD, Fett SL, Zinsmeister AR. Towards identifying optimal doses for alpha$_2$ adrenergic modulation of colonic and rectal motor and sensory function. Aliment Pharmacol Ther 2000; 14:783–793.
286. Cannon RO, Quyyumi AA, Mincemoyer R, et al. Imipramine in patients with chest pain despite normal coronary angiograms. N Engl J Med 1994; 330:1411–1417.
287. Tanum L, Malt UF. A new pharmacologic treatment of functional gastrointestinal disorder. A double-blind placebo-controlled study with mianserin. Scand J Gastroenterol 1996; 31:318–325.
288. Gray AM, Pache DM, Sewell RDE. Do alpha$_2$-adrenoceptors play an integral role in the antinociceptive mechanism of action of antidepressant compounds?. Eur J Pharmacol 1999; 378:161–168.
289. Su X, Gebhart GF. Effects of tricyclic antidepressants on mechanosensitive pelvic nerve afferent fibers innervating the rat colon. Pain 1998; 76:105–114.
290. Pertwee RG. Cannabinoid receptors and pain. Prog Neurobiol 2001; 63:569–611.
291. Hornby PJ, Prouty SM. Involvement of cannabinoid receptors in gut motility and visceral perception. Br J Pharmacol 2004; 141:1335–1345.
292. Hohmann AG, Herkenham M. Localization of central cannabinoid CB$_1$ receptor messenger RNA in neuronal subpopulations of rat dorsal root ganglia: a double-label in situ hybridization study. Neuroscience 1999; 90:923–931.
293. Ahluwalia J, Urban L, Capogna M, Bevan S, Nagy I. Cannabinoid 1 receptors are expressed in nociceptive primary sensory neurons. Neuroscience 2000; 100:685–688.
294. Lever IJ, Malcangio M. CB$_1$ receptor antagonist SR141716A increases capsaicin-evoked release of substance P from the adult mouse spinal cord. Br J Pharmacol 2002; 135:21–24.
295. Hohmann AG, Herkenham M. Cannabinoid receptors undergo axonal flow in sensory nerves. Neuroscience 1999; 92:1171–1175.
296. Piomelli D, Giuffrida A, Calignano A, Rodriguez de Fonseca F. The endocannabinoid system as a target for therapeutic drugs. Trends Pharmacol Sci 2000; 21:218–224.
297. Szallasi A, Di Marzo V. New perspectives on enigmatic vanilloid receptors. Trends Neurosci 2000; 23:491–497.
298. Hohmann AG. Spinal and peripheral mechanisms of cannabinoid antinociception: behavioral, neurophysiological and neuroanatomical perspectives. Chem Phys Lipids 2002; 121:173–190.
299. Rice AS, Farquhar-Smith WP, Nagy I. Endocannabinoids and pain: spinal and peripheral analgesia in inflammation and neuropathy. Prostaglandins Leukot Essent Fatty Acids 2002; 66:243–256.
300. Coutts AA, Izzo AA. The gastrointestinal pharmacology of cannabinoids: an update. Curr Opin Pharmacol 2004; 4:572–579.
301. Dinis P, Charrua A, Avelino A, et al. Anandamide-evoked activation of vanilloid receptor 1 contributes to the development of bladder hyperreflexia and nociceptive transmission to spinal dorsal horn neurons in cystitis. J Neurosci 2004; 24:11253–11263.
302. Jaggar SI, Hasnie FS, Sellaturay S, Rice ASC. The anti-hyperalgesic actions of the cannabinoid anandamide and the putative CB$_2$ receptor agonist palmitoylethanolamide in visceral and somatic inflammatory pain. Pain 1998; 76:189–199.
303. Izzo AA, Fezza F, Capasso R, et al. Cannabinoid CB$_1$-receptor mediated regulation of gastrointestinal motility in mice in a model of intestinal inflammation. Br J Pharmacol 2001; 134:563–570.
304. Blackshaw LA, Gebhart GF. The pharmacology of gastrointestinal nociceptive pathways. Curr Opin Pharmacol 2002; 2:642–649.

18 | Management of the Patient with Chronic Abdominal Pain and Clinical Pharmacology of Nonopioid Drugs

Michael Camilleri

Clinical Enteric Neuroscience Translational and Epidemiological Research (C.E.N.T.E.R.) Program, Mayo Clinic College of Medicine, Rochester, Minnesota, U.S.A.

INTRODUCTION

Much has been written about the prevalence, societal burden, and suffering of chronic abdominal pain. Reviews tend to focus on the particular expertise of the author and the literature is replete with scholarly treatises. These range from the perspective of the biopsychosocial model that considers chronic functional abdominal pain in a continuum of psychological disturbance with disturbances of the function of the sensory mechanisms and central interpretation of afferent input, to the surgical perspective: "A chance to cut is a chance to cure."

How does the busy clinician navigate the troubled waters when the patient reports experiencing chronic abdominal pain? This is the fundamental question that is addressed in this chapter. The goal is to provide a roadmap, to discuss the steps along the way, where evidence and guidance is available from the published literature to facilitate management and to review the effects of commonly used medications with focus on physiology and clinical trials (Fig. 1). In this field, there are no evidence-based, validated critical pathways, and hence one draws on the practical experience of three decades as a physician, as well as the desire, whenever possible, to apply evidence-based medicine in a scholarly fashion.

ESTABLISHING A ROADMAP
First Step: Is it Clearly Functional, Wall Pain, or Bloating?

Given the high prevalence of functional disorders, one could almost apply the assumption that patients presenting with abdominal pain are most likely to suffer a variant of functional gastrointestinal (GI) disorders, such as chronic functional abdominal pain or irritable bowel syndrome (IBS), when the pain is also associated with disturbance of bowel function. This approach is often pursued in primary care or office-based gastroenterology, and a therapeutic trial is started. Most often, this involves the use of a low-dose tricyclic antidepressant or a serotonin reuptake inhibitor at full dose, as well as a smooth muscle relaxant for acute exacerbations of pain. The roadmap, therefore, requires a fast track to the practical management of patients with chronic functional abdominal pain. Indeed, Drossman (1) has provided practical guidance on how to suspect chronic functional abdominal pain, as shown in Table 1 .

An important consideration in the evaluation of such patients is the possibility of chronic abdominal wall pain (CAWP), which often is misdiagnosed. Longstreth and coworkers evaluated CAWP patients regarding diagnosis accuracy, clinical features, comorbidity, referral frequency, use of care, and long-term outcome among all outpatients referred to a gastroenterologist in five years (2). Of 2709 patients, CAWP was diagnosed by physical examination (Carnett's test) in 137 patients. Carnett's test can help to distinguish visceral from somatic pain. After identifying the site of maximal abdominal pain, the patient is asked to tense the anterior abdominal musculature by having the patient attempt to sit up, while the physician applies pressure to the patient's forehead. A positive test result, i.e., increased pain with tensing of the abdominal musculature, would suggest an abdominal wall etiology (e.g., cutaneous nerve entrapment and hernia); whereas, a negative test result would be consistent with a visceral contribution to the pain. The diagnosis of CAWP remained unchanged after 47.3 ± 17.7 (mean $\pm$ SD) months in 133 (97.1%) patients. Women predominated over men four to one; pain

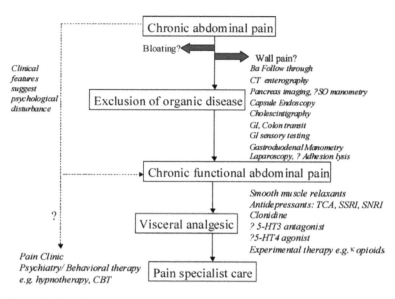

Figure 1 The chronic abdominal pain road map.

was usually upper abdominal and had lasted an average of over two years, and obesity and painful comorbidities [low back pain 30%, migraine 14%, fibromyalgia 10%, and IBS 22%] and depression (22%) were common. Postconsultation, primary care, emergency and specialist visits, and radiologic examinations markedly decreased, and estimated annual costs decreased from an average of $1133.87 to average $541.33 confirming the importance of considering and making this diagnosis. Over the long term, pain disappearance and persistence occurred in approximately equal proportions of patients but one could argue that a 50% success rate in pain disappearance is outstanding in this patient population (2).

Another important distinction in practice is to assess whether the patient's "chronic discomfort represents bloating," often with an element of constipation, or true pain. Clinical experience shows that many patients with predominantly gas-like distension, lower abdominal bloating, and delayed proximal colonic emptying on transit test can be relieved with symptomatic treatment of the delayed proximal colonic transit using simple laxatives, with or without addition of probiotic agents. Three studies have shown the potential symptomatic benefit of probiotics in the relief of bloating or flatulence (3,4) or the global relief of IBS symptoms including pain (5). Similarly, the potential for antibiotic therapy for presumed bacterial overgrowth deserves further evaluation (6).

Table 1 Evaluation of the Patient for Suspected Functional Abdominal Pain Syndrome

Psychosocial assessment
  What is the patient's life history of illness?
  Why is the patient coming now?
  Is there a history of traumatic life events?
  What is the patient's understanding of the illness?
  What is impact of the pain on quality of life?
  Is there an associated psychiatric diagnosis?
  What is the role of family or culture?
  What are the patient's psychosocial resources?
Physical examination
  No autonomic arousal
  Surgical scars
  Closed eyes sign
  Stethoscope sign
  Carnett's test

Note: Exclusion of other disease.

Table 2 Chronic Pain Features Suggestive of Structural or Organic Disease

More recent in onset (if undiagnosed)
Described in more sensory (e.g., sharp, crampy, and burning) rather than emotional terms
More variable or intermittent in intensity
More precise in locations conforming to neuroanatomic pathways
More responsive to antimotility agents and/or peripherally acting
  [e.g., nonsteroidal anti-inflammatory drugs (NSAIDs)] analgesics
Related to events that affect gut function
Usually associated with fewer difficulties in interpersonal relationships

Step 2: Exclusion of Organic Disease

Drossman has provided important indicators to suspect structural disease in patients with chronic pain. These features are listed in Table 2 .

As physicians, we are lulled into a false sense of security the longer the history, the absence of weight loss or rectal bleeding, the more prior tests have been unrevealing, and when there are no findings on examination (e.g., no abdominal mass or hepatomegaly) or on screening tests such as blood tests, sedimentation rate, or C-reactive protein, abdominal radiograph, and the inevitable abdominal imaging with ultrasound or computed tomography (CT) scan that most of these patients will have undergone prior to referral to the gastroenterologist. Yet there are certain investigations that are certainly worth considering in individual patients guided by the history and by clinical acumen.

The next section summarizes the clinical judgment and reasons for considering special investigations in individual patients in my practice. Seeking metabolic causes of chronic abdominal pain such as porphyria, hypercalcemia, or lead poisoning is usually indicated by indications in the family history or environmental exposure.

Imaging the Small Bowel

The advent of transaxial imaging has been a great boon for evaluating solid organs in the abdomen, but over the last three decades, the interest of radiologists in standard barium follow-through examinations seems to have decreased and with this comes the inevitable drop in interpretative skills. Standard follow-through examination or enteroclysis has been relegated to timed images because of costs, or replaced with CT enterography. These are probably complementary tests at the present time in my practice because sensitivity is not 100% for subtle lesions such as small mass lesions, short strictures (e.g., from NSAID enteropathy or Crohn's), and variability in technique and expertise may necessitate performance of both tests when there is a high index of suspicion for obstruction. A surgically or medically treatable lesion may be identified and treated.

Other times the diagnosis is clear, though the attribution of the chronic pain syndrome to the structural disorder may be less clear. This is often the case with patients with congenital nonrotation (often inappropriately termed malrotation) of the intestine. Midgut nonrotation is a congenital anomaly referring to either lack of or incomplete rotation of the fetal intestines around the axis of the superior mesenteric artery during fetal development. Most patients present with bilious vomiting in the first month of life because of duodenal obstruction or a volvulus. It is rare for this condition to present in adulthood. The true prevalence in adults is difficult to estimate because most patients are asymptomatic and are, therefore, never diagnosed. Patients who are symptomatic often present either acutely with bowel obstruction and intestinal ischemia with a midgut or cecal volvulus or chronically with vague abdominal pain. These symptoms are caused by peritoneal Ladd bands that run from the cecum to the right lateral abdominal wall (7).

Imaging the Pancreas

While spiral CT is often sufficient to investigate important lesions of the pancreas, further investigation may be necessary to characterize further the structural details including the correct identification of cystic lesions and their differentiation from intraductal pancreatic mucinous tumors. Thus, endoscopic ultrasound (EUS) with fine needle aspiration may be indicated to characterize lesions within the pancreas further (8).

The role of sphincter of Oddi manometry in the evaluation of chronic abdominal pain in the absence of elevated amylase/lipase or liver enzymes is the subject of continued debate, as is the role of sphincterotomy or stenting in the treatment of patients with so-called type III sphincter of Oddi dysfunction. Recent data suggest that patients were likely to respond to sphincterotomy if their pain was not continuous, if it was accompanied by nausea or vomiting, and if there had been a pain-free interval after cholecystectomy of at least one year (9). Some of these patients have a visceral hypersensitivity syndrome typical of chronic functional abdominal pain (10).

Other Small Bowel Imaging Using Novel Endoscopic Approaches
Capsule endoscopy and double-balloon endoscopy have enhanced our ability to image the small bowel and identify the cause of obscure GI bleeding. However, it appears that the yield in patients with chronic abdominal pain is low (11–13). It has, however, been claimed that capsule endoscopy may be superior to CT enterography and barium follow through examination (14). More formal controlled trials are needed.

Cholescintigraphy as a Predictor of Response to Cholecystectomy in Patients Without Gallstones
Our clinical experience in tertiary centers is often biased by the exposure to patients with persistent pain after cholecystectomy performed for acalculous disease, typically based on the poor ejection fraction of the gall bladder (GBEF) on cholescintigraphy. However, a thorough systematic review and meta-analysis suggests that, after cholecystectomy, 94% of the patients with reduced GBEF had a positive outcome compared to 85% among those with normal GBEF (15). The pooled Mantel-Haenszel odds ratio for positive outcome was 1.37 [95% confidence interval (CI) 0.56–3.34, $p = 0.56$]. These data do not support the use of GBEF to select patients with suspected functional biliary pain for cholecystectomy. Prospective randomized trials are required if this practice is to be evidence-based. Hence, I do not perform this test in my clinical practice.

Gastrointestinal and Colonic Transit
In our experience, the yield of upper GI transit tests in patients with chronic abdominal pain is low (16), in contrast to the situation in patients with symptoms more clearly suggestive of a motility disorder like postprandial fullness or constipation. This applies to experience in both adults (17) and children (18,19). However, clinical experience suggests that delayed proximal colonic transit is sometimes associated with chronic right-sided abdominal discomfort and mild constipation and patients may present with a main complaint of "chronic pain." Thus, the transit test and tests of anorectal evacuation are worth pursuing if the symptoms suggest irregular bowel pattern, examination reveals a large amount of palpable stool. Justification of this approach is based on the simplicity and safety of a therapeutic trial of laxatives to relieve the constipation and evaluation of the chronic pain after one month before pursuing further or invasive tests.

Visceral Sensory Tests
It has been proposed that visceral hypersensitivity is a biological marker of IBS (20); similar observations suggest that many of the functional GI disorders are associated with such hypersensitivity, and this likely is important in patients with chronic functional abdominal pain. A few centers measure viscus tone, compliance, and sensitivity regularly (20–22) with intubated methods as shown in Figure 2, but this is clearly still an area where there is not general expertise and standardization. Recently, noninvasive approaches to measure visceral hypersensitivity have been developed, mostly related to stomach sensation, and combinations of satiation testing (23) and measurements of gastric volume (24) may be developed to facilitate the identification of gastric hypersensitivity.

Gastroduodenal Manometry
Gastroduodenal manometry has been shown to be able to identify mechanical obstruction in rare instances where the radiographic examination of the small bowel is negative (25). However, this should never occur with the modern modalities of investigation including enteroclysis, CT enterography, and capsule endoscopy. Chronic intestinal pseudoobstruction may be associated with chronic pain, but the typical association with symptoms consistent with a motility disorder are dominant (26). Therefore, gastroduodenal manometry is not indicated for the evaluation of chronic abdominal pain when it is the sole symptom.

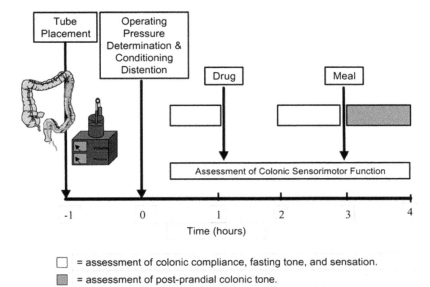

Figure 2 Experimental model for testing motor and sensory functions of candidate medications: A polyethylene bag with infinite compliance is placed in the viscus, and linked to an electronic barostat. The pressure of air in the bag is maintained at constant pressure, and sequential measurements of compliance, tone, and sensation are performed. This design facilitates the measurement of pharmacological actions on both sensory and motor functions, and can be used to assess dose-related efficacy of potential medications of interest.

Laparoscopy and Adhesiolysis

Despite the advances in imaging and endoscopy, there are clearly some diseases associated with chronic abdominal pain that cannot be identified and laparoscopy may be indicated (27). Examples include adhesions, internal herniation, or closed loop obstructions. Collaboration with a surgeon is key to the management of these patients.

Intestinal and abdominal adhesions may be responsible for a variety of clinical conditions, including chronic recurrent small-bowel obstruction, acute small-bowel obstruction, closed-loop bowel obstruction and, debatably, abdominal or pelvic pain. Experience in laparoscopic surgery has increased at a rapid pace in recent years, and adhesions are no longer considered a contraindication to treatment of these conditions (28,29). Other series show that laparoscopic adhesiolysis is a safe and effective management option for patients with prior abdominal surgery with chronic abdominal pain or recurrent bowel obstruction not attributed to other intra-abdominal pathology (30). However, a randomized controlled trial tested the hypothesis that laparoscopic adhesiolysis leads to substantial pain relief and improvement in quality of life in patients with adhesions and chronic abdominal pain. Of 116 patients enrolled for diagnostic laparoscopy, 100 were randomly allocated either to laparoscopic adhesiolysis ($n = 52$) or no treatment ($n = 48$). Both groups reported substantial pain relief and a significantly improved quality of life, but there was no difference between the groups (mean change from baseline of visual analog scale (VAS) score at 12 months: Difference of three points, $p = 0.53$; 95% CI: 7–13). This trial suggests that laparoscopic adhesiolysis cannot be recommended as a treatment for adhesions in patients with chronic abdominal pain (31).

The decision to pursue laparoscopy in my practice is based on the concern that the patient has organic disease that may have been missed despite the availability of sophisticated investigation. Hence this strategy is seldom pursued; when adhesions are clearly causing obstruction identified at laparoscopy, the decision is easy; however, in the absence of such findings of obstruction, we do not generally follow the surgical adage: "A chance to cut is a chance to cure"!

Step Three: Treatment of Chronic Functional Abdominal Pain

Much credit to the identification of effective management of patients in my practice is due to Drossman, who has outlined that the basis for treatment relies first on establishing an effective

Table 3 Treatment Approach For Patients with Chronic Functional Abdominal Pain

Establishing an effective patient–physician relationship
    Empathy
    Education
    Validation
    Reassurance
    Negotiate the treatment
    Set reasonable limits
The treatment plan
    Set reasonable treatment goals
    Help the patient take responsibility
    Base treatment on symptom severity and the degree of disability
    Medications
    Mental health referral
    Specific psychological treatments
    Multidisciplinary pain treatment center referral

Source: From Ref. 1.

physician–patient relationship and then providing a more specific plan that relies on several treatment options. The treatment approach is outlined in Table 3. Because this management plan is extensively reviewed elsewhere, the next section will focus on the clinical pharmacology of nonopioid drugs used in the treatment of chronic abdominal pain.

Medications: Clinical Pharmacology and Efficacy in Clinical Trials

The molecular targets for treatment of visceral pain are discussed in Chapter 13. This review will focus on applied clinical pharmacology in humans and evidence of efficacy from formal clinical trials.

Simple Analgesics

Most analgesics (e.g., aspirin and NSAIDs) offer little benefit because they act peripherally. Conversely, the use of these drugs was significantly associated with a greater number of upper GI symptoms and prescriptions for GI drugs, especially in the elderly (32). Given the risks of GI mucosal ulcers, intestinal stricturing, and other general adverse effects (e.g., renal impairment), especially with NSAIDs, and the lack of any evidence of efficacy, these medications are not used for chronic abdominal pain.

Narcotics

Narcotics should not be prescribed because of the potential for addiction and narcotic bowel syndrome, and this class of medication is reviewed in Chapter 16.

Benzodiazepines

IBS and psychiatric disorders are associated regardless of treatment-seeking status, and patients with psychiatric disorders may present to the clinician with chronic abdominal pain or IBS. Treatment of the associated anxiety or depression, panic attacks, or other psychiatric illness is clearly warranted. Most experts are of the opinion that benzodiazepines are of limited value and they might paradoxically lower pain threshold (33). However, they may play a secondary role in patients with general anxiety disorder (GAD) for the management of a wide array of complaints including headache, noncardiac chest pain, insomnia, or abdominal discomfort. Given the chronic, nonremitting, relapsing character of GAD, use of benzodiazepines, which confer short-term relief, is usually ill-advised in long-term treatment because these agents can impair cognitive and psychomotor function, interact with various central nervous system depressants (e.g., alcohol), and exhibit substantial potential for abuse, tolerance, dependence, and withdrawal effects. Buspirone and certain antidepressants, including the dual noradrenergic–serotonergic reuptake inhibitor, venlafaxine, represent first-line therapy for GAD (34).

Tricyclic Antidepressants

Clinical Pharmacology: Three studies have formally examined the effect of tricyclic agents on human GI sensitivity as a marker of experimental visceral pain: (i) A study in healthy volunteers showed that amitriptyline did not significantly alter visceral sensory thresholds in the esophagus or rectum (35). (ii) The University of California at Los Angeles (UCLA) group tested the effect of amitriptyline in patients with functional dyspepsia (36). Five of seven patients had evidence for altered perception of gastric balloon distension during placebo. However, the subjective symptom improvement on amitriptyline was not associated with a normalization of the perceptual responses to gastric distension. (iii). The Quebec group assessed rectal sensory threshold in patients with irritable bowel syndrome treated for four weeks with 25 mg amitriptyline (37). The pain threshold to rectal distension increased from 27.7 ± 1.0 to 33.7 ± 1.9 mmHg ($p < 0.01$) after drug treatment, but remained unchanged (30.6 ± 1.0 vs. 30.6 ± 1.1 mmHg) with psychotherapy. Evolution of the GI symptom index and rectal sensitivity were directly correlated ($r = -0.71$; $p < 0.01$) in amitriptyline patients, but not in those treated with psychotherapy ($r = -0.001$).

Clinical Efficacy: Tricyclic agents (e.g., amitriptyline, imipramine, and doxepin) are now frequently used to treat patients with IBS, particularly those with more severe or refractory symptoms, impaired daily function, and associated depression or panic attacks. Initially their use was based on the fact that a high proportion of patients with IBS reported significant depression. Antidepressants have neuromodulatory and analgesic properties, which may benefit patients independently of the psychotrophic effects of the drugs (38). It appears that the clinical effects of agents such as amitryptiline result from their central actions. Neuromodulatory effects may occur sooner and with lower dosages in IBS patients than the dosages used in the treatment of depression (e.g., 10–25 mg amitryptiline or 50 mg desipramine). Because antidepressants must be used on a continual rather than an as needed basis, they are generally reserved for patients having frequently recurrent or continual symptoms. A two- to three-month trial is usually needed before excluding a therapeutic benefit.

The placebo-controlled trials of antidepressants in IBS have been summarized elsewhere (39). In two large studies, trimipramine decreased abdominal pain, nausea, and depression, but did not alter stool frequency (40,41). The beneficial effect seems to be greater in those with abdominal pain and diarrhea. For example, desipramine improved abdominal pain and diarrhea (42), while in an earlier study (43) that combined patients with either diarrhea or constipation, there was no significant benefit for desipramine over placebo. Nortriptyline in combination with fluphenazine reduced abdominal pain and diarrhea in two studies (44,45).

As a therapeutic class, Jackson et al. (46) calculated a summary odds ratio for improvement with antidepressant therapy of 4.2 (95% CI: 2.3–7.9), and the average standardized mean improvement in pain was equal to 0.9 SD units (95% CI: 0.6–1.2 SD units). On average 3.2 patients needed to be treated (95% CI: 2.1–6.5 patients) to improve one patient's symptoms. However, there is considerable heterogeneity in the efficacy of the different medications and it is clear that an outlier result from a trial of mianserin in patients with functional dyspepsia or IBS biases the estimates reported. Thus, this trial of mianserin (which has actions other than being a tricyclic), which used a different experimental design with a placebo run-in with exclusion of responders, provided an odds ratio close to 22 (47). Interestingly, of the seven other trials in the meta-analysis, only one showed a significant advantage of the antidepressant, doxepin, over placebo (48).

The best trial of the effects of tricyclics was recently published from the North Carolina-Toronto groups (49). This randomized, comparator-controlled, multicenter trial enrolled 431 adults with moderate to severe symptoms of functional bowel disorders. Participants received psychological cognitive behavioral therapy vs. education (CBT vs. EDU) or antidepressant (DESipramine vs. PLAcebo) treatment for 12 weeks. Intention-to-treat analysis showed DES, did not show significant benefit over PLA ($p = 0.16$; responder rate, 60% DES vs. 47% PLA; NNT, 8.1), but did show a statistically significant benefit in the per protocol analysis ($p = 0.01$; responder rate, 73% DES vs. 49% PLA; number-needed-to-treat (NNT), 5.2), especially when participants with nondetectable blood levels of DES were excluded ($p = 0.002$). Because the per protocol analysis likely reflects more closely clinical practice in this setting, these data are indeed encouraging and suggest that, if patients stick to their treatment regimen, they are likely to benefit in the global response to desipramine. It is, however, unclear whether the benefit is the same in IBS as in patients with chronic functional abdominal pain.

There is also the additional challenge that patients might not tolerate the side effects (anticholinergic effects, hypotension, sedation, and cardiac arrhythmias) or might feel stigmatized by taking a "psychiatric" drug, leading to poor adherence with this class of drugs. Thus, it is important for the physician to help the patient properly understand its clinical value and to work with the patient to assure adherence.

Selective Serotonin, Combined Serotonin-Norepinephrine Reuptake Inhibitors, and Azapirones (Buspirone)

Clinical Pharmacology

While the effects of a selective serotonin (5-HT) reuptake inhibitor (SSRI), paroxetine, to accelerate small bowel transit is well known (50), five studies have recently reported, in greater detail, the effects of prototype SSRIs and serotonin–norepinephrine reuptake inhibitors (SNRIs):

1. Coulie et al. showed that the cat fundus relaxes with buspirone (51), and preliminary data confirm these findings in humans (52).
2. Chial et al. evaluated the effects of serotonergic psychoactive agents on GI functions in 51 healthy human participants, who received one of four regimens in a randomized, double-blind manner: Buspirone, a 5-HT (1A) receptor agonist (10 mg twice daily); paroxetine, a SSRI (20 mg daily); venlafaxine-XR, a selective serotonin and norepinephrine reuptake inhibitor (75 mg daily); or placebo for 11 days (53). Physiological testing performed on days 8 to 11 included scintigraphic assessment of GI and colonic transit, the nutrient drink test, and assessment of the postprandial change in gastric volume using a noninvasive measurement of the stomach using ^{99m}Tc-SPECT imaging. No effects on gastric emptying or colonic transit were identified with any agent. Small bowel transit of a solid meal was accelerated by paroxetine. Buspirone decreased postprandial aggregate symptom and nausea scores in response to a fully satiating meal. Venlafaxine-XR increased the postprandial change in gastric volume. The authors concluded that buspirone, paroxetine, and venlafaxine-XR affect upper GI functions in healthy humans and that the data support the need for clinical and physiological studies of these agents in functional GI disorders (53).
3. In a separate study, Chial et al. compared the effects of venlafaxine, buspirone, and placebo on colonic sensorimotor functions in 60 healthy adults with a randomized, double-blind, parallel-group, placebo-controlled trial (54). Oral venlafaxine, 150 mg; buspirone, 20 mg and placebo were tested. Venlafaxine significantly increased colonic compliance, decreased fasting colonic tone and the tonic response to a meal compared with placebo (Fig. 3A). Pressure thresholds for first sensation ($p = 0.1$) and gas ($p = 0.07$) were not statistically significant with venlafaxine. However, the increase in pain scores per unit pressure during phasic distensions was affected by treatment ($p = 0.02$), with the smallest changes on venlafaxine and the highest on placebo (Fig. 3B). Buspirone did not significantly alter colonic compliance, tone, or sensation relative to placebo. The authors suggested that these data support the need for further clinical and physiologic studies of venlafaxine in colonic disorders affecting motor and, possibly, sensory functions (54).
4. Kuiken et al. evaluated 40 nondepressed IBS patients, who underwent a rectal barostat study to assess the sensitivity to rectal distention before and after six weeks of treatment with fluoxetine, 20 mg, or placebo (55). Abdominal pain scores, individual GI symptoms, global symptom relief, and psychologic symptoms were assessed before and after the intervention. At baseline, 21 of 40 patients showed hypersensitivity to rectal distention. Fluoxetine did not significantly alter the threshold for discomfort/pain relative to placebo, either in rectal hypersensitive or normosensitive IBS patients. In contrast, in hypersensitive patients only, fluoxetine significantly reduced the number of patients reporting significant abdominal pain. They concluded that fluoxetine does not change rectal sensitivity in IBS patients and that possible beneficial effects on pain perception need to be confirmed in larger trials (55).
5. Finally, a preliminary report by Tack's group has also evaluated the effect of intravenous citalopram, an SSRI, and demonstrated effects on colonic tone and sensation in healthy individuals (56). A small crossover study of 14 patients suggested that citalopram, 20 mg, for six weeks reduced the number of days of abdominal pain and bloating in IBS, despite a single intravenous dose not altering colonic sensitivity (56).

Thus, it is unclear whether SSRIs, as a class, alter visceral sensation; more consistent results on viscus tone and sensation appear attributable to the SNRI class, where the effect on norepinephrine reuptake may be important for the potential peripheral pharmacological effects of SNRIs, as is evident from the pharmacological effects of clonidine (see below).

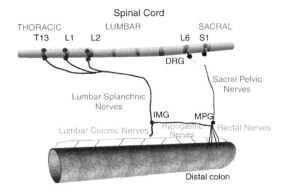

Figure 5.1 Extrinsic spinal innervation of the colon. (*See p. 47*)

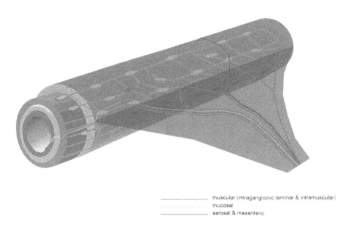

muscular (intraganglionic laminar & intramuscular)
mucosal
serosal & mesenteric

Figure 5.2 Several different classes of mechanoreceptor within the gastro-intestinal tract. (*See p. 48*)

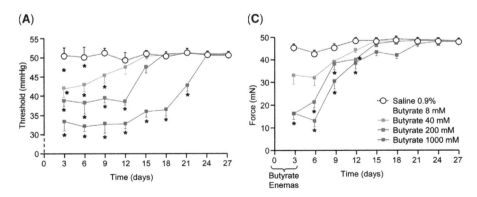

Figure 8.5 Intracolonic butyrate produces enhanced colonic sensitivity and referred hypersensitivity in the rat. The effect of six (twice daily) intracolonic infusions of 1 ml saline or butyrate solution (8, 40, 200 or 1000 mM) on the pressure thresholds inducing a specific behavior following colorectal distension (**A**), and on forces exerted by application of von Frey filaments to the lumbar abdominal skin required to induce a reaction (**C**). (*See p. 117*)

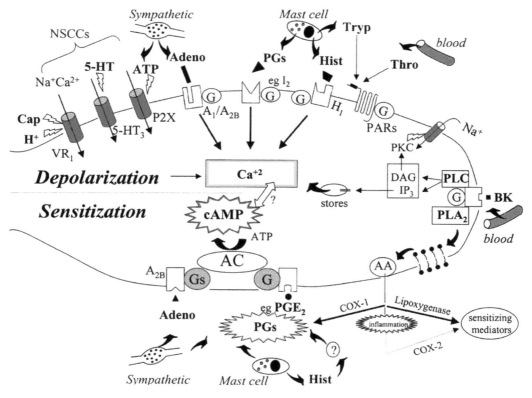

Figure 10.1 The potential receptor mechanisms mediating depolarization and sensitization of visceral afferent neurons. (*See p. 143*)

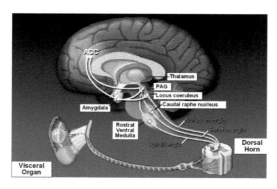

Figure 10.3 The principal components of descending pain modulatory pathways (*yellow lines*), which are activated in response to a painful visceral stimulus such as noxious balloon distension of the colon. (*See p. 145*)

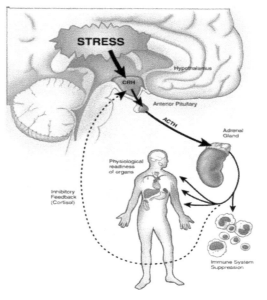

Figure 10.4 The functional anatomy of the hypothalamic-pituitary-adrenal axis. (*See p. 148*)

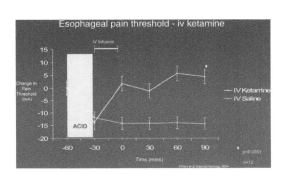

Figure 10.5 The effect of an *N*-methyl-D-aspartate receptor antagonist, ketamine, on proximal esophageal pain thresholds when given following a distal esophageal acid infusion. (*See p. 150*)

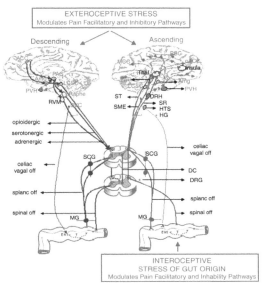

Figure 14.2 Schematic representation of ascending and descending visceral pain pathways and the stress-related neuronal circuitry that potentially modulates these pain pathways. (*See p. 207*)

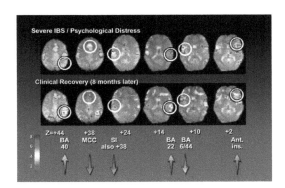

Figure 15.4 Cingulate activation in irritable bowel syndrome (IBS) before and after clinical recovery. (*See p. 227*)

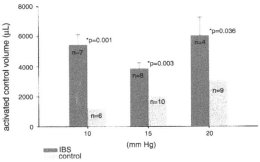

Figure 24.6 Total fMRI cortical activity volume response to three levels of subliminal rectal distention pressures in IBS patients and controls. (*See p. 346*)

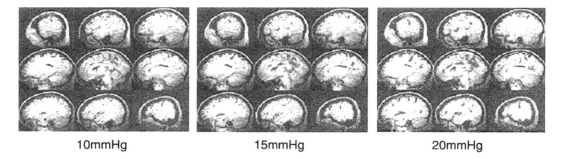

10mmHg   15mmHg   20mmHg

Figure 24.7 The anatomic location of composite fMRI activity associated with subliminal rectal distention in 10 diarrhea-predominant female IBS patients. fMRI activity can be characterized to exist in five broad cortical regions: the sensory/motor, the parietal/occipital, the cingulate gyrus, the prefrontal cortex, and the insula cortex. (*See p. 347*)

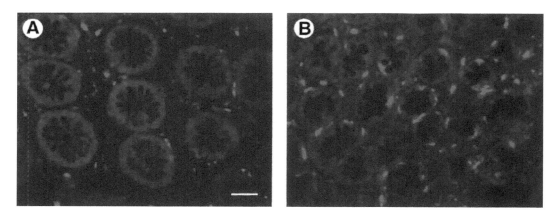

Figure 24.8 Representative photomicrographs showing tryptase-positive mast cells in the colonic mucosa of a healthy control (**A**) and an irritable bowel syndrome (IBS) patient (**B**). Note the higher number of positive mast cells in the IBS patient as compared with the control. (bar = 25 μm). (*See p. 349*)

(A)   (B)

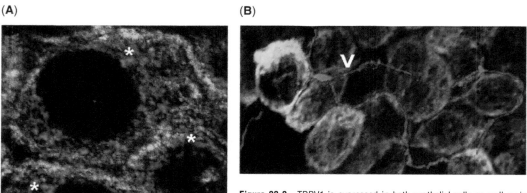

Figure 33.3 TRPV1 is expressed in both urothelial cells as well as in bladder afferents. (**A**) TRPV1-immunoreactivity (cy-3, red, *asterisks*) in basal epithelial cells (cyt 17, FITC green). (**B**) TRPV1-immunoreactivity in nerve fibers (*arrow*, cy-3, red) located in close proximity to basal cells (FITC, green). Punctate TRPV1 staining in urothelial cells was electronically subtracted to facilitate imaging of the TRPV1-immunoreactive nerve fiber. (*See p. 498*)

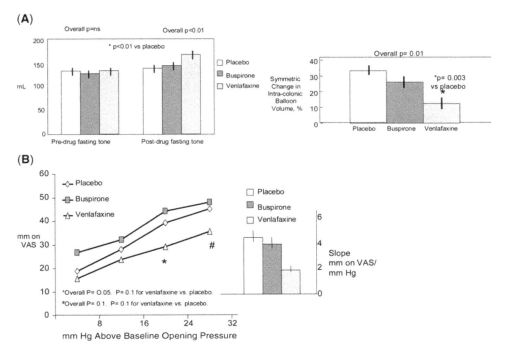

Figure 3 (**A**) Effects on fasting and postprandial colonic tone. Note the significant increase in intracolonic balloon volume after drug administration for venlafaxine, suggesting it relaxes the colon. "∗" indicates overall $p < 0.01$; $p = 0.003$ for venlafaxine versus placebo, unadjusted for three pairwise comparisons. (**B**) Overall effect of serotonergic psychoactive agents on sensation scores for pain in response to increasing pressures. "∗" indicates overall $p = 0.02$ for the linear trend over the four pressure levels. *Source*: From Ref. 54.

Clinical Efficacy

In the only placebo-controlled, randomized trial of the SSRI, paroxetine, to date, Tabas et al. compared 12-week's flexible dose treatment with paroxetine (10–40 mg/day) versus placebo in 81 IBS patients (57). Paroxetine treatment was associated with significantly higher improvement of overall well-being and patient preference compared to placebo. Abdominal pain and bloating were not significantly better after paroxetine (57).

Two open-label treatment studies with paroxetine in IBS have recently been published. Creed et al. randomized 257 subjects with severe IBS to the SSRI, paroxetine, 20 mg daily, individual psychotherapy, or usual care (58). At three months, the paroxetine group had a significantly larger reduction in days with pain compared with the treatment as usual arm, but the differences were relatively small, severity of pain was unchanged and, at one year, pain scores were similar in all groups. Quality of life improved, but this was sustained at the one-year follow up for only the physical component score of the short form 36 (SF-36) in the active treatment arms (58). Talley has discussed that the study had considerable weaknesses; it was not placebo controlled, subjects could not be blinded to the treatment received, it did not control for contact time with the study personnel, and only 50% allocated to the SSRI completed the 12-week treatment course (59). Moreover, the treatments given on follow up were poorly documented and may have confounded the results. Talley concluded that the data do not clearly define the efficacy of an SSRI in IBS (59).

Masand et al. documented improvements in overall pain, pain severity and frequency in 20 IBS patients treated for 12 weeks with paroxetine (mean dose 31 mg) (60). These results should be interpreted with caution due to the open-label design.

There are also negative aspects to the use of SSRIs, in view of their known propensity to cause agitation, sleep disturbance, vivid dreams, diarrhea, and sexual dysfunction (anorgasmia in women).

In summary, Drossman suggests that, although their efficacy for pain control is not well established, they have additional benefits, because they are anxiolytic and are helpful for patients with other comorbid conditions including social phobia (or agoraphobia), posttraumatic stress disorder, panic, and obsessional thoughts related to their condition (1). In some cases, when a single antidepressant is not helpful, augmentative therapy as used in psychiatry might be helpful. Examples of augmentative therapy include combining a low-dose tricyclic antidepressant with an SSRI, adding buspirone to an antidepressant, or combining an antidepressant with psychological treatment.

Clonidine, an Alpha-2 Adrenergic Agonist
Clinical Pharmacology
Clonidine relaxes the colon, enhances the compliance of the stomach and colon, and reduces sensation of pain during distension of the stomach, colon, or rectum in health and in IBS (61–67). On the basis of these dose-response studies, a clinical trial of clonidine was performed to assess the clinical efficacy in IBS.

Clinical Efficacy
A single-center study was performed to evaluate the efficacy and tolerability of clonidine in patients with diarrhea-predominant IBS (D-IBS) in a double-blind, randomized, parallel-group, placebo-controlled trial (68). Patients received 0.05, 0.1, or 0.2 mg clonidine or placebo twice a day for four weeks. The endpoints were satisfactory relief of IBS by weekly question and stool parameters with a daily diary and GI transit. Forty-four D-IBS patients participated. There were four treatment-related dropouts: 2/2 in the 0.2 mg and 2/12 in the 0.05 mg clonidine groups. The proportions with satisfactory relief of IBS were: 0.46, 0.42, and 0.67 with placebo, 0.05 mg, and 0.1 mg clonidine, respectively (Fig. 4). Relief was sustained through four weeks of treatment, and bowel dysfunction (firmer stools and easier stool passage) was significantly reduced with clonidine, 0.1 mg twice a day. Clonidine did not significantly alter GI transit. Drowsiness, dizziness, and dry mouth were the most common adverse events with the 0.1 mg dose; severity of adverse effects subsided after the first week of treatment. This study showed that a trial to replicate 20% or more responders with clonidine than placebo would require 95 patients per treatment arm (68).

In summary, clonidine may help relieve IBS symptoms in D-IBS, but the efficacy in chronic abdominal pain is unproven, the dose would likely need to be titrated up to be tolerated and long-term efficacy is unclear.

Serotonergic Agents: 5-HT$_3$ Antagonist and 5-HT$_4$ Agonist
Clinical Pharmacology
In humans, the *5-HT$_3$ antagonist, alosetron*, enhances colonic compliance and increases the volume but not the pressure threshold for pain in IBS with diarrhea (69). It also changes the regions of pain activated during rectal noxious distension suggesting that there are changes in control of central pain pathways (70,71).

There is only one study conducted in humans that demonstrates potential reduction of visceral pain in response to the *5-HT$_4$ agonist, tegaserod*. Coffin et al. showed that the medication changed the RIII reflex, a viscerosomatic nerve reflex, during rectal distension in healthy subjects (72).

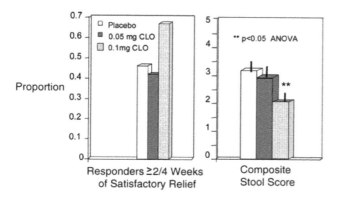

Figure 4 Effect of clonidine on satisfactory relief of irritable bowel syndrome (*left panel*) and overall stool score (*right panel*) in patients with diarrhea-predominant irritable bowel syndrome. Note the significant effect on stool score (derived from stool frequency, consistency, urgency, and ease of passage) and the 20% greater proportion of patients achieving satisfactory relief with 0.1 mg clonidine relative to placebo. *Source*: From Ref. 68.

Clinical Efficacy

Alosetron and tegaserod have been associated with significant improvement or induction of adequate relief of IBS symptoms. For both drugs, there is evidence that pain severity and number of pain-free days can improve as secondary endpoints in IBS trials. However, formal studies in patients with chronic abdominal pain have not been reported.

In a meta-analysis (73) of six studies of alosetron, the pooled odds ratio for adequate relief of pain or global symptoms improvement was 1.81 (95% CI 1.57–2.10). The average number of patients needed to treat with alosetron for one patient to achieve improvement over placebo treatment was seven (95% CI 5.74–9.43). The analysis showed that alosetron, 1 mg b.i.d., positively impacts global symptoms, pain and discomfort in nonconstipated IBS female patients, but efficacy in males was not evaluated (73). Kuo et al. (74) showed that alosetron was also associated with reduced upper GI symptom score in an experimental model of dyspepsia with the induction of postprandial symptoms with a fully satiating meal (Fig. 5). However, the main improvements were in nausea and (a trend) in bloating (74). A phase IIb trial of alosetron showed promising findings in the adequate relief of dyspepsia, which was defined using Rome criteria as upper abdominal pain and discomfort (75). Hence, these data suggest that 5-HT$_3$ antagonists may be efficacious in the treatment of chronic abdominal pain.

A Cochrane review on tegaserod (76) observed that at least 20 mm and 40% reduction in mean VAS score at endpoint compared to baseline for abdominal pain and discomfort in three tegaserod IBS trials showed disparate results and significant heterogeneity among the studies. Pooling all tegaserod doses compared with placebo ($n = 2521$) gave a relative risk of being a responder of 1.13 (95% CI, 0.85, 1.51), which was not statistically significant (76).

Formal clinical trials in patients with chronic abdominal pain have not been reported with either drug class.

Miscellaneous: Kappa-Opioid Agonist, Somatostatin Analog
Clinical Pharmacology

Clinical pharmacology data in humans suggest that these approaches may be promising, but the appropriate clinical trials in IBS or chronic abdominal pain have not been undertaken in sufficient numbers of patients to evaluate the clinical potential. Alternatively, when tried, the medication has not been observed to be clinically beneficial. For example, the kappa-opioid agonist, fedotozine, increases thresholds of perception of colonic distention in patients with IBS without modifying colonic compliance (77). Unpublished data suggest that fedotozine was not effective in the adequate relief of patients with IBS, though some efficacy was noted in small groups of patients with IBS and patients with dyspepsia (78,79). A newer agent in the class of kappa-opioid agonists, asimadoline, was shown to reduce postprandial symptoms in response to a fully satiation meal (80) and to reduce pain and gas scores in response to colonic distension at nonnoxious levels (81). In patients with IBS, there was a small reduction in pain of unclear significance (82). Results of clinical trials for the control of pain are awaited. Recent data suggest that its action may be at least partly through blockade of sodium channels. Several studies document the effects of octreotide to reduce rectal sensation in health and IBS (83–86); however, cost and inconvenience of administration by subcutaneous injection seem to have precluded further development for the treatment of functional GI disorders.

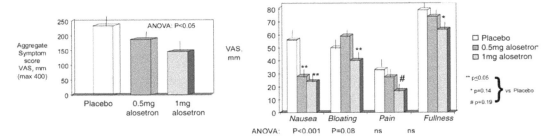

Figure 5 Effect of alosetron on aggregate postprandial symptom score and individual symptoms after a fully satiating meal in healthy volunteers. *Source*: From Ref. 74.

No.

Step 4: Seeking Specialist Care

Gastroenterologists often refer patients to specialty clinics such as pain clinics, behavioralists, or psychiatrists when such approaches do not suffice. Patients are often reluctant to see a psychologist or psychiatrist because they lack confidence in the benefits of referral, feel stigmatized for possibly having a psychiatric problem, or see referral as a rejection by the medical physician. Psychological interventions are best presented as ways to help manage pain and to reduce the psychological distress of the symptoms. There are now several lines of evidence that such approaches including hypnotherapy, cognitive behavioral therapy, and other psychotherapy are effective in managing such patients (49,58,87). Similarly, referral to a specialty or multidisciplinary pain clinic (88,89) can be very beneficial in children, adolescents, and adults, and these approaches are discussed elsewhere in this book.

CONCLUSION

Patients with chronic abdominal pain present a significant challenge to gastroenterologists and general clinicians. This approach has been developed based on clinical experience and the data in the literature. It is, nevertheless, a work in progress and it emphasizes the need for formal trials of novel medications for the treatment of this often-distressing condition. As physicians, we are always concerned that there may be something we are overlooking to explain the pain; experience, and empathy are needed to become an effective caregiver in this field.

ACKNOWLEDGMENTS

The author is supported by grants RO1-DK54681, RO1-DK67071 and K24-DK02638 from the National Institutes of Health. The excellent secretarial support of Mrs. Cindy Stanislav is gratefully acknowledged.

REFERENCES

1. Drossman DA. Functional abdominal pain syndrome. Clin Gastroenterol Hepatol 2004; 2:353.
2. Costanza CD, Longstreth GF, Liu AL. Chronic abdominal wall pain: clinical features, health care costs, and long-term outcome. Clin Gastroenterol Hepatol 2004; 2:395.
3. Nobaek S, Johansson ML, Molin G. Alteration of intestinal microflora is associated with reduction in abdominal bloating and pain in patients with irritable bowel syndrome. Am J Gastroenterol 2000; 95:1231.
4. Kim HJ, Kim, Camilleri, et al. A randomized, controlled trial of a probiotic, VSL#3, on gut transit and symptoms in diarrhea-predominant irritable bowel syndrome. Aliment Pharmacol Ther 2003; 17:895.
5. O'Mahony L, McCarthy, Kelly, et al. Lactobacillus and bifidobacterium in irritable bowel syndrome (IBS): symptom responses and relationship to cytokine profiles. Gastroenterology. 2005; 128:541.
6. Pimentel M, Chow EJ, Lin HC. Normalization of lactulose breath testing correlates with symptom improvement in irritable bowel syndrome. A double-blind, randomized, placebo-controlled study. Am J Gastroenterol 2003; 98:412.
7. Gamblin TC, Gamblin, Stephens, Johnson, Rothwell. Adult malrotation: a case report and review of the literature. Curr Surg 2003; 60:517.
8. Levy MJ, Clain JE. Evaluation and management of cystic pancreatic tumors: emphasis on the role of EUS FNA. Clin Gastroenterol Hepatol 2004; 2:639.
9. Topazian M, Topazian, Hong-Curtis, Li, Wells. Improved predictors of outcome in post-cholecystectomy pain. J Clin Gastroenterol 2004; 38:692.
10. Desautels SG, Desautels, Slivka, et al. Post-cholecystectomy pain syndrome: pathophysiology of abdominal pain in sphincter of Oddi type III. Gastroenterology 1999; 116:900.
11. Bardan E, Bardan, Nadler, Chowers, Fidder, Bar-Meir. Capsule endoscopy for the evaluation of patients with chronic abdominal pain. Endoscopy 2003; 35:688.
12. Fireman Z, Fireman, Eliakim, Adler, Scapa. Capsule endoscopy in real life: a four-centre experience of 160 consecutive patients in Israel. Eur J Gastroenterol Hepatol 2004; 16:927.
13. May A, May, Nachbar, Wardak, Yamamoto, Ell. Double-balloon enteroscopy: preliminary experience in patients with obscure gastrointestinal bleeding or chronic abdominal pain. Endoscopy 2003; 35:985.
14. Eliakim R, Eliakim, Suissa, Yassin, Katz, Fischer. Wireless capsule video endoscopy compared to barium follow-through and computerised tomography in patients with suspected Crohn's disease—final report. Dig Liver Dis 2004; 36:519.

15. Delgado-Aros S, Delgado-Aros, Cremonini, Bredenoord, Camilleri. Systematic review and meta-analysis: does gall-bladder ejection fraction on cholecystokinin cholescintigraphy predict outcome after cholecystectomy in suspected functional biliary pain? Aliment Pharmacol Ther 2003; 18:167.
16. Locke GR III, Locke, Camilleri, Kendall, Zinsmeister, Talley. The relationship between transit parameters and GI symptom complexes. Gastroenterology 2004; 126:A438.
17. Charles F, Charles, Camilleri, Phillips, Thomforde, Forstrom. Scintigraphy of the whole gut: clinical evaluation of transit disorders. Mayo Clin Proc 1995; 70:113.
18. Chitkara DK, Chitkara, Delgado-Aros, et al. Functional dyspepsia, upper gastrointestinal symptoms, and transit in children. J Pediatr 2003; 143:609.
19. Chitkara DK, Chitkara, Bredenoord, et al. The role of pelvic floor dysfunction and slow colonic transit in adolescents with refractory constipation. Am J Gastroenterol 2004; 99:1579.
20. Mertz H, Mertz, Naliboff, Munakata, Niazi, Mayer. Altered rectal perception is a biological marker of patients with irritable bowel syndrome. Gastroenterology 1995; 109:40.
21. Tack J, Tack, Piessevaux, Coulie, Caenepeel, Janssens. Role of impaired gastric accommodation to a meal in functional dyspepsia. Gastroenterology 1998; 115:1346.
22. Bouin M, Bouin, Plourde, et al. Rectal distention testing in patients with irritable bowel syndrome: sensitivity, specificity, and predictive values of pain sensory thresholds. Gastroenterology 2002; 122:1771.
23. Chial HJ, Chial, Camilleri, et al. A nutrient drink test to assess maximum tolerated volume and post-prandial symptoms: effects of gender, body mass index and age in health. Neurogastroenterol Mot 2002; 14:249.
24. De Schepper HU, De Schepper, Cremonini, Chitkara, Camilleri. Assessment of gastric accommodation: overview and evaluation of current methods. Neurogastroenterol Mot 2004; 16:275.
25. Frank JW, Sarr MG, Camilleri M. Use of gastroduodenal manometry to differentiate mechanical and functional intestinal obstruction: an analysis of clinical outcome. Am J Gastroenterol 1994; 89:39.
26. Coulie B, Camilleri M. Intestinal pseudo-obstruction. Annu Rev Med 1999; 50:37.
27. Parra JL, Reddy KR. Diagnostic laparoscopy. Endoscopy 2004; 36:289.
28. Reissman P, Spira RM. Laparoscopy for adhesions. Sem Laparoscopic Surg 2003; 10:185.
29. Onders RP, Mittendorf EA. Utility of laparoscopy in chronic abdominal pain. Surgery 2003; 134:549.
30. Shayani V, Siegert C, Favia P. The role of laparoscopic adhesiolysis in the treatment of patients with chronic abdominal pain or recurrent bowel obstruction. J Soc Laparoendoscopic Surg 2002; 6:111.
31. Swank DJ, Swank, Swank-Bordewijk, et al. Laparoscopic adhesiolysis in patients with chronic abdominal pain: a blinded randomised controlled multi-centre trial. Lancet 2003; 361:1247.
32. Pilotto A, Pilotto, Franceschi, Leandro, Di Mario. The Geriatric Gastroenterology Study Group (Societe Italiana Gerontologie Geriatria). NSAID and aspirin use by the elderly in general practice: effect on gastrointestinal symptoms and therapies. Drugs Aging 2003; 20:701.
33. King SA, Strain JJ. Benzodiazepines and chronic pain. Pain 1990; 41:3.
34. Lydiard RB. An overview of generalized anxiety disorder: disease state—appropriate therapy. Clin Ther 2000; 22:A3.
35. Gorelick AB, Gorelick, Koshy, et al. Differential effects of amitriptyline on perception of somatic and visceral stimulation in healthy humans. Am J Physiol 1998; 275:G460.
36. Mertz H, Mertz, Fass, et al. Effect of amitriptyline on symptoms, sleep, and visceral perception in patients with functional dyspepsia. Am J Gastroenterol 1998; 93:160.
37. Poitras P, Poitras, Riberdy Poitras, Plourde, Boivin, Verrier. Evolution of visceral sensitivity in patients with irritable bowel syndrome. Dig Dis Sci 2002; 47:914.
38. Hislop IG. Psychological significance of the irritable colon syndrome. Gut 1971; 12:452.
39. Drossman DA, Drossman, Camilleri, Mayer, Whitehead. AGA technical review on irritable bowel syndrome. Gastroenterology 2002; 123:2108.
40. Myren J, Myren, Groth, Larssen, Larsen. The effect of trimipramine in patients with the irritable bowel syndrome. Scand J Gastroenterol 1982; 17:871.
41. Myren J, Myren, Lovland, Larssen, Larsen. A double-blind study of the effect of trimipramine in patients with the irritable bowel syndrome. Scand J Gastroenterol 1984; 19:835.
42. Greenbaum DS, Greenbaum, Mayle, et al. The effects of desipramine on IBS compared with atropine and placebo. Dig Dis Sci 1987; 32:257.
43. Heefner JD, Wilder RM, Wilson JD. Irritable colon and depression. Psychosomatics 1978; 19:540.
44. Lancaster-Smith MJ, Lancaster-Smith, Prout, Pinto, Anderson, Schiff. Influence of drug treatment on the irritable bowel syndrome and its interaction with psychoneurotic morbidity. Acta Psychiatr Scand 1982; 66:33.
45. Ritchie JA, Truelove SC. Comparison of various treatments for irritable bowel syndrome. Br Med J 1980; 281:1317.
46. Jackson JL, Jackson, O'Malley, et al. Treatment of functional gastrointestinal disorders with antidepressant medications: a meta-analysis. Am J Med 2000; 108:65.
47. Tanum L, Malt UF. A new pharmacologic treatment of functional gastrointestinal disorder. A double-blind placebo-controlled study with mianserin. Scand J Gastroenterol 1996; 31:318.
48. Vij JG, Jiloha RC, Kumar N. Effect of antidepressant drug (doxepin) on irritable bowel syndrome patients. Indian J Psychiatr 1991; 33:243.

49. Drossman DA, Drossman, Toner, et al. Cognitive-behavioral therapy versus education and desipramine versus placebo for moderate to severe functional bowel disorders. Gastroenterology 2003; 125:19.

50. Gorard DA, Libby GW, Farthing MJ. Influence of antidepressants on whole gut and orocaecal transit times in health and irritable bowel syndrome. Aliment Pharmacol Ther 1994; 8:159.

51. Coulie B, Coulie, Tack, Sifrim, Andrioli, Janssens. Role of nitric oxide in fasting gastric fundus tone and in 5-HT1 receptor-mediated relaxation of gastric fundus. Am J Physiol 1999; 276:G373.

52. Tack J, Piessevaux H, Coulie B. A placebo-controlled trial of buspirone, a fundus-relaxing drug, in functional dyspepsia: effect on symptoms and gastric sensory and motor function. Gastroenterology 1999; 116:A325.

53. Chial HJ, Chial, Camilleri, et al. Selective effects of serotonergic psychoactive agents on gastrointestinal functions in health. Am J Physiol 2003; 284:G130.

54. Chial HJ, Chial, Camilleri, et al. Effects of venlafaxine, buspirone, and placebo on colonic sensorimotor functions in healthy humans. Clin Gastroenterol Hepatol 2003; 1:211.

55. Kuiken SD, Tytgat GN, Boeckxstaens GE. The selective serotonin reuptake inhibitor fluoxetine does not change rectal sensitivity and symptoms in patients with irritable bowel syndrome: a double blind, randomized, placebo-controlled study. Clin Gastroenterol Hepatol 2003; 1:219.

56. Broekaert D, Vos R, Gevers A-M. A double-blind randomized placebo-controlled crossover trial of citalopram, a selective 5-hydroxytryptamine reuptake inhibitor in irritable bowel syndrome. Gastroenterology 2001; 120:A641.

57. Tabas G, Tabas, Beaves, et al. Paroxetine to treat irritable bowel syndrome not responding to high-fiber diet: a double-blind, placebo-controlled trial. Am J Gastroenterol 2004; 99:914.

58. Creed F, Creed, Fernandes, et al. and The North of England IBS Research Group. The cost-effectiveness of psychotherapy and paroxetine for severe irritable bowel syndrome. Gastroenterology 2003; 124:303.

59. Talley NJ. SSRIs in IBS: sensing a dash of disappointment. Clin Gastroenterol Hepatol 2003; 1:155.

60. Masand PS, Masand, Gupta, et al. Does a preexisting anxiety disorder predict response to paroxetine in irritable bowel syndrome?. Psychosomatics 2002; 43:451.

61. Bharucha AE, Bharucha, Camilleri, Zinsmeister, Hanson. Adrenergic modulation of human colonic motor and sensory function. Am J Physiol 1997; 273:G997.

62. Malcolm A, Malcolm, Phillips, Camilleri, Hanson. Pharmacological modulation of rectal tone alters perception of distention in humans. Am J Gastroenterol 1997; 92:2073.

63. Thumshirn M, Thumshirn, Camilleri, Choi, Zinsmeister. Modulation of gastric sensory and motor functions by nitrergic and alpha$_2$-adrenergic agents in humans. Gastroenterology 1999; 116:573.

64. Malcolm A, Malcolm, Camilleri, et al. Towards identifying optimal doses for alpha-2 adrenergic modulation of colonic and rectal motor and sensory function. Aliment Pharmacol Ther 2000; 14:783.

65. Viramontes BE, Viramontes, Malcolm, et al. Effects of α_2 adrenergic agonist on gastrointestinal transit, colonic motility and sensation in humans. Am J Physiol 2001; 281:G1468.

66. Malcolm A, Camilleri M, Kellow JE. Clonidine alters rectal motor and sensory function in irritable bowel syndrome. Gastroenterology 1999; 116:A1035.

67. Malcolm A, Malcolm, Jones, Camilleri, Kellow. Clonidine reduces the rectal tone response to a meal in irritable bowel syndrome. Neurogastroenterol Mot 2000; 12:396.

68. Camilleri M, Camilleri, Kim, et al. A randomized, controlled exploratory study of clonidine in diarrhea-predominant irritable bowel syndrome. Clin Gastroenterol Hepatol 2003; 1:111.

69. Delvaux M, Delvaux, Louvel, Mamet, Campos-Oriola, Frexinos. Effect of alosetron on responses to colonic distension in patients with irritable bowel syndrome. Aliment Pharmacol Ther 1998; 12:849.

70. Berman SM, Berman, Chang, et al. Condition-specific deactivation of brain regions by 5-HT3 receptor antagonist alosetron. Gastroenterology 2002; 123:969.

71. Mayer EA, Mayer, Berman, et al. The effect of the 5-HT3 receptor antagonist, alosetron, on brain responses to visceral stimulation in irritable bowel syndrome patients. Aliment Pharmacol Ther 2002; 16:1357.

72. Coffin B, Coffin, Farmachidi, Rueegg, Bastie, Bouhassira. Tegaserod, a 5-HT4 receptor partial agonist, decreases sensitivity to rectal distension in healthy subjects. Aliment Pharmacol Ther 2003; 17:577.

73. Cremonini F, Delgado-Aros S, Camilleri M. Efficacy of alosetron in irritable bowel syndrome: a meta-analysis of randomized controlled trials. Neurogastroenterol Mot 2003; 15:79.

74. Kuo B, Kuo, Camilleri, et al. Effects of 5-HT$_3$ antagonism on postprandial gastric volume and symptoms in humans. Aliment Pharmacol Ther 2002; 16:225.

75. Talley NJ, Talley, Van Zanten, et al. A dose-ranging, placebo-controlled, randomized trial of alosetron in patients with functional dyspepsia. Aliment Pharmacol Ther 2001; 15:525.

76. Evans BW, Evans, Clark, Moore, Whorwell. Tegaserod for the treatment of irritable bowel syndrome. Cochrane Inflammatory Bowel Disease Group Cochrane Database of Systematic Reviews 2004:4.

77. Delvaux M, Delvaux, Louvel, et al. The kappa agonist fedotozine relieves hypersensitivity to colonic distention in patients with irritable bowel syndrome. Gastroenterology 1999; 116:38.

78. Dapoigny M, Abitbol JL, Fraitag B. Efficacy of peripheral kappa agonist fedotozine versus placebo in treatment of irritable bowel syndrome. A multicenter dose-response study. Dig Dis Sci 1995; 40:2244.

79. Read NW, Read, Abitbol, Bardhan, Whorwell, Fraitag. Efficacy and safety of the peripheral kappa agonist fedotozine versus placebo in the treatment of functional dyspepsia. Gut 1997; 41:664.
80. Delgado-Aros S, Delgado-Aros, Chial, et al. Effects of asimadoline, a kappa-opioid agonist, on satiation and postprandial symptoms in healthy humans. Aliment Pharmacol Ther 2003; 18:507.
81. Delgado-Aros S, Delgado-Aros, Chial, et al. Effects of a kappa-opioid agonist, asimadoline, on satiation and GI motor and sensory functions in humans. Am J Physiol 2003; 284:G558.
82. Delvaux M, Delvaux, Beck, et al. Effect of asimadoline, a kappa opioid agonist, on pain induced by colonic distension in patients with irritable bowel syndrome. Aliment Pharmacol Ther 2004; 20:237.
83. Hasler WL, Soudah HC, Owyang C. A somatostatin analogue inhibits afferent pathways mediating perception of rectal distention. Gastroenterology 1993; 104:1390.
84. Bradette M, Bradette, Delvaux, et al. Octreotide increases thresholds of colonic visceral perception in IBS patients without modifying muscle tone. Dig Dis Sci 1994; 39:1171.
85. Rasmussen OO, Rasmussen, Hansen, Zhu, Christiansen. Effect of octreotide on anal pressure and rectal compliance. Dis Colon Rect 1996; 39:624.
86. Plourde V, Plourde, Lembo, et al. Effects of the somatostatin analogue octreotide on rectal afferent nerves in humans. Am J Physiol 1993; 265:G742.
87. Gonsalkorale WM, Miller, Afzal, Whorwell. Long term benefits of hypnotherapy for irritable bowel syndrome. Gut 2003; 52:1623.
88. McGarrity TJ, McGarrity, Peters, Thompson, McGarrity. Outcome of patients with chronic abdominal pain referred to chronic pain clinic. Am J Gastroenterol 2000; 95:1812.
89. Eccleston C, Eccleston, Yorke, Morley, Williams, Mastroyannopoulou. Psychological therapies for the management of chronic and recurrent pain in children and adolescents. Cochrane Database of Systematic Reviews 2003; 1:CD003968.

19 | Pharmacology and Practice of Opioid Drugs for Visceral Pain

Jane C. Ballantyne[a]

Department of Anesthesia and Critical Care, Harvard Medical School, and Division of Pain Medicine, Massachusetts General Hospital, Boston, Massachusetts, U.S.A.

INTRODUCTION

Opioid drugs are the most effective analgesics we know, but their use is limited by several liabilities, including their propensity to produce addiction. Despite decades of search for therapeutic agents that might provide analgesia without tolerance, dependence, and addiction, or other adverse effects, standard opioids[b] remain the treatment of choice for severe pain of any origin. This supremacy persists because, unlike other drugs with analgesic properties, opioids can be titrated to achieve comfort, at least in the case of acute severe pain, with no strict ceiling dose. There is little debate about using opioids for visceral pain in hospitalized patients with pain of acute onset or an exacerbation of a chronic painful condition, and years of experience confirm that this practice is generally effective and safe, and bears minimal risk of addiction (1). The same is true of cancer-related pain treatment. However, long-term treatment of visceral pain with opioids is far from straightforward, not least because of a high risk of addiction that arises because many chronic visceral pain conditions share the comorbidities of addiction–depression, anxiety, posttraumatic stress disorder, somatoform disorder, personality disorder, and history of sexual abuse (2,3). Thus, while opioid therapy for acute visceral pain is relatively straightforward, the issues surrounding longer-term opioid therapy for visceral pain present a challenge in terms of balancing comfort and function in these complex patients.

PHARMACOLOGY
Pharmacodynamics

Opioid drugs achieve their effects through endogenous opioid receptors, mainly the three well-defined "classical" receptors μ, κ, and δ. These receptors are ubiquitous throughout the body, but are concentrated in distinct areas of the central nervous system (CNS) : the substantia gelatinosa of the spinal cord dorsal horn and the periaqueductal gray and related areas of the brain (analgesia), the mesocorticolimbic system (euphoria), and the locus ceruleus (physical dependence), with multiple and complex connections to each other and to other areas of the CNS. The μ-receptors are found abundantly in both peripheral and CNS sites, while κ-receptors are more prevalent in the periphery, and δ-receptors more prevalent in the CNS (Table 1) (4–6). The opioid receptors belong to the family of G-protein–coupled receptors. Activation results in inhibition of adenylate cyclase with subsequent reduction in cyclic adenosine monophosphate. At the membrane level they increase potassium permeability and inhibit voltage-gated calcium channels, thereby reducing neuronal excitability. Overall, their effects are inhibitory (7,8).

Physiologically, the endogenous opioid systems respond to injury and the threat of injury. Events that would otherwise be painful and distressing become bearable, even pleasurable;

---

[a] Dr. Ballantyne is the current Chief of the Division of Pain Medicine at the Massachusetts General Hospital and Associate Professor of Anesthesia, Harvard Medical School. Her clinical and research interests include outcomes measurement, meta-analysis, pharmacoeconomics, clinical trials of postoperative pain therapies, and assessment of the efficacy and safety of long-term opioids. She has been active in the field of pain management since 1986.

[b] Standard or commonly used opioids are the opium constituents morphine and codeine, derivatives of opium constituents oxycodone, hydromorphone and hydrocodone, and the synthetic opioids methadone, levorphanol, meperidine and fentanyl.

Table 1 Overview of the Endogenous and Exogenous Mediators of the Three Major Opioid Receptor Types, and Their Main Effects on Gut Physiology

	δ-Receptors	κ-Receptors	μ-Receptors
Preferred endogenous ligand	Enkephalin	Dynorphin	β-endorphin
Location	Myenteric plexus	Myenteric plexus	Myenteric and submucosal
	CNS	Afferent neurons	Plexus CNS and spinal cord
Agonists		Fedotozine	Morphine
		Asimadoline	Trimebutine
			Loperamide
Antagonists	Alvimopan		Naloxone
			Methylnaltrexone
			Alvimopan
Gastrointestinal effects	Delayed transit	Delayed transit	Delayed transit
		Visceral antinociception	Visceral antinociception

Source: Adapted from Ref. 8.

furthermore, there is a drive to repeat the inciting event, which has clear survival benefit. When exogenous opioids are given, their effects are less targeted and subtle, so that while they can be helpful, they can also be harmful. The importance of slowing the bowel and closing sphincters during "flight and fight" should not be forgotten, and it is not merely serendipitous that there are many opioid receptors in the Gastrointestinal (GI) tract, or that there are complex and numerous interactions between the limbic system and the bowel. The GI receptors have particular importance in the treatment of visceral pain.

Opioid actions are well known and listed in Table 2. Respiratory depression is the only adverse effect that can and does cause sudden death, and this effect provides a strong reason for caution in opioid prescribing. Euphoria can trigger addiction in susceptible individuals, but is notably absent during the treatment of severe pain, especially severe acute pain, as is the consequent development of addiction. Other adverse effects are common reasons for patients to abandon opioid therapy, even though tolerance to these effects (except bowel effects), as well as to analgesia, develops over time (9–12).

Pharmacokinetics

Pharmacokinetics differ widely between opioid drugs. Most are extensively metabolized, some having active and/or toxic metabolites. Most are excreted via the kidneys, and accumulation (especially of metabolites) may be an issue in patients with impaired renal function. Oral bioavailability varies according to lipophilicity and first-pass metabolism. The following considerations are of particular relevance in the treatment of pain with opioids. Most opioids have poor oral bioavailability and must be given in approximately a 3:1 ratio, oral to parenteral (Table 3). Methadone has relatively good oral bioavailability and does not need to be given at higher oral dose. Hydromorphone undergoes relatively little metabolic change, does not have active metabolites, and is therefore a good choice in patients with renal impairment. Meperidine, on the other hand, undergoes significant metabolic change, and high levels of its metabolite normeperidine cause seizure activity. Meperidine is therefore a poor

Table 2 Opioid Effects

Opioid effects
Analgesia
Respiratory depression
Cough suppression
Nausea
Euphoria
Dysphoria
Sedation
Pruritus
Meiosis
Direct bowel effects

Table 3 Standard Analgesic Doses of Commonly Used Opioids

Generic Name	Trade Name	Equianalgesic Doses		Typical First Dose	
		Oral	Parenteral	Oral	Parenteral
Codeine		200 mg	120 mg	30 mg q 3–4 hr	10 mg q 3–4 hr
Fentanyl patch	Duragesic	N/A	N/A	N/A	25 µg/hr patch q 72 hr[a]
Fentanyl oralet	Actiq	N/A	N/A	N/A	200 µg[b]
Hydrocodone	Vicodin[c], Lorcet[c], Lortab[c], Norco[c]	N/A	N/A	10 mg q 3–4 hr	N/A
Hydromorphone	Dilaudid	7.5	1.5 mg	2–4 mg q 3–4 hr	1.5 mg q 3–4 hr
Levorphano[c]	Levo-Dromoran	4 mg	2 mg	4 mg q 6–8 hr	2 mg q 6–8 hr
Meperidine	Demerol	300 mg	100 mg	100 mg q 3 hr	100 mg q 3 hr
Methadone[d]	Dolophine	2–4 mg	10 mg (acute) 2–4 mg (chronic)	5 mg q 8–12 hr	5 mg q 8–12 hr
Morphine		30 mg	10 mg	15 mg q 3–4 hr	10 mg q 3–4 hr
Morphine SR	MSContin	N/A	N/A	15 mg q 8–12 hr	N/A
Oxycodone	Percocet[c], Percodan[c]	N/A	N/A	5 mg q 3–4 hr	N/A
Oxycodone CR	Oxycontin	N/A	N/A	10 mg q 8–12 hr	N/A

[a]Lowest available dose. Risk of overdose in opioid-naïve patients. 25 µg/hr patch = 50–75 mg oral morphine per 24-hr. period. Conversions should be made conservatively (consult product literature) and titrated slowly.
[b]Lowest available dose. Contraindicated in opioid-naïve patients, especially children. Not for use in children < 10 kg. 200 µg oralet = 2 mg intravenous (IV) morphine. 800 µg oralet = 10 mg IV morphine.
[c]Combination formulations, with either acetaminophen or aspirin.
[d]Equianalgesic conversion dose for methadone decreases significantly with increasing dose of previous opioid. Caution guided by experience is mandatory.

choice for the elderly and renally impaired. Methadone has an exceptionally long elimination (β;) half-life, which confers advantage in terms of long action, but disadvantage in terms of potentially dangerous accumulation, especially knowing that its elimination is unpredictable and idiosyncratic (13,14). This makes methadone a less desirable choice for outpatient pain treatment, except in those already established on methadone treatment (15). One approach in the search for improved opioid analgesia for visceral pain seeks to achieve "peripheraliza-tion" of opioid agonists by pharmacokinetic manipulation in order to target bowel receptors that mediate visceral pain (16).

Opioid Responsiveness and the Gastrointestinal Effects of Opioids

The concept of opioid responsiveness was, to a large extent, born out of the observation that nociceptive pain seemed more responsive to opioids than neuropathic pain. We realize now that this was an issue of degree of responsiveness, not an all-or-none phenomenon, and that a better concept is that of "opioid-poorly-responsive pain" (17). Either the pain is less sensitive to opioids and a larger dose is needed (as in the case of neuropathic pain) (18–21), or adverse effects limit dose or efficacy, as may happen in some visceral pain states (22,23). Visceral pain can be considered poorly responsive to opioids, but for several different reasons. First, chronic visceral pain states tend to be refractory to all treatments, including opioid treatment. Addic-tion and other forms of problematic opioid use arise relatively often during opioid treatment of chronic visceral pain states[c], often obscuring the analgesic benefit in affected patients. Direct GI opioid effects can reduce opioid analgesic efficacy by worsening the underlying cause of the pain. This is particularly true when pain arises secondary to visceral distention because opioid drugs slow bowel mobility and produce distention in the presence of obstruc-tion or even partial obstruction. It is also the case when, as in chronic pancreatitis, biliary spasm or obstruction contributes to the pain. This is because opioid drugs cause biliary and other visceral sphincters to constrict (22–25).

In certain circumstances, the bowel-slowing effects of opioids aid rather than compro-mise pain relief. This is the case in hypermotility states such as irritable bowel disease and diarrhea, where excessive peristalsis becomes painful. The µ-opioid agonists loperamide

[c]True incidences of problematic opioid use are difficult to determine, and published estimates depend on uncertain definitions of problematic use and addiction. Rates appear to differ according to the disease; for example, opioid-treated chronic pancreatitis seems associated with a particularly high rate of addic-tion. The difficulties of assessing rates of prescription opioid abuse are discussed in Addiction.

(Imodium) and diphenoxylate (Lomotil) are most commonly used for this indication in the United States. There is minimal systemic absorption and therefore low abuse potential, although sedation can arise (8). These drugs are not controlled substances and are available over the counter, as well as by prescription. The κ-agonist fedotozine has also been used in hypermotility states to increase bowel muscular tone, with mixed success (8,26,27).

Kappa Opioid Receptors Mediate Visceral Pain

Visceral pain is not as easy to understand or as straightforward as somatic pain, and the fact that several chronic visceral pain states are not explained by structural or biochemical abnormalities, further complicates the clinical picture (2). Visceral pain is not evoked from all viscera and is not linked to visceral injury, reflecting the fact that many viscera are innervated by receptors whose activation does not evoke conscious perception and are not strictly sensory receptors (28). More recently, chronic functional abdominal pain has been characterized as a form of visceral hyper-sensitivity or hyperalgesia (2,29–32). The κ-opioid receptor has been implicated in the perception of visceral pain and hyperalgesia, with peripheral bowel receptors playing an important role (8,31–36). These receptors are not prevalent in the reward circuitry of the mesolimbic system; therefore the κ-receptor agonists would have the additional benefit of not being implicated in addiction. κ-opioid receptor agonists may also act by a nonopioid receptor–mediated effect (sodium channel blockade) (37,38). Currently available κ-agonists (butorphanol, nalbuphine, and pentazocine) have limited clinical utility because they are partial agonists (i.e., they are difficult to use in the presence of other opioids), and have dose-limiting central effects such as dysphoria, sedation, and hallucinations (39,40). In GI pain syndromes, the greatest experience to date has been with fedotozine, which is still regarded as investigational (8,26,27). The search for clinically useful κ-agonists continues (16,38,40), in the hope that they prove effective, especially in the treatment of functional abdominal pain.

Choice of Opioid

Standard opioids are listed in Table 3. The choice of opioid will depend on many of the pharmacological characteristics of these drugs that have already been described. Of particular relevance in the treatment of visceral pain are: (i) the theoretical consideration that morphine causes sphincter of Oddi constriction and (ii) the preference for addicts of meperidine.

The belief that morphine causes sphincter of Oddi constriction and should be avoided in biliary spasm has persisted and been perpetuated over many years, despite limited supporting data for the effect. Early studies that measured biliary pressures in animals and humans showed that all opioids increased biliary pressure, but morphine did so the most. Later studies, however, showed that the sphincter of Oddi is exquisitely sensitive to all opioids (22,24). Studies showing differences that may be clinically important are notably lacking (22). Avoidance of morphine in favor of other opioids when treating acute and chronic pancreatitis, and other conditions associated with biliary spasm, no longer seems justified, especially if the alternative is the traditional choice meperidine. Years of experience with meperidine treatment of chronic pain have taught the medical community that addicted patients often prefer meperidine, presumably due to its dominant euphoric effects. However, this has recently been questioned, and meperidine preference may be as much learned (for example, for decades meperidine was the opioid of choice for emergency room presentations of renal colic and headache) as due to true superiority in terms of euphoria. Despite this consideration, it is still preferable to avoid meperidine because of its association with improper use, as well as its toxic metabolite. Tramadol (a mixed mechanism analgesic with mild μ-opioid receptor actions) may be a useful alternative for the treatment of mild-to-moderate pain in chronic pancreatitis (or whenever biliary spasm contributes to the pain) (23).

Route of Administration

The choice of route for the administration of opioids is usually based on convenience, practicability, and limiting factors such as nil per os status. In general, the oral route is preferred for all but hospitalized patients. Lately, reliable transdermal preparations, notably transdermal fentanyl, have been developed that are useful for opioid treatment of chronic and cancer-related pain. Sometimes when treating visceral pain, particularly GI pain, it is desirable to avoid enteral administration so as to avoid direct bowel effects (unless the direct bowel effects are desirable as for hypermotility states). In this case, apart from intravenous (IV), intramuscular, and subcutaneous administration, which may be impracticable and/or uncomfortable, the transdermal, sublingual, or rectal routes may be used. These alternative routes of administration are particularly useful in the treatment of visceral pain because of cancer.

ACUTE VISCERAL PAIN

Acute severe visceral pain requiring hospitalization arises after surgery, as an acute inflammatory event (e.g., acute pancreatitis, acute cholecystitis, acute inflammatory bowel disease) or as an acute exacerbation of a chronic disease state (e.g., acute on chronic pancreatitis, Crohn's flare, cancer). In each case, opioid treatment is the analgesic treatment of choice, and IV patient-controlled analgesia (PCA), the preferred method of delivery. If PCA is not available, nurse administration of opioid by IV injection, or an alternative parenteral route, is also satisfactory. Acute severe visceral pain is likely to interfere with GI absorption; therefore the oral route may not provide satisfactory relief, although preexisting oral regimen can be maintained if the GI tract is functioning normally. PCA is chosen because of its inherent safety, easy titratability, preference by patients, ease of monitoring opioid usage, and comforting presence during weaning at the end of the acute event (41,42). While it may be advisable to plan the long-term treatment strategy during an acute event, the aggressive treatment of acute severe pain should not be compromised by longer-term considerations. Most acute exacerbations of visceral pain do not end as abruptly as they begin, and it may be necessary to continue opioid treatment, usually oral opioids, during a prolonged subacute phase. Nevertheless, the aim should be to avoid an insidious passage into chronic opioid treatment without due consideration of the commitment chronic opioid treatment entails.

Many less-severe acute visceral pain conditions such as acute cystitis can be managed without resort to opioids.

LONG-TERM OPIOID TREATMENT AND ITS LIABILITIES

Long-term opioid treatment differs from short-term treatment in that several liabilities interfere in the case of long-term opioid use. Because of this, a careful, structured approach during long-term treatment is needed, also recognizing that the treatment requires commitment from both physician and patient, and should never be embarked upon before careful consideration of this commitment. Physicians who wish to undertake the treatment of chronic nonterminal pain with opioids are well advised to familiarize themselves with one of several guidelines, which describe a structured treatment approach (15,43–45). These widely used guidelines all suggest similar treatment principles, which can be summarized as follows: include a comprehensive medical history and examination; firmly establish that nonopioid therapy has failed; develop an understanding between physician and patient about the true benefits and pitfalls of chronic opioid use; involve a single physician and pharmacy whenever possible; and ensure comprehensive follow-up comprising regular assessment of goal achievement, careful monitoring for signs of abuse (including toxicology screens in some cases), the use of adjunctive treatments whenever possible, and a willingness to end opioid treatment if goals are not met. These principles are summarized in Table 4.

Loss of Efficacy

Many patients receiving chronic opioid therapy appear to obtain satisfactory and sustained pain relief without dose escalation (43,46). This seems counter to our belief that the

Table 4 Management Principles for Long-term Opioid Treatment

Ensure that other options have been explored
Goal directed therapy; set limits and goals, and agree to these
Consider opioid therapy as an adjunct
Unless pain is occasional, base regime on long-acting opioid, and avoid breakthrough medications
Be prepared to treat side effects, particularly constipation
Sole opioid therapy is rarely successful
Careful and regular follow-up
Be prepared to wean and discontinue if treatment goals are not met
Provide good documentation

development of tolerance, a pharmacological phenomenon, is an inevitable consequence of prolonged opioid use. It is evident, nevertheless, that in many patients, tolerance "levels off," not only in the case of side effects, but also in the case of analgesia, and that these patients can derive adequate analgesia at a stable dose.

In other patients, the outcome is less favorable. Satisfactory analgesia is not sustained, and the patients request increasing doses. Tolerance develops to the analgesic and euphoric effects of opioids, as well as to their side effects (except direct bowel effects). Mechanisms of pharmacological tolerance to opioids have not been fully elucidated, but many mechanisms appear to be linked to the N-methyl-D-aspartate (NMDA) -receptor cascade (47). Alternatively, "apparent" tolerance could arise as a consequence of opioid-induced hyperalgesia, a phenomenon that has been largely forgotten for years, but that has been amply described, and could sometimes explain resistance to opioid treatment. Recently, the mechanism of opioid-induced hyperalgesia has been elucidated, and interestingly, it is also linked to the NMDA-receptor cascade and downregulation of glutamate transporters. This process may represent a form of neurotoxicity, considering that the NMDA-receptor is also implicated in the hyperalgesia associated with neuropathic pain (48,49). We are now presented with a quandary when a patient presents with escalating pain unresponsive to opioid therapy: do we, having eliminated the possibility of a change in disease state, assume that the cause is pharmacological tolerance and will be overcome by dose increase; or would dose increase make matters worse? The presence of whole-body allodynia (painful response to a nonpainful stimulus) can be suggestive of opioid-induced hyperalgesia.

Hormonal Effects

Opioids influence at least two major hormonal systems, the hypothalamic–pituitary–adrenal axis and the hypothalamic–pituitary–gonadal axis. The resultant increase in prolactin and decreases in plasma cortisol, follicular stimulating hormone, leutenizing hormone, testosterone, and estrogen may have deleterious clinical effects including male and female infertility, decreased libido and aggression, menstrual disorders, and galactorrhea (47,50–54). These opioid effects were observed long before they were chemically confirmed in heroin addicts (50,51,55). Later, testosterone depletion was demonstrated in male patients in methadone programs (56,57). Testosterone levels can be particularly low in patients receiving intrathecal opioids, to the extent that these patients often feel better and regain energy when they are treated with testosterone. The extent of hormonal changes in chronic patients treated with opioids, and the clinical significance of the change is unknown, but two recent study groups have demonstrated decrements in testosterone and cortisol in these patients (52,53,58,59). Whether or not hormonal replacement would improve the well-being of opioid-treated chronic non-terminal pain (CNTP) patients remains uncertain.

Immune Effects

Animal and human studies demonstrate the presence of opioid receptors on a wide range of immune cells, and the ability of opioids to alter the development, differentiation, and function of immune cells (60–62). Prolonged exposure to opioids appears more likely to suppress immune function than short-term exposure, while the abrupt withdrawal of opioids also seems to cause immunosuppression (63). Few studies have been conducted assessing immune function in chronic pain patients receiving opioids, but the direct evidence that opioids impair immune function does give rise to concern in these patients. On the other hand, preclinical studies have indicated a possible protective role of opioids against intestinal inflammation (64). Pain itself can produce immunosuppression; so the greatest concern is likely to pertain to patients receiving high doses of opioids without good pain relief (15).

Addiction

When one considers that three distinct sets of circumstances contribute to the development of addiction (Fig. 1), and that the risk of addiction is highest when these three circumstances collide, it is easy to understand why most patients treated with opioids do not become addicted. One of the real difficulties the medical community has had, however, since it started using opioids for chronic pain in the 1980s and 1990s, is determining the extent of the risk of

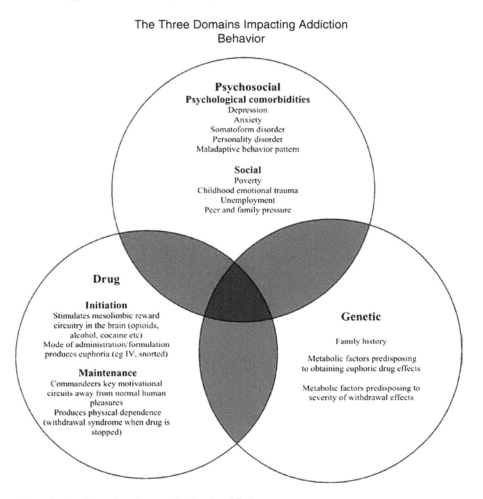

Figure 1 The three domains contributing to addiction.

addiction. Part of this difficulty stems from the fact that addiction in opioid-treated pain patients is not readily defined. Behaviors in this population do not appear like those in addicts using illicit substances (Table 5). The Diagnostic and Statistical Manual of Mental Disorders (DSM-IV) criteria for substance dependence (i.e., drug addiction[d]), incorporate physical dependence and tolerance as well as the behavioral features listed in Table 5 (66). But in pain practice, it is considered preferable to avoid the term "substance dependence" lest it confuse "psychological dependence" (a feature of addiction) with "physical dependence" (Table 6). This is because "physical dependence" and "tolerance" are inevitable consequences of chronic opioid use, and physically dependent patients are not necessarily considered addicted, i.e., they may not display the behavioral features of addiction. Confusion over addiction terminology has made it even more difficult to determine the risk of addiction in chronic pain patients treated with opioids. When we do not know how to define or recognize addiction, how can we quantify it? It is safe to say, nevertheless, that initial estimates of 0.5% to 8% (46) probably underestimated the problem, and higher estimates of 3% to 19% (67) are now accepted by many experienced practitioners. Further research should allow us to better define and better estimate the extent of the problem of prescription-opioid addiction (68–70).

---

[d] The term "drug addiction" is not used in the DSM-IV criteria but is often used synonymously with the psychiatrists' term "substance dependence" (65). The DSM-IV criteria for substance abuse and substance dependence are the criteria most commonly used by the medical community in the United States. Substance abuse arises before substance dependence and does not incorporate physical dependence and tolerance.

Table 5 Characteristic Behaviors in Prescription Opioid Abuse and Illicit Drug Abuse

Prescription Opioid Abuse	Illicit Drug Abuse
Self-escalation of dosage	The substance is often taken in larger amounts or over a longer period than intended
Repeated prescription loss with "classical" excuses:	There is a persistent desire or unsuccessful efforts to cut down or control substance use
"The pills fell into the toilet bowl"	A great deal of time is spent in activities necessary to obtain the substance, use the substance, or recover from its effects
"I left the prescription in the changing room"	Important social, occupational, or recreational activities are given up or reduced because of substance use
"The airline lost my luggage"	The substance use is continued despite knowledge of having a persistent physical or psychological problem that is likely to have been caused or exacerbated by the substance
"The dog ate it"	
"The vial was stolen from my medicine cabinet"	
"The pills were ruined in the laundry"	
Multiple prescribers	
Frequent telephone calls to the office	
Multiple drug intolerances described as "allergies"	
Focusing mainly on opioid issues during visits	
Visiting without an appointment	

Source: From Ref. 66,71.

Patients with chronic visceral pain present a particular challenge. Although there is no certainty about rates of addiction in this patient group, the addiction problem seems to be worsening[e] as physicians respond to pain advocacy and treat more of these patients with opioids (73–75). Because there is little scientific evidence to guide treatment choices, we rely on the knowledge we have acquired about addiction processes and risk factors (Fig. 1). We recognize that the comorbidities of chronic visceral pain and addiction are often shared (2,3), and that there is a strong biopsychosocial component to many chronic visceral pain syndromes. These factors alone suggest caution in opioid prescribing for chronic visceral pain.

PSYCHOSOMATIC GASTROINTESTINAL AND GENITOURINARY DISEASE

"Psychosomatic" is often considered a pejorative term; yet if one can see beyond the belief that psychosomatic illness is not a real disease and therefore not worthy of treatment, the term aptly describes pain states such as fibromyalgia, headache, chronic fatigue syndrome, irritable bowel disease, and chronic pelvic pain. In his biosocial model, Drossman (2) distinguishes illness (the patient's perception of ill health) from disease (externally verifiable evidence of a

Table 6 Definitions Related to the Use of Opioids for the Treatment of Pain

I	Addiction
	Addiction is a primary, chronic, neurobiologic disease, with genetic, psychosocial, and environmental factors influencing its development and manifestations. It is characterized by behaviors that include one or more of the following: impaired control over drug use, compulsive use, continued use despite harm, and craving
II	Physical Dependence
	Physical dependence is a state of adaptation that is manifested by a drug-class-specific withdrawal syndrome that can be produced by abrupt cessation, rapid dose reduction, decreasing blood level of the drug, and/or administration of an antagonist
III	Tolerance
	Tolerance is a state of adaptation in which exposure to a drug induces changes that result in a diminution of one or more of the drug's effects over time

Source: From Ref. 72.

---

[e] Personal observation.

pathological state). The biopsychosocial model differs from the traditional and dominant Western biomedical model, which assumes that all conditions can be reduced to a single etiology, and that illness and disease is either "organic" or "functional," but not both. In the biopsychosocial model, even in conditions with identifiable pathology (such as Crohn's disease, ulcerative colitis, gastroesophageal reflux, and pelvic inflammatory disease), as well as those without demonstrable structural or physiological disturbance (where symptoms are understood in terms of visceral hypersensitivity as modulated by CNS activity) (30,76–78), psychosocial and biological factors are seen to interact. Given the strong psychosocial component to all these conditions, it follows that behavioral treatments such as psychotherapy, biofeedback, relaxation, and hypnosis may be more successful and durable than symptom control by means of drug therapies (2,27). Certainly, pain treatment should be multidisciplinary and could include treatments such as acupuncture, transcutaneous electrical stimulation, and exercise. Treatment is always more successful if underlying psychopathology (and, indeed, structural pathology) is addressed and treated early in the course of treatment. There is a greater tendency to use opioids to treat pain when demonstrable pathology is present, as occurs in inflammatory bowel disease, pelvic inflammatory disease, and pancreatitis. At the same time, the presence of pathology provides a rationale for exploring specific treatment options such as surgery, steroids, sulfasalazines, antibiotics, and alcohol cessation before considering opioid treatment.

SPECIFIC CONDITIONS
Chronic Pancreatitis

Chronic pancreatitis is one of the few chronic pain conditions for which there are reliable objective markers of the causative disease such as biochemical and radiological abnormalities with reasonable correlation with severity of disease. One might think that this unusual ability to measure severity makes it easier to modulate the analgesic intervention. Yet, in practice, chronic pancreatitis is one of the most difficult and refractory of chronic pain conditions. The pain is severe and warrants opioid treatment; surgical intervention is often unsuccessful; and a high proportion of the population has underlying addiction (alcoholism), and is therefore at risk for prescription-opioid addiction (79). Given the frequency of acute exacerbations and the severity of the chronic pain, this is one condition where it may be impossible to wean patients off opioid treatment between acute exacerbations. Inevitably, addiction to the prescribed opioid arises frequently in this population. This is not to say that these patients should be denied opioid treatment for what is clearly a painful and distressing condition, but rather that the addiction risk should be faced squarely, and the patients should be given the benefit of appropriate treatment. This means providing the opioid treatment in a structured manner, as described under "Long-term Opioid Treatment," paying particular attention to watching for signs of addiction and including additional input from psychiatry or addiction medicine when necessary. Of course, this approach should also apply when addiction arises during the treatment of other conditions, but in many other conditions, it may be preferable not to embark on long-term opioid treatment in the first place, or it may be realistic to wean from opioid therapy as part of the approach to managing the addiction (15).

Childhood Abdominal Pain

Never is it more important to adhere to the principle that opioid treatment should be maximized during hospital treatment of acute pain, and minimized at home, than in the case of childhood abdominal pain. Nobody likes to see a child in pain, particularly the child's parents; on the other hand, there is a lot at stake if a child becomes addicted. In hospital practice, one sees increasing numbers of children who are treated with opioids for pain associated with inflammatory bowel disease, pelvic inflammation, and even unexplained abdominal pain. Some of these children become addicted, although there is always a great deal of reluctance to put the "addiction" label on a child. The literature does not help us determine whether addiction occurs at higher rate at young age, and the few studies that have looked at the issue have returned conflicting results (68,80). But even if one assumes that rates are the same as in adults (3–19%), this is still unacceptably high, given the importance of maintaining function in this population, so that emotional, educational, and physical development progresses as normally as possible. The treatment of chronic pain in children is always complicated and difficult, especially when parents, albeit unwittingly, unburden their own psychopathology on their child. Opioid treatment of chronic pain in children requires enormous patience, sensitivity, and dedication, and should not be undertaken casually.

Visceral Pain in Cancer

Opioids are the only effective treatment for severe visceral pain due to cancer, and their constipating effects must be recognized and treated. Constipation can usually be avoided by placing opioid-treated patients on a bowel regimen consisting of a stimulating laxative (e.g., Senokot), and a stool softener such as docusate. The bulk-forming laxatives do not help and may cause dehydration in susceptible patients. Naloxone can be given orally to reduce the opioids' effect on the GI mucosa. Dosing should be kept in the range of 1.6 to 2 mg per dose (usually given every six hours until effective) so as not to reverse the analgesia. Alternatively, methylnaltrexone, a less lipophilic quaternary ammonium derivative of naltrexone, less prone to CNS effects, can be used (81).

It is worth remembering that the principles of opioid treatment for cancer pain, particularly during terminal illness, differ markedly from those of opioid treatment for chronic nonterminal pain. In the treatment of terminal cancer pain, the primary goal is symptom control, while in the long-term treatment of pain, functional restoration is the most important goal of treatment. Some cancer patients, those who are cured or in remission, fall into the latter category and wish to lead fully functional lives. Opioids are used relatively liberally when treating terminal illness. If high doses are reached, it may become increasingly difficult to control the pain or the opioid side effects (particularly sedation, and possibly toxicity, including myoclonus). In this case, it may be helpful to switch to a different opioid. Because of incomplete cross-tolerance, 1/2 the equivalent dose is usually effective, or as little as 1/10 in the case of methadone (82,83).

CONCLUSION

Opioid treatment of severe, acute, and cancer pain improves lives, and makes patients less fearful of death. Although in some circumstances, visceral pain may be less responsive to opioid treatment than other types of pain, opioids remain the most effective analgesics for severe visceral pain. The popularization of opioid treatment for chronic pain has had mixed results—the treatment has helped many patients cope with perplexing and pervasive diseases; yet, too many have encountered the pitfalls of addiction, meaning that their lives have deteriorated rather than improved. The time has come for physicians to acknowledge the demands of chronic opioid therapy and avoid the casual use of prolonged opioid treatment.

In a landmark paper describing chronic opioid therapy published in 1986, Russell Portenoy and Katharine Foley made the following statement:

"It must be recognized . . . that the efficacy of [opioid] therapy and its successful management may relate as much to the quality of the personal relationship between physician and patient as to the characteristics of the patient, drug, or dosing regime" (46).

Unfortunately, the important principle they expressed has been rather lost under a barrage of commercial and other pressure to treat all of life's ills with medications. Their statement points out the importance of the physician–patient relationship to the success of chronic opioid treatment. It also reminds us that physicians who undertake to treat chronic pain with opioids must be committed to the long-term management of their patients. Few examples of iatrogenic harm are more blatant than the patients who trail from physician to physician, labeled and disparaged as addicts, who were started on opioid treatment by physicians who were ignorant of what chronic opioid treatment entails.

ACKNOWLEDGMENT

I would like to thank Tina Toland for her assistance in preparing this chapter.

REFERENCES

1. Porter J, Jick H. Addiction rare in patients treated with narcotics (letter). N Engl J Med 1980; 302.
2. Drossman DA. Gastrointestinal illness and the biopsychosocial model. Psychos Med 1998; 60:258.
3. Dersh J, Polatin PB, Gatchell RJ. Chronic pain and psychopathology: research finding and theoretical considerations. Psychom Med 2002; 64:773.
4. Kurz A, Sessler DI. Opioid-induced bowel dysfunction: pathophysiology and potential new therapies. Drugs 2003; 63:649.
5. Pasternak GW. Pharmacological mechanisms of opioid analgesics. Neuropharmacol 1993; 16:1.
6. Greenwald MK, Stitzer ML, Haberny KA. Human pharmacology of the opioid neuropeptide dynorphine. 1997; 281:1154.
7. Rang HP, Dale MM, Ritter JM. Analgesic drugs. In: Rang HP, ed. Pharmacology. 4th Ed., New York: Churchill Livingstone; 1999: 579.
8. De Schepper HU, et al. Opioids and the gut: pharmacology and current clinical experience. Neurogastroenterol Motil 2004; 16:383.
9. Huse E et al. The effect of opioids on phantom limb pain and cortical reorganization. Pain 2001; 90:47.
10. Attal NA et al. Effects of IV morphine in central pain. A randomized placebo-controlled study. Neurology 2002; 58:554.
11. Caldwell JR et al. Efficacy and safety of a once-daily morphine formulation in chronic, moderate-to-severe osteoarthritis pain: results from a randomized, placebo-controlled, double-blind trial and an open-label extension trial. J Pain Symptom Manage 2002; 23:278.
12. Watson CPN et al. Controlled-release oxycodone relieves neuropathic pain: a randomized controlled trial in painful diabetic neuropathy. Pain 2003; 105:71.
13. Fishman SM et al. Methadone reincarnated: novel clinical applications with related concerns. Pain Med 2002; 3:339.
14. Wilson PR. ASA statement to FDA committee. Opioid use and diversion: report on recent hearing by FDA and DEA. ASA Newslett 2002; 66:9.
15. Ballantyne JC, Mao J. Opioids for chronic pain. N Engl J Med 2003; 349:1943.
16. DeHaven-Hudkins DL, Dolle RE. Peripherally restricted opioid agonists as novel analgesic agents. Curr Pharma Des 2004; 10:743.
17. Hanks GW, Forbes K. Opioid responsiveness. Acta Anaesth Scand 1997; 41:154.
18. Rowbotham MC, Reisner-Keller LA, Fields HL. Both intravenous lidocaine and morphine reduce the pain of postherpetic neuralgia. Neurology 1991; 41:1024.
19. Dellemijn PL, Vanneste JA. Randomised double-blind active-placebo-controlled crossover trial of intravenous fentanyl in neuropathic pain. Lancet 1997; 349:753.
20. Rowbotham MD et al. Oral opioid therapy for chronic peripheral and central neuropathic pain. N Engl J Med 2003; 348:1223.
21. Foley KM. Opioids and chronic neuropathic pain. N Engl J Med 2003; 348:1278–1281.
22. Thompson DR. Narcotic analgesic effects on the sphincter of Oddi: a review of the data and therapeutic implications in treating pancreatitis. Am J Gastroenterol 2001; 96:1266.
23. Wilder-Smith CH et al. Effect of tramadol and morphine on pain and gastrointestinal motor function in patients with chronic pancreatitis. Digest Dis Sci 1999; 44:1107.
24. Lee F, Cundiff D. Meperidine vs. morphine in pancreatitis and cholecystitis. Arch Intern Med 1998; 158:2399.
25. Niemann T et al. Opioid treatment of painful chronic pancreatitis. Intern J Pancreatol 2000; 27:235.
26. Callahan MJ. Irritable bowel syndrome neuropharmacology. A review of approved and investigational compounds. J Clin Gastroenterol 2002; 35:S58.
27. Mach T. The brain-gut axis in irritable bowel syndrome–clinical aspects Med Sci Monitor 2004; 10:RA125.
28. Cervero F. Visceral pain-central sensitization. Gut 2000; 47(suppl 4):iv56–iv57; discussion iv58.
29. Whitehead WE, Engle BT, Schuster MM. Irritable bowel syndrome: physiological and psychological differences between diarrhea-predominant and constipation-predominant patients. Dig Dis Sci 1980; 25.
30. Mayer EA, Gebhart GF. Basic and clinical aspects of visceral hyperalgesia. Gastroenterology 1994; 107:271.
31. Gebhart GF. Visceral pain-peripheral sensitization Gut 2000; 47:(suppl 4):iv54–iv56; discussion iv58.
32. Gebhart GF. Pathobiology of visceral pain: molecular mechanisms and therapeutic implications IV. Visceral afferent contributions to the pathobiology of visceral pain. Am J Physiol Gastrointest Liver Physiol 2000; 278:G834.
33. Black D, Trevethick M. The kappa opioid receptor is associated with the perception of visceral pain. Gut 1998; 43:312.
34. Simonin F et al. Disruption of the kappa-opioid receptor gene in mice enhances sensitivity to chemical visceral pain, impairs pharmacological actions of the selective kappa-agonist U-50,488H and attenuates morphine withdrawal. EMBO J 1998; 17:886.

35. Su X, Wachtel RE, Gebhart GF. Inhibition of calcium currents in rat colon sensory neurons by κ- but not mu- or delta-opioids. J Neurophysiol 1998; 80:3112.
36. Gebhart GF et al. Peripheral opioid modulation of visceral pain. Ann N Y Acad Sci 2000; 909:41.
37. Su X et al. Sodium channel blocking actions of the kappa-opioid receptor agonist U50, 488 contribute to its visceral antinociceptive effects J Neurophysiol 2002; 87:1271.
38. Blackshaw LA, Gebhart GF. The pharmacology of gastrointestinal nociceptive pathways. Curr Opin Pharmacol 2002; 2:642.
39. Martin TJ, Eisenach JC. Pharmacology of opioid and nonopioid analgesics in chronic pain states. J Pharmacol Exp Ther 2001; 299:811.
40. Eisenach JC, Carpenter R, Curry R. Analgesia from a peripherally active kappa-opioid receptor agonist in patients with chronic pancreatitis. Pain 2003; 101:89.
41. Ballantyne JC et al. Postoperative patient-controlled analgesia: meta-analyses of initial randomized control trials. J Clin Anesth 1993; 5:182.
42. Walder B et al. Efficacy and safety of patient-controlled opioid analgesia for acute postoperative pain: a quantitative systematic review. Acta Anaesth Scand 2001; 45:795.
43. Portenoy RK. Opioid therapy for chronic nonmalignant pain: a review of the critical issues. J Pain Symptom Manage 1996; 11:203.
44. West JE et al. Model guidelines for the use of controlled substances for the treatment of pain. A policy document of the Federation of State Medical Boards of the United States Inc, 1998.
45. Haddox JD et al. The use of opioids for the treatment of chronic pain. A consensus statement from the American Academy of Pain Medicine and the American Pain Society. American Academy of Pain Medicine and American Pain Society, 1997.
46. Portenoy RK, Foley KM. Chronic use of opioid analgesics in non-malignant pain: report of 38 cases. Pain 1986; 25:171.
47. Mao J, Price DD, Mayer DJ. Mechanisms of hyperalgesia and opiate tolerance: a current view of their possible interactions. Pain 1995; 62:259–274.
48. Mao J, Price DD, Mayer DJ. Thermal hyperalgesia in association with the development of morphine tolerance in rats: roles of excitatory amino acid receptors and protein kinase C. J Neurosci 1994; 14:2301.
49. Mao J. Opioid induced abnormal pain sensitivity: implications in clinical opioid therapy. Pain 2002; 100:213.
50. Mendelson JH, Mendelson JE, Patch VD. Plasma testosterone levels in heroin addiction and during methadone maintenance. J Pharmacol Exp Ther 1975; 192:211.
51. Mendelson JH et al. Effects of heroin and methadone on plasma cortisol and testosterone. J Pharmacol Exp Ther 1975; 195:296.
52. Abs R et al. Endocrine consequences of long-term intrathecal administration of opioids. J Clin Endocrinol Metabol 2000; 85:2215.
53. Finch PM et al. Hypogonadism in patients treated with intrathecal morphine. Clin J Pain 2000; 16:251.
54. Daniell HW. Hypogonadism in men consuming sustained-action oral opioids. J Pain 2002; 3:377.
55. Daniell HW. Narcotic-induced hypogonadism during therapy for heroin addiction. J Addict Dis 2002; 21:47.
56. Bliesener N et al. Plasma testosterone and sexual function in men on buprenorphine maintenance for opioid dependence. J Clin Endocrinol Metab 2004.
57. Daniell HW. The association of endogenous hormone levels and exogenously administered opiates in males. Am J Pain Manage 2001; 11:8.
58. Rajagopal A et al. Symptomatic hypogonadism in male survivors of cancer with chronic exposure to opioids. Cancer 2004; 100:851.
59. Rajagopal A et al. Hypogonadism and sexual dysfunction in male cancer survivors receiving chronic opioid therapy. J Pain Symptom Manage 2003; 26:1055.
60. Roy S, Loh HH. Effects of opioids on the immune system. Neurochem Res 1996; 21:1375.
61. Risdahl JM et al. Opiates and infection. J Neuroimmunol 1998; 83:4.
62. Makman MH. Morphine receptors in immunocytes and neurons. Adv Neuroimmunol 1994; 4:69.
63. Rahim RT et al. Abrupt or precipitated withdrawal from morphine induces immunosuppression. J Neuroimmunol 2002; 127:88.
64. Philippe D et al. Anti-inflammatory properties of the mu opioid receptor support its use in the treatment of colon inflammation. J Clin Invest 2003; 111:1329.
65. Cami J, Farre M. Drug addiction. N Engl J Med 2003; 349:975.
66. Diagnostic and Statistical Manual of Mental Disorders. 4th ed. Washington, D.C.: American Psychiatric Association, 1994.
67. Fishbain DA, Rosomoff HL, Rosomoff RS. Drug abuse, dependence and addiction in chronic pain patients. Clin J Pain 1992; 8:77.
68. Passik SD et al. A pilot survey of aberrant drug-taking attitudes and behaviors in samples of cancer and AIDS patients. J Pain Symptom Manage 2000; 19:274.
69. Adams LL et al. Development of a self-report screening instrument for assessing potential opioid medication misuse in chronic pain patients. J Pain Symptom Manage 2004; 27:440.

70. Butler SF et al. Validation of a screener and opioid assessment measure for patients with chronic pain. Pain 2004; 112:65.
71. Wilsey BL, Fishman SM. Chronic opioid therapy, drug abuse and addiction. MGH Handbook of Pain Management. 3rd ed. Philadelphia: Lippincott, Williams and Wilkins, 2006: 513.
72. Savage S et al. Definitions related to the use of opioids for the treatment of pain. A Consensus Document from the American Academy of Pain Medicine. American Pain Society and the American Society of Addiction Medicine. 2001.
73. National Institute of Drug Abuse (NIDA), Info Facts, Prescription drugs and pain medications 1999. http://nida.nih.gov/Infofax/PainMed.html/http://www.gov/ResearchReports/Prescription7html.
74. CASA Report: missed opportunity. National survey of primary care physicians on patients with substance abuse. New York: National Center on Addiction and Substance Abuse. Columbia University, 2000.
75. DHHS, SAMHSA. National Household Survey on Drug Abuse Main Findings. Series H-11, 1998.
76. Karram MM. The painful bladder: urethral syndrome and interstitial cystitis. Curr Opin Obstet Gynecol 1990; 2:605.
77. Longstreth GF. Irritable bowel syndrome and chronic pelvic pain. Obstet Gynecol Survey 1994; 49:505.
78. Ghaly AFF, Chien PFW. Chronic pelvic pain: clinical dilemma of clinician's nightmare. Sex Transmit Infect 2000; 76:419.
79. Warshaw AL, Banks PA, Fernandez-Del Castillo C. AGA technical review: treatment of pain in chronic pancreatitis. Gastroenterology1998 ; 115:765.
80. Compton P, Darakjian J, Miotto K. Screening for addiction in patients with chronic pain with "problematic" substance use: evaluation of a pilot assessment tool. J Pain Symptom Manage 1998; 16:355.
81. Yuan CS, Foss JF. Oral methylnaltrexone for opioid-induced constipation. JAMA 2000; 284:1383.
82. Mercadante S. Opioid rotation for cancer pain. Cancer 1999; 86:1856.
83. Pasternak GW. The pharmacology of mu analgesics: from patients to genes. Neuroscientist 2001; 7:220.

20 | Clinical Approach to Visceral Cancer Pain

Sebastiano Mercadante

Anesthesia and Intensive Care Unit, Pain Relief and Palliative Care Unit, Law Maddalena Cancer Center, Palermo, Italy

MECHANISMS

Excluding pain directly originating from the abdominal wall, which has somatic characteristics, abdominal pain in cancer is due predominantly to a visceral involvement. Visceral cancer pain originates from a primary or metastatic lesion involving the abdominal or pelvic viscera. Mechanic stimuli, such as torsion or traction of mesentery, distension of hollow organs, stretch of serosal and mucosal surfaces, and compression of some organs produce pain in humans (1). These conditions are frequently observed in cancer patients with an abdominal diseases and intraperitoneal masses. Human studies have revealed that pain is produced when the intraluminal pressure of hollow organs is maintained above certain pressure thresholds. Obstruction or inflammation within the biliary tract or pancreatic duct induces pain directly related to an increased intraluminal pressure with consequent inflammation, and release of pain-producing substances (2). Distension or traction on the gallbladder leads to deep, epigastric pain, inspiratory distress, and vomiting. Spontaneous spasm of the sphincter of Oddi or that induced by morphine leads to increases in pain sensation, resulting in a paradoxical opioid-induced pain. On the other hand, morphine and other opioids increase the pressure threshold necessary to produce the sensation of pain due to distension of the biliary system. Renal colic is commonly secondary to ureteral obstruction and subsequent distension of ureter and renal pelvis. This may be evident in circumstances in which an abdominal-pelvic mass compresses or invades ureters, as often occurs in gynecological cancers.

Cancer in solid visceral organs can also be painful. For instance, capsular stretch of liver due to tumor growth produces pain. The etiology of pain from visceral tissues may also be related to ischemia, particularly in metastatic or recently damaged tissues (postsurgical). Ischemia may act as a modulator of mechanoreceptive visceral inputs. The variability in responses to ischemia may be due to the preexisting pathology or cancer-related mechanical distortion of the viscera secondary to local changes.

Chemical stimuli and algogenic tumor-mediated substances may produce serosal or mucosal irritation. However, these seem to act as modulators or costimulants of visceral sensory systems rather than as primary stimuli, as frank tissue damage (e.g., cutting and burning) does not reliably produce reports of visceral pain. However, if a viscus is inflamed, sensitization of nociceptors will result in pain from stimuli, which are normally nonpainful (allodynia, Chapter xx).

CLINICAL IMPLICATIONS IN CANCER PAIN

Initially, visceral pain is poorly localized and dull because of the wide divergence of visceral afferents in the spinal cord (Chapter xx). Better localization of a stimulus occurs when the disease extends to a somatically innervated structure such as the parietal peritoneum or when referred pain sets in due to sensitization of dorsal horn neurons sharing input from both visceral and somatic sites (Chapter xx). Common examples of referred pain in cancer patients include back pain, which occurs with pancreatic cancer, and right shoulder pain, which occurs with liver cancer or metastases. Somatic structures may also be involved indirectly. For example, diaphragmatic irritation due to abdominal distension produced by large subdiaphragmatic masses may induce shoulder pain, and may be associated with hiccup (3).

These concepts are useful in explaining the outcome of some neurolytic blocks for abdominal cancer pain and the response to analgesic drugs (4). Failure or partial success of celiac or hypogastric plexus block may be attributed to the fact the tumor has metastasized beyond the nerves that conduct pain via the celiac plexus. In such instances, pain may arise from parietal peritoneum and abdominal wall involvement as well as retroperitoneal nodal involvement or bone metastases. Other causes of pain in these patients may include postchemotherapy pain from mucositis, liver chemoembolization and/or injury from surgery or radiation (5).

TREATMENT

Most pain in cancer responds to pharmacological management using orally administered analgesics. The current treatment approach is based on an analgesic ladder, which is essentially a framework of principles rather than a rigid protocol (6). When patients with cancer experience severe pain, opioids are the mainstay of therapy. There are a large variety of options for the delivery of opioids in the management of cancer pain. In some instances, there are clear indications for using one preparation or delivery system over another, according to the ability of the patient to use a specific type of delivery system, the efficacy of that system to deliver acceptable analgesia, the ease of use by the patient and his or her family, and the potential or actual complications associated with that system. Cost is another important consideration for patients who must purchase their own medications.

Systemic Analgesics

Pharmacological studies of visceral pain have demonstrated that most analgesics are effective in this type of pain. Nonsteroidal anti-inflammatory drugs (NSAIDs) have been claimed to have a major role in the management of some specific cancer pain syndromes, including pain from bone metastasis, soft-tissue infiltration, arthritis, and recent surgery. In patients with cancer pain, NSAIDs were useful both for somatic and for visceral pain as the first step of the analgesic ladder, and were also useful in combination with opioids, regardless of the pain mechanism involved (7). Administration of analgesics resulted in an equal pain relief until death, although with more unpleasant adverse effects and deterioration of quality of life than when using celiac plexus block (8,9). There is some concern that morphine and other opioids may induce a spasm at a level of the intestinal valves and sphincters, and may paradoxically worsen the clinical picture in the presence of distended intestinal loops. Meperidine may be preferred in this setting as it is generally thought to be less spasmogenic.

Systemic analgesics can be given by many different routes. The oral route is the most common, least invasive, and easiest route for opioid administration for most patients with cancer pain. In all patients who can take oral medications, this route should be considered first. The main problem with the oral route is the first-pass biotransformation of opioids in the liver. This has a major impact on the systemic plasma concentrations of drugs. For example, the dose of an opioid given orally to a patient with cancer pain must be three times the intravenous or intramuscular dose of morphine and twice the parenteral dose of methadone, although large variations can be observed in individuals.

Morphine, the most commonly used medication in the world to treat cancer pain, has a terminal elimination plasma half-life of only about three hours. Although dose titration with the immediate release preparation is recommended, it is desirable to use extended-release preparations to provide longer-lasting analgesia. The bioavailability of these slow-release preparations is the same as that of immediate-release preparations, but time-to-peak plasma drug concentrations is longer, and peak plasma concentrations are decreased. Most of these preparations are recommended by the manufacturer to be administered every 12 hours. Clinicians occasionally use an eight-hour schedule, if necessary to provide adequate analgesia. If additional analgesia is needed for "breakthrough" pain, doses of a fast-onset, short-acting opioid preparation should be available to the patient. However, immediate-release oral opioid preparations usually require approximately 30 minutes to onset of analgesic action when taken on an empty stomach, and faster routes may be required. Oxycodone, methadone, and hydromorphone are possible alternatives to oral morphine (6). Opioid switching may be useful in improving the balance between analgesia and adverse effects in patients with a poor opioid response. This approach is based on the possible pharmacokinetic and pharmacodynamic differences existing among opioids, providing an asymmetric cross-tolerance.

This may allow the use of lower doses than expected according to equivalency tables (10). Many patients, even with abdominal masses, will develop tolerance to most of the undesirable side effects of opioids (such as nausea/vomiting or sedation) over a period of several days; therefore, a medication should not be labeled "intolerable" until a reasonable trial has been undertaken.

Certain patients may not be able to ingest oral medications because of swallowing difficulties, gastrointestinal obstruction, or nausea and vomiting. In these cases, an alternative form of analgesia must be used (6). Finally, the opioid response itself may improve after switching from the oral to the parenteral route (11). Alternative routes, including intravenous, subcutaneous, and transdermal ones, have been advocated in such circumstances. Various opioids are available for intravenous administration in the majority of countries, including morphine, hydromorphone, fentanyl, alfentanil, sufentanil, and methadone. The oral–parenteral ratio for morphine is 2:1 or 3:1 (6,12). Fentanyl is approximately 80 to 100 times more potent than morphine, and sufentanil is approximately 1000 times more potent. The main drawback to their use is their high cost compared with the cost of morphine. The major disadvantage of the intravenous route is that it is more complex to manage, especially at home, and requires some expertise. On the other hand, it provides the fastest delivery, allowing for an immediate effect in urgent conditions. Intravenous opioid infusions can be given as continuous infusions or by a patient-controlled analgesia (PCA) device, which provides continuous infusion plus on-demand boluses. Confused or uncooperative patients may not be the best candidates for PCA use (12).

For patients requiring parenteral opioids who do not have in-dwelling intravenous access, the subcutaneous route can be used. Most drugs used by intravenous route can also be used by subcutaneous infusion; the exception is methadone, which could induce local toxicity. This simple method of parenteral administration involves inserting a small plastic cannula on an area of the chest, abdomen, upper arms, or thighs and attaching the tubing to an infusion pump. The limiting factor is the volume of fluid that can be injected per hour, often requiring more concentrated solutions. The subcutaneous route can also be used in conjunction with a PCA device. The main advantage of subcutaneous over intravenous PCA is that there is no need for vascular access, changing sites can be easily accomplished, and problems associated with in-dwelling intravenous catheters are avoided.

For stable patients with abdominal cancer unable to take oral medications, the transdermal route is a noninvasive option of maintaining continuous plasma concentrations of opioids. A commonly used delivery system consists of a reservoir of fentanyl and alcohol, which contains a three-day supply of fentanyl. The patch releases fentanyl at a constant rate until the reservoir is depleted. Upon initial application of the patch, a subcutaneous "depot" is formed as fentanyl saturates the subcutaneous fat beneath the patch. After approximately 12 hours, steady-state plasma fentanyl concentrations are reached, which are maintained for about 72 hours. Fentanyl patches are currently available in 25, 50, 75, and 100 μg/hr dosages. The bioavailability of transdermal fentanyl is very high, approximately 90%. Several pharmacokinetic properties concerning transdermal fentanyl are of interest to the clinician. Because of the slow depot formation and slow rise in plasma concentrations, this system is not suitable for rapid titration of pain. Because of the prolonged elimination after removal of a system, the opioid side effects will take many hours to resolve. Thus, the transdermal fentanyl system is best suited for patients with stable pain in whom the 24-hour opioid requirement has already been determined. Vigorous exercise and elevation of body temperature secondary to fever or bathing will increase blood flow to the skin and increase drug diffusion into the systemic circulation. Adverse effects of the fentanyl patch include skin reactions and the typical opioid side effects, e.g., nausea/vomiting, constipation, somnolence, and confusion. In general, this delivery system is well tolerated by cancer patients with relatively constant pain who are on stable doses of opioids (13).

Transdermal buprenorphine is also available in release rates of 35, 52.5, and 70 mcg/hr, which correspond to daily doses of 0.8, 1.2, and 1.6 mg of buprenorphine, or approximately 60, 90, and 120 mg/day of oral morphine. Transdermal delivery of buprenorphine provides for a slower increase in serum concentration and no peak-and-trough effects as seen with the sublingual route of administration. As a result, there are fewer adverse events. The use of this drug has been considered as problematic, because of a possible antagonistic effect that might reduce analgesia or induce withdrawal symptoms when used with other opioids. However, clinically the combination of buprenorphine with morphine in the analgesic dose range results in a magnitude of effect compatible with an additive type of interaction (14).

Sublingual and transmucosal administration of opioids is particularly beneficial in the patient with cancer who is unable to tolerate oral administration because of nausea/vomiting or dysphagia. It may also be attractive in patients who cannot receive parenteral opioids because of lack of venous access or presenting typical contraindications for subcutaneous drug administration. Because sublingual venous drainage is systemic rather than portal, hepatic first-pass elimination can be avoided. On the other hand, the transmucosal or sublingual route also offers the potential for more rapid absorption and onset of action relative to the oral route. This is particularly useful for treating breakthrough pain. Lipophilic drugs are better absorbed via this route than are hydrophilic drugs. For these reasons, fentanyl and buprenorphine are commonly used by this route. Oral transmucosal fentanyl appears to be a safe and effective treatment for breakthrough pain and may have some advantages over currently available opioid formulations (15). Both the plasma fentanyl concentration and the bioavailability of fentanyl will vary depending on the fraction of the dose absorbed through the oral mucosa and the fraction swallowed. Approximately 25% of the total dose is rapidly absorbed from the buccal mucosa and becomes systemically available. The remaining 75% is swallowed, is slowly absorbed from the stomach, and then undergoes first-pass metabolism in the liver, with a bioavailability of 33%. Thus, the overall observed bioavailability of transmucosal fentanyl is approximately 50% of the total dose. The onset of action is within about 15 minutes. Transmucosal fentanyl is the only medication that has been found to be effective in the management of breakthrough pain in cancer patients in different controlled studies (16).

Finally, the rectal route may be a simple alternative when oral administration is not possible. Its principal advantage is that it is independent of gastrointestinal tract motility and rate of gastric emptying (17). However, there are several potential disadvantages. There may be a great deal of variation among individuals regarding the necessary dose, as the amount of drug drained from the rectum is highly variable. Absorption may be delayed or limited by the small surface area of the rectum and may be interrupted by defecation. Constipation may prevent contact of drug with rectal mucosa and cause subsequent absorption into feces. All these factors may affect bioavailability. Further, the rectal route is uncomfortable for prolonged use and contraindicated if the patient has painful anal conditions such as fissures or inflamed hemorrhoids. The usual recommendation for initial doses of morphine and most other opioids given rectally is the same dose as that which is given orally (12).

Spinal Analgesia

A small number of patients may still fail to obtain adequate analgesia despite large systemic opioid doses, or they may suffer from uncontrollable side effects such as nausea, vomiting, or oversedation. These patients may be candidates for the administration of a combination of opioids, local anesthetics, and clonidine via the spinal (epidural or intrathecal) route. The goal of spinal opioid therapy is to place a small dose of an opioid and/or local anesthetic close to the spinal opioid receptors located in the dorsal horn of the spinal cord to enhance analgesia and reduce systemic side effects by decreasing the total systemic daily opioid dose. The use of this route to deliver opioids requires placing a catheter into the epidural or intrathecal space and using an external or implantable infusion pump to deliver the medications. Deciding between epidural versus intrathecal placement or external versus implantable pumps to deliver the opioid is based on multiple factors including duration of therapy, type and location of the pain, disease extent and central nervous system involvement, opioid requirement, and individual experience. The daily epidural opioid requirement is approximately 10 times that of intrathecal administration. Intrathecal opioid administration has the advantage of allowing a higher concentration of drug to be localized at the receptor site while minimizing systemic absorption, thus possibly decreasing drug-related side effects. Morphine remains the drug of choice for the spinal route, because of its relatively low lipid solubility. It has a slow onset of action, but a long duration of analgesia when given via intermittent bolus. The starting dose is quite difficult to calculate and should take into consideration various factors, including the previous opioid dose, the age, and the pain mechanism. Adding a local anesthetic (bupivacaine or ropivacaine) to morphine via the spinal route has been successful in providing good analgesia in patients whose pain was resistant to epidural morphine alone, despite high doses.

Further clinical studies and trials will still be required to judge the safety, efficacy, and extended role of the spinal route in chronic cancer pain and, more importantly, to define in which patients this technique is best indicated. Clonidine, an alpha-adrenergic agonist that acts at the dorsal horn of the spinal cord to produce analgesia, has been used in cancer patients in combination with epidural (or intrathecal) morphine infusions. There is some evidence to suggest that neuropathic pain may be somewhat more responsive to the combination of clonidine/morphine than to morphine alone, although orthostatic hypotension is of concern. Procedural and surgical complications, system malfunction, and pharmacological adverse effects are the main categories of complications associated with spinal drug delivery (18).

In conclusion, for the patient with cancer pain, the oral route of opioid delivery should be the first choice. If the oral route cannot be used because of gastrointestinal obstruction and/or severe nausea/vomiting, the rectal is equivalent, although unsuitable for prolonged use. Another noninvasive alternative to the oral route is the transdermal route, which at present is available only for continuous administration of fentanyl and buprenorphine. For treatment of breakthrough pain in a patient unable to take oral or rectal medications, a transmucosal preparation of fentanyl is available. For those patients in whom oral or transdermal opioids are not appropriate, intravenous or subcutaneous administration is effective, the latter route being relatively easier to administer. The spinal route can be attempted when the oral and other parenteral routes have been unsuccessful. This route may be most successful when opioids, local anesthetics, and/or clonidine are used in combination. Whichever route is used, administration of opioids to manage cancer pain requires knowledge of potency relative to morphine and bioavailability of the route chosen. Dose-equivalent tables are only close approximations, and substantial interpatient variability is often observed. Therefore, patients should be closely followed and doses titrated to minimize side effects whenever the opioid, route, or dose is changed.

Neural Blockade

Interruption of visceral pain pathways has been applied widely to relieve oncologic pain. The classic targets of so-called sympatholysis in cancer pain are the celiac plexus, the superior hypogastric plexus, and the ganglion impar (Fig. 1).

Neurolytic celiac plexus block (NCPB) is indicated for abdominal pain from pancreatic cancer, painful retroperitoneal tumors or metastases, and chronic abdominal pain. This approach has been particularly used for pancreatic cancer, which is usually very painful and highly lethal. Controlled, randomized studies have reported prolonged efficacy of NCPB, and the use of neurolytic agents may provide long-term relief that could match the life expectancy of cancer patients. Sometimes, repeated blocks are performed when symptoms reemerge. However, this practice has never been rigorously assessed.

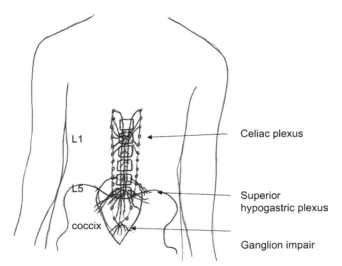

Figure 1 Sympathetic block areas.

TECHNIQUES

Various techniques differing in terms of anatomical approach, solution injected, instruments used, and radiologic guidance methods have been proposed in an attempt to improve the analgesic effects while avoiding complications. However, in practice, operator experience appears to be more important than the specific approach with respect to both of these outcomes (4,19). The choice of technique should therefore be individualized according to local expertise and available resources, as well as the patient's physical condition and extent of malignancy. In general, the retrocrural or deep splanchnic technique is among the best described. In this approach, needles are bilaterally inserted at the lower border of the 12th rib, about 7 cm from the spinous process of the L1 vertebra to the spine, advanced at an angle of about 45° from horizontal, and cephalad of about 15°, to contact the lateral part of the L1 vertebral body. The needle is withdrawn and then laterally redirected to walk-off the vertebral body 1 to 2 cm anteriorly. The position of the needle is checked using imaging in the posteroanterior and lateral position, during the procedure. When the position of the needle is deemed satisfactory, 3 to 5 mL of contrast medium is injected through each needle and its spread observed radiographically, after negative aspiration. This classical method allows for the bathing of the neurolytic agent at the celiac neural axis in addition to producing splanchnic neurolysis. However it is more likely to produce splanchnic nerve block, as the injectate appears to spread preferentially to the retroaortic celiac fibers and rostrally to the splanchnic nerves. The diaphragmatic crura may prevent the solution from extending around the celiac plexus, facilitating the involvement of the splanchnic nerves, although when high volumes of neurolytic solution are injected, it may diffuse caudad via the aortic hiatus of the diaphragm or flow through the gaps present in the diaphragmatic crura and spread anterior to the aorta to bathe the plexus.

An anterior abdominal approach provides a placement of the needle just anterior to the diaphragmatic crus at or between the levels of the celiac and superior mesenteric arteries. Although this technique involves the passage of fine needles through the liver, stomach, small and large bowel, and pancreas to reach the celiac ganglia, it is associated with very low rates of complications. The theoretic advantages of this approach include a reduced discomfort during the procedure avoiding a prolonged prone position and a lower risk of neurologic injury related to the spread of neurolytic solution to the somatic nerve roots. Ultrasound or computed tomography (CT) guidance are commonly used. The use of radiologic contrast medium is essential to enhance imaging capabilities, to better determine the correct needle localization and that the material to be injected spreads as expected, excluding an aberrant spread of injectate into areas not to be included in the block, such as vessels, somatic nerves, and organs. Although both fluoroscopic and CT-guided methods have been used, the latter is much more useful than fluoroscopy (20), as it allows an accurate placement of the needles and theoretically further reduces the risk of organ injury. It is preferred when the normal anatomy might be distorted and is particularly useful when the anterior and transcrural approach is planned.

In the transcrural approach, the needles are advanced another 1 to 2 cm with respect to the retrocrural technique, so that their points lie lateral to and approximately at the anterior wall of the aorta on the left, and at the same depth as the needle on the left, on the right. The transaortic approach is a single needle technique in which a needle is introduced on the left side intentionally to pierce the aorta until no blood can be aspirated to locate the center of the celiac plexus. A more specific technique for splanchnic nerve block differs from the classic approach above in that the needles are directed more cephalad, toward the anterolateral margin of the T12 vertebral body. Splanchnic neurolysis may last longer in patients with an upper abdominal malignancy. Moreover, a smaller volume of neurolytic solution is required than to block the celiac plexus. More recently, endoscopic ultrasound imaging has been used for the purpose of enhancing needle localization and spread of injectate. Larger, long-term, prospective, randomized-controlled trials that evaluate the cost and clinical outcomes are needed to identify advantages and disadvantages of this approach over conventional techniques (21).

Neurolytic Solutions

The principal neurolytic substances used for a NCPB are alcohol and phenol. Alcohol in concentrations from 50% to 100% has been the neurolytic agent most frequently used.

The extraction of cholesterol, phospholipid from neural membrane and by precipitation of lipoproteins, and mucoproteins are the main mechanisms of neurolysis from alcohol. Phenol 6% to 10% in water produces protein coagulation and necrosis of the neural structures.

Controlled comparisons between alcohol and phenol for a celiac plexus block have not been conducted. Alcohol may produce severe though transient pain on injection. This does not usually occur with phenol because phenol has an immediate local anesthetic effect. However, it is the general impression that alcohol produces more intense nerve destruction. Phenol seems to have a slightly slower onset of action, less efficacy, and a shorter duration (4). The amount of neurolytic solution depends on the localization of the needle and the ease of flow in the injected area.

Adverse Effects

The most common adverse effects, including local pain reported in 96% of patients, diarrhea in 44%, and hypotension in 38%, are transient. However the frequency of these effects is difficult to evaluate, due to the inconsistency in reporting them in several studies. Paraplegia following NCPB has been reported, due to vascular ischemia of spinal cord or unintentional spinal cord nerve damage (4,22).

Outcomes

Although NCPB has traditionally been regarded as an effective treatment for pancreatic cancer pain, critical analysis revealed major deficiencies in clinical noncontrolled studies. Often the real effectiveness of the NCPB was not known in relation to previous opioid consumption, and important data, such as pain level, pain characteristics, pain location and duration, the timing of the block, time from diagnosis to block, survival time, and follow-up until death, were omitted, as well as gender and age. The lack of consistent scientific evidence therefore prompted further controlled studies (23). In subsequent randomized-controlled studies, the effectiveness and the duration of the NCPB have been compared to traditional treatment with analgesics using, as a measure of efficacy, previous and subsequent consumption of opioids until the patient's death. The use of NCPB resulted in a reduced opioid consumption and less adverse effects when compared to the use of analgesics only (8,9,24). NCPB is effective in controlling pancreatic cancer pain in a higher percentage of cases if performed early after pain onset, when the pain is still only or mainly of a visceral type and local anatomy is not compromised (25,26). In a study focusing on the efficacy of NCPB in varying locations of pancreatic cancer, neurolysis was more effective in cases with tumor involving the head of the pancreas than in patients with cancer of the body and tail of the pancreas (27). This observation was not confirmed, however, by other studies (28). In another survey, patients with tumors in the head of the pancreas had less pain than patients with cancer in the body or tail of the pancreas, and this could not be explained by stage or size of the tumor (29).

Failure of the block may be attributable to tumor metastases, occurring generally in the later stages of pancreatic cancer. Concomitant pain of somatic origin, frequently observed in upper gastrointestinal cancer, due to large peritoneal involvement, requires other therapeutic measures, although it is difficult to differentiate between a somatic and visceral component in such circumstances. Other causes of the failure of NCPB include technical problems, the presence of tumor in the area of the celiac plexus preventing the spread of the neurolytic substance, or the presence of metastases. Simulated needle placement was more likely to fail in patients with pancreatic cancer than in patients without cancer, due to a reduction in the right retrocrural space (30) or distortion of the celiac area preventing an appropriate neurolytic spread (31,32). Thus, using NCBP early in the course of disease increases the chances of efficacy but does not necessarily guarantee a sustained response because of changes in pain mechanisms that may bypass the celiac plexus. Further, the assertion that neural block in pain-free patients may prevent the subsequent onset of pain as well as improve survival (25) has been not confirmed in other randomized, double-blind studies (8,9,24,26).

Patients with unsatisfactory pain relief after NCPB show massive growth of the tumor around the celiac axis with metastases (27). Additional intermittent administration of bupivacaine through a catheter previously placed near the celiac plexus provided prolonged pain relief in patients who had a substantial analgesic effect lasting three to four weeks after

NCPB (33). This may be because larger volumes are used with the local anesthetic, potentially facilitating action on involved somatic areas as well.

NCPB may offer other benefits in addition to analgesia. Increased weight gain has been reported, in part from decreasing the dose of opioids and a general increase in patient alertness. Suppression of sympathetic tone may also result in increased bowel motility with decreased constipation and less nausea with increased appetite.

Superior Hypogastric Block

Superior hypogastric plexus block has been claimed to be highly effective to control pelvic pain syndromes. Clinical problems concerning neurolytic superior hypogastric block are nearly the same as for celiac plexus block (34). Both control visceral pain. However, the less favorable results obtained with the hypogastric plexus block may be due to the greater tendency of pelvic tumors to infiltrate somatic structures and nerves compared to pancreatic tumors where the celiac plexus block is usually used. Although pain appears to be predominantly due to pressure on the sciatic nerve, pelvic cancers are also often associated with myofascial involvement. Buttock or rectal pain with or without posterior thigh pain, aggravated by sitting or activity, may be due to the compression of piriformis muscle. As a consequence, it may be associated with referred/localized pain of somatic origin. Motor reflexes may lead to muscle spasm and an additional component of somatic pain. In pelvic cancer, lumbar pain may also be due to iliopsoas muscle involvement. Nerve trunk pain often radiating to lower limbs may be observed, due to lumbosacral plexus involvement in the presacral area, or radiculopathy related to retroperitoneal spread. Pain may also result from surgery or radiotherapy directed at the tumor. The clinical picture is therefore often mixed and as a consequence, candidates for hypogastric plexus block have to be strictly selected.

Ganglion Impar Block

Visceral pain in the perineal area associated with malignancies may be treated with neurolysis of the ganglion impar. This ganglion, located at the level of sacrococcygeal junction, marks the end of the two sympathetic chains. The possible candidates who can benefit from this block are patients presenting a vague and poorly localized pain, associated with burning sensation and urgency. The best approach is in prone position. The needle is inserted through the sacrococcygeal ligament in the midline and then advanced 2 to 3 cm until the tip is placed posterior to the rectum (34). Long-term data on the effectiveness of this block is however limited.

CONCLUSION

The choice of performing neurolytic sympathetic blocks should be based on the preference of patients after correctly explaining the possible advantages and complications. These blocks should be considered as an adjuvant treatment to reduce opioid consumption and opioid-related adverse effects, and not as a last resort, when the advantages of the block seem to be minimal.

REFERENCES

1. Holzer-Petsche U, Brodacz B. Traction on the mesentery as a model of visceral nociception. Pain 1999; 80:319–328.
2. Cervero F, Laird JMA. Visceral pain. Lancet 1999; 353:2145–2148.
3. Payne R, Gonzales G. Pathophysiology of pain in cancer and other terminal diseases. In: Doyle D, Hanks GW, Cherny N, Calman K, eds. Oxford Textbook of Palliative Medicine. Oxford: Oxford Medical Publications, 2004:288–297.
4. Mercadante S. Celiac plexus block: a reappraisal. Reg Anesth Pain Med 1998; 23:37–48.
5. Caraceni A, Portenoy RK. Pain management in patients with pancreatic carcinoma. Cancer 1996; 78:639–653.
6. Hanks GW, Conno F, Cherny N, et al. Morphine and alternative opioids in cancer pain: the EAPC recommendations. Br J Cancer 2001; 84:587–593.
7. Colburn RW, Coombs DW, Degnen CC, Rogers LL. Mechanical visceral pain model: chronic intermittent intestinal distension in the rat. Physiol Behav 1989; 45:191–197.
8. Mercadante S. Celiac plexus block versus analgesics in pancreatic cancer pain. Pain 1993; 52:187–192.

9. Kawamata M, Ishitani K, Ishikawa K, et al. Comparison between celiac plexus block and morphine treatment on quality of life in patients with pancreatic cancer pain. Pain 1996; 64:597–602.
10. Mercadante S. Opioid rotation in cancer pain: rationale and clinical aspects. Cancer 1999; 86: 1856–1866.
11. Enting R, Oldenmenger W, van der Rijt C, et al. A prospective study evaluating the response of patients with unrelieved cancer pain to parenteral opioids. Cancer 2002; 94:3049–3056.
12. Mercadante S. Alternatives to oral morphine in cancer pain. Oncology 1999; 13:215–225.
13. Skaer TL. Practice guidelines for transdermal opioids in malignant pain. Drugs 2004; 64:2629–2638.
14. Atkinson R, Schofield P, Mellor P. The efficacy in sequential use of buprenorphine and morphine in advanced cancer pain. In: Doyle D, ed. "Opioids in the treatment of cancer pain". London: Royal Society of Medicine, 1990:81–87.
15. Hanks GW, Nugent M, Higgs C, Busch MA. Oral transmucosal fentanyl citrate in the management of breakthrough pin in cancer: an open, multicentre, dose-titration and long-term use study. Palliat Med 2004; 18:698–704.
16. Mercadante S, Radbruch L, Caraceni A, et al. Episodic (breakthrough) pain. Cancer 2002; 94:832–839.
17. De Conno F, Ripamonti C, Saita L, et al. Role of rectal route in treating cancer pain: a randomized crossover clinical trial of oral versus rectal morphine administration in opioid-naive cancer patients with pain. J Clin Oncol 1995; 13:1004–1008.
18. Mercadante S. Problems of long-term spinal opioid treatment in advanced cancer patients. Pain 1999; 79:1–13.
19. Ischia S, Ischia A, Polati E, Finco G. Three posterior percutaneous celiac plexus block techniques. Anesthesiology 1992; 76:534–540.
20. Moore DC. Computed tomography eliminates paraplegia and/or death from neurolytic celiac plexus block. Reg Anesth Pain Med 1999; 24:483–484.
21. Levy M, Wiersema M. EUS-guided celiac plexus neurolysis and celiac plexus block. Gastrointest Endosc 2003; 57:923–930.
22. Davies DD. Incidence of major complications of neurolytic coeliac plexus block. J R Soc Med 1993; 86:246–266.
23. Eisenberg E, Carr D. Chalmers TC: Neurolytic celiac plexus block for treatment of cancer pain: a meta-analysis. Anesth Analg 1995; 80:290–295.
24. Wong G, Schroeder D, Carns P, et al. Effect of neurolytic celiac plexus block on pain relief, quality of life, and survival in patients with unresectable pancreatic cancer. A randomized controlled trial. JAMA 2004; 291:1092–1099.
25. Lillemoe KD, Cameron JL, Kaufman HS, Yeo CJ, Pitt HA, Sauter PK. Chemical splanchnicectomy in patients with unresectable pancreatic cancer. A Prospective randomized trial. Ann Surg 1993; 217:447–457.
26. Polati E, Finco G, Gottin L, Bassi C, Pederzoli P, Ischia S. Prospective randomized double-blind trial of neurolytic celiac plexus block in patients with pancreatic cancer. Br J Surg 1998; 85:199–201.
27. Rykowski JJ, Hilgier M. Efficacy of neurolytic plexus block in varying locations of pancreatic cancer: influence on pain relief. Anesthesiology 2000; 92:347–354.
28. Mercadante S, Catala E, Arcuri E, Casuccio C. Celiac plexus block for pancreatic pain: factors influencing pain, symptoms and quality of life. J Pain Symptom Manage 2003; 26:1140–1147.
29. Graham AL, Andren-Sandberg A. Prospective evaluation of pain in exocrine pancreatic cancer. Digestion 1997; 58:542–549.
30. Weber JG, Brown DL, Stephens DH, Wong GY. Celiac plexus block. Retrocrural computed tomographic anatomy in patients with and without pancreatic cancer. Reg Anesth 1996; 21:407–413.
31. Di Cicco M, Matovic M, Balestreri L, et al. Single-needle celiac polexus block: is needle tip position critical in patients with no regional anatomic distortion? Anesthesiology 1997; 87:1301–1308.
32. Di Cicco M, Matovic M, Bortolussi R, et al. Celiac plexus block: injectate spread and pain relief in patients with regional anatomic distortions. Anesthesiology 2001; 94:561–565.
33. Vranken JH, Zuurmond WWA. Increasing the efficacy of a celiac plexus block in patients with severe pancreatic cancer pain. J Pain Symptom Manage 2001; 22:966–977.
34. De Leon Casasola O. Critical evaluation of chemical neurolysis of the sympathetic axis for cancer pain. Cancer Control 2000; 2:1242–1248.

21 | Neuromodulation Techniques for Visceral Pain from Benign Disorders

Charles D. Brooker and Michael J. Cousins
Pain Management Research Institute, Royal North Shore Hospital, St. Leonard's, New South Wales, Australia

INTRODUCTION

What is neuromodulation? It could be described as the ability of the nervous system to regulate impulses. Interventional neuromodulation, as applied to the treatment of pain, is any nondestructive and reversible therapy. This includes the use of implanted or nonimplanted electrical stimulation systems and chemical neuromodulation, the infusion of chemical agents directly into the cerebrospinal fluid.

In practice, for the treatment of pain, we use the term to include various techniques, transcutaneous electrical nerve stimulators (TENS), implanted spinal cord stimulators, nerve root stimulators, peripheral nerve stimulators, and intrathecal drug pumps. Of course, one could view any treatment that attempts to influence the amount of pain experienced by the patient as neuromodulation. For example, oral drug therapy or cognitive behavioral therapy could be entitled "neuromodulation," but this is not a convention.

For the purposes of this chapter, we have also included the discussion of "neurolytic" techniques. These are procedural interventions but not reversible, so we have included these to compare their use with neuromodulation.

From the interventionalist's point of view, there are some indications for neuromodulation in the field of visceral noncancer pain (VNCP). These indications have emerged with variable levels of evidence. With stimulation techniques, blinded studies cannot be used to establish efficacy. It is likely that these procedures have a strong placebo effect in view of the invasive nature of the intervention. With intrathecal drug infusions and neurolytic techniques, evidence is also poor despite the fact that blinded studies would be theoretically possible. The reasons for this are multiple, but they stem from the fear of withholding treatment from someone in severe pain. The evidence that is available in one condition is then used to infer that the technique may be effective in other related conditions. Patients in pain are desperate enough to demand a trial of "anything" to help relieve their symptoms. This can lead to inappropriate interventions with correspondingly poor results. Equally, trialing a treatment in a small number of patients can lead to a false negative response. False positive and negative responses are more likely if we are dealing with conditions that are known to have a fluctuating course or a strong relationship to stress, substance abuse, or generalized pain disorders. For example, patients with chronic pancreatitis have a poor response to neurolytic coeliac plexus block. Some series have noted that those with alcohol-related pancreatitis have a worse outcome than those with non–alcohol-related disease (1). However, looking at the number of patients, this is not conclusively proven and may just reflect the general bias of physicians against interventional procedures in patients with a tendency toward substance abuse.

It would be wise to reflect on clinical experience to some degree and be mindful of the need for both multidisciplinary assessment and treatment of patients whose pain is severe enough to justify invasive techniques. Those who have a long history of widespread chronic visceral symptoms or associated fibromyalgia or migraine would seem intuitively to be poor candidates for interventions, but they need to be assessed carefully. A severe focal problem may in fact improve with invasive management, allowing the patient to address their milder, more generalized symptoms through less invasive means. Equally, the patient may have a very good medical indication for an implant, but have very high pain scores and have adverse psychological factors contributing to this level of distress. The implant is likely to reverse only part of the problem. If it is thought that the implant will create more of a passive dependency profile, it may be a bad thing to do for that individual in the long term.

When attempting to apply these techniques in VNCP, it is common to try therapies known to be effective in nociceptive and neuropathic pain on an empiric basis. Is it appropriate to give the patients the benefit of the doubt? The answer is almost certainly "yes" because of the uncertainty of both the mechanism of VNCP and the true indications for these techniques.

There is some logic to the empiric application of analgesic techniques because some central convergence of mechanisms of severe chronic pain is likely. Animal models are lacking for many human chronic pain conditions, especially conditions with several underlying mechanisms. There is recognition that although the nervous system is apparently intact (and therefore the pain should be visceral nociceptive in type), there is some visceral hyperalgesia akin to the allodynia seen in peripheral neuropathic pain (2). In the absence of a true neuropathy, the post-surgery patient with pain may have visceral hyperalgesia, which has spread and intensified postoperatively. Can we confidently say which type of mechanism is operating in this case? Probably not, it may be that true peripheral–visceral "neuropathic" pain occurs and is caused by neuroma formation directly following surgery, trauma, or inflammation in patients who are susceptible. Although this is probably unusual, it does potentially allow us to apply neuropathic pain treatments with success. Degenerative conditions may also be associated with visceral neuropathic pain. A classic example is abdominal neuropathic pain associated with diabetes.

INTRATHECAL DRUG THERAPY
Principles and Scientific Basis

The administration of intrathecal opioids in the treatment of pain was stimulated in the 1970s by the discovery of spinal opioid receptors (3,4). The understanding that direct administration of opioids intrathecally gave profound analgesia with reduced side effects led to extensive use of spinal opioids in acute pain. In practice, this refers to intra- and postoperative and labor-ward analgesia. The particular pharmacokinetics of the hydrophilic opioids such as morphine, allow analgesia with a 100-fold reduction in dose compared with parenteral dosing. It was this combined with progress in implantable pump technology that led to the extensive use of implanted intrathecal pumps for the administration of opioids long term to patients with chronic pain.

With such a potent route, three things have become clear. Firstly, not all pain is opioid-responsive. Secondly, opioid tolerance is still a problem when the intrathecal route is used. Finally, a different and sometimes serious side-effect profile has been elucidated as well as potential neurological complications.

These three statements are all controversial to a degree. Certainly, the concept that all neuropathic pain is opioid-resistant has been challenged successfully (5,6); perhaps relatively resistant would be more appropriate. Opioid dose escalation has been observed in some series (7); however, published reviews tend to refute this (8). The side-effect profile includes some serious problems, which are probably related to the high dose in the central nervous system (CNS) relative to systemic administration. One complication that has recently become clearly related to the intrathecal route is the formation of an inflammatory mass, which is rare but may be serious if it presents with cord compression (9,10).

The search for details about the pathophysiology of pain has led to an understanding of the many cellular mechanisms involved in the transmission and processing of pain. Many of these occur in the dorsal horn of the spinal cord. This research has opened up possibilities for treatment. Several of the drugs that are effective at these receptor sites are effective when given intrathecally. This has led rapidly to clinical use of these drugs in an attempt to improve analgesia and reduce opioid-related side effects. Figure 1 indicates some of these sites at the dorsal horn and the relevant drug classes (11,12).

Current Practice and Evidence

The administration of opioids intrathecally has become well established in the treatment of pain. In acute and cancer pain, there is strong evidence of improved efficacy and reduced side

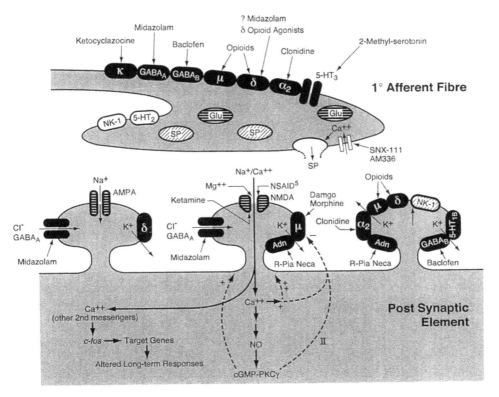

Figure 1   Possible arrangement of pre- and postsynaptic receptors on structures in the dorsal horn of the spinal cord and potential sites of action of opioid and nonopioid spinal analgesics. Presynaptic release of the neurotransmitter glutamate results in activation of the postsynaptic AMPA receptor, which controls a rapid release sodium (Na^+) channel. SP interacts with the NK-1 receptor and results in activation of second messengers. With prolonged activation, the NMDA receptor is primed, glutamate activates the receptor, the magnesium (Mg^{2+}) plug is removed, and the ion channel allows entry of Na^+ and calcium (Ca^{2+}) ions. The increase in intracellular Ca^{2+} then triggers a number of second messenger cascades. Production of NO increases via the Ca^{2+}/calmodulin-dependent enzyme NO synthase. NO may diffuse out of the neuron to have a retrograde action on primary afferents and also activates guanyl cyclase, leading to increases in intracellular cGMP and activation of cGMP-dependent protein kinases. Activation of the Ca^{2+}-dependent PKC-γ leads to phosphorylation of the NMDA receptor, which reduces the Mg^{2+} block (*dotted line II*) relating to the development of opioid tolerance. The increase in intracellular Ca^{2+} also results in the development of proto-oncogenes such as *c-fos*, with a presumed action on target genes of altering long-term responses of the cell to further stimuli. *Note*: SNX-111 and AM336 are omega-conopeptides that block neuronal Ca^{2+} channels; γ, μ, and δ are opioid receptors. *Abbreviations*: GABA, γ-aminobutyric acid; $\alpha 2$, $\alpha 2$ adrenoceptor; 5HT, serotonin; NSAID, nonsteroidal anti-inflammatory drug; DAMGO, D-Ala[2], N-Me-Phe[4], Gly-ol[5])-enkephalin; R-Pia, R-phenyl-isopropyl-adenosine; Neca, *N*-ethylcarboxamide-adenosine; AMPA, α-amino-3-hydroxy-5-methyl-4-isoxazolepropionic acid; NK, neurokinin; PKC-γ, protein kinase C-γ; cGMP, cyclic guanosine monophosphate; NMDA, *N*-methyl-D-aspartate; NO, nitric oxide; SP, substance P; Glu, glutamate; Adn, adenosine. *Source*: From Ref. (11).

effects over systemic opioids (11,13,14). Despite common use in chronic noncancer pain, the debate over efficacy is unresolved because of the lack of controlled studies and the frequent problems with ongoing pain, dose escalation, and side effects (see above). Several reviews of intrathecal opioid therapy for chronic noncancer pain have been published. These are mostly case series that may include a small proportion of patients with VNCP; so the level of evidence remains limited. Discussion with one author revealed two patients with VNCP out of a series of 39 patients. These two patients had very encouraging responses (15). The majority of patients in the published series appear to improve significantly in the medium term. It is likely that this is not just a placebo response because of the profoundly resistant nature of the patient's pain and the reasonably long follow-up period (7,8,16).

Side effects of nausea (25.2%), pruritus (13.3%), edema (11.7%), etc. are common. Weight gain and loss of libido are frequent (7). Pruritus is a temporary problem, but the others can be disabling, and necessitate abandoning the technique. One of these is hypogonadism, which is very frequent and requires routine prevention (17). This has also been noted in heroin addicts with systemic use. Fluid retention predominantly relates to opioids and it was not noted in a study of clonidine alone (18).

The current status of intrathecal pumps in visceral "cancer" pain is "fourth line" after the three steps of the World Health Organization (WHO) analgesic ladder. Neural ablation of major nerves is now usually reserved (see below) for cancer pain in view of its limited duration of effect.

It is common practice to use a trial of treatment prior to the decision to implant. This in itself carries some technical and resource allocation challenges. One of the unfortunate results of this is that the trial period is usually between one and five days. Many pain physicians recognize that this is not long enough to make a clear decision but is better than nothing.

In our practice, we have found that the decision should largely be made before the drug trial. The trial itself really only serves to confirm that the drugs do not cause too many side effects and at least show short-term efficacy.

Because of concerns about efficacy, tolerance, and side effects, many treating physicians have chosen to mix other analgesic drugs with opioids both to improve efficacy and to reduce side effects. Several classes of agents can be used in combination or alone for spinal analgesia. Many of these are ineffective systemically but work well when coming into direct contact with the dorsal horn of the spinal cord or supraspinal sites. They include local anesthetic drugs such as bupivacaine, alpha-2-agonists such as clonidine, benzodiazepines such as midazolam, and neuronal calcium antagonists such as ziconotide. The exact role of most of these drugs is yet to be delineated and should be further studied carefully to observe for local neurotoxicity.

Clonidine, for example, is effective intrathecally but has almost no direct analgesic effect when taken systemically. Hassenbusch et al. tried intrathecal clonidine alone for the treatment of cancer- and non–cancer-related pain with good results. The majority had complex regional pain syndrome and none of these patients complained of visceral pain (18).

A double-blind controlled test study on spinal cord injury patients with central neuropathic pain showed that some patients responded to intrathecal opioids and to intrathecal clonidine, but the combination of the two gave the best response (5). We should note here that many of these patients suffer from below-level neuropathic pain derived from cervical-level spinal injury. This frequently causes abdominal pain and is exacerbated by visceral pathology such as renal stones or constipation. It remains, in our view, a neuropathic pain phenomenon and as such, one should be careful about extrapolating findings from this study to patients with more conventional VNCP. In support of this, there seems to be very little evidence that vagotomy gives relief of visceral pain in humans (19). Sympathectomy on the other hand did seem successful at least in the short term (20).

Local anesthetics, especially bupivacaine, are commonly added to intrathecal pumps delivering opioids. The dose required initially is 5 mg per day, which does not appear to cause many side effects. The commercially produced maximum dose is 7.5 mg/mL; so, bearing in mind that the volume of these pumps is less than 40 mL, it can cause administration problems if higher doses are required. Some pharmacies are able to provide somewhat stronger solutions, which should be used under strict study conditions.

The other drug classes mentioned above are not currently in common clinical use for chronic noncancer pain because of uncertainty about their benefits and safety in this group of patients. Ziconotide is now approved and marketed for the treatment of neuropathic pain and may come into more common clinical use. Midazolam, however, while commonly used for relief in cancer pain, is generally avoided in noncancer pain because of conflicting reports about local neurotoxicity (14,21,22).

We have four patients under current management who are receiving intrathecal opioids for the management of VNCP. All have been well controlled in terms of the overall picture although this control has fluctuated in all. One patient with chronic renal pain has obtained a good result with opioid doses at the higher end of the normal spectrum, and clonidine has been used to try to reduce this unsuccessfully. Another has received hydromorphone and clonidine from initial implant with apparent good relief. Two are receiving opioids alone with stable dosing. Of these, one patient, with a history of probable irritable bowel syndrome (IBS) and multiple surgeries, is still complaining of poorly controlled pain but is more independent at least partly owing to greatly decreased hospital admissions for pain relief. Another, with nonalcoholic chronic pancreatitis, has been intolerant of all opioids except parenteral pethidine (meperidine) for years and is controlled on a small dose (0.34 mg/day) of intrathecal hydromorphone. However, in periods of stress, her pain worsens and she requests meperidine. This may represent poorly controlled pain but also may reflect the fact that intrathecal opioids are unlikely to reduce opioid craving and highlights the difficulties of treating such a subjective condition.

Technically, it is important to recognize the need for repeated pump replacements as well as the relatively common reoperation rate (10%–25%) for catheter problems or infection. This is more problematic in patients who have had multiple abdominal procedures because of the difficulty of siting the pump without causing skin ischemia and the increased rates of infection with a stoma present. If constant dosing has been achieved, a constant flow-rate pump should be inserted when the battery fails because this will last the lifetime of the patient.

In summary, the use of intrathecal opioids or opioid/clonidine or opioid/local anesthetic combinations is reasonably common in chronic noncancer pain. The vast majority of recorded cases have pain secondary to degenerative lumbar spine disease. Some have visceral chronic noncancer pain, especially chronic pancreatitis, and anecdotally have responded well. The technique has significant adverse effects, complications, and reoperation rates. The evidence remains of poor quality but the author's experience of a few resistant cases has been promising.

ELECTRICAL STIMULATION TECHNIQUES
Principles and Scientific Basis

Electrical stimulation includes TENS, spinal cord stimulation (SCS), and nerve root stimulation. Deep brain stimulation has never been used for visceral pain to our knowledge. The underlying principles of SCS are similar to TENS and nerve root stimulation.

When Melzack and Wall published their paper defining the "gate theory" of pain, they suggested that there was a "gate" in the dorsal horn that governed pain signals. The gate opened when increased small versus large afferent fiber activity occurred in the peripheral nervous system. Similarly, the gate was closed when there was increased large-diameter afferent fiber activity. Investigators have suggested that by selectively activating large afferent fibers through electrical stimulation, the "gate" can be closed.

This was the theory behind the first trials of stimulation techniques. It was validated to some extent by the observation that analgesia requires that stimulation be perceived by the patient to overlap the area of pain.

There are many uncertainties as to why SCS seems to work better for chronic pain than acute pain, why it takes some time to come on, why it takes some time to wear off after stimulation, and also why it is more effective for neuropathic pain than nociceptive pain.

The mode of action of spinal stimulation is as yet uncertain. TENS and nerve root stimulation probably recruit some of the same mechanisms as SCS. Linderoth has published an excellent review of the mechanisms involved (23).

These mechanisms probably include suppression of hyperexcitable "wide dynamic range" neurons in the dorsal horn, which will reduce transmission of large fiber mediated information. Also, a supraspinal effect is likely to be relevant as an experimental lesion rostral to the site of stimulation greatly reduces the effect. It is also known that activity in the pretectal nucleus is increased, which activates a descending inhibitory pathway. In addition, this activity outlasts the duration of the electrical stimulation, which is compatible with the observed response in humans (24). Importantly, it is not likely that a pure conduction block occurs because the clinically used stimulation intensities are not high enough to cause conduction block in small unmyelinated fibers.

Neurochemically, SCS is not inhibited or blocked by naloxone, implying that there is no endogenous opioid effect. An increase in dorsal horn gamma aminobutyric acid (GABA) has been correlated with successful SCS in an animal neuropathic pain model (25). A GABAergic mechanism has been suggested because the $GABA_A$ antagonist bicuculline inhibits the effect of SCS (26). Administration of adenosine acutely abolishes neuropathic pain in rats (27). Cui et al. have also shown that combining a GABA agonist (baclofen) with adenosine enhances the effect of SCS (28). Substance P and serotonin are released in association with SCS and are thought to be relevant in modulating pain (29).

During treatment of peripheral ischemia pain with SCS, vasodilatation occurs in peripheral vasculature. During SCS in angina pectoris, decreased demand for oxygen occurs in coronary ischemia. This is thought to occur due to inhibition of sympathetic outflow but also at high intensities of stimulation may be due to antidromic impulses releasing vasoactive peptides (e.g., Calcitonin-Gene Related Peptide, CGRP). More recently, (30) modification of the response of the intrinsic cardiac neurons to ischemia, and therefore the hemodynamic response to ischemia, has been shown to occur with SCS.

There is considerable evidence that nociceptive impulses are transmitted reliably, despite SCS, during coronary ischemia but only one study (31) showed the converse, that is, reduction of spinothalamic pain impulses by stimulation. This mechanism of analgesia is therefore not thought to be as important as the relief of ischemia in the treatment of angina pectoris. This is important when considering whether the technique is suitable for new indications such as visceral noncancer pain.

The use of vagal nerve stimulators for treatment of epilepsy is interesting in that it also appears to produce mood elevation and is being investigated for the treatment of depression (32). There is no suggestion that it could be used to treat visceral pain despite the fact that 80% of vagal fibers are afferent. However, experimentally it has been confirmed that vagal stimulation reduces "somatic" pain perception in human volunteers (33–38). Similarly, there have been conflicting suggestions that stimulation of the common peroneal nerve in humans gives relief of pelvic pain associated with interstitial cystitis (39). Currently, there appear to have been no attempts to use peripheral nerve or vagal nerve stimulation for treatment of visceral pain.

Description of Different Techniques

SCS comprises one or two percutaneously placed epidural wires, each containing four to eight electrodes. An alternative technique is to use a broad "paddle" with the electrode terminals all on the face of the paddle. The difference is that this requires a small laminotomy (and therefore a neurosurgeon) for insertion as opposed to a percutaneous puncture with a 13 g needle. A paddle electrode also has greater stimulation power, is less likely to migrate, but harder to remove. It is also harder to place under local anesthesia, which is considered essential. An incision is required with both techniques to anchor the leads in the paraspinal tissues. Having inserted this part of the device, it is connected to an implantable pulse generator sited subcutaneously in one of various sites. Some patients elect to have a radiofrequency receiver implanted. This necessitates an induction coil to be worn over the receiver during stimulation, but allows a wider variety of frequencies to be used and theoretically never needs replacing. In most patients, an implanted pulse generator with battery is used, so the need for replacement needs to be emphasized to the patient.

Generally, the procedure takes two to three hours and requires full operating facilities as well as image intensification and the usual aseptic and antibiotic precautions for implanting prostheses. The device placement requires a combination of local anesthesia and sedation or general anesthesia by an anesthesiologist experienced in such cases.

Strict attention must be paid to coexisting medical conditions, especially those predisposing to infection such as local infections, recurrent urinary tract infections, diabetes mellitus etc.

A recent review detailed a 21% revision rate and 6% removal rate of these devices (40) mainly because of lead migration, infection (4.5%), and failure of analgesia, which need to be included in the consent process.

One of the major parts of the percutaneous procedure is a trial period whereby the response is established without implanting the pulse generator. This is done with a temporary lead, which is secured to the skin for a number of days and then removed and discarded when the decision has been made. Some centers have a different protocol whereby the permanent lead is implanted and tunneled a small distance to one side with a temporary extension lead. If the decision is to keep the lead in place, a second, relatively straightforward procedure can remove the extension and implant the pulse generator.

For sacral nerve root stimulation, similar wires and anchoring techniques are used as for SCS. Three techniques exist. These are: cannulating the sacral epidural space via the sacrococcygeal hiatus, retrograde cannulation of the epidural space from above, and transforaminal epidural electrode placement through the posterior sacral foramina. All of them have technical issues although the transforaminal approach gives the most stable placement. It is however the least useful for pain syndromes and is generally only used for incontinence treatment (at S3).

In patients with pelvic pain, the usual current practice is to use the so-called "retrograde" cannulation of the epidural space to place wires from the L3/4 level in the epidural space and thread them inferiorly down to the sacral nerve roots. Most patients need bilateral stimulation using two wires and a suitably sophisticated pulse generator.

The use of peripheral and vagal nerve stimulators for the treatment of pain has not been reported and will not be discussed in detail. It seems likely to us that it will be attempted as vagal nerve stimulators have now been approved for resistant depression by the Food and Drug Administration The only difference in equipment is the attention paid to the design of the stimulation wire and the stimulation parameters used in the pulse generator. Insertion technique involves open surgical placement of the electrode on the relevant nerve.

TENS, although noninvasive, aims similarly to SCS at the dermatomes related to the pain. Generally, electrodes are applied directly to the area of pain or the same dermatome. Local stimulation is applied with a variety of frequencies and amplitudes to achieve a pleasant tingling sensation. Some persistence with placements is often required to achieve relief. For example, some of our patients with chronic pancreatic pain do use it to effect over the relevant part of the spine rather than directly over the pain site anteriorly.

Current Practice and Evidence
Spinal Cord Stimulation and Visceral Noncancer Pain
It has been usual clinical experience that neural pathology needs to be present before stimulation techniques are effective. This may also explain why the technique does not appear useful in acute pain. One exception to this is the treatment of ischemia, but in this situation, stimulation does induce vasodilatation and partially acts to prevent the nociceptive stimuli from being generated. In VNCP it would be expected that stimulation would be ineffective unless visceral neuropathy or ischemia is present. In fact it would seem likely that chronic visceral pain syndromes do respond partially, implying a mechanism closer to neuropathic pain than in acute visceral pain. In pelvic conditions, it is possible to implicate both visceral and somatic pathways in the pain e.g., interstitial cystitis (41). Thus it could be that enhanced central reflex activity exists and is an example of a neuropathic pain mechanism.

It is also notable that some intact sensation to the region is required for SCS to be effective implying that central lesions or complete deafferentation will not respond.

The commonest indication for SCS in North America and Australia is radicular pain following spinal surgery, but it is necessary for patients to have some intact sensation in the relevant dermatomes.

Stimulation is undoubtedly effective in refractory angina pectoris (42) for which it is used reasonably frequently in Europe. It may therefore be effective in visceral ischemia syndromes as one case report demonstrates (43).

In visceral pain, the anecdotal reports are conflicting. A recent case series (44) has described successful treatment of nine patients with visceral pain with SCS, which is somewhat surprising but encouraging. Another experienced practitioner reports trialing nine patients with chronic pancreatitis leading to permanent implantation in five, with good long-term relief (O' Keefe D—Personal Communication).

A single case report of its use in IBS has been published with reasonably positive results, especially in terms of the bowel habit (42). The resulting analgesia was less impressive, however.

On the other hand, an informal survey of the Australian chapter of the Neuromodulation Society revealed a small number of patients with chronic pancreatitis who had trialled SCS in whom the benefits were not clear. These individuals have all progressed to other forms of treatment at this stage (Sundaraj R—Personal Communication).

Spinal Cord Stimulation and Angina Pectoris
There are numerous reports of the benefits of SCS in this condition. The use of SCS in angina pectoris is restricted to those who are not suitable for a minimally invasive revascularization procedure or coronary artery graft surgery. In cases where surgery would be less straight forward, SCS may be a better option. Mannheimer's study and long-term followup show comparable results to Coronary Artery Bypass Graft (CABG) in terms of symptoms and morbidity. In fact the short-term CNS morbidity and mortality were much lower with SCS compared to CABG (45,46).

Sacral Nerve Root Stimulation

SCS rarely picks up the sacral dermatomes, so techniques for sacral nerve root stimulation (SNRS) have gradually emerged. This is used for the treatment of refractory interstitial cystitis including those with pelvic pain syndromes. The innervation of the bladder is complex and includes visceral and somatic fibers. Bladder pain could be viewed as nonvisceral pain, but this would be an oversimplification. Certainly, stimulation of nerve roots to inhibit the abnormal reflex activity is thought to work preferentially on somatic fibers (41). The level of evidence is currently still at the stage of case series although they are quite extensive and in some cases, multicenter (47–49).

The use of SNRS to treat other functional pelvic disorders includes intractable fecal incontinence and constipation. The emerging use, for these indications, will no doubt include some patients who have pain as part of their constipation (50).

Transcutaneous Electrical Nerve Stimulation

This originated as a practical application of the gate theory of pain. It was designed as a screen to decide whether a patient should have a trial of SCS.

It is essential for the patient to perceive the stimulation to obtain benefit. Again similar to SCS, TENS is also believed to create a sympathetic inhibition providing vasodilatation and relief of angina pectoris. Clinical experience suggests that most patients do not find it useful as a long-term analgesic technique. This is partly because of the skin irritation that occurs with long-term use. In angina pectoris, there is one long-term study of its use with documentation of reduced ischemia (51).

Evidence for its use generally is limited (52).

It is not recommended to use TENS with an implanted pacemaker or defibrillator although this may be overly conservative because even spinal stimulators have been used safely with implanted pacemakers (53).

In summary, the use of stimulators in the treatment of visceral pain remains unusual. Good controlled evidence exists for the efficacy of SCS in ischemia and this is relevant to some visceral pain syndromes, predominantly angina pectoris. Other visceral indications for SCS are based on case reports and one case series at this stage. TENS continues to be used because in a few patients it is highly effective and it is noninvasive. The use of SNRS for pelvic visceral pain requires a change in technique from that used for pure incontinence. Case series of patients with pelvic pain indicate that a high percentage of cases obtain analgesia from stimulation devices. Peripheral nerve and vagal nerve stimulation do not have an obvious role in the treatment of visceral pain at present. Because of the lack of evidence for the use of these devices, practitioners should proceed cautiously, preferably with a trial stimulation period, and a multidisciplinary assessment is certainly required to determine the other factors that may need addressing to obtain the best response.

NEUROLYTIC TECHNIQUES
Local Anesthetic Blocks and their Use as a Screening Tool

A visceral nerve block can be achieved by blocking the appropriate plexus. This may be temporary with local anesthesia or permanent with chemical or surgical means.

Sympathetic blocks have been largely abandoned in the treatment of reflex sympathetic dystrophy, largely because of some negative reviews of intravenous sympathetic blocks (54). However, the only randomized controlled study of stellate ganglion blocks (55) shows that local anesthetic block outlasts placebo by 48 hours even though the magnitude of the relief is the same.

It is interesting therefore to read the case report by Chester et al. of the patient with refractory angina pectoris who is treated by repeated stellate ganglion block with local anesthetic every three months (56).

Local anesthesia of the celiac and hypogastric plexi does not seem to have any long-term benefits. It is sometimes used as a prelude to a more permanent procedure, but this is an extremely unscientific test because of the confounding effects of placebo and nonspecific effects of injecting large amounts of local anesthetic into that region giving raised systemic levels (57).

Neurolytic Blocks-Current Practice and Evidence

Neurolytic stellate ganglion blocks are rarely used because of the proximity of somatic nerves, particularly the phrenic nerve. Mostly in VNCP, sympathetic blocks have been used as an attempted therapeutic procedure by way of a neurolytic celiac plexus block in chronic pancreatitis patients. The case series published always tend to have a majority of cancer pain patients. The universal experience is that the procedure is less effective in chronic noncancer pain and the duration is very limited. The evidence has been thoroughly reviewed (1).

Part of the reason for this may be the inability of the chemical sympathectomy technique to successfully denervate the plexus as evidenced by a post mortem study (58). Sympathetic fiber regrowth inevitably occurs in about six months; so this may be the predominant reason (59). It also may be because of less pain following the block, allowing the alcoholic patients to drink alchohol more easily and accelerating their disease, or because deafferentation allows a neuropathic pain syndrome to supervene.

Case series of a surgical splanchnicectomy seem to be showing somewhat longer-term results (60). Unfortunately, there is also a definite trend of complete return of pain in these patients eventually (61). The surgical procedure is minimally invasive using a thoracoscopic approach but still risks significant complications, for example a 9% thoracotomy rate for bleeding (60).

In summary, it is unlikely that diagnostic blocks with local anesthetic have much part to play in the treatment of VNCP except to confirm response in the rare case where neurolytic techniques are planned. Neurolytic techniques need to be planned with the knowledge that the pain will return eventually. They may still be appropriate in cases where lifespan is limited. They still have a prominent role in visceral cancer pain treatment where they have been shown to prolong life expectancy.

REFERENCES

1. Patt R, Cousins MJ. Techniques for neurolytic neural blockade. In: Cousins MJ, Bridenbaugh PO, eds. Neural Blockade in Clinical Anaesthesia and Management of Pain. 3rd ed. Philadelphia, U.S.A.: Lippincott-Raven, 1998:1007–1064.
2. Sullivan MA, Cohen S, Snape WJ Jr. Colonic myoelectrical activity in irritable-bowel syndrome. Effect of eating and anticholinergics. N Engl J Med 1978; 298(16):878–883.
3. Yaksh TL, Rudy TA. Studies on the direct spinal action of narcotics in the production of spinal analgesia in the rat. J Pharmacol Exp Ther 1977; 202:411.
4. Cousins MJ. History of the development of pain management with spinal opioid and nonopioid drugs. In: Meldrum ML, ed. Opioids and Pain Relief: a Historical Perspective. (Series: Progress in Pain Research and Management). Seattle: IASP Press, 2003; 25:141–155.
5. Siddall PJ, Molloy AR, Walker S, et al. The efficacy of intrathecal morphine and clonidine in the treatment of pain after spinal cord injury. Anesth Analg 2000; 91(6):1493–1498.
6. Rowbotham MC, Twilling L, Davies PS, Reisner L, Taylor K, Mohr D. Oral opioid therapy for chronic peripheral and central neuropathic pain. N Engl J Med 2003; 348(13):1223–1232.
7. Paice JA, Penn RD, Shott S. Intraspinal morphine for chronic pain: a retrospective, multicenter study. J Pain Symptom Manage 1996; 11(2):71–80.
8. Winkelmüller W, Burchiel K, Van Buyten JP. Intrathecal opioid therapy for pain: efficacy and outcomes. Neuromodulation 1999; 2(2):67–76.
9. Hassenbusch S, Burchiel K, Coffey RJ, et al. Management of intrathecal catheter tip masses: a consensus statement. Pain Med 2002; 3(4):313–323.
10. Yaksh, TL Hassenbusch S, Burchiel K, Hildebrand K, Page LM, Coffey RJ. Inflammatory masses associated with intrathecal drug infusion: a review of preclinical evidence and human data. Pain Med 2002; 3(4):300–312.
11. Walker SM, Goudas LC, Cousins MJ, Carr DB. Combination spinal analgesic chemotherapy: a systematic review. Anesth Analg 2002; 95:674–715.
12. Carr DB, Cousins MJ. Spinal route of analgesia: opioids and future options. In: Cousins MJ, Bridenbaugh PO, eds. Neural blockade in clinical anaesthesia and management of pain. 3rd ed. Philadelphia, U.S.A.: Lippincott-Raven, 1998:915–985.
13. Smith TJ, Staats PS, Deer T, et al. Randomized clinical trial of an implantable drug delivery system compared with comprehensive medical management for refractory cancer pain: impact on pain, drug-related toxicity, and survival [see comment]. J Clin Oncol 2002; 20(19):4040–4049.
14. Hassenbusch SJ, Portenoy RK, Cousins M, et al. Polyanalgesic Consensus Conference 2003: an update on the management of pain by intraspinal drug delivery—report of an expert panel. J Pain Symptom Manage 2004; 27(6):540–563.

15. Gay MLF. Spinal morphine in non-malignant chronic pain: a retrospective study in 39 patients. Neuromodulation 2002; 5:150–159.
16. Njee TB, Irthum B, Roussel P, Peragut J. Intrathecal morphine infusion for chronic non-malignant pain: a multiple center retrospective survey. Neuromodulation 2004; 7(4):249–259.
17. Finch PM, Roberts LJ, Price L, et al. Hypogonadism in patients treated with intrathecal morphine. Clin J Pain 2000; 16(3):251–254.
18. Hassenbusch SJ, Gunes S, Wachsman S, Willis KD. Intrathecal clonidine in the treatment of intractable pain: a phase I/II study. Pain Med 2002; 3(2):85–91.
19. Rack FJ, Elkins CW. Experiences with vagotomy and sympathectomy in the treatment of chronic recurrent pancreatitis. Arch Surg 1950; 61(5):937–943.
20. Bingham JR, Ingelfinger FJ, Smithwick RH. The effects of sympathectomy on abdominal pain in man. Gastroenterology 1950; 15(1):18–33.
21. Yaksh TL, Allen JW. Preclinical Insights into the implementation of intrathecal midazolam: a cautionary tale. Anesth Analg 2004; 98(6):1509–1511.
22. Yaksh TL, Allen JW. The use of intrathecal midazolam in humans: a case study of process. Anesth Analg 2004; 98(6):1536–1545.
23. Linderoth B, Foreman RD. Physiology of spinal cord stimulation: review and update. Neuromodulation 1999; 2(3):150–164.
24. Roberts MHT, Rees H. Physiological basis of spinal cord stimulation. Pain Rev 1994; 1:184–198.
25. Stiller C-O, Cui J-G, O'Connor WT, et al. Release of GABA in the dorsal horn and suppression of tactile allodynia by spinal cord stimulation in mononeuropathic rats. Neurosurgery 1996; 39:367–375.
26. Duggan AW, Fong FW. Bicuculline and spinal inhibition produced by dorsal column stimulation in the cat. Pain 1985; 22:249–259.
27. Cui J-G, Sollevi A, Linderoth B, et al. Adenosine receptor activation suppresses tactile hypersensibility and potentiates effect of spinal cord stimulation in mononeuropathic rats. Neurosci Lett 1997; 223:173–176.
28. Cui J-G, Meyerson BA, Sollevi A, et al. Effects of spinal cord stimulation on tactile hypersensitivity in mononeuropathic rats is potentiated by GABA B and adenosine receptor activation. Neurosci Lett 1998; 247:183–186.
29. Linderoth B, Gazelius B, Franck J, et al. Dorsal column stimulation induces release of serotonin and substance P in the cat dorsal horn. Neurosurgery 1992; 31:289–297.
30. Foreman RD, Linderoth B, Ardell JL, et al. Modulation of intrinsic cardiac neurons by spinal cord stimulation: implications for its therapeutic use in angina pectoris. Cardiovasc Res 2000; 47(2):367–375.
31. Chandler MJ, Brennan TJ, Garrison DW, et al. A mechanism of cardiac pain suppression by spinal cord stimulation: implications for patients with angina pectoris. Eur Heart J 1993; 14(1):96–105.
32. Rosenbaum JF, Heninger G. Vagus nerve stimulation for treatment-resistant depression. Biol Psychiatry 2000; 47:273–275.
33. Ness TJ, et al. Left vagus nerve stimulation suppresses experimentally induced pain. *Neurology* 2001; 56:985–986.
34. Birklein F. Kirchner A. Stefan H, et al. Left vagus nerve stimulation suppresses experimentally induced pain. Neurology 2001; 56(7):986.
35. Kirchner A, Birklein F, Stefan H, Handwerker HO. Left vagus nerve stimulation suppresses experimentally induced pain. Neurology 2000; 55:1167–1171.
36. Ness TJ, Fillingim RB, Randich A, et al. Low intensity vagal nerve stimulation lowers human thermal pain thresholds. Pain 2000; 86:81–85.
37. Randich A, Gebhart GF. Vagal afferent modulation of nociception. Brain Res Rev 1992; 17:77–99.
38. Sedana O, Sprecherb E, Yarnitsky D. Vagal stomach afferents inhibit somatic pain perception. Pain 2005; 113(3):354–359.
39. Zhao J, Nordling J. Posterior tibial nerve stimulation in patients with intractable interstitial cystitis. BJU Int 2004; 94(1):101–104.
40. Turner JA, Loeser JD, Deyo RA, Sanders S. Spinal cord stimulation for patients with failed back surgery syndrome or complex regional pain syndrome: a systematic review of effectiveness and complications. Pain 2004; 108:137–147.
41. Chancellor MB, Chartier-Kastler EJ. Principles of sacral nerve stimulation (SNS) for the treatment of bladder and urethral sphincter dysfunctions. Neuromodulation 2000; 3(1):15–26.
42. Krames E, Demian DG. Spinal cord stimulation reverses pain and diarrhoeal episodes of irritable bowel syndrome: a case report. Neuromodulation 2004; 7(2):82.
43. Ceballos A, Cabezudo L, Bovaira M, et al. Spinal cord stimulation: a possible therapeutic alternative for chronic mesenteric ischaemia. Pain 2000; 87:99–101.
44. Khan YN, Raza SS, Khan EA. Application of spinal cord stimulation for the treatment of abdominal visceral pain syndromes: case reports. Neuromodulation 2005; 8(1):14–21.
45. Mannheimer C, Eliasson T, Augustinsson LE, et al. Electrical stimulation versus coronary artery bypass surgery in severe angina pectoris: the ESBY study. Circulation 1998; 97(12):1157–1163.
46. Mannheimer C, Camici P, Chester, et al. The problem of chronic refractory angina report from the ESC joint study group on the treatment of refractory angina. Eur Heart J 2002; 23:355–370.

47. Whitmore KE, Payne CK, Diokno AC, Lukban JC. Sacral neuromodulation in patients with interstitial cystitis: a multicentre clinical trial. Int Urogynecol J 2003; 14:305–309.
48. Feler CA, Whitworth LA, Brookoff D, Powell R. Recent advances: sacral nerve root stimulation using a retrograde method of lead insertion for the treatment of pelvic pain due to interstitial cystitis. Neuromodulation 1999; 2(3):211–216.
49. Alo K, McKay E. Selective nerve root stimulation for the treatment of intractable pelvic pain and motor dysfunction: a case report. Neuromodulation 2002; 4(1):19.
50. Kenefick NJ, Vaizey CJ, Cohen CR, Nicholls RJ, Kamm MA. Double-blind placebo-controlled crossover study of sacral nerve stimulation for idiopathic constipation. Br J Sur 2002; 89(12):1570–1571.
51. Mannheimer C, Carlsson C-A, Vedin A, Wilhelmsson C. Transcutaneous electrical nerve stimulation (TENS) in angina pectoris. Pain 1986; 26:291–300.
52. Fargas-Babjak A. Acupuncture, transcutaneous electrical nerve stimulation, and laser therapy in chronic pain. Clin J Pain 2001; 17(suppl 4):S105–S113.
53. Pyatt JR, Trenbath D, Chester M, Connelly DT. The simultaneous use of a biventricular implantable cardioverter defibrillator (ICD) and transcutaneous electrical nerve stimulation (TENS) unit: implications for device interaction. Europace 2003; 5(1):91–93.
54. Jadad AR, Carroll D, Glynn CJ, McQuay HJ. Intravenous regional sympathetic blockade for pain relief in reflex sympathetic dystrophy: a systematic review and a randomized, double-blind crossover study. J Pain Symptom Manage 1995; 10(1):13–20.
55. Price DD, Long S, Wilsey B, Rafii A. Analysis of peak magnitude and duration of analgesia produced by local anesthetics injected into sympathetic ganglia of complex regional pain syndrome patients. Clin J Pain 1998; 14(3):216–226.
56. Chester M, Hammond C, Leach A. Long-term benefits of stellate ganglion block in severe chronic refractory angina. Pain 2000; 87(1):103–105.
57. Hogan QH, Abram S. Diagnostic and prognostic neural blockade. In: Cousins MJ, Bridenbaugh PO, eds. Neural Blockade in Clinical Anaesthesia and Management of Pain. 3rd ed. Philadelphia, U.S.A.: Lippincott-Raven, 1998:837–878.
58. Vranken JH, Zuurmond WW, Van Kemenade FJ, Dzoljic M. Neurohistopathologic findings after a neurolytic celiac plexus block with alcohol in patients with pancreatic cancer pain. Acta Anaesthesiol Scand 2002; 46(7):827–830.
59. Cousins MJ, Reeve TS, Glynn CJ, Walsh JA, Cherry DA. Neurolytic lumbar sympathetic blockade: duration of denervation and relief of rest pain. Anaesth Intensive Care 1979; 7:121–135.
60. Maher JW, Johlin FC, Pearson D. Thoracoscopic splanchnicectomy for chronic pancreatitis pain. Surgery 1996; 120(4):603–610.
61. Maher JW, Johlin FC, Heitshusen D. Long-term follow-up of thoracoscopic splanchnicectomy for chronic pancreatitis pain. Surg Endosc 2001; 15(7):706–709.

22 | Psychological Interventions for Patients with Chronic Abdominal and Pelvic Pain

Luis F. Buenaver, Robert Edwards, and Jennifer A. Haythornthwaite
Department of Psychiatry and Behavioral Sciences, Johns Hopkins University School of Medicine, Baltimore, Maryland, U.S.A.

INTRODUCTION

Psychological factors associated with the onset, maintenance, and treatment of chronic pain have long been established. However, much of this literature focuses on specific pain disorders including low back pain, headache, and arthritis. In recent years, a significant literature has developed examining psychological variables in abdominal and pelvic pain, and to a lesser degree, noncardiac chest pain (NCCP). Because psychological variables have been shown to influence each of these painful conditions, there is potential value to including psychological treatments in the management of these complex disorders. Following a brief discussion of the psychological factors associated with these disorders, we will review the different psychological treatments studied in each condition. The focus of our discussion of abdominal pain will be primarily on psychological treatments for irritable bowel syndrome (IBS) because it is the most common and commonly studied type of chronic abdominal pain in adults. Similarly, studies that examine a broad diagnosis of pelvic pain related to menstruation or the reproductive organs will be reviewed. A separate literature has developed examining vulvodynia, or chronic vulvar discomfort, which has recently been conceptualized as a chronically painful condition [chronic pelvic pain (CPP)] that requires a shift in paradigm from an acute, infection-focused model to a more comprehensive, interdisciplinary conceptualization (1). The psychological treatment of NCCP will also be included in our discussion, though this body of literature is not well developed.

Initially, it is important to note that many selection factors influence our understanding of the psychiatric and psychological comorbidities seen in these painful conditions. While most studies of IBS and CPP are conducted on samples of patients seeking treatment through tertiary care clinics, symptoms of these disorders are extremely common in the general population. For example, the majority (75–90%) of individuals who meet criteria for IBS do not see physicians for treatment (2,3). Drossman, as well as several other groups of investigators, have compared samples of patients with IBS referred for treatment (i.e., "consulters") to demographically matched samples of individuals in the community meeting criteria for IBS but not seeking treatment for their symptoms [i.e., "nonconsulters"; (3)]. Collectively, the findings suggest that distress, rather than the severity of gastrointestinal (GI) symptomatology, differentiates treatment-seeking IBS patients from nonconsulters (3–5). In general, nonconsulters with IBS do not differ from normal controls on measures of psychological symptomatology, while IBS patients seeking treatment show higher rates of depression, anxiety, and life stress. Although not as thoroughly studied, CPP nonconsulters and consulters likely differ in pain, pain-related disability, sleep disturbance, and poor health status (6).

Similar to IBS and CPP, population-based studies on the prevalence of NCCP are limited. Data suggest that only 25% of individuals with chest pain actually seek treatment (7) and approximately 75% of treatment-seeking patients with normal or near-normal coronary arteries have some type of psychiatric diagnosis (8), including panic disorder, anxiety, or depression (9,10). Compared to patients with ischemic heart disease, NCCP patients have been found to be significantly more anxious, more concerned about pain, more preoccupied with bodily sensations and more likely to experience hypochondriacal beliefs (11). However, whether these factors differentiate patients with NCCP who seek treatment from those who do not has not been studied.

A variety of psychosocial factors including depression, anxiety, life stress, somatization, hypervigilance, coping style, learning history, and abuse history have been shown to be involved in the onset, course, and treatment of IBS (12). Studies have documented relationships between these factors and such IBS-related variables as reported GI symptomatology, treatment-seeking behavior, health care utilization, pain sensitivity, and GI function. NCCP also has been associated with panic disorder, anxiety, and depression, which affect the presentation, course, and treatment of NCCP. Similarly, CPP has long been associated clinically with psychiatric comorbidity, a history of sexual abuse, and severe psychological sequela. Although carefully controlled studies do seem to indicate a higher prevalence of physical and sexual abuse history, more recent studies comparing women with CPP to appropriate control groups indicate that those with known versus unknown etiologies are not different on psychological functioning and that women with CPP are analogous to those with other chronic pain conditions with regard to psychiatric comorbidity and psychosocial adjustment.

These psychological factors (i.e., stress, anxiety, depression, somatization, and hypochondriasis), in addition to the pain-related suffering many of these patients experience, suggest that psychological treatment might be helpful in managing these complex conditions. Unfortunately, with only a few notable exceptions, there are not many well-designed studies evaluating the potential benefits of psychological interventions for these persistent pain conditions. Although the IBS literature is quite sophisticated in both conceptualizing and integrating psychological components into treatment and the NCCP outcome literature on the benefits of cognitive-behavioral treatments is growing nicely, the CPP literature has been criticized for its dearth of methodologically sound, randomized, controlled treatment trials (13,14).

BIOFEEDBACK

Biofeedback was one of the earliest behavioral interventions used with chronically painful conditions and comprises a set of techniques designed to teach patients to monitor and subsequently control a physiologic function. This is generally accomplished by representing either an involuntary response (e.g., skin temperature) or a voluntary response (e.g., muscle tension) as an easily perceived signal (e.g., visual) that patients can learn to modify using a variety of cognitive and behavioral processes. Although not always, biofeedback typically includes training in relaxation procedures. There is a small IBS-related literature on biofeedback, which has shown promise in some studies, though a recent review indicated that there was insufficient evidence to support the use of biofeedback for some GI conditions (15). Electromyographic (EMG) biofeedback has shown benefits in the reduction of constipation (16–18), but a multicomponent behavioral intervention for IBS that included thermal biofeedback was not more effective than an attention–control intervention (19). For women with vulvodynia, EMG biofeedback has been shown to reduce pain and allow women to resume sexual intercourse (20), as well as improve psychological adjustment (21). A case series of 19 males with prostatitis found reduced pain and urgency following pelvic floor reeducation (22), and a more recent case series found that EMG biofeedback reduced pelvic floor muscle tone by approximately 65%, paralleling robust reductions in the report of pelvic pain and its impact on function (23). These results and recent findings that greater stress is prospectively associated with greater pain and disability in men with CPP (24) suggest that biofeedback may be particularly beneficial for CPP.

HYPNOSIS

While no universally accepted definition of hypnosis exists, researchers generally describe hypnotic analgesic interventions as including the induction of relaxed states of focused attention and inner absorption, with a relative suspension of peripheral awareness, combined with suggestions for analgesia (25). Hypnotherapy has been tested in several studies with IBS patients, yielding encouraging outcomes. Blanchard and Scharff (26) suggest that hypnotherapy and cognitive therapy have the strongest support as psychological interventions for IBS with at least three separate randomized controlled trials supporting their efficacy in reducing symptomatology and improving quality of life. A more recent review evaluated 14 published studies on the efficacy of hypnosis in treating IBS, concluding that hypnosis consistently produces significant results and improves the cardinal symptoms of IBS in the majority of patients, as well as positively affecting noncolonic symptoms (27). For example, hypnotherapy normalized visceral pain thresholds in IBS patients, and treatment-associated changes in pain threshold correlated highly with improvement in clinical symptoms (28). In addition, hypnotherapy has reduced the sensory and motor component of the gastrocolonic response in patients with IBS. That is, increases in muscle tone and reductions in sensory thresholds observed after infusion of duodenal lipids were eliminated after hypnotherapy (29). One of the principal drawbacks to hypnosis can be the intensive time requirement; however, although hypnosis may not be a feasible option for most practicing physicians, audiotapes employing hypnotic induction techniques, a less time-intensive alternative, may provide benefits as well (30). Interestingly, hypnosis appears to maintain its long-term benefits quite well, with 81% of IBS patients who improved following hypnosis maintaining their reductions on IBS symptoms scores, psychological distress, and health care utilization, for five years following the completion of hypnotherapy (31).

COGNITIVE BEHAVIOR THERAPY

Cognitive-behavioral therapies (CBT) are widely used in the management of a variety of chronic pain syndromes, and they show promise in IBS, CPP, and NCCP specifically. These therapies blend specific skills training (e.g., relaxation and pain coping skills training) with cognitive therapy (e.g., restructuring negative cognitions such as catastrophizing) (32) to reduce pain, pain-related disability, and distress, as well as to increase self-efficacy.

IBS. In IBS, both progressive muscle relaxation training (33) and cognitive therapy (34) reduce GI symptoms more than self-help control interventions. The addition of a multicomponent behavioral therapy (expanding progressive muscle relaxation training to include coping strategies and problem-solving training) to standard treatment resulted in greater IBS symptom reduction and larger increases in quality of life although rectovisceral perception remained unchanged (35). Group CBT reduced pain and GI symptoms, increased use of successful coping strategies, and decreased avoidance behavior among IBS patients for a period of up to four years following treatment (36). Group psychotherapy combined with low-dose amitriptyline (25 mg) resulted in improvements in GI symptoms, though only drug treatment increased rectal pain thresholds (37). In a recent well-designed multisite trial of CBT for severe functional bowel disorder, Drossman et al. (38) reported that CBT was more effective than education for reduction of IBS symptoms across IBS subtypes, whereas desipramine was only superior to placebo for particular clinical subgroups, suggesting a wide applicability of psychosocial and behavioral interventions.

Recent modifications to standard CBT protocols for IBS include a shortening of intervention length in order to make these treatments more practical to implement on a large scale. For example, an eight-session CBT program was compared to a single-session version of CBT and to a usual care group (39). Both CBT treatments enhanced, relative to usual care, quality of life for up to 12 months posttreatment. The eight-session intervention produced more robust outcomes, and reduced GI symptoms and psychological distress in addition to increasing quality of life, suggesting that brief CBT interventions can harness some, but not all, of the benefits of longer-term CBT treatments (40).

Changes in psychological distress appear to parallel changes in GI symptoms during treatment. IBS patients successfully treated with CBT show significant reductions in symptoms of depression and anxiety whereas those with no reductions in GI symptoms do not (26), and direct pharmacological treatment of comorbid axis I psychiatric disorders in IBS patients improves GI symptoms concurrently with psychiatric symptoms (41). Moreover, the benefits of psychologically based therapies may increase over time. Following a cognitive therapy treatment (34), improvements in GI symptoms were maintained and even increased at three-months followup (42) and significant additional reductions in pain and bloating have been shown at 3- to 12-month followup (43). Patients also showed significant reductions in depression and anxiety (42), and GI symptom reductions were associated with increases in positive and decreases in negative automatic thoughts (34).

CPP. In a case series of 138 men with CPP, Anderson et al. (44) combined a technique referred to as "paradoxical relaxation training" with myofascial trigger-point release therapy. Patients received eight sessions of instruction and practice with a psychologist, supplemented by home practice for six months. Patients engaged in diaphragmatic breathing and were directed to accept their muscle tension as a way of relieving it. Collectively, 72% of patients showed a moderate or marked decrease in pain and urinary symptom scores over the course of treatment. Although not technically a cognitive-behavioral intervention, a recently randomized controlled trial of written emotional disclosure recently demonstrated an intriguing reduction in evaluative pain in a group of women with CPP (45). Women were asked to write for at least 20 minutes each day for three days about the impact CPP has had on their lives. This type of simple intervention has been shown to reduce pain in rheumatoid arthritis (46) and fibromyalgia patients (47), although these effects are inconsistent across studies (48) and the benefits of emotional disclosure may be moderated by important factors related to emotions and emotional expression (45).

   NCCP. A multicomponent exercise/biofeedback/CBT intervention that included education, breathing retraining (i.e., hyperventilation prevention), physical exercise, graded exposure, cognitive restructuring, and relaxation training supplemented by the use of relaxation tapes, galvanic skin response biofeedback devices, and alarm watches to cue rapid relaxation exercises has been studied using an uncontrolled small group format in patients with NCCP (49). This multicomponent treatment was associated with a significant reduction in chest pain frequency, anxiety, depression, and disability ratings as well as improved exercise tolerance, and treatment effects were maintained six months posttreatment (49). Randomized controlled trials of CBT specifically demonstrate decreased symptom severity and frequency, improved mental state and quality of life, and increased participation in social activities (50) as well as significant reductions in autonomic symptoms, chest pain, and disruption to daily life with treatment benefits being maintained four to six months posttreatment (51). In addition to improved quality of life and mental state, CBT interventions for NCCP increase the likelihood of patients being pain-free six months following treatment (52).

MULTIDISCIPLINARY TREATMENT

The multidisciplinary care that has been consistently shown to be successful in treating other chronic pain conditions (53) has been adapted for the treatment of CPP. This approach was first piloted by Rapkin and Kames (54) and has since been shown to be superior to standard care in a randomized clinical trial. Peters et al. (55) demonstrated that significantly more women randomized to receive an integrated approach of combined medical evaluation, psychological treatment, and physical therapy improved more on general pain, disturbance in daily activities and symptoms associated with CPP than those receiving standard care. Surprisingly however, despite ongoing reviews and editorials highlighting the effectiveness of multidisciplinary interventions that include CBT and physical therapy (56), randomized clinical trials have not continued this line of work to determine the necessary components of treatment.

FUTURE DIRECTIONS

As this review highlights, the quality of the empirical literature for psychological treatments for abdominal and pelvic pain is quite variable and includes many critical gaps. Given the well-established role for psychological factors in these persistent pain conditions and the generally refractory nature of these conditions to standard medical care, the development of effective psychological interventions that can be integrated into the management of these patients is imperative.

   Two dimensions of the psychological treatments as they are typically administered may contribute to the lack of translation from research-based academic specialty settings into general practice: the specialized expertise required of providers and the substantial time commitment required from patients. These factors may be ameliorated by developing interventions that require less professional involvement and allow patients to pursue them at convenient times outside the constraints of the usual professional schedule. As mentioned above, the use of audiotapes employing hypnotic induction techniques shows some benefit in treating symptoms of IBS (30). A brief, single-session CBT intervention yielded partial improvement, although an eight-session CBT intervention produced greater reductions in psychological distress and improvements in quality of life (39). Telephone technology may provide additional strength to such brief interventions by supplementing them with interactive voice systems that remind patients and reinforce them for using cognitive and behavioral pain management strategies (57). Use of the internet to provide and test self-management interventions is growing (58), and internet-based relaxation training produces reductions in headaches (59). Whether these types of convenient intervention techniques—audiotapes, written or computer-driven materials—provide a viable and effective alternative to the usual labor-intensive and time-demanding psychological interventions typically investigated remains to be determined. Because lay people accomplish as good, if not better, outcomes with arthritis self-management programs (60), the potential for these interventions to yield widespread dissemination, if shown to be effective, is likely greater than the limited dissemination seen with the typical psychological interventions in recent years.

And finally, a recent functional neuroimaging study illustrates another important direction for studies of psychological treatments for abdominal and pelvic pain. IBS participants were treated in small groups with 10 weekly sessions of cognitive therapy targeting improved problem-solving and the identification and correction of maladaptive beliefs and information processing errors (61,62). Treatment resulted in improvements in pain severity and psychological distress. Consistent with these changes, resting neural activity in portions of the limbic system including the amygdala and part of the anterior cingulate cortex were also reduced (61). These brain regions are intimately involved in pain perception and self-regulation, and such findings provide further validation of the value of these psychological interventions in altering dysregulated central nervous system processing of pain-related information from visceral structures. Furthermore, such translational studies emphasize the importance of refining biopsychosocial approaches to the understanding and management of persistent abdominal and pelvic pain, as well as pain in the context of other "functional" pain disorders.

REFERENCES

1. Masheb RM, Nash JM, Brondolo E, et al. Vulvodynia: an introduction and critical review of a chronic pain condition. Pain 2000; 86:3–10.
2. Camilleri M. Management of the irritable bowel syndrome. Gastroenterology 2001; 120:652–668.
3. Drossman DA. Do psychosocial factors define symptom severity and patient status in irritable bowel syndrome. Am J Med 1999; 107:41S–50S.
4. Drossman DA, McKee DC, Sandler RS, et al. Psychosocial factors in the irritable bowel syndrome. A multivariate study of patients and nonpatients with irritable bowel syndrome. Gastroenterology 1988; 95:701–708.
5. Whitehead WE, Bosmajian L, Zonderman AB, et al. Symptoms of psychologic distress associated with irritable bowel syndrome. Comparison of community and medical clinic samples. Gastroenterology 1988; 95:709–714.
6. Zondervan KT, Yudkin PL, Vessey MP, et al. The community prevalence of chronic pelvic pain in women and associated illness behaviour. Br J Gen Pract 2001; 51:541–547.
7. Eslick GD, Jones MP, Talley NJ. Non-cardiac chest pain: prevalence, risk factors, impact and consulting—a population-based study. Aliment Pharmacol Ther 2003; 17:1115–1124.
8. Bass C, Cawley R, Wade C, et al. Unexplained breathlessness and psychiatric morbidity in patients with normal and abnormal coronary arteries. Lancet 1983; 1:605–609.
9. Beitman BD, Basha I, Flaker G, et al. Atypical or nonanginal chest pain. Panic disorder or coronary artery disease. Arch Intern Med 1987; 147:1548–1552.
10. Katon W, Hall ML, Russo J, et al. Chest pain: relationship of psychiatric illness to coronary arteriographic results. Am J Med 1988; 84:1–9.
11. Tew R, Guthrie EA, Creed FH, et al. A long-term follow-up study of patients with ischaemic heart disease versus patients with nonspecific chest pain. J Psychosom Res 1995; 39:977–985.
12. Camilleri M, Heading RC, Thompson WG. Clinical perspectives, mechanisms, diagnosis and management of irritable bowel syndrome. Aliment Pharmacol Ther 2002; 16:1407–1430.
13. Howard FM. An evidence-based medicine approach to the treatment of endometriosis-associated chronic pelvic pain: placebo-controlled studies. J Am Assoc Gynecol Laparosc 2000; 7:477–488.
14. Stones RW, Selfe SA, Fransman S, et al. Psychosocial and economic impact of chronic pelvic pain. Baillieres Best Pract Res Clin Obstet Gynaecol 2000; 14:415–431.
15. Coulter ID, Favreau JT, Hardy ML, et al. Biofeedback interventions for gastrointestinal conditions: a systematic review. Altern Ther Health Med 2002; 8:76–83.
16. Bassotti G, Chistolini F, Sietchiping-Nzepa F, et al. Biofeedback for pelvic floor dysfunction in constipation. BMJ 2004; 328:393–396.
17. Chiarioni G, Salandini L, Whitehead WE. Biofeedback benefits only patients with outlet dysfunction, not patients with isolated slow transit constipation. Gastroenterology 2005; 129:86–97.

18. Battaglia E, Serra AM, Buonafede G, et al. Long-term study on the effects of visual biofeedback and muscle training as a therapeutic modality in pelvic floor dyssynergia and slow-transit constipation. Dis Colon Rectum 2004; 47:90–95.

19. Blanchard EB, Schwarz SP, Suls JM, et al. Two controlled evaluations of multicomponent psychological treatment of irritable bowel syndrome. Behav Res Ther 1992; 30:175–189.

20. Glazer HI, Rodke G, Swencionis C, et al. Treatment of vulvar vestibulitis syndrome with electromyographic biofeedback of pelvic floor musculature. J Reprod Med 1995; 40:283–290.

21. Bergeron S, Binik YM, Khalife S, et al. A randomized comparison of group cognitive—behavioral therapy, surface electromyographic biofeedback, and vestibulectomy in the treatment of dyspareunia resulting from vulvar vestibulitis. Pain 2001; 91:297–306.

22. Clemens JQ, Nadler RB, Schaeffer AJ, et al. Biofeedback, pelvic floor re-education, and bladder training for male chronic pelvic pain syndrome. Urology 2000; 56:951–955.

23. Cornel EB, van Haarst EP, Schaarsberg RW, et al. The effect of biofeedback physical therapy in men with chronic pelvic pain syndrome type III. Eur Urol 2005; 47:607–611.

24. Ullrich PM, Turner JA, Ciol M, et al. Stress is associated with subsequent pain and disability among men with nonbacterial prostatitis/pelvic pain. Ann Behav Med 2005; 30:112–118.

25. Kupers R, Faymonville ME, Laureys S. The cognitive modulation of pain: hypnosis- and placebo-induced analgesia. Prog Brain Res 2005; 150:251–269.

26. Blanchard EB, Scharff L. Psychosocial aspects of assessment and treatment of irritable bowel syndrome in adults and recurrent abdominal pain in children. J Consult Clin Psychol 2002; 70:725–738.

27. Tan G, Hammond DC, Joseph G. Hypnosis and irritable bowel syndrome: a review of efficacy and mechanism of action. Am J Clin Hypn 2005; 47:161–178.

28. Lea R, Houghton LA, Calvert EL, et al. Gut-focused hypnotherapy normalizes disordered rectal sensitivity in patients with irritable bowel syndrome. Aliment Pharmacol Ther 2003; 17:635–642.

29. Simren M, Ringstrom G, Bjornsson ES, et al. Treatment with hypnotherapy reduces the sensory and motor component of the gastrocolonic response in irritable bowel syndrome. Psychosom Med 2004; 66:233–238.

30. Forbes A, MacAuley S, Chiotakakou-Faliakou E. Hypnotherapy and therapeutic audiotape: effective in previously unsuccessfully treated irritable bowel syndrome. Int J Colorectal Dis 2000; 15:328–334.

31. Gonsalkorale WM, Houghton LA, Whorwell PJ. Hypnotherapy in irritable bowel syndrome: a large-scale audit of a clinical service with examination of factors influencing responsiveness. Am J Gastroenterol 2002; 97:954–961.

32. Sullivan MJ, Thorn B, Haythornthwaite JA, et al. Theoretical perspectives on the relation between catastrophizing and pain. Clin J Pain 2001; 17:52–64.

33. Blanchard EB, Greene B, Scharff L, et al. Relaxation training as a treatment for irritable bowel syndrome. Biofeedback Self Regul 1993; 18:125–132.

34. Greene B, Blanchard EB. Cognitive therapy for irritable bowel syndrome. J Consult Clin Psychol 1994; 62:576–582.

35. Heymann-Monnikes I, Arnold R, Florin I, et al. The combination of medical treatment plus multicomponent behavioral therapy is superior to medical treatment alone in the therapy of irritable bowel syndrome. Am J Gastroenterol 2000; 95:981–994.

36. van Dulmen AM, Fennis JF, Bleijenberg G. Cognitive-behavioral group therapy for irritable bowel syndrome: effects and long-term follow-up. Psychosom Med 1996; 58:508–514.

37. Bouin M, Plourde V, Boivin M, et al. Rectal distention testing in patients with irritable bowel syndrome: sensitivity, specificity, and predictive values of pain sensory thresholds. Gastroenterology 2002; 122:1771–1777.

38. Drossman DA, Toner BB, Whitehead WE, et al. Cognitive-behavioral therapy versus education and desipramine versus placebo for moderate to severe functional bowel disorders. Gastroenterology 2003; 125:19–31.

39. Heitkemper MM, Jarrett ME, Levy RL, et al. Self-management for women with irritable bowel syndrome. Clin Gastroenterol Hepatol 2004; 2:585–596.

40. Heitkemper M, Jarrett M, Bond EF. Irritable bowel syndrome in women: a common health problem. Nurs Clin North Am 2004; 39:69–81.

41. Lydiard RB. Irritable bowel syndrome, anxiety, and depression: what are the links. J Clin Psychiatry 2001; 62(Suppl 8):38–45.

42. Payne A, Blanchard EB. A controlled comparison of cognitive therapy and self-help support groups in the treatment of irritable bowel syndrome. J Consult Clin Psychol 1995; 63:779–786.

43. Keefer L, Blanchard EB. A one year follow-up of relaxation response mediation as a treatment for irritable bowel syndrome. Behav Res Ther 2002; 40:541–546.

44. Anderson RU, Wise D, Sawyer T, et al. Integration of myofascial trigger point release and paradoxical relaxation training treatment of chronic pelvic pain in men. J Urol 2005; 174:155–160.

45. Norman SA, Lumley MA, Dooley JA, et al. For whom does it work? Moderators of the effects of written emotional disclosure in a randomized trial among women with chronic pelvic pain. Psychosom Med 2004; 66:174–183.

46. Smyth JM, Stone AA, Hurewitz A, et al. Effects of writing about stressful experiences on symptom reduction in patients with asthma or rheumatoid arthritis: a randomized trial (see comments). JAMA 1999; 281:1304–1309.

47. Broderick JE, Junghaenel DU, Schwartz JE. Written emotional expression produces health benefits in fibromyalgia patients. Psychosom Med 2005; 67:326–334.
48. Kelley JE, Lumley MA, Leisen JC. Health effects of emotional disclosure in rheumatoid arthritis patients. Health Psychol 1997; 16:331–340.
49. Potts SG, Lewin R, Fox KA, et al. Group psychological treatment for chest pain with normal coronary arteries. QJM 1999; 92:81–86.
50. Mayou RA, Bryant BM, Sanders D, et al. A controlled trial of cognitive behavioural therapy for non-cardiac chest pain. Psychol Med 1997; 27:1021–1031.
51. Klimes I, Mayou RA, Pearce MJ, et al. Psychological treatment for atypical non-cardiac chest pain: a controlled evaluation. Psychol Med 1990; 20:605–611.
52. Peski-Oosterbaan AS, Spinhoven P, van Rood Y, et al. Cognitive-behavioral therapy for noncardiac chest pain: a randomized trial. Am J Med 1999; 106:424–429.
53. Flor H, Fydrich T, Turk DC. Efficacy of multidisciplinary pain treatment centers: a meta-analytic review. Pain 1992; 49:221–230.
54. Rapkin AJ, Kames LD. The pain management approach to chronic pelvic pain. J Reprod Med 1987; 32:323–327.
55. Peters AA, van Dorst E, Jellis B, et al. A randomized clinical trial to compare two different approaches in women with chronic pelvic pain. Obstet Gynecol 1991; 77:740–744.
56. Greco CD. Management of adolescent chronic pelvic pain from endometriosis: a pain center perspective. J Pediatr Adolesc Gynecol 2003; 16:S17–S19.
57. Naylor MR, Helzer JE, Naud S, et al. Automated telephone as an adjunct for the treatment of chronic pain: a pilot study. J Pain 2002; 3:429–438.
58. Ritter P, Lorig K, Laurent D, et al. Internet versus mailed questionnaires: a randomized comparison. J Med Internet Res 2004; 6:e29.
59. Strom L, Pettersson R, Andersson G. A controlled trial of self-help treatment of recurrent headache conducted via the Internet. J Consult Clin Psychol 2000; 68:722–727.
60. Lorig K, Feigenbaum P, Regan C, et al. A comparison of lay-taught and professional-taught arthritis self-management courses. J Rheumatol 1986; 13:763–767.
61. Lackner JM, Lou CM, Mertz HR, et al. Cognitive therapy for irritable bowel syndrome is associated with reduced limbic activity, GI symptoms, and anxiety. Behav Res Ther 2005; 44:621–638.
62. Lackner JM, Jaccard J, Blanchard EB. Testing the sequential model of pain processing in irritable bowel syndrome: a structural equation modeling analysis. Eur J Pain 2005; 9:207–218.

23 | Complementary and Integrative Medicine Approaches to Visceral Pain

Victor S. Sierpina and Indumathi Kuncharapu
University of Texas Medical Branch, Galveston, Texas, U.S.A.

INTRODUCTION

Patients may inquire as to the use of complementary therapies, when conventional medical or surgical therapies do not alleviate symptoms of visceral pain syndromes. Such alternatives are generally utilized in combination with conventional therapy, not replacing conventional treatment. The rational blending of conventional and complementary therapies has been referred to as integrative medicine. Findings from various studies and case reports provide a spectrum from high-to-low quality of evidence for the use of integrative medicine to manage pain.

It is essential to determine the cause of visceral pain as precisely as possible through a thorough history, physical exam, and diagnostic workup. This allows the clinician to rule out acute conditions and arrive at the most specific diagnostic category possible. Repeated re-evaluations are often necessary to verify that the symptoms are either related or not to the visceral pain syndrome or are an exacerbation of the patient's condition. A wide variety of visceral pain syndromes include thoracic (pulmonary, cardiac, mediastinal, and esophageal), abdominal (hepatobiliary, pancreatic, gastric, intestinal, and genitourinary), and pelvic (adnexal, uterine, genitourinary, and muscular).

This chapter will summarize what evidence is available for the treatment of abdominal visceral pain and related pain disorders using the most common alternative therapies. We provide evidence for their application, give case studies, and offer therapeutic approaches to two common visceral pain problems, irritable bowel syndrome (IBS) and recurrent abdominal pain (RAP) in children. Because these topics have been widely studied, we hope that information about them can be applied to the treatment of other visceral pain syndromes and guide future research. Physicians must have a collaborative discussion with the patient, which weighs the risks and benefits, levels of evidence, safety, efficacy, and patient preference before suggesting any therapy, whether conventional or alternative. Documentation of such discussion should be entered into the medical record. This type of patient-centered informed discussion is intrinsic to the very definition of "integrative medicine."

> "*Integrative medicine* is the practice of medicine that reaffirms the importance of the relationship between practitioner and patient, focuses on the whole person, is informed by evidence, and makes use of all appropriate therapeutic approaches to achieve optimal health and healing."
> ...definition from the Consortium of Academic Health Centers for Integrative Medicine (1)

In integrative medicine, emphasis is placed on several components of the healing process: (i) the *therapeutic relationship* itself, a well-known source of the nonspecific aspects of the healing response and the placebo effect, (ii) *patient-centered care*, which encourages the patient to be an active participant in choosing and deploying various therapeutic modalities, (iii) *holistic view of healing*, which emphasizes the importance of mind, body, and spirit in the relief of pain and suffering, the treatment of illness, and the promotion of wellness. Other significant aspects of integrative medicine that are relevant to the treatment of the visceral pain syndrome are the *concepts of homeostasis and self-healing*, i.e., that the body primarily heals itself and that therapeutic interventions are implemented to assist in this process.

An example is the use of mind–body therapies in pain control. Autogenic training, biofeedback, hypnosis, and various relaxation therapies such as meditation and imagery assist the person in reinterpreting pain and experiencing it at a lower level of anxiety.

Table 1 Categories of Complementary and Alternative Medicine from National Institutes of Health's National Center for Complementary and Alternative Medicine

Biological therapies
Botanical and herbal medicine, nutritional supplements, special dietary programs

Mind–body therapies
Relaxation therapies, meditation, biofeedback, hypnosis, autogenics, psychoeducational approaches, yoga, tai chi

Manual therapies
Massage, chiropractic, osteopathy, other physical modalities

Alternative systems of care
Traditional Chinese medicine, Ayurveda, kampo, native African or native American medicine, homeopathy, naturopathy, anthroposophic medicine

Bioenergetic therapies
Healing touch, therapeutic touch, magnet therapy, Reiki

This self-regulation then downregulates the sympathetic nervous system, allowing painful stimuli to be perceived at a higher threshold.

So what are the specific therapies in the integrative medicine field that are available to the patient with visceral pain or to the physician or other health-care practitioner caring for them? The National Institutes of Health's National Center for Complementary and Alternative Medicine has defined five domains of so-called complementary and alternative therapies for the purposes of clinical and research purposes (Table 1). We will examine the applicability and evidence for each of these areas in the treatment of visceral pain. This will familiarize the reader with additional options for care along with the evidence to support them.

CASE STUDY

Perhaps the simplest way to illustrate *the process of an integrative medicine approach* to a visceral pain syndrome is the description of a case of a woman with IBS. This condition is often difficult both to diagnose and treat. Dietary, psychosocial, and other nonspecific factors all play a major role in its fluctuating course.

Ashley A, a 34-year-old attorney comes in for her annual well-woman examination. She feels healthy except for recurrent feelings of abdominal bloating, gas, diarrhea, and colicky abdominal pain. She had abdominal colic as newborn. She continued to have abdominal symptoms through teenage years and later. She was fully worked up in the past and was diagnosed with IBS.

After her annual exam, Ms. A asked, "What can I do about this abdominal pain? It is really affecting my life. I've missed days of work, I have to run to the bathroom a lot and I have embarrassing stomach rumbling and gas. I am ready to try anything. This is no way to live."

She has tried metoclopramide in the past and it helped her to some extent but had made her mouth dry and made her feel drowsy. Dairy products, caffeine, most sweets, alcohol, and some grains made her symptoms worse. In addition, her stress related to her work and relations with her boyfriend, Jack, made her symptoms worse from time to time.

> Ashley was offered an integrative treatment, which included increasing dietary fiber, eliminating allergenic foods, using enteric-coated peppermint oil, and controlling psychological factors through stress reduction and exercise (2).

> A treatment plan was negotiated. Psyllium seed powder (3) was started with one teaspoon twice a day and was advised to be increased gradually. We eliminated milk, cheese, and ice cream, but advised that she could take yogurt a couple of times a week. We explained that yogurt contains helpful bacteria (probiotics) for her gut. Because caffeine and sweets seemed to aggravate her problem, we switched her to herbal teas or decaffeinated beverages and cut out soft drinks, refined sugars, and desserts.

> "Giving up milk is one thing, but coffee and ice cream ... that may be hard!" she said.

> We encouraged her to be patient with the process of change, doing as much as she felt able to reasonably accomplish. We also prescribed 300 mg capsules of enteric-coated peppermint oil three times a day before meals. This antispasmodic has been found useful in some clinical trials (4–7).

"I'll be happy for relief of the painful spasms," she says. "Is that it?"

We discussed that people with IBS often find it is aggravated by stress, as it had been in her case. We took a history of her coping and relaxation techniques and offered to teach her some new mind–body techniques. Other options were increasing her regular exercise by going to the gym and working out three to four times a week instead of once or twice. Ashley expressed concerns about her time schedule. But she agreed to look into options. We advised counseling and referred her to a psychologist who could teach relaxation and biofeedback.

"I'll think about it," she said warily.

A month later Ashley returned. She had an exacerbation of her abdominal symptoms. Her issues with her boyfriend had escalated. Acute abdominal conditions were ruled out. At this visit, she agreed to see a psychologist. At her next visit, a month later, Ashley came in smiling. "Dr. Borstein was great. He suggested some ways to handle issues. He also taught me some deep breathing exercises and showed me some relaxation exercises that have really helped.

I am also learning to handle stress better at work. Except for when I slipped and ate a pint of icecream, my stomach really is doing better."

Dietary changes and regular exercise were reinforced. Chamomile tea at bedtime was suggested as a substitute for coffee and also for its antispasmodic effect (8).

In ensuing months, she continued to have discomfort from time to time but nothing that she could not handle. These episodes have been less intense than before and do not last as long.

As this case illustrates, a variety of modalities can be employed that integrate conventional and complementary care options. Such an approach does not shun any reasonable therapy nor does it insist on a single approach as suitable for every patient. Multiple therapeutic interventions may be tried simultaneously with the chief goal of enhancing the patient's quality of life and reducing symptoms.

In addition to the mind–body, dietary, and botanical approaches described in this case, other therapies that a holistic practitioner might consider could include probiotics administered in higher doses than available in yogurt, acupuncture, biofeedback, alternative systems of care such as homeopathy, and even bioenergetic therapies such as healing touch. Some similarities in approach can be found in treating RAP in children, a condition that often is a prelude to IBS in adults. In the case of children, an intensified focus on mind–body and family dynamic approaches is often helpful. An overview of therapeutic regimens for IBS and for abdominal pain in children is given in Table 2. Dosing of herbs and supplements can be located in references provided.

BIOLOGICAL THERAPIES

Pharmaceutical approaches such as analgesics, opiates, antispasmodics, antidepressants, neuroleptics, and others are familiar examples of biological therapies to clinicians. For the purposes of this chapter, we would like to limit our survey of biologic therapies to those in the complementary and alternative medicine (CAM) domain such as herbal medicines, nutritional supplements, and specialized dietary approaches.

In treatment with botanicals (phytotherapy), there is a traditional emphasis on normalizing the functions of the digestive system (10). Examples here include such approaches as following:

- Antidiarrheals: blackberry, blueberry, and raspberry
- Antispasmodics, Matricaria (chamomile), Mentha (peppermint), Melissa (lemon balm), Achillea (yarrow), *Nepeta cataria* (catmint) Petroselinum (parsley root), and Thymus spp. (thyme)
- Aromatic digestives to improve gastric acid secretions: *Angelica archangelica*, Cinnamomum (Cinnamon), and *Coleus forskohlii*
- Bitters to improve most aspects of upper digestive function: *Gentiana lutea* and Taraxacum (dandelion)

Table 2

Integrative therapeutic approach to irritable bowel syndrome
Diet: eliminate any foods that could be provoking an allergic response; common offenders are dairy and wheat. Consider an elimination diet followed by a reintroduction diet for trial of potentially offending foods (caffeine, sweets, citrus, corn)
High fiber diet, psyllium, flax, bran
Nutritional supplements: probiotics, *Lactobacillus, Acidophilus* spp.
Botanicals: enteric-coated peppermint oil, ginger, fennel, chamomile, caraway, bitters (gentian, goldenseal, angelica) diarrhea predominant irritable bowel syndrome: blackberry, blueberry, raspberry
Mind–body approaches to reduce stress and improve coping behaviors such as progressive muscle relaxation, imagery, meditation
Alternative systems: acupuncture, traditional Chinese herbal mixtures; classical homeopathy
Manual methods for improved function and relaxation, massage, osteopathy
Pharmaceutical therapies, antispasmodics, antidiarrheals, osmotic agents

Integrative therapeutic approach to recurrent abdominal pain in children
Dietary modification: avoid caffeine, high-fructose corn syrup, sorbitol; 2–4 wk trial off all dairy products if suspected lactose intolerance
Fiber should be increased to at least 10 g/day with fruits, vegetables, whole grains, legumes; psyllium if needed
Behavior modification: encourage school attendance, avoid reinforcing or rewarding illness behavior; examine family systems patterns, stress and communication issues in family
Botanical medicines: chamomile, peppermint tea or enteric-coated capsules, ginger
Mind–body therapies: progressive muscle relaxation, biofeedback, hypnosis, imagery
Pharmaceuticals: antacids, H2-receptor antagonists or proton pump inhibitors for dyspepsia

Source: From Ref. 9.

- Bulking: Linseed (flax), psyllium, and wheat bran
- Carminatives to reduce flatulence and colic; peppermint, ginger, fennel, chamomile, and caraway
- Demulcents to coat mucosal surfaces and decrease inflammation: marshmallow and slippery elm
- Osmotics: cascara, senna, and aloe
- Pungent herbs to stimulate gastric acid, Zingiber (ginger), and Capsicum (cayenne)

Botanical medicines are best thought of in terms of their mechanism of action in the same way pharmaceuticals are. So, for example, peppermint and chamomile all have components useful in the therapy of abdominal and pelvic pain problems through antispasmodic activity. Ginger, devil's claw, and willow bark (from which aspirin was originally derived) block cyclooxygenase and thus modulate inflammatory processes. Many traditional herbal mixtures from alternative systems of care such as Ayurveda (tumeric, curcumin) exert their activity through mediating anti-inflammatory pathways.

Similarly, certain dietary approaches and supplements, particularly those emphasizing high intake of omega-3 fatty acids, mediate and reduce the production of inflammatory prostaglandins and leukotrienes through the arachidonic acid pathway. Fish oil and flaxseed oil are rich as a source of omega-3 fatty acids and competitively inhibit the enzyme (delta-6-desaturase), which produces inflammatory mediators via the omega-6 fatty acid metabolic pathway (11). Calcium can be useful in relieving premenstrual syndrome and magnesium for smooth muscle relaxation. It has also been used for other conditions such as IBS in which spasm of smooth muscle plays an important role. Such nutritional supplements may serve a dual role because they are normally prescribed for other indications such as osteoporosis prevention. Let us look into the evidence we have for biological therapies. There is a paucity of literature on clinical studies in use of botanicals specifically related to visceral pain; however, several studies have been done to show usefulness of different botanicals for various symptoms like nausea, vomiting, epigastric pain secondary to hyperacidity, bloating and flatulence, diarrhea, and constipation.

The most widely used agents for IBS are ginger, aloe, and peppermint oil. Pooled analysis of several methodologically sound studies on ginger has shown benefit for nausea and vomiting (12–17). Aloe commonly used in constipation-dominant IBS is considered a safe natural remedy with its active ingredients being anthraquinones. Presently no data exist regarding the use of aloe alone. In combination with celandin, aloe helped with constipation but not with reducing pain scores (18). Peppermint oil, an antispasmodic with its active ingredient menthol, relaxes smooth muscle by blocking calcium influx. Several randomized, controlled trials showed that peppermint was superior to placebo in improving symptoms. The duration of treatment in these studies ranged from two to four weeks (4,6,7,19–23).

Use of the probiotic Lactobacillus plantarum for four weeks in patients with IBS reduced flatulence and abdominal pain significantly in a randomized, placebo-controlled, double blind study (23). Probiotics, oligofructose and inulin, are being evaluated for their use in consti-pation-predominant IBS patients. Bulking agents for adults with IBS appear to be helpful for constipation but had little efficacy for the entire IBS complex (24).

For children with RAP, there is a lack of high-quality evidence on the effectiveness of dietary interventions. Fiber supplements are not effective in the management of RAP. The trials from lactose-restricting diets are as yet wholly inconclusive. There is a need for well-designed trials of all recommended dietary interventions for children with RAP (25).

MIND–BODY THERAPIES

Mind–body therapy can be introduced to patients as complementary therapy to ongoing medical care. A wide variety of mind–body therapies has been studied for pain of different types. While it is clear that stress precipitates or exacerbates pain, having a chronically painful condition is in itself highly stressful. Therefore, application of therapies to alleviate stress, promote relaxation, peace, and well-being is broadly useful in the visceral pain syndromes. While more clinical trials are needed, implications from a number of clinical trials, reviews, and consensus statements all suggest the need for consideration of these therapies in any integrative therapeutic approach.

If relief can be found from cancer-related pain, certainly the application of mind–body therapies to visceral pain is entirely credible. A great advantage of mind–body therapies is their safety, cost-efficiency, and ease of application. Simple and even advanced techniques can be taught to patients, either individually or in group settings. When practiced regularly, patients not only gain relief of symptoms but also an enhanced sense of self-efficacy and control over their condition (26–35).

Biofeedback therapy in functional disorders seeks to normalize the abnormalities of physiological functioning that is believed to underlie the symptom production. Cognitive and cognitive behavioral therapies help by identifying maladaptive thoughts and perceptual biases that affect symptoms and impact of symptoms on life. Psychodynamic and interpersonal therapy approaches aim to ameliorate the symptoms caused by difficulties in interpersonal relationships. Stress management training such as progressive muscle relaxation is often combined with other specific interventions: cognitive therapy, hypnosis, or biofeedback. This combination of therapies helps to neutralize the sympathetic arousal that may amplify or trigger symptoms and may improve overall well-being (36).

Several randomized, controlled trials have shown that multimodal mind–body therapies as well as individual therapies are effective in various visceral pain conditions like IBS and RAP in children. A recent report provides an excellent review of evidence for mind–body therapies in gastrointestinal (GI) conditions (37). Biofeedback with cognitive stress management and progressive muscle relaxation showed overall decrease in physical symptoms of IBS, but only biofeedback and relaxation caused decrease in psychological symptoms (38). Individual therapies for IBS like cognitive therapy (39), stress management (40), relaxation training (41), and hypnotherapy (42–44) have been shown to be very effective in reducing symptoms of IBS.

In children and adolescents, there is currently no evidence for the effectiveness of psychological therapies for managing chronic pain (other than headache,) and there is little evidence for the effectiveness of psychological therapies in improving pain in other conditions (45,46).

MANUAL THERAPIES

A popular therapy for pain relief is massage. While this is used widely for musculoskeletal pain, fibromyalgia, injuries, back pain and so on, rather less is known about massage for visceral pain. Its effects, if any, can most likely be attributed to the nonspecific effects of relaxation, increased endorphin and serotonin release, altering sympathetic nervous system tone, and so on. Other forms of bodywork such as Shiatsu, Feldenkrais, Rolfing, and Alexander are widely used for musculoskeletal pain though, even for those indications, few controlled trials exist and also the practitioners are variously trained and regulated. Similarly, popular manual and manipulative therapies such as osteopathy and chiropractic have historically mainly been applied to somatic pain. While mostly used for the management of back pain, significant controversy exists in the literature as to their efficacy. Each, however, offers their form of manipulation of soft and deep tissue, of spinal segments, of their impact on spinal ganglia, as well as neural stimulation through peripheral afferents as potentially beneficial for internal problems such as visceral pain syndromes. These also require further validation by clinical trials, such trials being challenged as in all hands-on therapies with the difficulty of creating a credible placebo control and adequate blinding.

ALTERNATIVE SYSTEMS OF CARE

When conventional Western medical therapies have not relieved visceral pain, a patient may seek diagnostic and therapeutic approaches from another paradigm. There is little training about these alternative systems provided in most medical schools and the context of other Western medical health care training. This makes the proper utilization of these approaches and appropriate referrals challenging.

However, often another view is noted looking through a different window. As Sir William Osler once said, "It is more important to know what kind of patient has the disease rather than what disease the patient has."

One pervading characteristic of alternative systems of care, be it the traditional Chinese medicine (TCM), Ayurveda, naturopathy, classical homeopathy, and the like is the individualization of therapy. A visceral syndrome, e.g., the neurocardiogenic syndrome, might have several entirely separate diagnostic and therapeutic categories. This highly individualized approach has made research, which is typically based on epidemiological or statistical group analysis, problematic. However, as the ultracontemporary fields of genomics, pharmacogenomics, nutrigenomics, and proteomics are revealing, such biological individualization is the norm rather than the exception. We are as different as our fingerprints on a genomic level. Hence, individualized therapies as has been propounded for millennia by some of the ancient alternative systems of care such as TCM and Ayurveda are making more sense in the validity of new science.

Acupuncture, perhaps the best known of the alternative therapies, is simply a part of the greater whole of TCM. Treatments for pain syndromes will evolve according to the patient's evolving clinical response, rather than repeating a fixed combination of points. This has made the validation of classical acupuncture treatment for any condition, including pain, suggestive but not ultimately "evidence-based." The NIH Consensus Development Panel concluded that acupuncture is promising but not proven in the management of pain (47).

In order to illustrate another approach to visceral pain, we describe an actual case from our files:

AT, a 38 year of age Latin-American female presented to the clinic seeking alternative therapy for recurrent visceral abdominal pain. Her problem began 10 years previously following gall bladder colic when an ERCP was done. The contrast dye injected resulted in a severe case of pancreatitis, with frequent recurrences in the ensuing years. She has required hospitalization two to three times annually for periods of up to six weeks for pain control, stenting of the pancreatic duct, and work-up for potential surgical complications, and has frequently required intravenous and patient-controlled analgesia. She is now insulin dependent.

Her last hospitalization was over a year ago. In addition to her abdominal pain, at that time she suffered a major pulmonary embolus requiring continuous oxygen therapy and prolonged anticoagulation. Her pain was unremitting despite intravenous hydromorphone per PCA and 100 mg fentanyl patch. In the fourth week of her last hospitalization, she received electroacupuncture three times and was able to be discharged home off all pain medications except for hydromorphone as needed, which she used about once weekly.

In consultation with a physician acupuncturist and a TCM practitioner, the patient has been treated for two years utilizing acupuncture on a weekly or biweekly basis. In addition to acupuncture, she is following a dietary plan prescribed by the TCM practitioner in relation to her "spleen and kidney deficiencies" and "liver heat" syndromes. She reports substantial relief of abdominal pain, relief of nausea, and most importantly to her, an improved quality of life and ability to remain out of the hospital.

This case illustrates the difficulty encountered by an iatrogenically caused condition that responds poorly to the usual supportive measures. The patient was on a revolving door of hospital admissions every three to four months but has now been stable for over a year and a half under acupuncture treatment.

The evidence that is available for some of these alternative systems is as follows:

A review of studies from both the Western and the Chinese literature supports the efficacy of acupuncture in the regulation of GI motor activity and secretion through opioid and other neural pathways. However, because of the lack of properly randomized, controlled trials, no firm conclusion can be drawn about the effectiveness of acupuncture in the treatment of certain specific GI disorders (48). In a double-blind, controlled study on 24 patients with IBS, acupuncture on an acupoint on the large colon meridian (LI-4) showed improvement in symptoms but these were not statistically significant (49). Acupuncture has been found to be useful in elderly patients with epigastric pain (Acupoint Zusanli ST 36), patients with enterospasm (Acupoint Jimai LIV12) for relief of symptoms in patients with digestive disorders (Acupoint Tianshu ST 25). Moxibustion, the application of heat from a smoldering herb at certain acupoints, was found useful in a study of 97 patients with GI spasm (50).

BIOENERGETIC THERAPIES

Without doubt the most controversial category of CAM therapies is the arena of the human biofield. This area advocates provocative ideas about the nature of human anatomy and physiology extending to an aura of energy, of *prana*, *qi*, or other concepts taken as de facto from other systems of medicine. The general concept, as elucidated in TCM, is that disturbance in the body's energy field (qi), results in blockage, excess, deficiency, or other imbalance. The consequence of this imbalance results in illness.

Therapeutic touch, healing touch, and other approaches allege to smooth, shift, or reorganize this field so that healing can occur. These approaches are widely exercised in the nursing field where there is an extensive literature. Other related therapies such as Reiki, qi gong, and advanced meditation techniques can be directed specifically to raising or manipulating energy through various centers in the body. In systems such as Ayurveda, these centers are referred to as chakras, sequential energy centers arising from the base of the spine to the crown of the head. Practitioners of these systems assess energy balance or imbalance in others through their hands, vision, or even intuition. Using a variety of techniques such a brushing or cleansing, often done directly on the energy field without physical contact with the patient, therapeutic intervention is performed to alter the field and to open up access to healing and homeostasis (51). Reiki is a commonly practiced nontouch therapy that uses a spiritual orientation in which the practitioner acts to channel divine healing energy from a universal source and direct it toward physical healing of the person with whom they are working.

Additionally, the use of applied stationary magnets to the surface of the body or pulsed magnetic fields has been found to be useful in a number of pain syndromes including chronic pelvic pain, renal colic, postpolio syndrome, and promoting the healing of bones. These effects are speculated to be mediated through a variety of mechanisms: increased blood flow, ionic changes, alteration in cytokines, enhanced endorphin production, anti-inflammatory and antiedema activity, reduction in spasms, changes in membrane transport, and gene expression. Other nonthermal, nonionizing bioelectromagnetics are applied using laser and radiofrequency, sometimes to acupuncture points for several pain indications. Finally, music and music vibrations can be useful for pain relief by acting as a distracter, by stimulating endorphins, inducing relaxation, and inducing mechanical vibration within Pacinian corpuscles and other vibrotactile elements resulting in decreased perception of pain and decreased analgesic use (52).

SUMMARY

Perhaps the most intriguing question about the use of integrative approaches in visceral pain syndromes is how much of the evidence regarding the treatment of somatic pain is applicable?

More research is certainly needed as we have reviewed above. Clues from existing research offer a rich and broad array of future possibilities.

For now, the least harmful and most promising are the mind–body therapies. With some increased emphasis in training and clinical application, physicians and other health care providers have the potential to significantly increase the quality of life of patients with visceral pain by teaching mind–body methods. Certain botanical and nutritional therapies, manual methods, and bioenergetic therapies all have evolving roles, which require further investigation to determine their place, if any, in the standard of care. Alternative systems of care, which can include therapies such as acupuncture, likewise deserve consideration in view of treatment failures using standard methods.

The thoughtful clinician of the future will be prepared to survey the literature to first establish safety. Efficacy, cost factors, patient preference all need to be taken into consideration as decisions are made in the patient-centered model. The therapeutic relationship must respect all traditions of healing to allow the widest range of possible therapies to patients with chronic and challenging pain syndromes.

REFERENCES

1. http://www.imconsortium.org.
2. Murray M, Pizzorno J. Rocklin, CA. Encyclopedia of Natural Medicine Prima Publishing, 1998.
3. Hotz J, Plein K. The effectiveness of plantago seed husks in comparison with wheat grain on stool frequency and manifestations of irritable colon syndrome with constipation. Med Klin 1994; 89:645.
4. Dew M et al. Peppermint oil for irritable bowel syndrome: a multi-center trial. Br J Clin Pract 1989; 38:394.
5. Blumenthal et al. Herbal Medicine-expanded Commission E Monographs, 2000.
6. Liu J et al. Enteric-coated peppermint-oil capsules in the treatment of irritable bowel syndrome: a prospective, randomized trial. J Gastroenterology 1997; 32:765.
7. Rees W et al. Treating irritable bowel syndrome with peppermint oil. BMJ 1979; 2:835.
8. Robbers J, Tyler V. Tyler's Herbs of Choice—The Therapeutic Use of Phytomedicinals. New York: Haworth Press, 1999.
9. Rakel D. Integrative Medicine. Saunders, 2004.
10. Mills S, Bone K. Herbal approaches to system dysfunctions. In: Principles and Practice of Phytotherapy: Modern Herbal Medicine. United Kingdom: Churchill Livingstone, 2000:161–182.
11. Rakel D. The anti-inflammatory diet. In: Rakel, ed. Integrative Medicine. Philadelphia: Saunders, 2003:667.
12. Arfeen Z et al. A double-blinded randomized controlled trial of ginger for the prevention of postoperative nausea and vomiting. Anaesth Intensive Care 1995; 23:449.
13. Visalyaputra S et al. The efficacy of ginger root in the prevention of postoperative nausea and vomiting after outpatient gynaecological laparoscopy. Anaesthesia 1998; 53:506.
14. Phillips C et al. Zingiber officinale (ginger)—an antiemetic for day case surgery. Anaesthesia 1993; 48:715.
15. Bone M et al. Ginger root—a new antiemetic: the effect of ginger root on postoperative nausea and vomiting after major gynaecological surgery. Anaesthesia 1990; 45:669.
16. Ernst E, Pittler M. Efficacy of ginger for nausea and vomiting: a systematic review of randomized clinical trials. Br J Anaesth 2000; 84:367.
17. Fischer-Rasmussen W et al. Ginger treatment of hyperemesis gravidarum. Eur J Obstet Gynecol Reprod Biol 1991; 38:19.
18. Odes H, Madar Z. A double-blind trial of a celandin, aloe vera and psyllium laxative preparation in adult patients with constipations. Digest 1991; 49(2):65.
19. Kline R et al. Enteric-coated peppermint-oil capsules for the treatment of irritable bowel syndrome in children. J Pediatrics 2001; 138:125.
20. Carling I et al. Short-term treatment of the irritable bowel syndrome: a placebo-controlled trial of peppermint oil against hyoscyamine. Opusc Med 1989; 34:55.
21. Nash P et al. Peppermint oil does not relieve the pain of irritable bowel syndrome. Br J Clin Pract 1986; 40:292.
22. Lawson M et al. Failure of enteric-coated peppermint in the irritable bowel syndrome: a randomized, double-blind crossover study. J Gastroenterol Hepatol 1988; 3:235.
23. Nobaek S et al. Alteration of intestinal microflora is associated with reduction in abdominal bloating and pain in patients with irritable bowel syndrome. Am J Gastroenterol 2000; 95:1231.
24. Akehurst R, Kaltenthaler E. Treatment of irritable bowel syndrome: a review of randomized, controlled trials. Gut 2001; 48:272.
25. Huertas-Ceballos A et al. Dietary interventions for recurrent abdominal pain (RAP) in childhood. Cochrane Database Syst Rev 2004.

26. Jacobs G. Clinical applications of the relations response and mind-body interventions. J Altern Comp Med 2001; 7(suppl):S93–S101.
27. Cole B, Brunk Q. Holistic interventions for acute pain episodes: an integrative review. J Holistic Nurs 1999; 17(4):384.
28. Hoffart M, Keene E. The benefits of visualization. Am J Nurs 1998; 98(12):44.
29. Carroll D, Seers K. Relaxation for the relief of chronic pain: a systematic review. J Adv Nurs 1998; 27(3):476.
30. Carroll D, Seers K. Relaxation techniques for acute pain management: a systematic review. J Adv Nurs 1998; 27(3):466.
31. NIH. State-of-the-Science Conference Statement on Symptom Management in Cancer: Pain, depression and fatigue, 2002.
32. Bauer-Wu S. Psychoneuroimmunology. Part II. Clin J Oncol Nurs 2002; 6(4):243.
33. Luebbert K et al. The effectiveness of relaxation training in reducing treatment-related symptoms and improving emotional adjustment in acute non-surgical cancer treatment: a meta-analytical review. Psycho-oncology 2001; 10(6):490.
34. Wallace K. Analysis of recent literature concerning relaxation and imagery interventions for cancer pain. Cancer Nurs 1997; 20(20):79.
35. Syrjala K et al. Relaxation and imagery and cognitive-behavioral training reduce pain during cancer treatment: a controlled clinical trial. Pain 1995; 63(2):189.
36. Dillard J. Integrative approach to pain. In: Integrative Medicine: Principles for Practice. : McGraw-Hill, 2004:591–608.
37. AHRQ. Mind-Body Interventions for Gastrointestinal Conditions: Summary of Evidence Report, No. 40, 2001.
38. Bergeron CN. Comparison of cognitive stress management, progressive muscle relaxation, and biofeedback in the treatment of irritable bowel syndrome. 1983.
39. Greene B, Blanchard E. Cognitive therapy for irritable bowel syndrome. J Consult Clin Psychol 1994; 62(3):576.
40. Shaw G et al. Stress management for irritable bowel syndrome: a controlled trial. Digestion 1991; 50(1):36.
41. Blanchard E et al. Relaxation training as a treatment for irritable bowel syndrome. Biofeedback Self Regul 1993; 18(3):125–132.
42. Whorwell P et al. Controlled trial of hypnotherapy in severe refractory irritable-bowel syndrome. Lancet 1984; 2(2):1232.
43. Galvoski T, Blanchard E. The treatment of irritable bowel syndrome with hypnotherapy. Appl Psychophysiol Biofeedback 1998; 212–232.
44. Forbes A et al. Hypnotherapy and therapeutic audiotape: effective in previously unsuccessfully treated irritable bowel syndrome? Int J Colorectal Dis 2000; 15(5–6):328.
45. Huertas-Ceballos A et al. Pharmacological interventions for recurrent abdominal pain (RAP) in childhood. Cochrane Database Syst Rev 2004.
46. Eccleston C et al. Psychological therapies for the management of chronic and recurrent pain in children and adolescents. Cochrane Database Syst Rev 2005:1.
47. NIH Consensus Development Panel on Acupuncture. JAMA 1998; 280(17):1–34.
48. Li Y et al. The effect of acupuncture on gastrointestinal function and disorders. Am J Gastroenterol 1992; 87(10):1372.
49. Fireman Z, Segal A, Kopelman Y, Sternberg A, Carasso R. Acupuncture treatment for irritable bowel syndrome. A double-blind controlled study. Digestion 2001; 64:100–103.
50. Song Z, Zhu D. 97 cases of gastrointestinal spasm treated with moxibustion. J of Trad Chin 1991; 11(2):110.
51. Blodgett D et al. Bio-electromagnetic therapies. Integrative Health Care: Complementary and Alternative Therapies for the Whole Person. Sierpina V, ed. Philadelphia: F.A. Davis Company, 2001:194–207.
52. Taylor A. Complementary/alternative therapies in the treatment of pain. In: Complementary/Alternative Medicine: An Evidence Based Approach. St. Louis: Mosby, 1999:282–339.

24 | Irritable Bowel Syndrome and Functional Abdominal Pain Syndromes: Pathophysiology

Andrew W. DuPont

Department of Medicine, Division of Gastroenterology and Hepatology, University of Texas Medical Branch, Galveston, Texas, U.S.A.

Pankaj Jay Pasricha

Department of Internal Medicine, Division of Gastroenterology and Hepatology, and Enteric Neuromuscular Disorders and Pain Center, University of Texas Medical Branch, Galveston, Texas, U.S.A.

INTRODUCTION AND NATURE OF THE PROBLEM

Irritable bowel syndrome (IBS), a chronic episodic medical condition associated with abdominal pain or discomfort and altered bowel habits, is the most common reason for referral to gastroenterologists and is responsible for combined direct and indirect costs of up to $30 billion per year in the United States (1,2). Despite the fact that pain is the defining element of this syndrome, much of the earlier literature dealt predominantly with the disturbances in bowel function. It is only recently that pain itself has come in focus, and several plausible theories have been put forward based on experimental and phenomenological studies. As will be apparent from this chapter, we are still not close to forming any definitive conclusions. In part, this is due to the nature of the subject itself—pain is perhaps the most subjective of the various symptom components in IBS and has been incompletely and/or inaccurately characterized in this syndrome (3). Thus, it is conceivable that there are several different types (qualitatively as well as quantitatively) of pain in patients with IBS, each with its own causative phenomena. This is in all probability a reflection of the heterogeneous nature of the syndrome itself. It is hoped that with increasing mechanistic insight, we will be able to cull out distinct disorders from the "mixed bag" that we call IBS today. This in turn will allow us to discriminate between those instances when pain (or discomfort) is a secondary (and perhaps relatively minor) accompaniment to diarrhea, constipation, or bloating that results from a primary bowel problem (such as one caused by persistent "microinflammation" or small bowel bacterial overgrowth) or when changes in central circuitry (such as those induced in a vulnerable nervous system by stress) result in pain being as prominent a symptom, if not more, than disturbed bowel function. Another way of framing this question is by analogy to the classification of somatic pain, based on putative neurophysiologic mechanisms. According to this, pain can be either *nociceptive* or *neuropathic*, the former due to persistent stimulation of peripheral nociceptors by local injury and/or inflammation, while the latter is independent of nociceptor stimulation, implying changes in the pain pathways (either peripheral or central) that result in persistent, aberrant signaling.

While a search for the neurobiological substrate for pain in patients with IBS is clearly a major objective of current research efforts, it is also important not to equate pain with nociception. The latter is the physiological process that detects tissue damage by specialized transducers attached to C and Aδ fibers and is neither sufficient nor necessary for pain *perception*, which can occur in the absence of tissue injury due to alterations in the peripheral or central nervous system (CNS). Equally important in this context are two other phenomena: *suffering* (a combination of anxiety, fear, stress, uncertainty, and loss of loved objects), which inevitably accompanies clinically significant pain and *illness behavior*, which results from a complex mixture of physiological (e.g., pain intensity/severity or associated features), psychological (mental state, stress, mood, coping style, prior memories of experiences with pain, etc.), and social factors (concurrent negative life events, attitudes and behavior of family and friends, perceived benefits such as avoidance of unpleasant duties, etc). The patient with chronic pain represents a dysregulation or dysfunction of a system that is in effect a continuum of biopsychosocial factors and in any given patient, the primary disturbance may disproportionately affect one component of the spectrum. Unless this is recognized, therapy may be directed to inappropriate targets leading to futility and frustration. These issues are discussed in greater detail in Chapter 15.

IS PAIN SECONDARY TO MOTILITY ABNORMALITIES IN IBS?

This is perhaps the simplest level of inquiry into the pathogenesis of pain in IBS. IBS has traditionally been considered as a "motility disorder" based on the association with altered bowel movements and early research showing colonic motor abnormalities that occurred in response to stress and food ingestion and potentially associated with symptoms (4). Even though our understanding of the pathophysiology of this syndrome has matured considerably since then, this view continues to play a prominent role in directing therapy, in part, because of its intuitive appeal. Significant alterations in small or large intestinal motility can clearly result in changes in bowel movements; further, excessive contractility may result in pain due to either increases in intraluminal pressure or wall tension. Adding support for these hypotheses is the fact that antispasmodic agents are modestly effective in temporary relief of acute exacerbations of pain at least in some patients with IBS.

Since the initial reports, several other motility abnormalities have been documented in patients with IBS, including accelerated whole gut and colonic transit times in diarrhea-predominant IBS (5–7) and decreased migrating motor complexes (MMC) in constipation-predominant IBS compared to controls (8). Other studies have also found that patients with IBS may have increased discrete clustered contractions in the small intestine, and in some patients, these clusters have been associated with the onset of abdominal discomfort (9–11). However, other researchers have failed to reproduce these findings (12–16), and others have documented clusters in several other disorders (17,18).

Finally, another emerging area of research deals with alterations of gas transport in patients with IBS. Patients with IBS often attribute their symptoms, particularly abdominal distention and discomfort, to retained gas. Recent studies suggest that both gas production (19,20) and handling (21–23) may be altered in patients (Fig. 1). Voluntary gas retention can also reproduce many of the symptoms of IBS in healthy volunteers, thus lending credibility to a potential role for impaired gas handling in their pathogenesis (24).

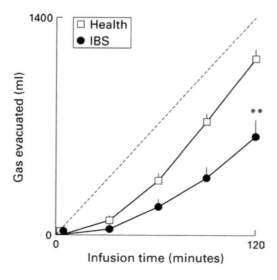

Figure 1 Evacuation of intestinal gas in patients with irritable bowel syndrome (IBS)($n = 20$) and healthy subjects ($n = 20$). Gas was infused into the intestine at a constant rate (represented by the broken line) for two hours and collected via an anal cannula. Note that IBS patients expelled a significantly lower volume of gas. Values are means (SEM)($p < 0.01$). *Source*: From Ref. 23.

A recently reemerging area of research is the potential role of small intestinal bacterial overgrowth (SIBO) in the pathogenesis of IBS. It has been suggested that the symptoms of abdominal distention or bloating may be a result of SIBO (25). In an uncontrolled study of 202 IBS patients meeting Rome I criteria, Pimentel et al. (26) documented abnormal lactulose breath testing suggestive of SIBO in 78% of patients. In this population, normalization of breath test results after antibiotic treatment was associated with reduction of symptoms to the extent that only half still met diagnostic criteria for IBS. In a subsequent double-blind, randomized, placebo-controlled trial (neomycin vs. placebo), normalization of global symptoms within one week was 11% for placebo, 37% for antibiotic-treated patients with persistently abnormal lactulose breath testing, and 75% for patients treated with antibiotics who had normalization of breath testing demonstrating a graded response to treatment (27). In further work from this group, patients with IBS and abnormal lactulose breath test have been shown to have a diminished frequency and duration of phase III of the MMC compared to controls (28). Also, methane production on lactulose breath testing appears to be associated with constipation-predominant IBS (29). This subgroup also was found to have decreased postprandial serotonin levels, compared to patients with a predominant hydrogen production (30).

It remains to be proven that any one of these disturbances can completely explain the pathogenesis of pain in patients with IBS. Although multiple patterns of abnormal intestinal motility have been described in IBS, no single motility disturbance is pathognomonic of IBS. Also, intestinal dysmotility does not appear to be the primary cause of pain in IBS, although it may result in the predominant symptom of diarrhea or constipation. For example, the number of high-amplitude propagated contractions has been shown to be decreased in constipation-predominant IBS compared to controls but not compared to patients with slow-transit constipation (31). Thus, the observed changes in motility are neither very specific nor have a predictable relationship to pain perception. It is unlikely therefore that such disturbances can explain the entire spectrum of pain in IBS. Nevertheless, they may conceivably be important in the pathogenesis of some phenomena in selected patients, e.g., postprandial cramping due to an exaggerated gastrocolonic motor response (32).

IS PAIN SECONDARY TO DISTURBANCES IN SENSORY PROCESSING (VISCERAL HYPERSENSITIVITY)?

Enhanced perception of visceral stimuli has emerged as an important phenomenon in IBS. Multiple studies have shown that a significant proportion (but not all) of patients with IBS have altered thresholds to pain within the gastrointestinal (GI) tract compared to healthy individuals (33–35). Patients with IBS have been found to perceive pain and abnormal sensation with intestinal contractions or balloon distention of the small intestine (9,36–38) and rectosigmoid (39–43) at pressures and volumes significantly lower than in non-IBS individuals; indeed, some investigators have even suggested that this physiological hallmark is useful in clinical diagnosis, with a positive and negative predictive value of 85% and 90%, respectively

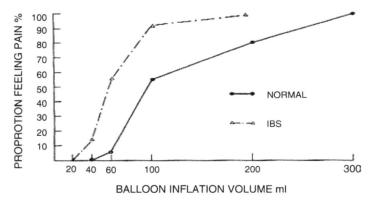

Figure 2 Onset of pain at different volumes of balloon inflation. *Abbreviation*: IBS, irritable bowel syndrome. *Source*: From Ref. 39.

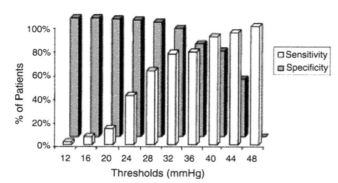

Figure 3 Sensitivity and specificity of barostat rectal distention in irritable bowel syndrome (IBS) ($n = 86$) and non-IBS ($n = 103$) subjects. Values are depicted at each distention level (pressure distention in mm Hg) tested. *Source*: From Ref. 43.

(Figs. 2 and 3). Further, even though other studies have suggested that only about 50% to 60% of patients may have reduced thresholds for painful distention of the colon, many more have altered viscerosomatic referral patterns, with IBS patients showing extension of referred pain to a significantly broader somatic area than controls (Fig. 4) (44–46). Further, apart from an occasional exception (45), most studies report that such hypersensitivity is specific to visceral stimulation and that patients with IBS appear to have similar, if not greater, somatic pain thresholds when compared with healthy controls (36,39,42,47–49).

Further support for a role of visceral hypersensitivity in the genesis of pain comes from studies in patients showing temporal correlation of variation in rectal thresholds to distention with clinical symptoms (Fig. 5) (42).

Finally, there are reports of therapeutic interventions directed principally at pain, such as the tricyclic antidepressant amitriptyline, which can cause improvement in symptoms accompanied by appropriate changes in rectal sensitivity (50).

By analogy to somatic pain states, it has been suggested that visceral hypersensitivity causes patients with IBS to experience pain at distension pressures or volumes that produce, at best, normal internal sensation in healthy volunteers (allodynia); they can also experience more severe discomfort at noxious distention pressures or volumes (hyperalgesia). Thus, it has been shown that postprandial colonic contractions, unnoticed by controls, are associated with pain in patients with IBS (51).

While it can be argued that the term "allodynia" strictly does not apply to visceral pain since visceral organs are normally insensate, such concepts are useful in helping understand how sensitization can lead to symptoms in a variety of functional bowel syndromes including IBS. Indeed, this theme recurs prominently in several other chapters in this book dealing with painful conditions affecting other organs. It is still not fully clear to what extent regional specificity of visceral hypersensitivity plays a role in determining the predominant clinical phenotype when it comes to functional pain syndromes of the viscera. Evidence in humans is somewhat conflicting, with some reports indicating that hypersensitivity is restricted to

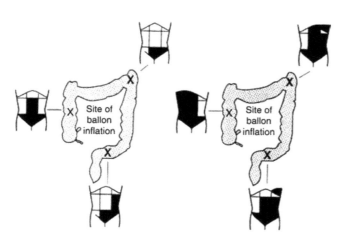

Figure 4 Balloon distension in different parts of the human colon results in increased and atypical somatic referral areas in patients with irritable bowel syndrome (*right*) compared to healthy subjects (*left*). The figure shows a schematic abdomen divided into different regions. X indicates the sight of balloon distension. Black areas indicate abdominal sites to which subjects referred the sensations in response to colonic distension. *Source*: From Ref. 46.

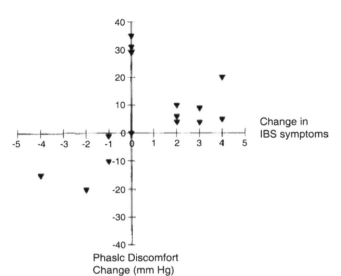

Figure 5 Intestinal sensitivity correlates with symptoms in irritable bowel syndrome (IBS). Rectal discomfort thresholds change in parallel with symptoms of IBS. When symptoms are worse, thresholds for discomfort in the rectum are lower. *Source*: From Ref. 42.

the organ in question (52), and others that suggest substantial overlap, with patients with IBS demonstrating decreased thresholds for esophageal and small bowel distention and conversely, patients with functional dyspepsia also manifesting hypersensitivity to rectal stimulation (38,53). However, experimental evidence in animals increasingly validates the concept of cross-sensitization. Two recent papers suggest cross-sensitization between bladder and rectum (54,55). This could not only explain the common association of interstitial cystitis with IBS, but also potentially provide an explanation for the gender bias, because urinary tract infections are far more common in women.

VISCERAL HYPERSENSITIVITY: CENTRAL OR PERIPHERAL?

The biological basis of visceral hypersensitivity in IBS or other functional bowel syndromes is not known. Nevertheless, it is reasonable to postulate an underlying sensitization of the nociceptive system in these patients. Such sensitization can occur at any level along the pain pathway. Most peripheral stimuli that cause significant, persistent pain also produce tissue injury or inflammation; this in turn, results in the local accumulation of several factors that amplify the activity of peripheral nociceptors, a phenomenon referred to as peripheral sensitization. An increase in the responsiveness of neurons upstream from the primary nociceptor (at the spinal cord level or higher) is called central sensitization and can result from either repetitive stimulation by "afferent barrage" from the periphery or also reflect a primary disturbance at that level. In either case, the gain of the entire system is therefore reset upwards, with the result that noxious stimuli now elicit a pain response that is excessive (hyperalgesia) and even innocuous stimuli may be perceived as painful (allodynia).

The relative contributions of central and peripheral factors in IBS remain unknown, although there is evidence for both as reviewed below.

Changes in Central Perception and Modulation of Pain in IBS

Given the prominence of psychosocial factors in health-care seekers with this syndrome (see Chapter 15), IBS has always been regarded as the archetypal disorder involving the brain–gut axis. These aspects are reviewed thoroughly in other chapters in this book (see Chapter 14) and will only be briefly discussed here. Ascending pathways from the spinal cord relay pain from the viscera to the thalamus and other subcortical organs (see Chapter 4), and then to higher centers. From a functional perspective, these circuits can be viewed as either "sensory-discriminative" or "affective-cognitive." The former is responsible for precisely characterizing the noxious stimuli according to their location and nature. The latter is responsible for autonomic and emotional responses accompanying pain including arousal, fear, and escape and is part of what has been termed the "emotional motor system" (EMS). The EMS has many other components including ascending monoaminergic pathways, the hypothalamic-pituitary adrenal axis, the autonomic nervous system, and endogenous pain modulatory centers such as the periaqueductal gray (PAG) region (56). In a chronic setting, the EMS modulates several important aspects of the clinical pain experience such as mood, attention, memory, ability to cope and tolerate, as well as the characteristic feeling of unpleasantness, and emotions about the long-term consequences of pain.

With advances in functional brain imaging, such as positron-emission tomography and functional magnetic resonance imaging (fMRI), a number of studies have recently demonstrated differences between IBS patients and normal subjects in how the CNS functions, particularly the components, described as constituting the "EMS" (57–59). Some (but not all) studies suggest that, compared to controls, IBS patients may have increased activation of the dorsal anterior cingulate cortex (ACC) and inhibition of the PAG region (59). The ACC occupies a critical position in the emotional-behavioral response to perceived threats (internal or external). Through various connecting pathways, it can integrate information about the immediate environmental threat from the parietal cortex with the emotional and behavioral response plans originating in the prefrontal cortex and, subsequently, directing attention and response priorities to noxious stimuli. It also provides input to both inhibitory and facilitatory pain modulation pathways. Thus, activation of the ACC along with inhibition of the PAG could lead to enhanced perception of visceral stimuli. Further, this pattern appears relatively specific to the viscera and is not reproduced with somatic stimulation in most patients with IBS (60). On the other hand, in IBS patients who also had fibromyalgia, somatic stimulation results in greater activation of the dorsal ACC subregion than in patients with IBS alone (49). Both disorders overlap substantially in their clinical and biopsychosocial profiles, providing support for a role for the dorsal ACC in the pathogenesis of chronic pain and suffering in these conditions.

A critical question for brain imaging research in IBS is whether patients have increased signaling from a truly "irritable" bowel or do their symptoms arise from changes in the CNS response to a relatively normal signal. Our present state of knowledge does not allow this question to be answered definitively, with some studies showing conflicting results and others suggesting possible overlap of these hypotheses. Thus, as reviewed by Naliboff and Mayer (61), there are at least three possibilities, with none of them being mutually exclusive. First, visceral stimulation in patients with IBS does not necessarily lead to increased (as compared with controls) activation of visceral sensory regions in the brain. Instead, as discussed above, IBS patients may simply have increased arousal and attention/vigilance for viscera-related stimuli (including increased activation of the dorsal ACC during stimulation and its anticipation). On the other hand, it is also possible that IBS patients show increased activity in ascending afferent processing (62). A third, and perhaps additional, possibility is that IBS patients have altered descending modulation of pain input. It has been difficult to distinguish these possibilities until recently. Thus, it is not clear whether stimulus-evoked activity on brain imaging is enhanced in patients with IBS because of sensitization of nociceptive circuitry or because of an aberrant cognitive-emotional response to the stimulus. In a recent report, Lawal et al. (63) provide evidence of significantly greater fMRI activity in response to subliminal

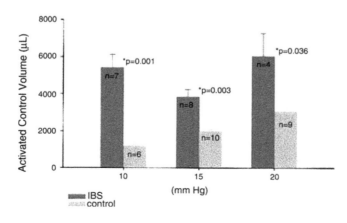

Figure 6 (*See color insert*) Total fMRI cortical activity volume response to three levels of subliminal rectal distention pressures in IBS patients and controls. In all three subliminal distention pressures, the fMRI activity volumes in IBS patients were significantly larger than those of controls. Furthermore, fMRI cortical activity volumes showed a stimulus intensity–dependent relationship in controls ($p<0.001$), but not in IBS patients for the three analyzed pressure levels. *Abbreviations*: fMRI, functional magnetic resonance imaging; IBS, irritable bowel syndrome. *Source*: From Ref. 63.

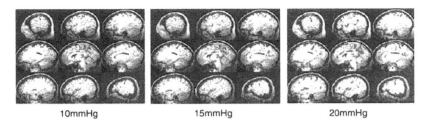

10mmHg   15mmHg   20mmHg

Figure 7 (*See color insert*) The anatomic location of composite fMRI activity associated with subliminal rectal distention in 10 diarrhea-predominant female IBS patients. fMRI activity can be characterized to exist in five broad cortical regions: the sensory/motor, the parietal/occipital, the cingulate gyrus, the prefrontal cortex, and the insula cortex. *Abbreviations*: fMRI, functional magnetic resonance imaging; IBS, irritable bowel syndrome. *Source*: From Ref. 63.

(unperceived) rectal distention in IBS patients compared with controls (Figs. 6 and 7). Thus, it is possible that both nociceptive sensitization and abnormal cognitive-emotional processing may be found in patients with IBS and could account for pain in these patients.

Clearly, brain imaging has significantly advanced our understanding of the pathophysiology of IBS pain and further insight will be forthcoming as technology and techniques become more sophisticated. We still do not know what is cause and effect, and further, if nociceptive sensitization exists, whether it is primarily central or, as speculated below, due to ongoing peripheral stimulation.

Changes in the Periphery
Intestinal Inflammation
There is convincing experimental evidence that inflammation, either acute or chronic, can result in peripheral sensitization. This is also true for the viscera with reports showing that acute inflammation (e.g., colitis or gastritis) in animals causes a reduction in the threshold for inducing pain-like behavior in response to distention (see Chapter 8). Many of the products of inflammation can induce peripheral sensitization by inducing early posttranslational changes in nociceptors as well as later transcription-dependent changes in effector genes (see chapters for a detailed discussion of these factors). Traditionally, such mechanisms were not thought to be important in IBS, as it was presumed that peripheral inflammation did not exist in the intestine of these patients. Recent studies, some of which are summarized in Table 1 below suggest, however, that an inflammatory component may be prominent in at least a subset of these patients.

Tibble et al. (76) have documented that 15% to 20% of patients with IBS had increased fecal calprotectin levels consistent with low-grade inflammation. Chadwick et al. (70) recently

Table 1 Studies Describing Low-Grade Inflammation in Irritable Bowel Syndrome

Clinical Setting	No. of Patients	Diagnostic Criteria	Type of Inflammatory Cells	Intestinal Tract Assessed	Intestinal Layer Assessed	References
Irritable colon	4	–	Mast cells	Colon	Muscularis propria	64
IBS	51	–	Unspecified	Right colon	Lamina propria	65
D-IBS	20	Manning	Mast cells	Ileum	Lamina propria	66
PI-IBS	10	Rome I	Chronic infiltrate	Left colon	Lamina propria	67
D-IBS	14	Rome I	Mast cells	Right colon	Lamina propria	68
PI-IBS	10	Rome I	T-lymphocytes	Rectum	Lamina propria	69
IBS	77	Rome I	Activated T-lymphocytes	Colon	Lamina propria	70
IBS	10	Rome I	Lymphocytes	Proximal jejunum	Myenteric plexus	71
IBS	75	Rome I	T-lymphocytes Mast cells	Rectum	Lamina propria	72
PI-IBS	30	Rome I	T-lymphocytes	Rectum	Lamina propria	73
IBS	44	Rome II	Mast cells	Left colon	Lamina propria	74

Abbreviations: C-IBS, constipation-predominant irritable bowel syndrome; D-IBS, diarrhea-predominant irritable bowel syndrome; PI-IBS, postinfectious- irritable bowel syndrome. *Source*: From Ref. 75.

evaluated 77 IBS patients (55% diarrhea predominant) by colonic biopsies who had a history of insidious onset of symptoms without documented infectious enteritis and found 49% had normal conventional histology and 40% had evidence of microscopic inflammation with increased lamina propria cellularity, frequently with focal neutrophil infiltration (8% met diagnostic criteria for lymphocytic colitis). However, among patients with normal histology, immunohistochemistry revealed increased intraepithelial lymphocytes, in addition to increased CD3$^+$ and CD25$^+$ cells, and therefore, all showed evidence of immune activation.

There is also evidence of extension of the inflammatory process beyond the mucosal level. Tornblom et al. (71) performed full-thickness jejunal biopsies during laparoscopy on 10 patients with severe IBS and found 90% had low-grade infiltration of lymphocytes in the myenteric plexus; four had an increase in intraepithelial lymphocytes; six were found to have evidence of neuronal degeneration; nine had longitudinal muscle hypertrophy; and seven had abnormal numbers or morphology of interstitial cells of Cajal.

It can be argued that the patients described in the above studies are not suffering from IBS but should be treated as variants of other disorders such as microscopic inflammatory bowel disease (IBD) or chronic idiopathic intestinal pseudo-obstruction. At the very least, these findings support the concept of heterogeneity in IBS. Further studies are needed to determine whether the presence or absence of peripheral inflammation affects the natural history of the illness in patients with the IBS clinical phenotype. In addition, it is also very important to determine if patients with microscopic inflammation respond to immunosuppressive or anti-inflammatory treatment. In the only controlled trial of its kind, Dunlop et al. treated post-infectious-IBS (PI-IBS) patients with a three-week course of prednisolone (30,30) and found no symptomatic benefit (77). The results of this trial can be interpreted in many different ways. First, peripheral inflammation may not be contributing at all to symptom genesis, but is simply a marker for the syndrome. Secondly, inflammation may have been an inciting factor, but left in its wake a permanent sensitization of the sensory nervous system that is either no longer reversible or would take considerably longer than the short duration of observation in the trial. It is also possible that the treatment itself was ineffective in suppressing inflammation (either because of dose, duration, or intrinsic lack of efficacy), since there was no significant reduction in the number of enterochromaffin cells and relative reduction in T-lymphocytes or mast cells. Clearly, further studies are needed to address this issue.

Potential Molecular Mechanisms of Pain in IBS at the Peripheral Level

Apart from general speculation on inflammatory cytokines such as tumor necrosis factor (TNF) and the interleukins (ILs), there is very little information on specific molecules involved in the pathogenesis of pain in IBS. Of these, serotonin or 5-HT has received the most attention for several reasons. First, it is an important player in the normal peristaltic reflex (78) and can also sensitize visceral nociceptors and facilitate transient receptor potential family V receptor 1 (TRPV1) function (79). Secondly, even if developed empirically, several drugs for IBS have targeted serotonin receptors (80) Finally, there is some evidence from clinical studies implicating abnormalities in enterochromaffin cell number and function in patients with IBS, as summarized in Table 2 (75).

Table 2 Changes in Enterochromaffin Cells, Serotonin and Serotonin Reuptake Transporter in Irritable Bowel Syndrome

Condition	Site	EC Cells	5-HT Content	SERT	References
IBS	Rectum	↑	–	–	81
D-IBS	Serum	–	↑	–	82
Constipation	Colon	↓	–	–	83
PI-IBS	Rectum	↑	–	–	69
C-IBS	Rectum	–	↑	–	84
D-IBS	Serum	–	↑	–	85
IBS	Rectum	⇌	⇌(release)	↓ (mRNA)	86

Abbreviations: EC, enterochromaffin; C-IBS, constipation-predominant irritable bowel syndrome, D-IBS, diarrhea-predominant irritable bowel syndrome; EC, enterochromaffin; SERT, serotonin reuptake transporter. ↑, increase; ↓, decrease; ⇌ no change; –, not assessed.
Source: From Ref. 75.

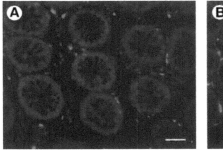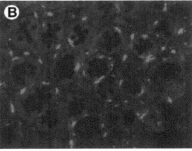

Figure 8 (*See color insert*) Representative photomicrographs showing tryptase-positive mast cells in the colonic mucosa of a healthy control (**A**) and an irritable bowel syndrome (IBS) patient (**B**). Note the higher number of positive mast cells in the IBS patient as compared with the control. (bar = 25 μm). *Source*: From Ref. 74.

5-HT is produced by enterochromaffin (EC) cells lining the mucosa, released upon stimulation and then is removed by the serotonin reuptake transporter (SERT) terminating its effects. Theoretically, overproduction of 5-HT by increased numbers of enteroendocrine cells, in the setting of altered 5-HT reuptake by SERT, leading to stimulation of enteric secretions and increased visceral hypersensitivity by activation of visceral afferents, may at least partly explain the postinfectious symptoms of persistent diarrhea and abdominal discomfort. However, as can be seen from the table, there is conflicting data on these changes in patients with IBS; further, some of these studies are difficult to reconcile (similar changes are seen in constipation and diarrhea subtypes).

One of the most intriguing cell types noted to be prominent in the mucosa of patients with IBS is the mast cell (Table 1). In animal models, mast cell degranulation has been shown to influence intestinal muscle contraction and enteric nerve excitability (87), as well as pain behavior in response to colorectal distention (88,89). Increased mast cells have been identified in ileal and colonic mucosal biopsies in patients with both diarrhea- and constipation-predominant IBS (66,68,74,90). Barbara et al. (74) studied 44 patients with IBS and found two- to threefold increases in mucosal mast cell counts (females greater than males) as compared with controls. Most importantly, mast cells located within 5 μm of nerve fibers were increased about threefold and this finding correlated significantly with the severity and frequency of abdominal pain/discomfort (Figs. 8 and 9).

The association of changes in mast cell number and function in patients with IBS has also led to speculation about the nature of their products that may be important in pain. These

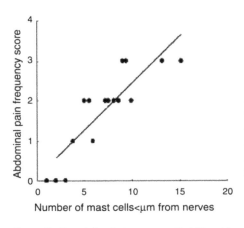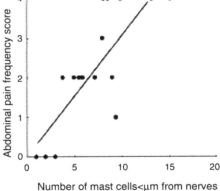

Figure 9 Correlation between severity (**A**) and frequency (**B**) of abdominal pain and the number of mast cells located within 5 μm of nerves in the colonic mucosa of irritable bowel syndrome patients ($r = 0.75$, $p = 0.001$ and $r = 0.70$, $p = 0.003$, respectively). The number of mast cells is relative to 10 electron microscopy fields. *Source*: From Ref. 74.

cells are chemical powerhouses and capable of producing a variety of enzymes, neurotrophic factors, and other biologically active peptidergic and nonpeptidergic substances. Thus, histamine, the prototypical mast cell product, is capable of sensitizing nociceptors, via H1 receptors (91). More recently studied neuromediators include tryptase, an enzyme capable of, amongst other things, activating the protease-activated receptor, PAR-2. This receptor has been shown to be important in nociception in experimental models of both somatic and visceral pain, and its activation can cause release of neurotransmitters from nociceptors as well as sensitize the responses to stimulation of the vanilloid receptor, TRPV1 (92–94). Both histamine and tryptase release have been shown to be enhanced in mucosal specimens from patients with IBS, although this did not correlate with abdominal pain severity or frequency (74).

Mast cells also produce the nerve growth factor (NGF) (95–98), and this can function both as a chemoattractant for other mast cells, as well as itself trigger mast cell degranulation (99). More importantly, it is a potent sensitizer of nociceptive neurons in the setting of inflammation acting via its high affinity receptor, tyrosine kinase A (trkA), through both transcription-dependent and -independent mechanisms to increase the activity and expression of proalgesic receptors such as the vanilloid receptor, TRPV1 (previously known as VR1) and neurotransmitters such as substance P and calcitonin gene–related peptide (CGRP). In a small cohort of patients with severe rectal hypersensitivity and fecal urgency, nerve fibres immunoreactive for TRPV1 were increased in muscle, submucosal, and mucosal layers of full-thickness biopsies of the rectum (100). These changes correlated significantly with the decrease in rectal heat and the distension sensory thresholds. In addition, expression of the trkA receptor was also increased, setting the stage for a role for NGF.

ETIOPATHOGENESIS OF VISCERAL HYPERSENSITIVITY
Susceptibility Factors

Regardless of the predominant site of sensitization, it is reasonable to assume that multiple factors are operative in determining who develops IBS. Thus, it is clear that only a minority of patients with infectious colitis or even IBD will develop IBS. In a two-hit hypothesis, IBS will develop only if a particular inciting factor occurs on a background of host susceptibility. The inciting factor could be directed peripherally (e.g., infectious colitis) or centrally (e.g., significant acute psychological stress). Even if this initiating event was transient, it can leave persistent changes in its wake that result in peripheral and/or central hyperalgesia. Host factors and genetic susceptibility may determine which patients are vulnerable to these changes. In some patients, vulnerability lies in the regulation of the immune system, resulting in persistent, albeit subtle, inflammation with secondary changes in nociceptive signaling. In yet others, susceptibility to permanent neuronal plasticity itself is the vulnerability factor, even in the absence of ongoing inflammation. Finally, in some patients, there may be impairment of the normal mechanisms to counteract upregulation of sensitizing factors (e.g., a deficiency in SERT, the SERT required for terminating the action of serotonin).

In an effort to identify potential genetic variants in IBS, investigators have begun to directly evaluate DNA sequences in individuals with IBS. Recent studies suggest that genetic factors may play a role in decreased levels of the anti-inflammatory cytokine IL-10 in some IBS patients, suggesting a subset of patients may have an inflammatory component. Gonsalkorale et al.(101) found that IBS patients had significantly reduced frequencies of the high producer genotype for IL-10 compared to healthy, ethnically matched controls (21%vs. 32%; $p < 0.05$). It was speculated that individuals with this polymorphism (-1082) might produce lesser amounts of IL-10 and would be more likely to develop IBS, due to an inappropriate inflammatory response after an episode of acute infectious gastroenteritis. The same IL-10 polymorphism was evaluated in a separate cohort; however, no difference was seen compared to controls (102).

G-protein polymorphisms, associated with diminished signal transduction, and α_2-adrenoreceptor polymorphisms, postulated to result in loss of normal synaptic autoinhibitory feedback and enhanced presynaptic release of norepinephrine, have also been recently evaluated in IBS. G-protein polymorphisms (wild-type C allele) have been shown to occur more commonly in individuals with chronic upper abdominal symptoms and functional dyspepsia compared to healthy blood donors; however, no significant association was seen in individuals with IBS symptoms compared to healthy controls (103). In an evaluation of α_2-adrenoreceptor polymorphisms, Kim et al. (104) found no association with IBS compared to controls, although an association was observed between the α_2c del 322–325 polymorphism and the α_2a-1291C/G polymorphism with constipation-predominant IBS.

The most studied polymorphism in IBS is located in the promoter region of the serotonin transporter gene (serotonin transporter protein, SERT). There are no extracellular enzymes that catabolize 5-HT, thus reuptake of 5-HT mediated by SERT is required for the termination of its action (105,106). SERT polymorphisms leading to altered reuptake of 5-HT in IBS have been evaluated in several studies (104,107–109). However, thus far no association between SERT polymorphism and IBS patients as a whole has been found, although associations have been suggested in specific IBS subtypes.

Genetic studies have also not yet disclosed any definite mechanism for susceptibility to IBS. It is not unusual for patients with IBS to have family members with symptoms of functional GI disorders or a diagnosis of IBS, which has been validated in several studies (110,111). For example, among 100 consecutive outpatients with IBS, Whorwell et al.(110) reported 33% of patients had a family history of IBS compared with only 2% of controls matched for age, gender, and socioeconomic status. Based on these results and other similar studies demonstrating familial aggregation, research was initiated to evaluate for a potential role of genetic predisposition in the development of IBS. In 1998, Morris-Yates et al. (112) published the first twin study of functional bowel disorders reporting concordance in 33% of monozygotic twins versus 13% for dizygotic twins among 343 twin pairs ($p < 0.05$). The Virginia Twin Study involving 6060 twin pairs found that concordance rates for self-reported IBS diagnosis were 17% for monozygotic twins compared to 8% for dizygotic twins ($p < 0.05$) (113). Although these two twin studies support a genetic contribution to the development of IBS, a definite genetic predisposition is difficult to conclude based on these results due to their methods of defining IBS cases. In addition, the Virginia Twin Study found having a mother with IBS was more common than having a co-twin with IBS (17% vs 7% for monozygotic twins and 15% vs. 7% for dizygotic twins), implying social learning is at least as important as genetic predisposition. In contrast to these first two reports, a third twin study evaluating 4480 twin pairs using Rome II criteria for identification of IBS cases found no increased concordance in monozygotic twins compared to dizygotic twins (16% monozygotic vs 17% dizygotic) (114). Therefore, based on these studies, genetic factors may play a limited role in the development of IBS; however, the exact extent of genetic predisposition, irrespective of environment, cannot be determined from these results.

Apart from genotype, another susceptibility factor may be developmental age. It is well known that the symptoms of many, if not most, patients with IBS may date back to childhood. Animal studies have suggested a unique vulnerability of the neonatal period to the development of an IBS-like syndrome (115). Stressors during this period could include a variety of factors commonly seen in early life, including changes in colonic pH due to carbohydrate malabsorption, noninvasive infections, and food allergies.

Inciting Factors
Infection and Postinfectious IBS
Over 40 years ago, Chaudhary and Truelove (116) reported that a portion of IBS patients first developed their symptoms after an episode of acute gastroenteritis. Recently, multiple other studies have found that PI-IBS develops in 7% to 31% patients after acute infection (117–121), with the majority developing diarrhea-predominant IBS. Risk factors for subsequent PI-IBS include female gender, prolonged episode of gastroenteritis, and higher scores for anxiety, depression, somatization, and neurosis (119).

Several studies have also suggested that symptoms of PI-IBS result from immune mechanisms. The presence of microinflammation in the intestines of some patients with IBS has been proposed possibly to represent a response to an initial bacterial infection among individuals susceptible due to a relative deficiency of anti-inflammatory cytokines (122). Patients with PI-IBS after documented infectious enteritis have been found to have an increased number of intraepithelial lymphocytes, lamina propria lymphocytes, and increased enteroendocrine cells on rectal biopsy that persisted for up to one year and were associated with increased gut permeability (69). Compared to individuals whose symptoms resolved after acute enteritis, those who developed PI-IBS have been shown to have higher IL-1 mRNA

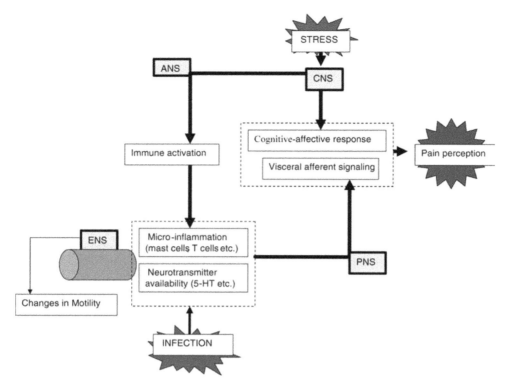

Figure 10 Current and emerging pathophysiological concepts on pain in IBS. The figure assumes a vulnerable background (genetic, developmental phase) that is predisposed to developing a persistent state of activation in response to two major inciting factors, stress and infection, acting initially at central and peripheral sites, respectively. Subgroups of IBS patients may differ in the nature of the inciting factor, as well as activity of the various components that eventually lead to pain perception. Although changes in motility are shown separately, it is possible that in some instances they may also contribute to increased afferent signaling and discomfort. *Abbreviations*: IBS, irritable bowel syndrome; ANS, autonomic nervous system; CNS, central nervous system; ENS, enteric nervous system; PNS, peripheral nervous system (spinal afferents).

expression in rectal biopsies (123). Elevated IL-1 levels have also been associated with structural changes in enteric nerves and increased mast cells in biopsies from patients with PI-IBS (124). Increased IL-1, a proinflammatory cytokine, suggests persistence of symptoms may be a result of a failure to downregulate the acute inflammatory response.

As discussed above, mast cell proximity to sensory nerves has been shown to correlate with abdominal pain in patients with IBS. Although mast cell activation has traditionally been thought to be an allergic phenomenon, it is clear that there are several non–immunoglobulin E (IgE)-dependent mechanisms that may recruit mast cells as well. The exact factors responsible for increased mast cell numbers and activity in IBS are not known. A role for food allergies, always a suspect in patients' minds, has been difficult to prove, but at least one study excluded this by a careful history and food-specific IgE antibodies (74). Infection, particularly bacterial, is clearly another important potential factor (67), as is stress (see discussions below). However, it is also theoretically possible that mast cells (and other inflammatory cells as well) are being recruited and activated because of increased activity of spinal sensory neurons, a concept known as "neurogenic inflammation" (125). Sensory neuron contain neuroeffector molecules and upon activation release factors such as substance P that are potent degranulators of mast cells. In such a model, mast cell activity is an effect and not the cause of increased afferent activity.

A recent study examined the role of inflammation and in particular, T-lymphocytes, in a postinfectious murine model of visceral hypersensitivity (*Trichinella spiralis* infection). The effects of steroid treatment and the T-cell dependence of the observed responses were assessed by infection of hydrocortisone-treated or T-cell receptor knock out [s(βxδ) KO] animals. Infection increased EC density and reduced jejunal SERT expression. Specific deficiencies in all T-cells reduced EC hyperplasia and abrogated infection-induced mastocytosis (126).

Stress

The role of stress in the pathogenesis of visceral pain and sensitivity is discussed in great detail in Chapter 14 and is clearly an important and perhaps critical factor. Significant psychological and physical stress can activate central and peripheral signaling mechanisms that can result in most of the phenomena described in experimental and clinical studies of IBS including activation of the EMS, visceral hypersensitivity, and changes in colonic permeability and degranulation of mast cells (56,127,128). As reviewed by Tache (129), corticotrophin release factor is emerging as a master molecule that is capable of mediating all these effects, acting via specific receptors on a variety of target cells.

CONCLUSIONS

The pathophysiology and pathogenesis of pain in IBS is complex. Visceral hypersensitivity is clearly a key feature but the anatomic sites, physiologic derangements, cellular mediators, and molecular mechanisms are incompletely understood. It is likely that multiple factors will be involved, and their relative importance will vary from patient to patient, as is to be expected in a diverse and heterogeneous syndrome. Figure 10 summarizes some of the key concepts discussed in this chapter.

REFERENCES

1. American Gastroenterological Association. The Burden of Gastrointestinal Diseases. Bethesda, MD: American Gastroenterological Association, 2001.
2. Sandler RS, Everhart JE, Donowitz M, et al. The burden of selected digestive diseases in the United States. Gastroenterol 2002; 122:1500–1511.
3. Tougas G. The nature of pain in irritable bowel syndrome. J Clin Gastroenterol 2002; 35(suppl 1): S26–S30.
4. Quigley EMM. Disturbances of motility and visceral hypersensitivity in irritable bowel syndrome: biological markers or epiphenomenon. Gastroenterol Clin N Am 2005; 34:221–233.
5. Cann PA, Read NW, Brown C, et al. Irritable bowel syndrome. Relationship of disorders in the transit of a single solid meal to symptom patterns. Gut 1983; 24:405–411.
6. Bazocchi G, Ellis J, Villaneuva-Meyer J, et al. Colonic scintigraphy and manometry in constipation, diarrhea, and inflammatory bowel disease. Gastroenterol 1988; 94:A29.
7. Vassallo M, Camilleri M, Phillips SF, et al. Transit through the proximal colon influences stool weight in the irritable bowel syndrome. Gastroenterol 1992; 102:102–108.
8. Bazocchi G, Ellis J, Villaneuva-Meyer J, et al. Postprandial colonic transit and motor activity in chronic constipation. Gastroenterol 1990; 98:686–693.
9. Kellow JE, Miller LJ, Phillips SF, et al. Dysmotility of the small intestine in irritable bowel syndrome. Gut 1988; 29:1236–1243.
10. Kellow JE, Phillips SF. Altered small bowel motility in irritable bowel syndrome is correlated with symptoms. Gastroenterol 1987; 92:1885–1893.
11. Kellow JE, Gill RC, Wingate DL. Prolonged ambulant recordings of small bowel motility demonstrate abnormalities in the irritable bowel syndrome. Gastroenterol 1990; 98:1208–1218.
12. Gorard DA, Libby GW, Farthing MJ. Ambulatory small bowel motility in diarrhoea-predominant irritable syndrome. Gut 1994; 35:203–210.
13. Quigley EMM, Donovan JP, Lane MJ. Antroduodenal manometry—usefulness and limitations as an outpatient study. Dig Dis Sci 1992; 37:20–28.
14. Schmidt T, Hackelsberger N, Widmer R. Ambulatory 24-hour jejunal motility in diarrhea-predominant irritable bowel syndrome. Scand J Gastroenterol 1996; 31:581–589.
15. Small PK, Loudon MA, Hau CM. Large-scale ambulatory study of postprandial jejunal motility in irritable bowel syndrome. Scand J Gastroenterol 1997; 32:39–47.
16. Gorard DA, Vesselinova-Jenkins CK, Libby GW. Migrating motor complex in sleep in health and irritable bowel syndrome. Dig Dis Sci 1995; 40:2383–2389.
17. McKee DP, Quigley EMM. Intestinal motility in irritable bowel syndrome: Is IBS a motility disorder? Part 2: motility of the small bowel, esophagus, stomach and gall bladder. Dig Dis Sci 1993; 38:1763–1782.
18. Quigley EMM. Disturbances in small bowel motility. Baillieres Best Pract Res Clin Gastroenterol 1999; 13:385–395.
19. Haderstorfer B, Pscholgin D, Whitehead WE, et al. Intestinal gas production from bacterial fermentation of undigested carbohydrate in irritable bowel syndrome. Am J Gastroenterol 1989; 84:375–378.
20. King TS, Elia M, Hunter JO. Abnormal colonic fermentation in irritable bowel syndrome. Lancet 1998; 352:1187–1189.

21. Serra J, Azpiroz F, Malagelada JR. Impaired transit and tolerance of intestinal gas in the irritable bowel syndrome. Gut 2001; 48:14–19.
22. Serra J, Salvioli B, Azpiroz F, et al. Lipid-induced intestinal gas retention in irritable bowel syndrome. Gastroenterology 2002; 123:700–706.
23. Caldarella MP, Serra J, Azpiroz F, et al. Prokinetic effects in patients with intestinal gas retention. Gastroenterology 2002; 122:1748–1755.
24. Hebden JM, Blackshaw E, D'Amato M, et al. Abnormalities of GI transit in bloated irritable bowel syndrome: effect of bran on transit and symptoms. Am J Gastroenterol 2002; 97:2315–2320.
25. Lin HC. Small intestinal bacterial overgrowth: a framework for understanding irritable bowel syndrome. JAMA 2004; 292:852–858.
26. Pimentel M, Chow EJ, Lin HC. Eradication of small intestinal bacterial overgrowth reduces symptoms of irritable bowel syndrome. Am J Gastroenterol 2000; 95:3503–3506.
27. Pimentel M, Chow EJ, Lin HC. Normalization of lactulose breath testing correlates with symptom improvement in irritable bowel syndrome: a double-blind, randomized, placebo-controlled study. Am J Gastroenterol 2003; 98:412–419.
28. Pimentel M, Soffer EE, Chow EJ, et al. Lower frequency of MMC is found in IBS subjects with abnormal breath test, suggesting bacterial overgrowth. Dig Dis Sci 2002; 47:2639–2643.
29. Pimentel M, Mayer AG, Park S, et al. Methane production during lactulose breath test is associated with gastrointestinal disease presentation. Dig Dis Sci 2003; 48:86–92.
30. Pimentel M, Kong Y, Park S. IBS subjects with methane on lactulose breath test have lower postprandial serotonin levels than subjects with hydrogen. Dig Dis Sci 2004; 49:84–87.
31. Bassotti G, Chistolini F, Marinozzi G, et al. Abnormal colonic propagated activity in patients with slow-transit constipation and constipation-predominant irritable bowel syndrome. Digestion 2003; 68:178–183.
32. Cremonini F, Talley NJ. Treatments targeting putative mechanisms in irritable bowel syndrome Nat Clin Pract Gastroenterol Hepatol. 2005; 2:82–88.
33. Ritchie J. Pain from distention of the pelvic colon by inflating a balloon in the irritable colon syndrome. Gut 1973; 14:125–132.
34. Thompson WG, Creed F, Drossman DA, et al. Functional bowel disorders and functional abdominal pain. Gastroenterol Int 1992; 5:75–91.
35. Thompson WG, Longstreth GF, Drossman DA, et al. Functional bowel disorders and functional abdominal pain. Gut 1999; 45:43–47.
36. Accarino AM, Azpiroz F, Malagelada JR. Selective dysfunction of mechanosensitive intestinal afferents in irritable bowel syndrome. Gastroenterol 1995; 108:636–643.
37. Evans PR, Bennett EJ, Bak YT. Jejunal sensorimotor dysfunction in irritable bowel syndrome: clinical and psychosocial features. Gastroenterology 1996; 110:393–404.
38. Holtmann G, Goebell H, Talley NJ. Functional dyspepsia and irritable bowel syndrome: Is there a common pathophysiological basis?. Am J Gastroenterol 1997; 92:954–959.
39. Whitehead WE, Holtkotter B, Enck P. Tolerance for rectosigmoid distention in irritable bowel syndrome. Gastroenterol 1990; 98:1187–1192.
40. Naliboff BD, Munakata J, Fullerton S. Evidence for two distinct perceptual alterations in irritable bowel syndrome. Gut 1997; 41:505–512.
41. Munakata J, Naliboff B, Harraf F. Repetitive sigmoid stimulation induces rectal hyperalgesia in patients with irritable bowel syndrome. Gastroenterology 1997; 112:55–63.
42. Mertz H, Naliboff B, Munakata J. Altered rectal perception is a biological marker of patients with irritable bowel syndrome. Gastroenterology 1995; 109:40–52.
43. Bouin M, Plourde V, Boivin M. Rectal distension testing in patients with irritable bowel syndrome: sensitivity, specificity, and predictive values of pain sensory thresholds. Gastroenterology 2002; 122:1771–1777.
44. Swarbrick ET, Hegarty JE, Bat L, et al. Site of pain from the irritable bowel syndrome. Lancet 1980; 2:443–446.
45. Verne GN, Robinson ME, Price DD. Hypersensitivity to visceral and cutaneous pain in the irritable bowel syndrome. Pain 2001; 93:7–14.
46. Mayer EA, Gebhart GF. Basic and clinical aspects of visceral hyperalgesia. Gastroenterol 1994; 107:271–293.
47. Cook IJ, Van Eeden A, Collins SM. Patients with irritable bowel syndrome have greater pain tolerance than normal subjects. Gastroenterology 1987; 93:727–733.
48. Zighelboim J, Talley NJ, Phillips SF, et al. Visceral perception in irritable bowel syndrome. Dig Dis Sci 1995; 40:819–827.
49. Chang L, Mayer EA, FitzGerald L, et al. Differences in somatic perception in patients with irritable bowel syndrome with and without fibromyalgia. Pain 2000; 84:297–307.
50. Poitras P, Poitras M, Plourde V, Boivin M, Verrier P. Evolution of visceral sensitivity in patients with irritable bowel syndrome. Dig Dis Sci 2002; 47:914–920.
51. Chey WY, Jin HO, Lee MH, et al. Colonic motility abnormality in patients with irritable bowel syndrome exhibiting abdominal pain and diarrhea. Am J Gastroenterol 2001; 96:1499–1506.
52. Coffin B, Azpiroz F, Guarner F, et al. Selective gastric hypersensitivity and reflex hyporeactivity in functional dyspepsia. Gastroenterology 1994; 107:1345–1351.

53. Trimble KC, Farouk R, Pryde A, et al. Heightened visceral sensation in functional gastrointestinal disease is not site-specific: evidence for a generalized disorder of gut sensitivity. Dig Dis Sci 1995; 40:1607–1613.
54. Qin C, Malykhina AP, Akbarali HI, Foreman RD. Cross-organ sensitization of lumbosacral spinal neurons receiving urinary bladder input in rats with inflamed colon. Gastroenterology 2005; 129:1967–1978.
55. Pezzone MA, Liang R, Farser MO. A model of neural cross-talk and irritation in the pelvis (implications for the overlap of chronic pelvic pain disorders). Gastroenterology 2005; 128:1953–1964.
56. Schwetz I, Bradesi S, Mayer EA. The pathophysiology of irritable bowel syndrome. Minerva Med 2004; 95:419–426.
57. Silverman DHS, Munakata JA, Ennes H, et al. Regional cerebral activity in normal and pathological perception of visceral pain. Gastroenterol 1997; 112:64–72.
58. Mertz H, Morgan V, Tanner G, et al. Regional cerebral activation in irritable bowel syndrome with painful and nonpainful stimuli. Gastroenterol 2000; 118:842–888.
59. Naliboff BD, Derbyshire SWG, Munakata J, et al. Cerebral activation in irritable bowel syndrome patients and control subjects during rectosigmoid stimulation. Psychosom Med 2001; 63:365–375.
60. Chang L. Brain Responses to visceral and somatic stimuli in irritable bowel syndrome: a central nervous system disorder? Gastroenterol Clin N Am 2005; 34:271–279.
61. Naliboff BD, Mayer EA. Brain imaging in IBS: drawing the line between cognitive and non-cognitive processes. Gastroenterology 2006; 130:267–270.
62. Verne GN, Himes NC, Robinson ME, et al. Central representation of visceral and cutaneous hypersensitivity in the irritable bowel syndrome. Pain 2003; 103:99–110.
63. Lawal A, Kern M, Sidhu H, et al. Novel evidence for hypersensitivity of visceral sensory neural circuitry in irritable bowel syndrome patients. Gastroenterology 2006; 130:26–33.
64. Hiatt RB, Katz L. Mast cells in inflammatory conditions of the gastrointestinal tract. Am J Gastroenterol 1962; 37:541–555.
65. Salzmann JL, Peltier-Koch F, Bloch F, et al. Morphometric study of colonic biopsies: a new method of estimating inflammatory diseases. Laboratory Invest 1989; 60:847–851.
66. Weston AP, Biddle WL, Bhatia PS, et al. Terminal ileal mucosal mast cells in irritable bowel syndrome. Dig Dis Sci 1993; 38:1590–1595.
67. Gwee KA, Leong YL, Graham C, et al. The role of psychological and biological factors in postinfective gut dysfunction. Gut 1999; 44:400–406.
68. O'Sullivan M, Clayton N, Breslin NP, et al. Increased mast cells in the irritable bowel syndrome. Neurogastroenterol Motil 2000; 12:449–457.
69. Spiller RC, Jenkins D, Thornley JP, et al. Increased rectal mucosal enteroendocrine cells, T lymphocytes, and increased gut permeability following acute Campylobacter enteritis and in post-dysenteric irritable bowel syndrome. Gut 2000; 47:804–811.
70. Chadwick VS, Chen W, Shu D, et al. Activation of the mucosal immune system in irritable bowel syndrome. Gastroenterol 2002; 122:1778–1783.
71. Tornblom H, Lindberg G, Nyberg B, et al. Full-thickness biopsy of the jejunum reveals inflammation and enteric neuropathy in irritable bowel syndrome. Gastroenterology 2002; 123:1972–1979.
72. Dunlop SP, Jenkins D, Spiller RC. Distinctive clinical, psychological, and histological features of postinfective irritable bowel syndrome. Am J Gastroenterol 2003; 98:1578–1583.
73. Dunlop SP, Jenkins D, Neal KR, et al. Relative importance of enterochromaffin cell hyperplasia, anxiety, and depression in postinfectious IBS. Gastroenterol 2003; 125:1651–1659.
74. Barbara G, Stanghellini V, De Giorgio R, et al. Activated mast cells in proximity to colonic nerves correlate with abdominal pain in irritable bowel syndrome. Gastroenterol 2004; 126:693–702.
75. Barbara G, De Giorgio R, Stanghellini V, et al. New Pathophysiological mechanisms in irritable bowel syndrome. Aliment Pharmacol Ther 2004; 20:(suppl 2):1–9.
76. Tibble JA, Sigthorsson G, Foster R, et al. Use of surrogate markers of inflammation and Rome criteria to distinguish organic from nonorganic intestinal disease. Gastroenterol 2002; 123:450–460.
77. Dunlop SP, Jenkins D, Neal KR, et al. Randomized, doubleblind, placebo-controlled trial of prednisolone in postinfectious irritable bowel syndrome. Aliment Pharmacol Ther 2003; 18:77–84.
78. Hansen MB. Neurohumoral control of gastrointestinal motility. Physiol Res 2003; 52:1–30.
79. Sugiuar T, Bielefeldt K, Gebhart GF. TRPV1 function in mouse colon sensory neurons is enhanced by metabotropic 5-hydroxytryptamine receptor activation. J Neurosci 2004; 24:9521–9530.
80. Crowell, MD. Role of serotonin in the pathophysiology of the irritable bowel syndrome. Br J Pharmacol 2004; 141:1285–1293.
81. Kyosola K, Penttila O, Salaspuro M. Rectal mucosal adrenergic innervation and enterochromaffin cells in ulcerative colitis and irritable colon. Scand J Gastroenterol 1977; 12:363–367.
82. Bearcroft CP, Perrett D, Farthing MJ. Postprandial plasma 5-hydroxytryptamine in diarrhoea predominant irritable bowel syndrome: a pilot study. Gut 1998; 42:42–46.
83. El Salhy M, Norrgard O, Spinnell S. Abnormal colonic endocrine cells in patients with chronic idiopathic slow-transit constipation. Scand J Gastroenterol 1999; 34:1007–1011.
84. Miwa J, Echizen H, Matsueda K, et al. Patients with constipation-predominant irritable bowel syndrome (IBS) may have elevated serotonin concentrations in colonic mucosa as compared with diarrhea-predominant patients and subjects with normal bowel habits. Digestion 2001; 63:188–194.

85. Houghton LA, Atkinson W, Whitaker RP, et al. Increased platelet depleted plasma 5-hydroxytryptamine concentration following meal ingestion in symptomatic female subjects with diarrhoea predominant irritable bowel syndrome. Gut 2003; 52:663–670.

86. Coates MD, Mahoney CR, Linden DR, et al. Molecular defects in mucosal serotonin content and decreased serotonin reuptake transporter in ulcerative colitis and IBS. Gastroenterology 2004; 126:1657–1664.

87. Barbara G, Vallance BA, Collins SM. Persistent intestinal neuromuscular dysfunction after acute nematode infection in mice. Gastroenterol 1997; 113:1224–1232.

88. Coelho AM, Fioramonti J, Bueno L. Mast cell degranulation induces delayed rectal allodynia in rats: role of histamine and 5-HT. Dig Dis Sci 1998; 43:727–737.

89. La JH, Kim TW, Sung TS, et al. Role of mucosal mast cells in visceral hypersensitivity in a rat model of irritable bowel syndrome. J Vet Sci 2004; 5:319–324.

90. Park CH, Joo YE, Choi SK, et al. Activated mast cells infiltrate in close proximity to enteric nerves in diarrhea-predominant irritable bowel syndrome. J Korean Med Sci 2003; 2:204–210.

91. Fu LW, Pan HL, Longhurst JC. Endogenous histamine stimulate isochemically sensitive abdominal visceral afferents through H1 receptors. Am J Physiol 1997; 273:H2726–H2737.

92. Coelho AM, Vergnolle N, Guiard B, et al. Proteinases and proteinase-activated receptor 2: a possible role to promote visceral hyperalgesia in rats. Gastroenterol 2002; 122:1035–1047.

93. Hoogerwerf WA, Zou L, Shenoy M, et al. The proteinase-activated receptor 2 is involved in nociception. J Neuroscience 2001; 21:9036–9042.

94. Amadesi S, Nie J, Vergnolle N, et al. Protease-activated receptor 2 sensitizes the capsaicin receptor transient receptor potential vanilloid receptor 1 to induce hyperalgesia. J Neuroscience 2004; 24:4300–4312.

95. Shu XQ, Mendell LM. Neurotrophins and hyperalgesia. Proc Natl Acad Sci U S A 1999; 96: 7693–7696.

96. Zhang YH, Nicol GD. NGF-mediated sensitization of the excitability of rat sensory neurons is prevented by a blocking antibody to the p75 neurotrophin receptor. Neurosci Lett. 2004; 366: 187–192.

97. Skaper SD, Pollock M, Facci L. Mast cells differentially express and release active high molecular weight neurotrophins. Brain Res Mol Brain Res 2001; 97:177–185.

98. Theodosiou M, Rush RA, Zhou XF, et al. Hyperalgesia due to nerve damage: role of nerve growth factor. Pain 1999; 81:245–255.

99. Florenzano F, Bentivoglio M. Degranulation, density, and distribution of mast cells in the rat thalamus: a light and electron microscopic study in basal conditions and after intracerebroventricular administration of nerve growth factor. J Comp Neurol 2000; 424:651–669.

100. Chan CLH, Facer P, Davis JB, et al. Sensory fibres expressing capsaicin receptor TRPV1 in patients with rectal hypersensitivity and faecal urgency. Lancet 2003; 361:385–391.

101. Gonsalkorale WM, Perrey C, Pravica V, et al. Interleukin 10 genotypes in irritable bowel syndrome: evidence for an inflammatory component? Gut 2003; 52:91–93.

102. van der Veek P, de Kroon Y, Verspaget H, et al. Tumor necrosis factor alpha and interleukin 10 gene polymorphisms in irritable bowel syndrome. Gastroenterol 2004; 126:A53.

103. Holtmann G, Siffert W, Haag S, et al. G-protein beta 3 subunit 825 CC genotype is associated with unexplained (functional) dyspepsia. Gastroenterology 2004; 126:971–979.

104. Kim HJ, Camilleri M, Carlson PJ, et al. Association of distinct alpha(2) adrenoceptor and serotonin transporter polymorphisms with constipation and somatic symptoms in functional gastrointestinal disorders. Gut 2004; 53:829–837.

105. Fuller RW, Wong DT. Serotonin uptake and serotonin uptake inhibition. Ann N Y Acad Sci 1990; 600:68–80.

106. Iversen L. Neurotransmitter transporters: fruitful targets for CNS drug discovery. Mol Psychiatry 2000; 5:357–362.

107. Pata C, Erdal ME, Derici E, et al. Serotonin transporter gene polymorphism in irritable bowel syndrome. Am J Gastroenterol 2002; 97:1780–1784.

108. Lee DY, Park H, Kim WH, et al. Serotonin transporter gene polymorphism in healthy adults and patients with irritable bowel syndrome. Korean J Gastroenterol 2004; 43:18–22.

109. Yeo A, Boyd P, Lumsden S, et al. Association between a functional polymorphism in the serotonin transporter gene and diarrhoea predominant irritable bowel syndrome in women. Gut 2004; 53:1452–1458.

110. Whorwell PJ, McCallum M, Creed FH, et al. Non-colonic features of irritable bowel syndrome. Gut 1986; 27:37–40.

111. Locke GR III, Zinsmeister AR, Talley NJ, et al. Familial association in adults with functional gastrointestinal disorders. Mayo Clin Proc 2000; 75:907–912.

112. Morris-Yates A, Talley NJ, Boyce PM, et al. Evidence of a genetic contribution to functional bowel disorder. Am J Gastroenterol 1998; 93:1311–1317.

113. Levy RL, Jones KR, Whitehead WE, et al. Irritable bowel syndrome in twins: hereditary and social learning both contribute to etiology. Gastroenterol 2001; 121:799–804.

114. Mohammed I, Cherkas L, Riley SA, et al. Genetic influence in irritable bowel syndrome: a twin study. Gut 2002; 50:A1.

115. Al-Chaer ED, Kawasaki M, Pasricha PJ. A new model of chronic visceral hypersensitivity in adult rats induced by colon irritation during postnatal development. Gastroenterol 2000; 119: 1276–1285.
116. Chaudhary NA, Truelove SC. The irritable colon syndrome: a study of the clinical features, predisposing causes, and prognosis in 130 cases. Q J Med 1962; 123:307–322.
117. McKendrick MW, Read MW. Irritable bowel syndrome-post salmonella infection. J Infect 1994; 29:1–3.
118. Gwee KA, Graham JC, McKendrick MW, et al. Psychometric scores and persistence of irritable bowel after infectious diarrhea. Lancet 1996; 347:150–153.
119. Neal KR, Hebden J, Spiller R. Prevalence of gastrointestinal symptoms six months after bacterial gastroenteritis and risk factors for the development of the irritable bowel syndrome: postal survey of patients. BMJ 1997; 314:779–782.
120. Rodriguez LA, Ruigomez A. Increased risk of irritable bowel syndrome after bacterial gastroenteritis: cohort study. BMJ 1999; 318:565–566.
121. Parry SD, Stansfield R, Jelley D, et al. Does bacterial gastroenteritis predispose people to functional gastrointestinal disorders? A prospective, community-based, case-control study. Am J Gastroenterol 2003; 98:1970–1975.
122. Spiller RC. Neuropathology of IBS? Gastroenterol 2002; 123:2144–2147.
123. Gwee KA, Collins SM, Read NW, et al. Increased rectal mucosal expression of interleukin 1beta in recently acquired postinfectious irritable bowel syndrome. Gut 2003; 52:523–526.
124. Wang LH, Fang XC, Pan GZ. Bacillary dysentery as a causative factor of irritable bowel syndrome and its pathogenesis. Gut 2004; 53:1096–1101.
125. Black PH. Stress and the inflammatory response: a review of neurogenic inflammation. Brain Behav Immun 2002; 16:622–653.
126. Wheatcroft J, Wakelin D, Smith A, Mahoney CR, Mawe G, Spiller R. Enterochromaffin cell hyperplasia and decreased serotonin transporter in a mouse model of postinfectious bowel dysfunction. Neurogastroenterol Motil 2005; 17:863–870.
127. Mayer EA. The neurobiology of stress and gastrointestinal disease. Gut 2000; 47:861–869.
128. Mayer EA, Naliboff BD, Chang L, et al. Stress and the gastrointestinal tract: V. stress and irritable bowel syndrome. Am J Physiol Gastrointest Liver Physiol 2001; 280:G519–G524.
129. Tache Y, Millioni M, Nelsono AG, et al. Role of corticotropin-releasing factor pathways in stress-related alterations of colonic motor function and viscerosensibility in female rodents. Gend Med 2005; 2:146–154.

Irritable Bowel Syndrome and Functional Abdominal Pain Syndromes: Clinical Features and Management

Lin Chang
Center for Neurovisceral Sciences and Women's Health, Division of Digestive Diseases, Department of Medicine, David Geffen School of Medicine at UCLA, and VA, Greater Los Angeles Healthcare System, Los Angeles, California, U.S.A.

Lucinda Harris
Division of Gastroenterology and Hepatology, Mayo Clinic, Scottsdale, Arizona, U.S.A.

INTRODUCTION

Functional gastrointestinal disorders (FGIDs) are very common and are estimated to account for up to 40% of diagnoses made by gastroenterologists (1). One of the main consistent symptoms among FGIDs is the presence of abdominal pain and/or discomfort. The most common FGID is irritable bowel syndrome (IBS), which is found in 10% to 20% of the population and is characterized by the presence of abdominal pain and/or discomfort associated with altered bowel habits (2). Another FGID, which presents with chronic abdominal pain and may be confused with IBS, is functional abdominal pain syndrome (FAPS) (3). One of the main differences between IBS and FAPS is that abdominal pain does not have to be associated with changes in bowel habits in FAPS, e.g., diarrhea and/or constipation, as it does in IBS. In this chapter, IBS and FAPS will be discussed in terms of their epidemiology, diagnosis, and treatment. However, because there are many more studies conducted in IBS than in FAPS, and IBS is much more common than FAPS, IBS will be discussed in greater depth.

IRRITABLE BOWEL SYNDROME
Epidemiology

IBS has worldwide prevalence rates of 9% to 23% in the general population (4) and accounts for 12% of diagnoses made by primary care physicians and 36% of diagnoses made by gastro-enterologists (5). IBS patients may present with diarrhea and/or constipation and, therefore, are often subgrouped by predominant bowel habit. These subgroups are referred to as diarrhea-predominant IBS (IBS-D), constipation-predominant IBS (IBS-C), and IBS associated with alternating diarrhea and constipation (IBS-A). Some studies have reported a higher prevalence of IBS in the young and a decrease in prevalence with age (6),(7), but another study did not find age to have an impact on prevalence (8). IBS symptom severity can range from mild and intermittent to severe and continuous. Recent data suggest that severity is a multidimensional concept that is not fully explained by intensity of symptoms and has important clinical implications including diagnosis, treatment, health-care utilization, and health-related quality of life (HRQoL). While there are no current consensus criteria for symptom severity in IBS, studies have used various measurement scales and have reported the prevalence of severe or very severe IBS to be higher than previously estimated with a range from 3% to 69% (9).

This condition appears to have a female predominance, but the female-to-male ratio is higher in the health-seeking patient population than in the community. A female-to-male ratio of 1–2:1 has been reported in population studies, while a higher ratio of 2–4:1 has been demonstrated in clinic settings (10–12). It is well established that a greater number of women seek health-care services for symptoms of IBS than men. In addition, there appears to be a female predominance in greater symptom severity, particularly gastrointestinal (GI) and extraintestinal symptoms, in IBS patients. Two studies have reported increased symptom severity in women with IBS compared to men with IBS surveyed in the outpatient clinic population (13,14). While one study found that men and women with IBS similarly reported pain-related symptoms (15), there have been other studies, which found that nausea, bloating, constipation, and extraintestinal symptoms (e.g., urinary urgency and muscle stiffness) were more prevalent in women with IBS than in men (13,16,17). Furthermore, recent clinical trials suggest that gender differences in response to pharmacological treatments also occur (18–21).

There are likely many factors that influence these gender differences in clinical presentation and physiologic responses in IBS and include biological, hormonal, behavioral, psychological, and sociocultural differences between men and women (10). Several studies indicate that the menstrual cycle influences GI symptoms, which are reportedly increased immediately before and during menses (22–24). In addition, brain imaging studies have reported gender differences in the central processing of aversive information originating from pelvic viscera in IBS (25). Further studies are needed to provide additional insight into gender differences in the epidemiology, pathophysiology, symptom expression, and response to treatment in IBS.

A large proportion of patients with IBS or other functional bowel disorders have concurrent psychological disturbances, particularly those with severe symptoms or those seen in tertiary care referral centers. In tertiary care centers, the prevalence of psychiatric disorders in IBS patients ranges from 40% to 90% (4). Psychosocial factors have been recognized to modify the illness experience and influence health-care utilization and treatment outcome. Factors that adversely affect health status and clinical outcome include a history of emotional, sexual, or physical abuse, stressful life events, chronic social stress, anxiety disorders, or maladaptive coping styles. Studies have demonstrated that IBS patients report a higher prevalence of sexual, physical, and emotional abuse compared to healthy individuals (26,27). In addition, patients with FGID report a higher prevalence of severe abuse (i.e., life-threatening or sexual penetration) compared to those with organic GI conditions (28).

Studies have demonstrated elevated health-care costs of IBS patients compared to non-IBS patients with indirect and direct annual costs, estimated to be a total of up to 30 billion dollars (29,30). Three recently published studies, two performed in health maintenance organizations (31,32) and one in two different Medicaid populations (33), found that the total costs for health care were approximately 50% higher in patients with IBS compared to those for non-IBS controls. These studies similarly found that health-care costs were increased particularly with regard to outpatient rather than inpatient services (32–34). Two other studies measured the prevalence of surgeries in IBS patients and found an increased prevalence of cholecystectomy and hysterectomy in population and referral settings (35) and higher rates of cholecystectomy, appendectomy, hysterectomy, and back surgery compared to non-IBS controls in a HMO setting (36).

The high prevalence of extraintestinal symptoms in IBS, such as fatigue, somatic pain, sleep, and sexual disturbances (37), has clinical relevance with regard to health-care costs and utilization. One study found that the majority of excess total health-care costs were due to non–lower GI-related services (31). This finding is supported by the increased physician visits by IBS patients not only for GI symptoms, but also for non-IBS related reasons (6). IBS patients are twice as likely as comparison groups to be diagnosed with a non-GI chronic pain disorder (37). These non-GI chronic disorders include fibromyalgia, chronic fatigue syndrome, chronic pelvic pain, and interstitial cystitis (38,39). In particular, fibromyalgia and IBS share many clinical and physiological features suggesting that there may be shared pathophysiological mechanisms (37,40,41). Although the pathophysiology of IBS and fibromyalgia are incompletely understood, several observations suggest that a similar pathophysiological model integrating neurobiological, behavioral, and psychological factors is operative in both (42,43).

Several studies have demonstrated reductions in HRQoL measures as well as general well-being in patients with IBS with moderate-to-severe symptoms relative to healthy controls, particularly those seen in referral settings. In addition, HRQoL has been found to be lower than those with gastroesophageal reflux disease and asthma (44), and similar (and lower in some domains) compared to other chronic illnesses such as diabetes mellitus or end-stage renal disease (45). Spiegel et al. recently evaluated determinants that predicted both mental and physical components of HRQoL in IBS patients recruited from both advertisement and a tertiary referral clinic at a university-based center (46). Both physical and mental HRQoL shared an association with symptoms of chronic stress (lack of energy and tiredness), and neither was determined by traditionally elicited GI symptoms, including stool frequency, stool characteristics, or IBS bowel habit subtype. However, the IBS symptom-specific factors that affected HRQoL (the physical and not mental composite score) were severe, predominantly painful, and flares greater than 24 hours. The literature also suggests that HRQoL can be improved with effective treatments for IBS (47). Based on these findings, a recent American College of Gastroenterology (ACG) guideline suggests routine HRQoL screening in patients with IBS and recommends initiating treatment when the symptoms of IBS are found to reduce functional status and diminish overall HRQoL (48).

Diagnosis

A thorough medical history and physical examination are essential to make a proper diagnosis of IBS. The diagnosis is based on the Rome II symptom criteria for IBS (Table 1) (49). These criteria require the presence of chronic or recurrent abdominal pain and/or discomfort associated with altered bowel habits. The approach to diagnosing IBS is to identify the dominant symptom complex and then eliminate "red flag" signs and symptoms that may indicate an organic disorder and not IBS. Organic conditions, which may present with IBS-like symptoms include colon cancer, inflammatory bowel disease, malabsorption disorders (e.g., celiac sprue), endocrine disorders (e.g., thyroid disease), and medication-related side effects. When "alarm signs" such as weight loss, fever, anemia, GI bleeding, family history of colon cancer, or onset of disease late in life are excluded, the Rome criteria reach a sensitivity of 65%, specificity of 100%, and a positive predictive value of 100%. Vanner et al. found that 93% of patients diagnosed based on Rome I criteria, and the absence of red flags were found to be true-positive cases after two years (50). Hence, if the diagnosis of IBS is made properly, the risk of missing organic disease is low, and most patients have no change in diagnosis after initial evaluation (51–53).

Recent guidelines by the American Gastroenterological Association have advocated the following diagnostic tests be considered: (i) complete blood count, (ii) thyroid-stimulating

Table 1 Rome II Diagnostic Criteria for Irritable Bowel Syndrome

At least 12 wk or more, which need not be consecutive, in the preceding 12 mo of abdominal discomfort or pain that has 2 out of 3 features
Relieved with defecation; *and/or*
Onset associated with a change in frequency of stool; *and/or*
Onset associated with a change in form (appearance) of stool
Supportive symptoms (present at least 25% of the time)
Abnormal stool form
Passage of mucus
Bloating or distention
Abnormal stool passage (feeling of strain, urgency, or feeling of incomplete evacuation)
Altered stool frequency (>3 bowel movements/wk or <3 bowel movements/day)

Source: Frome Ref. 54.

hormone, (iii) complete metabolic profile, (iv) erythrocyte sedimentation rate or C-reactive protein, (v) stool for ova and parasites, (vi) fecal occult blood testing, (vii) stool culture examination, and (viii) celiac sprue panel (4). Other diagnostic tests including barium enema, flexible sigmoidoscopy or colonoscopy as well as hydrogen breath tests for bacterial overgrowth can be considered on an individualized basis. However, it is important that in the medical evaluation of patients with IBS symptoms that practitioners take an evidence-based medicine approach. The decision to perform many of the tests mentioned above must be made with a certain amount of discrimination. Evidence from studies of reasonably good quality has suggested that the diagnostic yield is not very high particularly in the absence of alarm signs. In fact, for many, the yield of the tests is less than 2% (55). The presence of "red flag" symptoms would suggest a higher pretest probability of the presence of an organic disorder. Performing colonoscopy has resulted in identifying organic disease in only 1% to 2% of cases in patients with IBS-like symptoms (55). However, it has been recommended by the ACG that patients ≥ 50 years of age should undergo a routine colon examination (e.g., colonoscopy or barium enema with a flexible sigmoidoscopy) for screening purposes similar to the general healthy population (48). The threshold is lowered to 40 years of age, if there is a significant family history of colon cancer.

Two medical conditions, which have a relatively high pretest probability in IBS patients, are lactose intolerance and celiac sprue. In the case of lactose intolerance, the prevalence is approximately 22% to 26% and is similar to that of the general population, which is 25% (55). In fact, documentation of lactase deficiency seldom leads to improvement in IBS symptoms (56). Furthermore, up to one-third of patients with reported lactose intolerance actually absorbs lactose normally (57), and some people with lactose malabsorption may consume moderate quantities of lactose without symptoms (e.g., 12.5 g/day) (58).

The prevalence of celiac sprue in patients with IBS-like symptoms ranges from 0% to 11.4% (59–63). A study done in the United Kingdom demonstrated a sevenfold increase in occurrence of celiac disease in patients suspected of having IBS that were seen in a gastroenterology practice (59). In general, the studies reporting a relatively higher prevalence of celiac sprue were performed in a GI specialty setting (59,63), while the other studies with the lower prevalence rates evaluated primary care patients (60–62) who probably had less severe GI symptoms. Cash et al. (55) found that the pretest probability for the presence of celiac disease in patients with IBS symptoms was significantly higher than that found in the general population (4.67% vs. 0.25–0.5%). Therefore, screening with celiac sprue–associated antibodies (e.g., antiendomysial antibody and antitissue transglutaminase) may be indicated. Additionally 5% to 7% of patients with celiac disease are immunoglobulin A (IgA) -deficient and, therefore, the clinician may want also to measure IgA levels. A recent study by Spiegel et al. used decision analysis to determine if initial testing for celiac sprue might be a cost-effective diagnostic strategy in IBS compared to empirical IBS treatment (64). Testing for celiac sprue in patients with IBS has an acceptable cost when the prevalence of celiac sprue is above 1% and is the dominant strategy when the prevalence exceeds 8%. The decision to test should be based upon a consideration of the population prevalence of underlying celiac sprue, the operating characteristics of the screening test employed, and the cost of proposed therapy for IBS (64).

Another condition to consider excluding in a patient with IBS symptoms is bacterial overgrowth. It has recently been proposed that many IBS patients have symptoms due to the presence of small intestinal bacterial overgrowth (SIBO) measured by the lactulose breath test, which had been detected in up to 78% to 84% of patients (65,66). There has been considerable debate regarding the accuracy of the lactulose breath test compared to small bowel aspirates for bacteria, which has been considered the gold standard for SIBO (67). Other institutions have found much lower prevalence of SIBO in patients presenting with IBS-like symptoms using the different diagnostic tests, e.g., lactulose hydrogen breath test, glucose hydrogen breath test, and small bowel aspirates for bacteria. The prevalence of SIBO in these patients appears to vary widely depending on the patient population and type of methodology used. Treatment of SIBO in patients with symptoms of IBS is discussed below.

Treatment

The foundation of successful treatment is the establishment of a good physician–patient relationship. Addressing the patient health concerns about their symptoms and providing reassurance and education about IBS are important (4). While patients need to be informed that this disorder may be associated with increased morbidity (i.e., impact on HRQoL), it is not associated with increased mortality and does not lead to more serious disorders such as cancer or inflammatory bowel disease. In patients with more severe and complex symptoms, a multidisciplinary approach including pharmacotherapy and psychosocial intervention should be considered.

Dietary Factors

A dietary history and a two-week symptom diary may help determine if significant correlations exist between diet, daily activities, emotional factors, and the symptoms of IBS. Meal-induced symptoms are common. Careful analysis of potential food triggers can be aided by a one- to two-week food and symptom diary. While most patients cannot completely control symptoms through diet alterations alone, diet-related exacerbations may be minimized. Common food triggers include high fat foods, raw fruits and vegetables, and caffeinated beverages. Certain intolerances to lactose, fructose, and sorbitol may play a role in symptoms, and decreases in these dietary substances may help with diarrhea and bloating. Recent evidence by Atkinson et al. supports the involvement of dietary antigens in symptom production (68). This study showed that removing foods from the diet for which patients had specific immunoglobulin G (IgG) antibodies reduced the IBS symptom severity score by 10% to 26%, compared to a sham diet. Wheat, milk, yeast, egg, and cashew nuts were the most commonly eliminated foods. The patients who were highly compliant with the true diet had a greater reduction in symptom severity than those who were not, but unfortunately many patients were not able to be highly compliant during the course of the study. Patients with constipation-predominant symptoms may benefit from an increase of 20 to 25 g of fiber per day. Exercise, adequate sleep, and stress reduction may also help to modulate symptoms of IBS.

Traditional IBS Treatment

While some therapeutic agents may benefit patients regardless of their bowel habit subtype, others are specifically indicated for a certain IBS bowel habit subtype due to their facilitatory or inhibitory effects on GI function, e.g., motility and secretion. Traditional pharmacologic agents for the treatment of IBS include bulking agents, antispasmodics, tricyclic antidepressants (TCAs) and other psychotropic agents, and laxatives. Several excellent systematic reviews evaluating controlled treatment trials for IBS have been performed (69–71). The ACG Functional GI Disorders Task Force evaluated many of the available treatments in terms of the evidence available to support their use and their ability to alleviate the symptoms of IBS (71). Therapies were given a grade of A, B, or C depending on the level of evidence available to support their use. Four levels of evidence were identified: (i) level I data was based on high-quality, randomized, placebo-controlled studies (Grade A), (ii) level II data was based on intermediate quality randomized, controlled trials (Grade B), (iii) level III data was based on nonrandomized studies (Grade C), and (iv) level IV data was based on case controls or anecdotal experience (Grade C). The therapies based on the highest quality of data were given a grade A recommendation. Unfortunately, the majority of therapies studied, including antispasmodic agents, bulking agents and fiber supplementation, antidiarrheal agents such as loperamide and TCAs, and behavioral therapy were not shown to be more effective than placebo in treating the *global* symptoms of IBS and, therefore, were given a grade B recommendation. However, most of these treatment options may relieve *individual* symptoms of IBS and, therefore, they may be useful in select patients depending on their predominant symptom. Antispasmodic agents are commonly prescribed to treat abdominal pain (70), but may cause side effects such as dry mouth, blurred vision, and urinary retention. Fiber supplementation may help relieve constipation by improving ease of stool passage and stool form, but can cause bloating and abdominal cramps. Although antidiarrheal agents may not improve abdominal pain, they help decrease stool frequency and improve stool consistency. Dosing should be adjusted to avoid constipation. TCAs are prescribed for the treatment of several chronic pain disorders. These agents have been shown to be effective when used at low doses for the treatment of abdominal pain via their visceral analgesic effects in patients with FGIDs. Higher doses are used when treating comorbid affective symptoms such as depression and anxiety. However, since this review, there has been a recently published study by Drossman et al. which demonstrated the efficacy of the TCA, desipramine, in treating moderate-to-severe functional bowel disorders in a large, randomized, 12-week placebo-controlled trial (72). This is discussed in greater detail below.

Serotonergic Agents

The regulation of peristalsis and secretion within the gut is primarily under the control of the enteric nervous system, although gut function is also significantly influenced by extrinsic neural input from the parasympathetic and sympathetic nervous systems. Many neuropeptides are involved in the regulation of motility, sensation, and secretion. A key mediator of both of these functions is serotonin (73,74), 95% of which is in the gut. The discovery of serotonergic molecular targets has led to the development of novel medications and review of older pharmacologic agents that also act on the serotonin system. Thus far, two drugs have been given Grade A recommendations because they were studied in high-quality, multicenter clinical trials. Each of these therapies targets different serotonergic receptors and, therefore, different aspects of bowel function.

5-HT$_3$ Receptor Antagonists

The first clinically available 5-HT$_3$ antagonists were ondansetron and granisetron, which were approved for the treatment of chemotherapy- and radiotherapy-induced nausea and vomiting. Alosetron is the only medication currently approved in the United States for the treatment of women with severe IBS-D. Alosetron is a very potent 5-HT$_3$ antagonist that can slow colonic transit, particularly in the left colon (75). It also decreases chloride and water secretion and seems to affect mechanoelastic properties of the colon by increasing colonic compliance (76). There have been multiple clinical trials in almost 2500 patients comparing the drug to placebo (18,77–80) and one trial comparing alosetron to a smooth muscle relaxant, mebeverine (81). All studies found that alosetron effectively relieved IBS symptoms, including decreasing abdominal pain, urgency, and stool frequency and consistency. The therapeutic gain has ranged from 12% to 27%. These studies used adequate relief of abdominal pain and discomfort as their primary efficacy end point. Alosetron was also demonstrated to improve stool frequency, stool consistency, and urgency in women with nonconstipated IBS. While the pivotal phase III clinical studies on which the Food and Drug Administration (FDA) approval was established did not show efficacy in men (most likely due to small sample sizes of men), benefit in men with IBS has been recently reported, although the beneficial effect was not to the extent as seen in women (82). There is also a recently published study that demonstrated long-term efficacy of alosetron in women with severe IBS-D (83). Interestingly, the decrease in IBS symptoms seen with alosetron correlated with decreased activation of brain regions associated with central autonomic processing as measured by functional magnetic resonance imaging, indicating a central as well as a peripheral effect of the drug (84).

Alosetron is currently prescribed at a dose of 0.5 to 1.0 mg twice a day. The drug is metabolized via the cytochrome P-450 system and has a half-life of 6 to 10 hours. No clinically significant drug interactions are known, but it should be avoided in patients with severe hepatic and renal failure. Alosetron is currently under a restricted use program, requiring physician attestation, and patient and physician education, due to potentially serious adverse events reported after its initial FDA approval. These events included severe constipation, serious complications of constipation in 1 in 1000 (ileus, bowel obstruction, toxic megacolon, fecal impaction, and perforation), and ischemic colitis ($\leq$ 1 in 1000) (85). Seventy-four percent of these cases occurred during the first month of therapy. The medication is currently indicated for women with severe IBS-D who have chronic IBS symptoms that have been present for at least six months, for whom structural and biochemical abnormalities have been ruled out and who have failed to respond to conventional therapy. IBS is considered severe when there is at least one of the following features: (i) frequent bowel urgency or fecal incontinence, (ii) frequent and/or severe pain, and (iii) disability or restriction of daily activities due to IBS.

The efficacy of another 5-HT$_3$ antagonist, cilansetron, has been assessed in two large, randomized, placebo-controlled multicenter trials. These trials showed that cilansetron was efficacious in the treatment of both men and women with IBS-D (86,87). The dose was 2 mg three times a day. This medication has not yet been approved for use by the FDA and is therefore not currently available. Similar to alosetron, the chief side effect of cilansetron was constipation.

5-HT$_4$ Receptor Agonists

Tegaserod is a partial 5-HT$_4$ agonist that is currently available in the United States for women with IBS-C and in men and women less than 65 years of age with chronic constipation less than 65 years of age. Tegaserod exerts its effects by stimulating the peristaltic reflex and accelerating oral cecal transit (88). Tegaserod also increases intestinal chloride secretion, and by this mechanism increases fluid in the stool and improves stool consistency. The effect of tegaserod on visceral sensitivity in human experimental studies is less clear. Five large, multicenter, randomized, double-blind, placebo-controlled phase III clinical trials have evaluated the efficacy of tegaserod in IBS patients with constipation (19–21,89–91). A measure of global symptom relief was the primary efficacy end point, and individual GI symptoms such as abdominal pain, bloating, and stool frequency/consistency were the secondary efficacy end points. There were significantly greater responses on all of these outcome measures with tegaserod compared to placebo. The therapeutic gain of the global end point ranged from 5% to 19%. Tegaserod has a half-life of 11 ± 5 hours and is taken 30 minutes before breakfast and dinner for the best results. It has no significant drug–drug interactions. Dose adjustment is not needed in the elderly, and it is contraindicated in patients with severe renal or hepatic failure.

Tegaserod is a safe and well-tolerated medication. The two side effects, which occurred more often in patients taking tegaserod compared to placebo, were diarrhea and headache (92). Diarrhea often dissipates with continued use of the drug. There have been no reported associated electrocardiographic effects such as QT prolongation or cardiac arrhythmias with this medication. There is no evidence to suggest an increased incidence of ischemic colitis in patients taking tegaserod compared to the background incidence in the general population or an IBS population (93). There have been an insufficient number of male patients enrolled in clinical trials to assess the efficacy of this agent in the IBS patient population, although it has been shown to relieve constipation symptoms effectively in men as well as women with chronic constipation (i.e., without predominant pain as in IBS-C).

Combination 5-HT$_4$ Agonist and 5-HT$_3$ Antagonist

Renzapride is a combined 5-HT$_4$ agonist and 5-HT$_3$ antagonist, which has shown promise as a treatment for IBS in both men and women. In one study of renzapride in IBS-C patients (94), this medication was shown to increase the frequency of bowel movements and improve stool consistency, but there was no overall significant benefit in terms of relief of abdominal pain and discomfort. In another study, 48 patients with IBS-C, who did not have any evidence of pelvic outlet obstruction but did have normal or slow baseline colonic transit, were randomized in a double-blind, parallel-group, two-week study to renzapride at a dose of 1, 2, or 4 mg, or placebo (95). Renzapride was associated with acceleration of colonic transit and improvement in bowel function scores. Gastric emptying and small bowel transit were not affected by renzapride. In a clinical trial with patients with IBS-A, renzapride at doses of 1, 2, and 4 mg were given to 168 patients, of whom 78% were women (96). Satisfactory relief of overall IBS symptoms for the 2-mg dose was 57% compared with a placebo response of 43%, but this difference failed to reach statistical significance. Phase III clinical trials evaluating the efficacy of renzapride in IBS are currently ongoing.

Antidepressants

Both TCAs and selective serotonin reuptake inhibitors (SSRIs) have been used in the treatment of IBS. They likely exert their beneficial effects via several different actions. Firstly, they are effective agents in treating psychological symptoms such as depression, anxiety, and somatization, which affect many IBS patients (97), particularly those with more severe symptoms and who are seen in tertiary care referral centers. Secondly, these agents may have modulating effects either through local gut action (98) or through a centrally mediated action (99) that changes visceral or motor activity or both. Lastly is the fact that both drugs seem to have central modulating effects on pain. Low-dose TCAs (e.g., amitriptyline, desipramine, and nortriptyline at a starting dose of 10–25 mg at bedtime) are now frequently used in the treatment of IBS, particularly in patients with more severe or refractory symptoms, impaired daily function, and associated depression and anxiety. The temporal effects of TCAs on GI function precede those that relate to improvement in mood, which suggests that the therapeutic actions are unrelated to improvement in mental state. A recent systematic review found seven randomized, placebo-controlled trials evaluating the effect of TCAs in the treatment of IBS. It was found that none of these studies were of high quality due to relatively small sample sizes and that there were poorly defined primary and secondary end points (71). However, a recently published study by Drossman et al.(72), which is not included in the systematic review, evaluated the efficacy of the TCA, desipramine, in treating moderate-to-severe functional bowel disorders in a large, randomized, 12-week placebo-controlled trial. Patients taking desipramine were started on a dose of 50 mg/day and then increased in one week to 100 mg/day and then to 150 mg/day from week 3 to week 12 as tolerated. Desipramine was shown to have a statistically significant benefit over placebo in the per protocol analysis which included only those patients who completed treatment (responder rate 73% vs. 49%), but not in the intention-to-treat analysis. The lack of benefit in the intention-to-treat analysis may have been related to a substantial (28%) drop out primarily due to symptom side effects, thus attesting to the value of carefully monitoring dosage and helping the patient stay on the medication long enough to achieve a treatment response. Desipramine was found to be more effective in the subgroup of patients with less severe symptoms and a history of abuse.

The benefits of SSRIs in the treatment of IBS have not been well studied and their potential central and peripheral effects are less clear. A possible mechanism of SSRIs is through their central effects in reducing the vicious cycle of anxiety and pain. They may also have the peripheral effect of decreasing orocecal transit time, which is presumably the mechanism responsible for the side effect of diarrhea. However, the most beneficial effect of SSRIs appears to be improving overall well-being than specifically decreasing particular GI symptoms of IBS, such as abdominal pain. There is a published study comparing the efficacy of SSRIs (paroxetine) to treatment as usual in reducing abdominal pain, HRQoL and health-care costs in a relatively large group of severe IBS patients at three months of treatment and one year later (100). Between 40% and 48% of the patients had a psychiatric disorder, and 12% reported a history of sexual abuse. Paroxetine did not significantly reduce abdominal pain scores, although it did decrease days of pain compared to the treatment as usual group. While paroxetine was significantly superior to treatment as usual in improving HRQoL, there was no difference between patients with and without a depressive disorder. In a second study that compared the efficacy of a high fiber diet alone and in combination with fluoxetine or placebo in IBS, overall well-being improved more with paroxetine than with placebo (63.3% vs. 26.3%), but abdominal pain, bloating, and social functioning did not (101). These studies provide some preliminary evidence that SSRIs may have some overall efficacy in IBS patients with moderate-to-severe symptoms. It is still not clear if they are effective in patients with milder symptoms, and if they exert their beneficial effect by specifically relieving GI symptoms such as abdominal pain versus decreasing psychological symptoms.

Other Pharmacologic Agents

In a preliminary study, the effects of clonidine, which is an α_2-adrenergic receptor agonist, on GI symptoms, gut transit and fasting and postprandial gastric volumes were evaluated in patients with IBS-D in a double-blind, randomized, parallel-group, placebo-controlled trial (102). Clonidine, at a dose of 0.1 mg twice a day for four weeks, relieved altered bowel habits but not abdominal pain; however, these effects were not associated with significant alterations in transit. Clonidine did not significantly alter GI transit or gastric volumes. Drowsiness, dizziness, and dry mouth were the most common adverse events with the 0.1 mg dose, but severity of adverse effects subsided after the first week of treatment. Clinical trials with larger sample sizes will be required to assess more completely the effect of clonidine in IBS.

There are only two placebo-controlled trials assessing the efficacy of eradicating SIBO and relieving IBS symptoms. Pimental et al. have reported that those patients with bacterial overgrowth that were treated with neomycin had a $\geq 35\%$ reduction (i.e., improvement in symptoms) compared with an 11% reduction in patients on placebo (66). However, these studies had methodological limitations that prohibit routine hydrogen breath testing for bacterial overgrowth from being generally advocated. Pimental et al. are currently conducting a two-center, randomized, placebo-controlled trial assessing the efficacy of a 10-day course of the nonabsorbable broad-spectrum antibiotic, rifaximin, at a dose of 400 mg p.o. t.i.d.(103). A seven-day stool diary, questionnaires, and lactulose breath test for SIBO are being administered before and after treatment. The primary efficacy end point is global improvement in IBS with clinical responders defined as having greater than 50% improvement overall. Preliminary data has reported that 43 patients have randomized to rifaximin, and 43 were randomized to placebo. The intention-to-treat analysis demonstrated a $37.7 \pm 5.8\%$ overall improvement with rifaximin compared to $23.4 \pm 4.3\%$ with placebo ($p < 0.05$). Rifaximin was also associated with a significantly higher responder rate of 37% compared to 16% with placebo. Patients with diarrhea showed a greater clinical response with rifaximin (49%) than placebo (23%), but patients with constipation did not.

Complementary Alternative Treatment

Herbal treatments are used throughout the world and have been used by individuals for conditions of chronic pain conditions. However, there are only two placebo-controlled trials, which have evaluated herbal remedies in relieving the symptoms of IBS (104,105). The effect of Chinese herbal medicine (CHM) in the treatment of IBS was assessed in a randomized, double-blind, placebo-controlled trial (104). A total of 116 IBS patients were randomized to one of three treatment groups: individualized Chinese herbal formulations ($n = 38$), a standard Chinese herbal formulation ($n = 43$), or placebo ($n = 35$). Compared with patients in the placebo group, patients in the active treatment groups (standard and individualized CHM) had significant improvement in bowel symptom scores, global improvement, and reduction in the degree of interference with life caused by IBS symptoms. Chinese herbal formulations individually tailored to the patient proved no more effective than standard CHM treatment. On follow-up 14 weeks after completion of treatment, only the individualized CHM treatment group maintained improvement. In another treatment trial, the efficacy and safety of a commercially available herbal preparation, STW 5 (nine plant extracts), and the research herbal preparation, STW 5-II (six plant extracts), were found to be significantly better than placebo in reducing the total abdominal pain score and the IBS symptom score at four weeks in 208 patients with IBS (105).

Probiotics are live, microbial food supplements that are thought to exert beneficial effects by improving intestinal microbial balance and immune modulation. The beneficial effect of probiotics appears to be dependent on the particular strain. Studies have looked at single strains of *Lactobacillus* or *Bifidobacteria*, mixtures of *Bifidobacteria* and *Lactobacillus*, and one probiotic additionally mixed with *Streptococcus* (VSL# 3). In a 10-week treatment study, the effects of a probiotic formulation, VSL# 3 (450 billion lyophilized bacteria/day), on GI transit and symptoms were compared to placebo in 25 IBS-D patients (106). There were no significant differences in mean GI transit measurements, bowel function scores, or satisfactory global symptom relief between the two treatment groups, pre- or post-therapy. However, VSL# 3 reduced abdominal bloating compared to placebo. A follow up placebo-controlled study was recently conducted by the same investigators in 48 IBS patients with bloating (107). Treatment with VSL# 3 was associated with reduced flatulence over the entire treatment period. The proportions of responders for satisfactory relief of bloating, stool-related symptoms, abdominal pain, and bloating scores were not different. Colonic transit was measured using scintigraphy and was slowed with VSL# 3 relative to placebo. Thus, VSL# 3 reduced flatulence scores and retarded colonic transit without altering bowel function in patients with IBS and bloating.

The efficacy of the probiotic, *Bifidobacterium infantis* 35624, in relieving IBS symptoms has been demonstrated in a recently published eight-week randomized, placebo-controlled trial conducted in 77 patients with IBS (108). Compared to patients who received placebo, those randomized to *B. infantis* 35624 experienced a greater reduction in symptom scores including those for abdominal pain/discomfort, bloating/distention, and bowel movement difficulty. However, there was no significant effect with the other probiotic *Lactobacillus salivarius* UCC4331. At baseline, patients with IBS demonstrated an abnormal interleukin (IL) -10/ IL-12 ratio, indicative of a proinflammatory state. This ratio was normalized by *B. infantis* 35624 feeding alone. The authors suggested that *B. infantis* 35624 relieved symptoms in IBS possibly by its beneficial effects on immune modulation by normalizing the ratio of anti-inflammatory to proinflammatory cytokine levels.

There are very limited data on the efficacy of acupuncture in IBS. A recent study found a small numeric, but nonsignificant, difference between the therapeutic response rate of IBS symptoms in patients receiving acupuncture (40.7%) and sham treatment (109). Another study evaluated the effect of both electroacupuncture and placeboacupuncture on rectal distensibility, perception, and spatial summation (110). Electroacupuncture had no effect on rectal sensation, elastance, and cutaneous referral when compared to placeboacupuncture. In contrast, a third study found that transcutaneous electrical acustimulation reduced rectal sensitivity in seven IBS-D patients compared to control and sham stimulation conditions, but that the effect was not modulated by changes in rectal tone or compliance (111). Further studies are needed to assess this potentially therapeutic modality on IBS symptoms, their mechanisms of action, and safety.

Behavioral and Psychological Treatment

Psychological treatments used to treat FGIDs include psychotherapy (dynamic and cognitive-behavioral therapy), relaxation therapy, hypnotherapy, and biofeedback therapy. Psychological treatments can also be combined. Psychological treatments are generally recommended in patients with moderate-to-severe IBS, when patients fail medical treatment options, or when there is evidence that stress or psychological factors are contributing to symptom onset or exacerbation (4). Although studies have been criticized for their small sample sizes, use of an inactive (waiting list) control group, and various other methodological flaws, a recent meta-analysis of psychological treatments found an overall benefit (112). This meta-analysis also suggests that psychological therapies are efficacious not only for psychological symptoms of anxiety and depression, but may have a larger effect on visceral or somatic symptoms. A review by the ACG Functional GI Disorders Task Force of the psychological treatment studies of IBS supports the superiority of psychological treatment over conventional medical therapy for individual symptoms of IBS (71). There are two recent studies that have shown the beneficial effects of psychotherapy (100) and cognitive-behavioral therapy (CBT) (72) in moderate-to-severe IBS patients compared to controlled conditions. Drossman et al. randomized 215 patients with moderate to severe FGID (most had IBS and a small number had FAPS) to CBT or an education control (72). In an intention-to-treat and per-protocol analysis, CBT was found to have a significantly beneficial response in 70% of patients versus 37% of control patients, with the least benefit from IBS patients with depression. CBT is a widely available modality of psychological treatment and should be considered for patients with moderate-to-severe symptoms who have an inadequate response to medical management, even in the absence of an overt psychological disorder. Unfortunately, most psychologists are not trained specifically to treat IBS symptoms, thus comparable results to clinical trials may not be achieved in a community setting.

Hypnotherapy has been shown to improve overall IBS symptoms after an initial treatment course (symptoms "much better" or "moderately better" in 71%) with retained benefit in 81% at follow-up over one year later (113). While this may be a good alternative to CBT for some patients, qualified hypnotherapists may not be widely accessible in most practice settings. Studies have shown that hypnotherapy has beneficial effects that are long lasting, with most patients maintaining improvement, and with decreased consultation and medication needs in the long term (114). While the mechanisms by which hypnotherapy improves IBS symptoms is not completely understood, it is thought that changes in central processing of visceral stimuli, colonic motility, and rectal sensitivity as well as psychological effects are likely (114–116).

Table 2   Rome II Diagnostic Criteria for Functional Abdominal Pain Syndrome

At least 6 mo of
Continuous or nearly continuous abdominal pain; *and*
No or only occasional relationship of pain with physiological events (e.g., eating, defecation, or menses); *and*
Some loss of daily functioning; *and*
The pain is not feigned (e.g., malingering); *and*
Insufficient criteria for other functional gastrointestinal disorders which would explain the abdominal pain

Source: From Ref. 54.

FUNCTIONAL ABDOMINAL PAIN SYNDROME
Epidemiology

FAPS is much less prevalent than IBS and has been estimated to occur in 1.7% of the community. These patients have also been shown to miss 11.8 workdays from illness compared to 4.2 days for those without bowel symptoms. Patients with FAPS also made 7.2 physician visits in the previous year compared to 1.9 visits in those without bowel symptoms (6). Patients with FAPS, who were followed over a seven-year period, were found to be referred to an average of 5.7 consultants, underwent 6.4 endoscopic or radiological procedures, and had 2.7 major surgeries (e.g., hysterectomy and exploratory laparotomy) (117). Similar to IBS, FAPS is more common in women than men.

Diagnosis

The diagnosis of FAPS is currently based on Rome II symptom criteria as shown in Table 2. The absence of associated bowel dysfunction with abdominal pain distinguishes FAPS from IBS. A careful medical history and physical examination should be performed to exclude other medical conditions, which could explain the symptoms as well as identifying clinical, emotional, and behavioral features that may aid in the management of these patients. The pain in FAPS is often described in more emotional terms than those used to describe structural disease, e.g., "agonizing" and "sickening" rather than "crampy," "sharp," or "stabbing" (118). Diagnostic tests should be limited unless there are alarm signs or "red flags" (e.g., unexplained weight loss, blood in the stool, anemia, and fever) similar to those used to evaluate IBS patients to suggest organic disease.

Treatment

The basic principles of managing FAPS are similar to IBS with regard to establishing a successful patient–physician relationship, education, and reassurance. Few clinical trials have been performed in FAPS. However, the Rome committees support the following general therapeutic principles: (i) single supervising physician; (ii) listening, empathy, explanation, and reassurance; (iii) seek psychosocial factors; (iv) legitimize symptoms; (v) judicious use of tests and consultations; (vi) confident diagnosis; (vii) regular visits or telephone calls; (viii) patient responsibility; (ix) focus on life effects of symptoms; (x) belief in reality of condition and patient improvement; (xi) individualize drug therapy; (xii) consider behavioral therapy; and (xiii) coping instead of curing (119).

Therapy for FAPS should be directed at central rather than peripheral mechanisms because their symptoms may not be explained by bowel disturbances (119). In general, narcotics are not recommended because of their potential for dependency and GI side effects including impaired motility and increased pain sensitivity (narcotic bowel syndrome) (54). Psychotropic agents and psychological and behavioral therapies are frequently used. The discussion of these therapeutic modalities for IBS can be applied to patients with FAPS.

CONCLUSION

IBS and FAPS are FGIDs characterized by chronic or recurrent abdominal pain. The association of pain with altered bowel habits distinguishes IBS from FAPS. These conditions are more prevalent in women and are associated with a considerable health care and economic burden and decreased HRQoL. Due to the lack of a diagnostic biologic marker for both conditions, these conditions are diagnosed by symptom-based diagnostic criteria and excluding organic disease. The management of IBS and FAPS includes nonpharmacologic (e.g., education and reassurance and psychological treatment) and pharmacologic approaches and should be based on predominant symptoms, symptom severity, and presence of comorbid psychological features. While treatment of IBS can be directed toward peripheral (GI) and/or central mechanisms, the management of FAPS is directed centrally. The presence of extraintestinal symptoms may be due to comorbidity of other chronic functional disorders such as fibromyalgia. Similar clinical characteristics between IBS and these other syndromes have raised the possibility of a common underlying mechanism.

REFERENCES

1. Mitchell CM, Drossman DA. Survey of the AGA membership relating to patients with functional gastrointestinal disorders. Gastroenterology 1987; 92:1282–1284.
2. Thompson WG, Longstreth GF, Drossman DA, et al. C. Functional bowel disorders and functional abdominal pain. In: Drossman DA, Corazziari E, Talley NJ, et al., eds. Rome II. The Functional Gastrointestinal Disorders, Diagnosis, Pathophysiology and Treatment: A Multinational Consensus. McLean: Degnon Associates, 2000: 351–432.
3. Drossman DA. The functional gastrointestinal disorders and the Rome II process. In: Drossman DA, Corazziari E, Talley NJ, et al., eds. Rome II: The Functional Gastrointestinal Disorders: Diagnosis, Pathophysiology, and Treatment. A Multinational Consensus. McLean, VA: Degnon Associates, 2000: 1–29.
4. Drossman DA, Camilleri M, Mayer EA, et al. AGA technical review on irritable bowel syndrome. Gastroenterology 2002; 123:2108–2131.
5. Sandler RS. Epidemiology of irritable bowel syndrome in the United States. Gastroenterology 1990; 99:409–415.
6. Drossman DA, Li Z, Andruzzi E, et al. U.S. householder survey of functional gastrointestinal disorders. Prevalence, sociodemography and health impact. Dig Dis Sci 1993; 38:1569–1580.
7. Talley NJ, Zinsmeister AR, Melton LJ III. Irritable bowel syndrome in a community: symptom subgroups, risk factors, and health care utilization. Am J Epidemiol 1995; 142:76–83.
8. Talley NJ, O'Keefe EA, Zinsmeister AR, et al. Prevalence of gastrointestinal symptoms in the elderly: a population-based study. Gastroenterology 1992; 102:895–901.
9. Lembo A, Ameen VZ, Drossman DA. Irritable bowel syndrome: toward an understanding of severity. Clin Gastroenterol Hepatol 2005; 3:717–725.
10. Chang L, Heitkemper MM. Gender differences in irritable bowel syndrome. Gastroenterology 2002; 123:1686–1701.
11. Saito YA, Locke GR, Talley NJ, et al. A comparison of the Rome and Manning criteria for case identification in epidemiological investigations of irritable bowel syndrome. Am J Gastroenterol 2000; 95:2816–2824.
12. Saito YA, Talley NJ, Melton L, et al. The effect of new diagnostic criteria for irritable bowel syndrome on community prevalence estimates. Neurogastroenterol Motil 2003; 15:687–694.
13. Coffin B, Dapoigny M, Cloarec D, et al. Relationship between severity of symptoms and quality of life in 858 patients with irritable bowel syndrome. Gastroenterol Clin Biol 2004; 28:11–15.
14. van der Horst HE, van Dulmen AM, Schellevis FG, et al. Do patients with irritable bowel syndrome in primary care really differ from outpatients with irritable bowel syndrome? Gut 1997; 41:669–674.
15. Taub E, Cuevas JL, Cook EW, et al. Irritable bowel syndrome defined by factor analysis. Gender and race comparisons. Dig Dis Sci 1995; 40:2647–2655.
16. Talley NJ, Boyce P, Jones M. Identification of distinct upper and lower gastrointestinal symptom groupings in an urban population. Gut 1998; 42:690–695.
17. Lee OY, Mayer EA, Schmulson M, et al. Gender-related differences in IBS symptoms. Am J Gastroenterol 2001; 96:2184–2193.
18. Camilleri M, Mayer EA, Drossman DA, et al. Improvement in pain and bowel function in female irritable bowel patients with alosetron, a 5-HT$_3$ receptor antagonist. Aliment Pharmacol Ther 1999; 13:1149–1159.
19. Kellow J, Lee OY, Chang FY, et al. An Asia-Pacific, double blind placebo controlled, randomised study to evaluate the efficacy, safety, and tolerability of tegaserod in patients with irritable bowel syndrome. Gut 2003; 52:671–676.
20. Müller-Lissner SA, Fumagalli I, Bardhan KD, et al. Tegaserod, a 5-HT(4) receptor partial agonist, relieves symptoms in irritable bowel syndrome patients with abdominal pain, bloating and constipation. Aliment Pharmacol Ther 2001; 15:1655–1666.
21. Nyhlin H, Bang C, Elsborg L, et al. A double-blind, placebo-controlled, randomized study to evaluate the efficacy, safety and tolerability of tegaserod in patients with irritable bowel syndrome. Scand J Gastroenterol 2004; 39:119–126.
22. Heitkemper MM, Jarrett M. Patterns of gastrointestinal and somatic symptoms across the menstrual cycle. Gastroenterology 1992; 102:505–513.

23. Whitehead WE, Cheskin LJ, Heller BR, et al. Evidence for exacerbation of irritable bowel syndrome during menses. Gastroenterology 1990; 98:1485–1489.
24. Heitkemper MM, Cain KC, Jarrett ME, et al. Symptoms across the menstrual cycle in women with irritable bowel syndrome. Am J Gastroenterol 2003; 98:420–430.
25. Naliboff BD, Berman S, Chang L, et al. Sex-related differences in IBS patients: central processing of visceral stimuli. Gastroenterology 2003; 124:1738–1747.
26. Talley NJ, Fett SL, Zinsmeister AR, et al. Gastrointestinal tract symptoms and self-reported abuse: a population-based study. Gastroenterology 1994; 107:1040–1049.
27. Longstreth GF, Wolde-Tsadik G. Irritable bowel-type symptoms in HMO examinees Prevalence, demographics, and clinical correlates. Dig Dis Sci 1993; 38:1581–1589.
28. Drossman DA, Li Z, Leserman J, et al. Health status by gastrointestinal diagnosis and abuse history. Gastroenterology 1996; 110:999–1007.
29. Talley NJ, Gabriel SE, Harmsen WS, et al. Medical costs in community subjects with irritable bowel syndrome. Gastroenterology 1995; 109:1736–1741.
30. Sandler RS, Everhart JE, Donowitz M, et al. The burden of selected digestive diseases in the United States. Gastroenterology 2002; 122:1500–1511.
31. Levy RL, Von Korff M, Whitehead WE, et al. Costs of care for irritable bowel syndrome patients in a health maintenance organization. Am J Gastroenterol 2001; 96:3122–3129.
32. Longstreth GF, Wilson A, Knight K, et al. Irritable bowel syndrome, health care use, and costs: a U.S. managed care perspective. Am J Gastroenterol 2003; 98:600–607.
33. Martin BC, Ganguly R, Pannicker S, et al. Utilization patterns and net direct medical cost to medicaid of irritable bowel syndrome. Curr Med Res Opin 2003; 19:771–780.
34. Aston-Jones G, Rajkowski J, Kubiak P, et al. Role of the locus coeruleus in emotional activation. Prog Brain Res 1996; 107:379–402.
35. Hasler WL, Schoenfeld P. Systematic review: abdominal and pelvic surgery in patients with irritable bowel syndrome. Aliment Pharmacol Ther 2003; 17:997–1005.
36. Longstreth GF, Yao JF. Irritable bowel syndrome and surgery: a multivariable analysis. Gastroenterology 2004; 126:1665–1673.
37. Whitehead WE, Palsson O, Jones KR. Systemic review of the comorbidity of irritable bowel syndrome with other disorders: what are the causes and implications?. Gastroenterology 2002; 122:1140–1156.
38. Whitehead WE, Winget C, Fedoravicius AS, et al. Learned illness behavior in patients with irritable bowel syndrome and peptic ulcer. Dig Dis Sci 1982; 27:202–208.
39. Whorwell PJ, Lupton EW, Erduran D, et al. Bladder smooth muscle dysfunction in patients with irritable bowel syndrome. Gut 1986; 27:1014–1017.
40. Chang L. The association of functional gastrointestinal disorders and fibromyalgia. Eur J Surg 1998; 583:32–36.
41. Chang L. Extraintestinal manifestations and psychiatric illness in IBS: is there a link? In: Holtmann G, Talley NJ, eds. Gastrointestinal Inflammation and Disturbed Gut Function: The Challenge of New Concepts. Dordrecht, The Netherlands: Kluwer Academic, 2003:10–16.
42. Mayer EA. Emerging disease model for functional gastrointestinal disorders. Am J Med 1999; 107:12S–19S.
43. Clauw DJ, Crofford LJ. Chronic widespread pain and fibromyalgia: what we know, and what we need to know. Best Pract Res Clin Rheumatol 2003; 17:685–701.
44. Frank L, Kleinman L, Rentz A, et al. Health-related quality of life associated with irritable bowel syndrome: comparison with other chronic diseases. Clin Ther 2002; 24:675–689.
45. Gralnek IM, Hays RD, Kilbourne A, et al. The impact of irritable bowel syndrome on health-related quality of life. Gastroenterology 2000; 119:654–660.
46. Spiegel BM, Gralnek IM, Bolus R, et al. Clinical determinants of health-related quality of life in patients with irritable bowel syndrome. Arch Intern Med 2004; 164:1773–1780.
47. El-Serag HB. Impact of irritable bowel syndrome: prevalence and effect on health-related quality of life. Rev Gastroenterol Disord 2003; 3:S3–S11.
48. American College of Gastroenterology Functional Gastrointestinal Disorders Task Force. Evidence-based position statement on the management of irritable bowel syndrome in North America. Am J Gastroenterol 2002; 97:S1–S5.
49. Drossman DA, Corazziari E, Talley NJ, et al. ROME II. The Functional Gastrointestinal Disorders. Diagnosis, Pathophysiology and Treatment: A Multinational Consensus. McLean, VA: Degnon Associates, 2000.
50. Vanner SJ, Depew WT, Paterson WG, et al. Predictive value of the Rome Criteria for diagnosing the irritable bowel syndrome. Am J Gastroenterol 1999; 94:2912–2917.
51. Svendsen JH, Munck LK, Andersen JR. Irritable bowel syndrome: prognosis and diagnostic safety. A 5-year follow-up study. Scand J Gastroenterol 1985; 20:415–418.
52. Harvey RF, Mauad EC, Brown AM. Prognosis in the irritable bowel syndrome: a 5-year prospective study. Lancet 1987; 1:963–965.
53. Owens DM, Nelson DK, Talley NJ. The irritable bowel syndrome: long term prognosis and the physician-patient interaction. Ann Intern Med 1995; 122:107–112.

54. Thompson WG, Longstreth GF, Drossman DA, et al. Functional bowel disorders and functional abdominal pain. Gut 1999; 45:II43–II47.
55. Cash BD, Schoenfeld P, Chew WD. The utility of diagnostic tests in irritable bowel syndrome patients: a systematic review. Am J Gastroenterol 2002; 97:2812–2819.
56. Tolliver BA, Jackson MS, Jackson KL, et al. Does lactose maldigestion really play a role in the irritable bowel? J Clin Gastroenterol 1996; 23:15–17.
57. Newcomer AD, McGill DB, Thomas PJ, et al. Tolerance to lactose among lactase-deficient American Indians. Gastroenterology 1978; 74:44–46.
58. Suarez FL, Savaiano DA, Levitt MD. A comparison of symptoms after the consumption of milk or lactose-hydrolyzed milk by people with self-reported severe lactose intolerance. N Engl J Med 1995; 333:1–4.
59. Sanders DS, Carter MJ, Hurlstone DP, et al. Association of adult coeliac disease with irritable bowel syndrome: a case-control study in patients fulfilling ROME II criteria referred to secondary care. Lancet 2001; 358:1504–1508.
60. Hin H, Bird G, Fisher P, et al. Coeliac disease in primary care: case finding study. BMJ 1999; 318:164–167.
61. Holt R, Darnley SE, Kennedy T, et al. Screening for coeliac disease in patients with clinical diagnosis of irritable bowel syndrome. Gastroenterology 2001; 120:A-757.
62. Sanders DS, Patel D, Stephenson TJ, et al. A primary care cross-sectional study of undiagnosed adult coeliac disease. Eur J Gastroenterol Hepatol 2003; 15:407–413.
63. Shahbazkhani B, Forootan M, Merat S, et al. Coeliac disease presenting with symptoms of irritable bowel syndrome. Aliment Pharmacol Ther 2003; 18:231–235.
64. Spiegel BM, DeRosa VP, Gralnek IM, et al. Testing for celiac sprue in irritable bowel syndrome with predominant diarrhea: a cost-effectiveness analysis. Gastroenterology 2004; 126:1721–1732.
65. Pimentel M, Chow EJ, Lin HC. Eradication of small intestinal bacterial overgrowth reduces symptoms of irritable bowel syndrome. Am J Gastroenterol 2000; 95:3503–3506.
66. Pimentel M, Chow EJ, Lin HC. Normalization of lactulose breath testing correlates with symptom improvement in irritable bowel syndrome A double-blind, randomized, placebo-controlled study. Am J Gastroenterol 2003; 98:412–419.
67. Walters B, Vanner SJ. Dectection of bacterial overgrowth in IBS using the lactulose H2 breath test: comparison with 14C-D-xylose and healthy controls. Am J Gastroenterol 2005; 100:1566–1570.
68. Atkinson W, Sheldon TA, Shaath N, et al. Food elimination based on IgG antibodies in irritable bowel syndrome: a randomised controlled trial. Gut 2004; 53:1459–1464.
69. Klein KB. Controlled treatment trials in the irritable bowel syndrome: a critique. Gastroenterology 1988; 95:232–241.
70. Jailwala J, Imperiale TF, Kroenke K. Pharmacologic treatment of the irritable bowel syndrome: a systematic review of randomized, controlled trials. Ann Intern Med 2000; 133:136–147.
71. Brandt LJ, Bjorkman D, Fennerty MB, et al. Systematic review on the management of irritable bowel syndrome in North America. Am J Gastroenterol 2002; 97:S7–S26.
72. Drossman DA, Toner BB, Whitehead WE, et al. Cognitive-behavioral therapy versus education and desipramine versus placebo for moderate to severe functional bowel disorders. Gastroenterology 2003; 125:19–31.
73. Gershon MD. Review article: roles played by 5-hydroxytryptamine in the physiology of the bowel. Aliment Pharmacol Ther 1999; 13:15–30.
74. Camilleri M. Serotonergic modulation of visceral sensation: lower gut. Gut 2002; 51:i81–i86.
75. Clemens CH, Samsom M, van Berge Henegouwen GP, et al. Effect of alosetron on left colonic motility in non-constipated patients with irritable bowel syndrome and healthy volunteers. Aliment Pharmacol Ther 2002; 16:993–1002.
76. Delvaux M, Louvel D, Mamet JP, et al. Effect of alosetron on responses to colonic distension in patients with irritable bowel syndrome. Aliment Pharmacol Ther 1998; 12:849–855.
77. Camilleri M, Northcutt AR, Kong S, et al. Efficacy and safety of alosetron in women with irritable bowel syndrome: a randomised placebo-controlled trial. Lancet 2000; 355:1035–1040.
78. Camilleri M, Chey WY, Mayer EA, et al. A randomized controlled clinical trial of the serotonin type 3 receptor antagonist alosetron in women with diarrhea-predominant irritable bowel syndrome. Arch Intern Med 2001; 161:1733–1740.
79. Lembo T, Wright RA, Bagby B, et al. Alosetron controls bowel urgency and provides global symptom improvement in women with diarrhea-predominant irritable bowel syndrome. Am J Gastroenterol 2001; 96:2662–2670.
80. Lembo AJ, Olden KW, Ameen VZ, et al. Effect of alosetron on bowel urgency and global symptoms in women with severe, diarrhea-predominant irritable bowel syndrome: analysis of two controlled trials. Clin Gastroenterol Hepatol 2004; 2:675–682.
81. Jones RH, Holtmann G, Rodrigo L, et al. Alosetron relieves pain and improves bowel function compared with mebeverine in female nonconstipated irritable bowel syndrome patients. Aliment Pharmacol Ther 1999; 13:1419–1427.
82. Chang L, Ameen VZ, Dukes GE, et al. A dose-ranging, phase II study of the efficacy and safety of alosetron in men with diarrhea-predominant IBS. Am J Gastroenterol 2005; 100:115–123.

83. Chey WD, Inadomi JM, Booher AM, et al. Primary-care physicians' perceptions and practices on the management of GERD: results of a national survey. Am J Gastroenterol 2005; 100:1237–1242.
84. Berman SM, Chang L, Suyenobu B, et al. Condition-specific deactivation of brain regions by 5-HT$_3$ receptor antagonist alosetron. Gastroenterology 2002; 123:969–977.
85. Chang L, Chey WD, Harris L, et al. Incidence of ischemic colitis and serious complications of constipation among patients using alosetron: systematic review of clinical trials and post-marketing surveillance data. Am J Gastroenterol 2006. In press.
86. Bradette M, Moennikes H, Carter F, et al. Cilansetron in irritable bowel syndrome with diarrhea predominance (IBS-D): efficacy and safety in a 6 month global study. Gastroenterology 2004; 126:A-42.
87. Coremans G, Clouse RE, Carter F, et al. Cilansetron, a novel 5-HT$_3$ antagonist, demonstrated efficacy in males with irritable bowel syndrome with diarrhea-predominance (IBS-D). Gastroenterology 2004; 126:A-643.
88. Prather CM, Camilleri M, Zinsmeister AR, et al. Tegaserod accelerates orocecal transit in patients with constipation-predominant irritable bowel syndrome. Gastroenterology 2000; 118:463–468.
89. Novick J, Miner P, Krause R, et al. A randomized, double-blind, placebo-controlled trial of tegaserod in female patients suffering from irritable bowel syndrome with constipation. Aliment Pharmacol Ther 2002; 16:1877–1888.
90. Appel-Dingemanse S, Horowitz A, Campestrini J, et al. The pharmacokinetics of the novel promotile drug, tegaserod, are similar in healthy subjects - male and female, elderly and young. Aliment Pharmacol Ther 2001; 15:937–944.
91. Lefkowitz M, Ruegg P, Dunger-Baldauf C, et al. Validation of a global relief measure in clinical trials of irritable bowel syndrome with tegaserod. Gastroenterology 2000; 188:A145.
92. Tougas G, Snape WJ Jr., Otten MH, et al. Long-term safety of tegaserod in patients with constipation-predominant irritable bowel syndrome. Aliment Pharmacol Ther 2002; 16:1701–1708.
93. Cole JA, Cook SF, Sands BE, et al. Occurrence of colon ischemia in relation to irritable bowel syndrome. Am J Gastroenterol 2004; 99:486–491.
94. Meyers NL, Palmer RMJ, George A. Efficacy and safety of renzapride in patients with constipation-predominant IBS: a phase IIb study in the UK primary healthcare setting. Gastroenterology 2004; 126:A-640.
95. Camilleri M, McKinzie S, Fox J, et al. Renzapride accelerates colonic transit and improves bowel function in constipation-predominant irritable bowel syndrome (C-IBS). Gastroenterology 2004; 126:A-642.
96. Henderson JC, Palmer RMJ, Meyers NL, et al. A phase IIb clinical study of renzapride in mixed symptom (alternating) irritable bowel syndrome. Gastroenterology 2004; 126:A-644.
97. Talley NJ, Boyce PM, Jones M. Predictors of health care seeking for irritable bowel syndrome: a population based study. Gut 1997; 41:394–398.
98. Su X, Gebhart GF. Effects of tricyclic antidepressants on mechanosensitive pelvic nerve afferent fibers innervating the rat colon. Pain 1998; 76:105–114.
99. Morgan V, Pickens D, Gautam S, et al. Amitriptyline reduces rectal pain related activation of the anterior cingulate cortex in patients with irritable bowel syndrome. Gut 2005; 54:601–607.
100. Creed F, Fernandes L, Guthrie E, et al. The cost-effectiveness of psychotherapy and paroxetine for severe irritable bowel syndrome. Gastroenterology 2003; 124:303–317.
101. Tabas G, Beaves M, Wang J, et al. Paroxetine to treat irritable bowel syndrome not responding to high-fiber diet: a double-blind, placebo-controlled trial. Am J Gastroenterol 2004; 99:914–920.
102. Camilleri M, Kim DY, McKinzie S, et al. A randomized, controlled exploratory study of clonidine in diarrhea-predominant irritable bowel syndrome. Clin Gastroenterol Hepatol 2003; 1:111–121.
103. Pimentel M, Park S, Kong Y, et al. Rifaximin, a non-absorbable antibiotic, improves the symptoms of irritable bowel syndrome: a double-blind randomized controlled study. Am J Gastroenterol 2005; 100:S324.
104. Bensoussan A, Talley NJ, Hing M, et al. Treatment of irritable bowel syndrome with Chinese herbal medicine: a randomized controlled trial. JAMA 1998; 280:1585–1589.
105. Madisch A, Holtmann G, Plein K, et al. Treatment of irritable bowel syndrome with herbal preparations: results of a double-blind, randomized, placebo-controlled, multi-centre trial. Aliment Pharmacol Ther 2004; 19:271–279.
106. Kim HJ, Camilleri M, McKinzie S, et al. A randomized controlled trial of a probiotic, VSL#3, on gut transit and symptoms in diarrhoea-predominant irritable bowel syndrome. Aliment Pharmacol Ther 2003; 17:895–904.
107. Kim HJ, Vazquez Roque MI, Camilleri M, et al. A randomized controlled trial of a probiotic combination VSL# 3 and placebo in irritable bowel syndrome with bloating. Neurogastroenterol Motil 2005; 17:687–696.
108. O'Mahony L, McCarthy J, Kelly P, et al. Lactobacillus and bifidobacterium in irritable bowel syndrome: symptom responses and relationship to cytokine profiles. Gastroenterology 2005; 128:541–551.
109. Forbes A, Jackson S, Walter C, et al. Acupuncture for irritable bowel syndrome: a blinded placebo-controlled trial. World J Gastroenterol 2005; 11:4040–4044.

110. Rohrbock RB, Hammer J, Vogelsang H, et al. Acupuncture has a placebo effect on rectal perception but not on distensibility and spatial summation: a study in health and IBS. Am J Gastroenterol 2004; 99:1990–1997.

111. Xing J, Larive B, Mekhail N, et al. Transcutaneous electrical acustimulation can reduce visceral perception in patients with the irritable bowel syndrome: a pilot study. Altern Ther Health Med 2004; 10:38–42.

112. Lackner JM, Mesmer C, Morley S, et al. Psychological treatments for irritable bowel syndrome: a systematic review and meta-analysis. J Consult Clin Psychol 2004; 72:1100–1113.

113. Gonsalkorale WM, Miller V, Afzal A, et al. Long-term benefits of hypnotherapy for irritable bowel syndrome. Gut 2003; 52:1623–1629.

114. Gonsalkorale WM, Whorwell PJ. Hypnotherapy in the treatment of irritable bowel syndrome. Eur J Gastroenterol Hepatol 2005; 17:15–20.

115. Simren M, Ringstrom G, Bjornsson ES, et al. Treatment with hypnotherapy reduces the sensory and motor component of the gastrocolonic response in irritable bowel syndrome. Psychosom Med 2004; 66:233–238.

116. Lea R, Houghton LA, Calvert EL, et al. Gut-focused hypnotherapy normalizes disordered rectal sensitivity in patients with irritable bowel syndrome. Aliment Pharmacol Ther 2003; 17:635–642.

117. Maxton DG, Whorwell PJ. Use of medical resources and attitudes to health care of patients with "chronic abdominal pain". Br J Med Econ 1992; 2:75–79.

118. Matthews PJ, Aziz Q. Functional abdominal pain. Postgrad Med J 2005; 81:448–455.

119. Longstreth GF, Drossman DA. Severe irritable bowel and functional abdominal pain syndromes: managing the patient and health care costs. Clin Gastroenterol Hepatol 2005; 3:397–400.

25 | Noncardiac Chest Pain: Pathophysiology

Premjit S. Chahal and Satish S. C. Rao
Department of Internal Medicine, University of Iowa Carver College of Medicine, Iowa City, Iowa, U.S.A.

INTRODUCTION

Noncardiac or functional chest pain of esophageal origin is characterized by episodes of unexplained chest pain that are usually midline and of visceral quality (1). The diagnostic criteria include at least 12 weeks in the preceding 12 months of midline chest pain or discomfort that is not burning in quality, and with an absence of pathologic gastroesophageal reflux, achalasia, or other motility disorder with a recognized pathologic basis (1). This chapter explores the evolving research in the pathophysiology of chest pain, with a particular emphasis on the role of sensory and afferent neuronal dysfunction.

Most patients with functional chest pain receive a thorough yet negative cardiac evaluation, and estimates suggest an annual incidence of 450,000 new cases in the United States (2). The quality of life is often severely affected in these individuals, and considerable time and expense is invested in seeking medical evaluation and treatment (3). Noncardiac chest pain (NCCP) has been reviewed in journals spanning numerous disciplines, including cardiology (4), internal medicine (5), gastroenterology (6–8), emergency medicine (9), and psychiatry (10). This clearly implies the complex and overlapping nature of this problem.

Functional Anatomy of the Esophagus

The esophagus is a muscular tube, which extends approximately 25 cm from the pharynx to the stomach. Although uniform in appearance, the esophagus has several sections, and each possesses unique biomechanical and sensory characteristics (11). Once past the cricopharyngeus muscle [also termed the "upper esophageal sphincter" (UES)], the esophagus is divided into three gross regions identified by their location: cervical, thoracic, and abdominal esophagus. The cervical esophagus extends from the UES, behind the trachea to the carina. At this point, the thoracic esophagus will pass behind the left mainstem bronchus and lies next to the left atrium as it terminates at the diaphragmatic hiatus. The abdominal esophagus, also termed the "lower esophageal sphincter" (LES), is approximately 2 to 4 cm in length and is the conduit to the stomach. Additionally, there are three areas of luminal narrowing due to extrinsic compression, including the UES constriction (due to the cricoid cartilage, the lumen narrows to 14 mm in diameter), the bronchoaortic constriction (due to left mainstem bronchus and crossing aortic arch, the lumen narrows to 15–17 mm in diameter), and the diaphragmatic constriction (at the diaphragmatic hiatus, the lumen narrows to 16–19 mm in diameter). These areas of constriction are prone to dysphagia and strictures lending to a variety of esophageal sensations, including pain (12).

Histologically, the esophageal wall is composed of four discrete layers: an outer fibrous adventitia (without a serosa), the muscularis, the submucosa, and a squamous mucosal epithelium. Directly underneath the adventitia, two muscular layers exist composed of an outer, longitudinal layer, and an inner, circular layer. The composition of these muscular layers is variable, but typically in the upper third of the esophagus, there is a predominance of striated (skeletal) muscle compared to the lower two-thirds of the esophagus, which is primarily nonstriated (smooth) muscle. Sympathetic and parasympathetic nerve bundles innervating the esophagus are located in the two regions. The myenteric, or Auerbach's plexus, can be found between the muscularis layers while a smaller collection of nerve fibers known as the Meissner's plexus is located in the submucosa. Loss of ganglion cells and neuronal degeneration of these plexi results in esophageal dysmotility, particularly achalasia (13).

Sensory innervation of the esophagus arises from both branches of the vagus nerve (CN X), which originate in the nodose ganglia and project centrally to the tractus solitarus (14) as well as from spinal nerves. It is currently believed that most pain sensation is relayed by the latter; these nerve fibers receive viscerosensory input from two physiological classes of nociceptor receptors: "high-threshold" and "low-threshold" receptors. The high-threshold receptors respond to mechanical stimulation within a noxious range while the low-threshold encode for a stimulus intensity corresponding to the magnitude of the innocuous stimuli into the noxious range (15). It also proposed that visceral organs contain "silent" spinal nociceptive afferent fibers, which are sensitized by chronic inflammation (16).

An assessment of the biomechanical and sensory parameters of the esophagus at four discrete levels showed that the LES had the smallest cross-sectional area (CSA) followed by the proximal esophagus, and both these segments displayed greater wall tension and less deformability than the mid or distal esophagus (11). Sensory thresholds were also significantly lower in the proximal compared with the mid- to distal esophagus. Thus, the striated muscle segments of the esophagus are more sensitive and less compliant than the smooth muscle portion. Furthermore, gender did not seem to influence the esophageal sensory or biomechanical properties, but in both the striated and smooth muscle segments, the CSA was significantly larger ($p < 0.05$), the esophageal was less distensible ($p < 0.05$), and the median thresholds for discomfort and pain were higher in older subjects. Thus, aging but not gender influences esophageal function (17).

Recently esophageal function has also been shown to vary at the striated and smooth muscle segments in NCCP patients. During balloon distentions at 5 cm below the UES (skeletal muscle) and 10 cm above the LES (smooth muscle) in 20 patients with NCCP and 15 healthy subjects (18), balloon distention reproduced chest pain in 85% of patients. Furthermore, 20% of patients reported pain only in the smooth muscle section (compared to 10% in the skeletal portion) and had significantly lower CSA and esophageal wall stiffness than at the striated muscle level in both patients and controls ($p < 0.01$). This suggests that care should be taken when interpreting results of balloon distention studies because some patients may be uniformly hypersensitive but a small proportion may have more localized hypersensitivity causing their symptoms (18).

Mechanisms of Pain

A discomfort or pain arising from the thoracic region, extending from the epigastric region to the clavicles, is often described as chest pain, which may either be somatic or visceral in origin. Somatic pain, often due to musculoskeletal ailments, tends to be well localized, whereas visceral pain arising from internal organs tends to be poorly localized and difficult to describe.

Perturbations in Nociceptors and Afferent and Efferent Signaling

The exact mechanism of NCCP is unclear and several mechanisms have been proposed (Figs. 1 and 2). Gilbert's original studies (19) showed that esophageal balloon distention induced coronary artery vasoconstriction in a canine model, and this response was eliminated by either atropine or vagotomy. This response, termed the "viscerocardiac reflex," established a common neural pathway shared by cardiac and esophageal plexi. However, there is a lack of study evaluating these pain pathways. It is also unknown if this pain syndrome is primarily a peripheral disorder of esophageal chemoreceptors, mechanoreceptors, or thermoreceptors (11,20) or a perturbation of the central modulation of pain pathways.

Recent work has provided some intriguing concepts regarding the potential pathways and modulation of chronic pain (21). In this model, chronic pain is composed of three distinct, yet interrelated, phases. In Phase 1, activation of primary nociceptors causes direct transmission of noxious stimuli to the central pain centers via afferent A-delta (thinly myelinated) and C-fibers (unmyelinated) that ascend in the sensory tracts. Due to reflex withdrawal protective mechanisms, Phase 1 activation is often not associated with tissue injury. In Phase 2, the noxious signal is associated with inflammation or tissue injury. The damaged tissue releases bradykinin, serotonin, prostaglandins, cytokines, and growth factors (22). These nociceptor

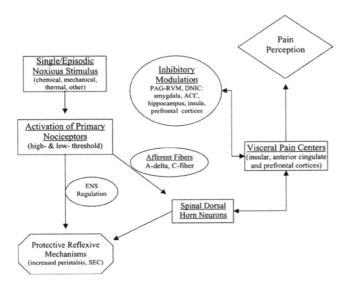

Figure 1 Proposed model of esophageal pain perception with noxious signals. *Abbreviations*: PAG-RVM, periaqueductal grey-rostroventral medulla; DNIC, diffuse noxious inhibitory control; SEC, sustained esophageal contraction.

sensitizing mediators cause greater afferent firing. With the onset of afferent sensitization and central modulation, other features of chronic pain syndromes such as *allodynia* (painful sensation to non-noxious stimuli), *primary hyperalgesia* (increased response to noxious stimuli in injured area), and *secondary hyperalgesia* (increased response to noxious stimuli from the surrounding uninjured area) (23) may become manifest. Long-term sensitization of primary visceral afferents induced by chronic inflammation is supported by several models, including chronic visceral pain induced in the colons of rats (24). It is also speculated that plasticity in chronic visceral pain of the colon is sustained by feedback loops ascending in the dorsal column and engaging the thalamus (25). In Phase 3, there may be direct injury to the peripheral or central nerves. This causes spontaneous neuropathic pain (26), which is independent of any stimulus (27).

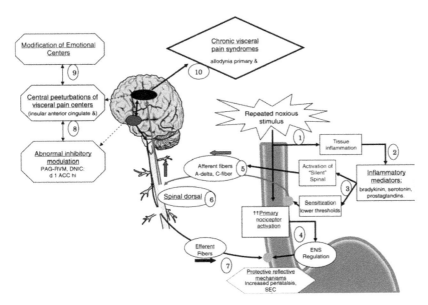

Figure 2 Proposed model of chronic esophageal chest pain and development of visceral hypersensitivity secondary to repeated noxious insult and sensitization of viscera. *Abbreviations*: PAG-RVM, periaqueductal grey-rostroventral medulla; DNIC, diffuse noxious inhibitory control; SEC, sustained esophageal contraction.

Inhibitory pathways serve to counter stimulatory pathways and facilitate endogenous analgesia (28). Although studies have yet to evaluate inhibitory esophageal pain modulation, counterirritation studies (the modulation of a painful stimulus by a second heterotopically applied nociceptive stimulus) in rectal pain have shown perturbations in several cerebral regions, including the periaqueductal grey (PAG) -rostroventral medulla (RVM) network and the spino-bulbo-spinal diffuse noxious inhibitory controls (DNIC) pathways, which become abnormally modified in several pain syndromes (29,30). Because these areas promote the inhibitory feedback loops and the intrinsic communication with the anterior cingulate cortex, the insular cortex, and the prefrontal cortex, they potentially modulate somatic, autonomic, and antinociceptive responses (31).

Esophageal origins of functional chest pain span a spectrum of disorders that include acid reflux, motility disorders, and visceral hypersensitivity, likely with considerable overlap. A possible unifying hypothesis is that a noxious stimulus such as reflux of acid or bile may not only induce pain via esophageal chemosensitive receptors, but also cause protective or reactive motility phenomena that in turn causes pain. With repeated and chronic insult, modulation of this visceral pain pathway may occur either peripherally or centrally. A proposed model is shown in Figure 2.

Role of Visceral Hypersensitivity: Peripheral Versus Central

The concept of esophageal hypersensitivity was first reported by Richter et al. (32). Using the esophageal balloon distention test, they found that a higher percentage of patients reported chest pain compared to healthy controls (60% vs. 20%). A larger study of 50 patients with NCCP and 30 healthy volunteers showed that balloon distention induced chest pain in 56% of patients and 20% of volunteers giving a diagnostic yield of 48% (33). The balloon distention test remains controversial because of mixed results (34,35). Without appreciating the changes in the biomechanical properties of the esophageal wall and without excluding patients with acid reflux or motility disorders, the interpretation of data during the balloon distention test may be inexact (36).

The development of impedance planimetry, a technique that allows simultaneous assessment of esophageal sensory, biomechanical, and motor properties during graded, intraluminal balloon distention, has provided evidence implicating visceral hypersensitivity in patients with unexplained chest pain (33,38). Using this technique, patients with NCCP were shown to have 50% lower sensory thresholds together with a hyperreactive and poorly compliant esophagus when compared to controls (39). Typical chest pain was reproduced in 80% of individuals. To determine further whether hypersensitivity or motor dysfunction plays a predominant role, Rao et al. used the balloon distention test before and after administration of intravenous atropine (to relax the esophageal wall and decrease the motor component) in 16 patients and five volunteers (40). Balloon distentions reproduced chest pain in 81% of patients compared to inducing chest pain in 20% of controls at baseline and the sensory thresholds did not change after esophageal wall relaxation (40). This study confirms, albeit indirectly, an important role for visceral hyperalgesia in the pathogenesis of functional chest pain.

Recent developments in neuroimaging have led to the exploration of central mechanisms of chest pain in these patients. By monitoring cortical blood flow as a marker of cortical activity during esophageal balloon distention, Aziz et al. identified paralimbic and limbic structures such as the insular, anterior cingulate, and prefrontal cortices as visceral pain centers (41). Shaker et al. compared functional magnetic resonance imaging (fMRI) changes during infusion of acid or saline compared to balloon distention of the esophagus in 10 healthy volunteers (42). They confirmed similar cortical activation patterns that were concentrated in the mesial parieto-occipital and frontal lobes, and adjacent to or within the cingulate gyrus (43). Interestingly, the cerebral fMRI response to acid perfusion displayed a longer latency period compared to balloon distention, suggesting a possible delay in processing or interpreting the afferent signal. Aziz et al. also suggested that pain perception may be due to central sensitization. This was defined as an activity-dependent amplification of the transfer of sensory signals in the central nervous system (44). Electrical stimulation of the proximal and distal esophagus, before and after acid exposure in seven patients with NCCP and 19 healthy volunteers, showed that the NCCP group had lower esophageal pain thresholds that decreased further and persisted for a longer duration when exposed to acid instillation. This suggests a central enhancement of sensory input (45). The theory of central sensitization is further supported by a study involving duodenal acidification resulting in esophageal hypersensitivity. As the visceral afferents of numerous organs of the gastrointestinal tract converge on spinal dorsal horn neurons, activation of visceral afferents in the duodenum resulted in hypersensitivity of the esophagus to acid infusion but not to saline (46). Recent work by this group also suggests that an activity-dependent increase in spinal cord neuronal excitability is dependent on the *N*-methyl-d-aspartate (NMDA) receptor as the induction and maintenance of acid-induced esophageal hypersensitivity is prevented and reversed by ketamine (NMDA receptor antagonist) (43). Also, cortical evoked potential (CEP) studies suggested that some patients with chest pain and visceral hypersensitivity have sensitized esophageal afferents while others are hypervigilant to esophageal sensations, further suggesting a central perturbation of pain regulation (47).

Central endogenous pain modulating mechanisms, including the PAG-RVM network and the spino-bulbo-spinal DNIC pathways may regulate pain perception and contribute to endogenous inhibitory pain mechanisms (48). Applying fMRI during painful heterotopic rectal stimulation, increased cerebral activation of the amygdala, anterior cingulate cortex, hippocampus, insula, PAG, and prefrontal cortex was observed (49). These brain regions govern the emotional responses to pain such as fear, depression, and anxiety (50). This could explain the altered psychosocial behavior in many of these patients.

Role of Motility Disorders

In 1892, Sir William Osler first described "pseudo-angina" and attributed this to esophageal dysmotility (51). Since then, esophageal spasm has been promoted as a cause of chest pain (52). Several motility disorders have also been implicated including diffuse esophageal spasm (DES), "nutcracker esophagus," achalasia, scleroderma, and nonspecific motility disorders (53,54). Esophageal dysmotility has been reported in 12% to 33% of patients with unexplained chest pain (55). Among these, approximately 30% to 50% have nutcracker esophagus, 30% have nonspecific motility disorders, and 15% have DES (52,56,57). In a group of seven patients, abnormally high amplitude peristaltic contractions were associated with unexplained chest pain that may provide indirect evidence of esophageal mechanoreceptor activation producing chest pain (58).

However, the evidence for a motility disorder in NCCP is conflicting. Richter's group evaluated 100 patients with NCCP, and although 32% had an abnormal esophageal manometry, they experienced no pain episodes during the abnormal manometric periods (59). Likewise, another large study of 248 patients found that motility dysfunction was uncommon (60). An American Gastroenterology Association (AGA) technical review concluded that there was insufficient evidence to implicate dysmotility as a cause of chest pain and therefore did not recommend the use of esophageal manometry for routine assessment of functional chest pain (61). Recently, 10 patients with NCCP were evaluated with endoluminal ultrasonography and were found to have sustained esophageal contractions (SEC) during episodes of spontaneous chest pain (62). However, this activity occurred only in a subset of patients and only during some of the pain episodes. In a subsequent investigation, the same investigators found that the SEC was correlated with heartburn and acid reflux (63). Therefore, SEC may be a pathophysiologic marker of chest pain but not causally related. This observation is further corroborated by a recent study, which showed that 90% of patients with chest pain and nutcracker esophagus demonstrate esophageal hypersensitivity (64). Thus, it seems that an esophageal motility disorder is less likely to cause chest pain, but pain is associated with an altered sensation and biomechanical changes of the esophageal wall.

Role of Gastroesophageal Reflux Disease

In a typical outpatient setting, atypical chest pain of noncardiac origin is often presumed to be due to gastroesophageal reflux disease (GERD). Demeester et al. showed that 46% of patients with chest pain had symptoms associated with acid reflux based on prolonged ambulatory pH studies (65). Another study of 100 patients with unexplained chest pain showed that pH testing yielded a combined positive symptom index and/or pathological acid reflux in approximately 50% of individuals (59). Recent studies by Fass et al. (66) have shown that acid reflux may cause chest pain in 30% to 60% of patients. Acid or bile reflux may also stimulate esophageal chemoreceptors (20), and indeed, in a small ($n = 36$), placebo-controlled trial of NCCP patients with documented GERD, omeprazole significantly decreased chest pain compared to placebo (67).

The literature on GERD and NCCP, however, is not consistent. In one study, exercise testing, edrophonium provocation, and esophageal acid perfusion showed no significant differences between 63 NCCP patients and 22 controls (68), similar to findings by other investigators (60). In another study of patients with NCCP, those with acid reflux were more likely to respond to proton pump inhibitors than those without (66). Additionally, nonerosive reflux represents 70% of the GER population, and 50% of these individuals may have functional heartburn (heartburn without acid reflux) (69). Thus, at least one-third of the presumed symptomatic acid reflux population has physiologically normal levels of acid refluxate. These individuals may be hypersensitive to normal amounts of acid reflux, implicating either altered afferent receptor dysfunction or aberrant central modulation of pain. Undoubtedly, acid reflux plays a role in NCCP, but is only one of the many components of this complex, multifactorial process.

Role of Psychiatric or Behavioral Disorders

In 1871, DaCosta described his observation on soldiers having functional chest pain and attributed this to "disordered innervation" (70). More recently, Clouse and Lustman (71) performed manometric and psychiatric evaluations in 50 patients and found that 25 (50%) had nonspecific, abnormal esophageal manometry; among these, 21 (84%) had a psychiatric diagnosis. In contrast, only eight (31%) subjects with normal manometry had a psychiatric diagnosis. Trials of an antidepressant, trazadone, administered at low doses improved chest pain in patients with a psychiatric diagnosis (72). Another study by Cannon and Benjamin showed that 38 of 60 (63%) patients with NCCP had one or more psychiatric disorders as well as a significant decrease in chest pain after treatment with low-dose imipramine (73). A panic disorder has also been reported by several investigators (74). In a study of 441 patients with functional chest pain, the prevalence of panic disorder was 24.5% (74). Although these studies provide indirect evidence, the precise role of psychiatric or behavioral disorders in the pathogenesis of chest pain is unclear. Whether they are a primary cause, a predisposing factor, a comorbid illness, or sequelae to chronic intermittent and unexplained symptoms is unknown.

CONCLUSION

The pathophysiology of esophageal chest pain continues to evolve (Figs. 1 and 2). There has been a significant paradigm shift from the considerations of a panic disorder and psychosomatic causes to that of a motility disorder and currently GERD or altered visceral sensation. We believe that alterations in the sensory receptors and in the gut-brain-gut regulatory mechanisms play a pivotal role in the pathogenesis of this syndrome, as shown in Figures 1 and 2. Considerable interest and research activity is currently focused on the investigation of cerebral activity and modulation with the application of a variety of stimulation and imaging studies, including magnetic encephalogram, CEP, and fMRI. Further research should help to characterize the precise roles of neurotransmitters, and their receptors such as adenosine and serotonin, gamma amino butyric acid (GABA) and NMDA receptors, and the ascending, central, and descending pathways, including stimulatory and inhibitory pain modulation.

ACKNOWLEDGMENT

This work was supported in part by grant 1RO1 DK57100–0141 from the National Institutes of Health, Bethesda.

REFERENCES

1. Clouse R, Richter J, et al. Functional esophageal disorders. In: Rome II: The Functional Gastrointestinal Disorders. 2nd ed. Lawrence: Allen Press, 2000:264–274.

2. Katz P, Codario R, Castell D. Approach to the patient with unexplained chest pain. Comprehensive Therapy 1997; 23:249.
3. Achem S, DeVault K. Recent developments in chest pain of undetermined origin. Curr Gastroenterol Rep 2000; 2:201.
4. Cannon R. Cardiac pain. In: Visceral Pain, Progress in Pain Research and Management. Vol. 5. Seattle: IASP Press, 1995.
5. Langdon DE. Empiric therapy for noncardiac chest pain. Arch Int Med 2000; 160:3331.
6. Shrestha S, Pasricha P. Update on noncardiac chest pain. Dig Dis 2000; 18:138.
7. Fang J, Bjorkman D. A critical approach to noncardiac chest pain: pathophysiology, diagnosis and treatment. Am J Gastroenterol 2001; 96:958.
8. Botoman AV. Noncardiac chest pain. J Clin Gastroenterol 2002; 34:6.
9. Murphy P, Colwell C, Bryan T. Noncardiac chest pain. Emerg Med Serv 2001; 30:66.
10. Fleet R, Beitman B. Unexplained chest pain: when is it panic disorder? Clin Cardiol 1997; 20:187.
11. Patel RS, Rao SSC. Biomechanical and sensory parameters of the human esophagus at four levels. Am J Physiol 1998; 275:G187–G191.
12. Wo JM, Waring JP. Medical therapy of gastroesophageal reflux and management of esophageal strictures. Surg Clin North Am 1997; 77:1041.
13. Long JD, Orlando RC. Anatomy, histology, embryology, and developmental anomalies of the esophagus. In: Sleisenger & Fordtran's Gastrointestinal and Liver Disease. 7th ed. Philadelphia: Saunders, 2002:551–560.
14. Al-Chaer ED, Traub RJ. Biological basis of visceral pain: recent developments. Pain 2002; 96:221.
15. Sengupta JN, Gebhart GF. Characterization of mechanosensitive pelvic nerve afferent fibers innervating the colon of the rat. J Neurophysiol 1994; 71:2046.
16. Gebhart GF. J.J. Bonica Lecture–2000: physiology, pathophysiology, and pharmacology of visceral pain. Reg Anesth Pain Med 2000; 25:632.
17. Rao SSC, Mudipalli RS, Mujica VR, Patel RS, Zimmerman B. Effects of gender and age on esophageal biomechanical properties and sensation. Am J Gastroenterol 2003; 98:1688.
18. Rao SSC, Hayek B, Mudipalli R, Gregersen H. Does esophageal function vary at the striated and smooth muscle segments in functional chest pain? Am J Gastroenterol 2002; 97:2201.
19. Gilbert NC, LeRoy GV, Fenn GK. The effect of distention of abdominal viscera on the blood flow of the circumflex branch of the left coronary artery of the dog. Am Heart J 1940; 20:519.
20. Lynn R. Mechanisms of esophageal pain. Am J Med 1992; 92:S11–S19.
21. Cervero F, Laird J. From acute to chronic pain: mechanisms and hypothesis. In: Zimmerman GCM, ed. Progress in Brain Research. Amsterdam: Elsevier, 1996:3–16.
22. Kidd B, Urban L. Mechanisms of inflammatory pain. Br J Anaesth 2001; 87:3.
23. Cervero F, Laird J, Garcia-Nicas E. Secondary hyperalgesia and presynaptic inhibition: an update. Eur J Pain 2003; 7:345.
24. Al-Chaer ED, Kawasaki M, Pasricha PJ. A new model of chronic visceral hypersensitivity in adult rats induced by colon irritation during postnatal development. Gastroenterology 2000; 119:1276.
25. Saab CY, Park YC, Al-Chaer ED. Thalamic modulation of visceral nociceptive processing in adult rats with neonatal colon irritation. Brain Res 2004; 1008:186.
26. Zimmerman M. Pathobiology of neuropathic pain. Eur J Pharmacol 2001; 429:23.
27. Takaishi K, Eisle J, Carstens E. Behavioral and electrophysiological assessment of hyperalgesia and changes in dorsal horn responses following partial sciatic nerve ligation in rate. Pain 1996; 66:297.
28. Lautenbacher S, Rollman GB. Possible deficiencies of pain modulation in fibromyalgia. Clin J Pain 1997; 13:189.
29. Willer JC, De Brouker T, Le Bars D. Encoding of nociceptive thermal stimuli by diffuse noxious inhibitory controls in humans. J Neurophysiol 1989; 62:1028.
30. Willer JC, Bouhassira D, Le Bars D. Neurophysiological basis of the counterirritation phenomenon: diffuse control inhibitors induced by nociceptive stimulation. Neurophysiol Clin 1999; 29:379.
31. Keay KA, Clement CI, Owler B, Depaulis A, Bandler R. Convergence of deep somatic and visceral nociceptive information onto a discrete ventrolateral midbrain periaqueductal gray region. Neuroscience 1994; 61:727.
32. Richter J, Barish C, Castell D. Abnormal sensory perception in patients with esophageal chest pain. Gastroenterology 1986; 91:845.
33. Barish C, Castell D, Richter J. Graded esophageal balloon distention. A new provocative test for noncardiac chest pain. Dig Dis Sci 1986; 31:1292.
34. Cherian P, Smith L, Bardham K, et al. Esophageal tests in the evaluation of non-cardiac chest pain. Dis Esoph 1995; 8:129.
35. Lasch H, DeVault K, Castell D. Intraesophageal balloon distention in the evaluation of sensory thresholds: studies on reproducibility and comparison of balloon composition. Am J Gastroenterol 1994; 89:1185.
36. Chahal PS, Rao SSC. Functional chest pain: nociception and visceral hyperalgesia. J Clin Gastroenterol 2005; 39:S204–S209.
37. Gregersen H, Djurhuus J. Impedance planimetry: a new approach to biomechanical intestinal wall properties. Dig Dis Sci 1991; 9:332.

38. Rao SSC, Hayek B, Summers R. Impedance planimetry: an integrated approach for assessing sensory, active and passive biomechanical properties of the human esophagus. Am J Gastroenterol 1995; 90:431.
39. Rao SSC, Gregersen H, Hayek B, et al. Unexplained chest pain: the hypersensitive, hyperreactive, and poorly compliant esophagus. Ann Int Med 1996; 124:950.
40. Rao SSC, Hayek B, Summers R. Functional chest pain of esophageal origin: hyperalgesia or motor dysfunction. Am J Gastroenterol 2001; 96:2584.
41. Aziz Q, Andersson J, Valind S, Thompson D. Identification of human brain loci processing esophageal sensation using positron emission tomography. Gastroenterology 1997; 113:50.
42. Shaker R, Kern M, Arndorfer R, Jesmanowicz A, Hyde J. Cerebral cortical fMRI responses to esophageal acid exposure and distention: a comparative study [abstr]. Gastroenterology 1996:A395.
43. Willert R, Woolf C, Hobson A, Delaney C, Thompson D, Aziz Q. The development and maintenance of human visceral pain hypersensitivity is dependent on the N-methyl-D-aspartate receptor. Gastroenterology 2004; 126:683.
44. Aziz Q, Schnitzler A, Enck P. Functional neuroimaging of visceral sensation. J Clin Neurophysiol 2000; 17:604.
45. Sarkar S, Aziz Q, Woolf C, Hobson A, Thompson D. Contribution of central sensitisation to the development of non-cardiac chest pain. Lancet 2000; 356:1154.
46. Hobson AR, Khan RW, Sarkar S, Furlong PL, Aziz Q. Development of esophageal hypersensitivity following experimental duodenal acidification. Am J Gastroenterol 2004; 99:813.
47. Hobson AR, Aziz Q. Brain processing of esophageal sensation in health and disease. Gastroenterol Clin North Am 2004; 33:69.
48. Silverman DH, Munakata J, Enees H, et al. Regional cerebral activation in normal and pathological perception of visceral pain. Gastroenterology 1997; 112:64.
49. Wilder-Smith CH, Schindler D, Lovblad K, et al. Brain functional magnetic resonance imaging of rectal pain and activation of endogenous inhibitory mechanisms in irritable bowel syndrome patient subgroups and healthy controls. Gut 2004; 53:1595.
50. Davidson RJ, Abercrombie H, Nitschke JB, Putnam K. Regional brain function, emotion and disorders of emotion. Curr Opin Neurobiol 1999; 9:228.
51. Osler W. The principles and practice of medicine. New York: Appleton, 1892.
52. Herrington J, Burns T, Balart L. Chest pain and dysphagia in patients with prolonged peristaltic contractile duration of the esophagus. Dig Dis Sci 1984; 29:134.
53. Rao SSC. Esophageal (noncardiac) chest pain: visceral hyperalgesia, motor disorder, or reflux disease? In: Visceral Pain, Progress in Pain Research and Management. Vol. 5. Seattle: IASP Press, 1995.
54. Gregersen H, Kassab G. Biomechanics of the gastrointestinal tract. Neurogastroenterol Mot 1996; 8:1.
55. Peters L, Maas L, Petty D, et al. Spontaneous noncardiac chest pain. Evaluation by 24-hour ambulatory esophageal motility and pH monitoring. Gastroenterology 1988; 94:878.
56. Katz P, Dalton C, Richter J, Wu W, Castell D. Esophageal testing of patients with non-cardiac chest pain or dysphagia–results of three years of experience with 1161 patients. Ann Int Med 1987; 106:593.
57. Richter J, Bradley L, Castell D. Esophageal chest pain: current controversies in pathogenesis, diagnosis and therapy. Ann Int Med 1989; 110:66.
58. Benjamin S, Gerhardt D, Castell D. High amplitude peristaltic contractions associated with chest pain and/or dysphagia. Gastroenterology 1979; 77:478.
59. Hewson E, Sinclair J, Dalton C, Richter J. 24-hour esophageal pH monitoring: the most useful test for evaluating noncardiac chest pain. Am J Med 1991; 90:576.
60. Nevens F, Janssens J, Piessens J, et al. Prospective study on prevalence of esophageal chest pain in patients referred on an elective basis to a cardiac unit for suspected myocardial ischemia. Dig Dis Sci 1991; 36:229.
61. Kahrilas P, Clouse R, Hogan W. American Gastroenterological Association technical review on the clinical use of esophageal manometry. Gastroenterology 1994; 107:1865.
62. Balaban D, Yamamoto Y, Mittal R, et al. Sustained esophageal contraction: a marker of esophageal chest pain identified by intraluminal ultrasonography. Gastroenterology 1999; 116:29.
63. Pehlivanov N, Liu J, Mittal R. Sustained esophageal contraction: a motor correlate of heartburn symptom. Am J Physiol Gastrointest Liver Physiol 2001; 281:G743.
64. Mujica V, Mudipalli R, Rao SSC. Pathophysiology of chest pain in patients with nutcracker esophagus. Am J Gastroenterol 2001; 96:1371.
65. Demeester TR, O'Sullivan G, Bermudez G, et al. Esophageal function in patients with angina-type chest pain and normal coronary angiograms. Ann Surg 1982; 196:488.
66. Fass R, Fennerty B, Ofman J, et al. The clinical and economical value of a short course of omeprazole in patients with noncardiac chest pain. Gastroenterology 1998; 115:42.
67. Achem S, Kolts B, MacMath T, et al. Effects of omeprazole versus placebo in treatment of noncardiac chest pain and gastroesophageal reflux. Dig Dis Sci 1997; 42:2138.
68. Frobert O, Funch-Jensen P, Bagger J. Diagnostic value of esophageal studies in patients with angina-like chest pain and normal coronary angiograms. Ann Int Med 1996; 124:959.
69. Fass R, Tougas G. Functional heartburn: the stimulus, the pain, and the brain. Gut 2002; 51:885.

70. DaCosta J. On irritable heart: a clinical study of a form of functional cardiac disorder and its consequences. Am J Med Sci 1871; 61:17.
71. Clouse R, Lustman P. Psychiatric illness and contraction abnormalities of the esophagus. N Engl J Med 1983; 309:1337.
72. Clouse R, Lustman P, Eckert T, et al. Low dose trazadone for symptomatic patients with esophageal contraction abnormalities: a double-blind placebo-controlled trial. Gastroenterology 1987; 92:1027.
73. Cannon RO III, Benjamin SB. Chest pain as a consequence of abnormal visceral nociception. Dig Dis Sci 1993; 38:193.
74. Fleet R, Dupuis G, Marchand A, et al. Panic disorder in emergency department chest pain patients: prevalence, comorbidity, suicidal ideation and physician recognition. Am J Med 1996; 101:371.

Noncardiac Chest Pain: Clinical Features and Management

Ronnie Fass

The Neuro-Enteric Clinical Research Group, Section of Gastroenterology, Department of Medicine, Southern Arizona VA Health Care System, and University of Arizona Health Sciences Center, Tucson, Arizona, U.S.A.

Ram Dickman

The Neuro-Enteric Clinical Research Group, Southern Arizona VA Health Care System, and University of Arizona Health Sciences Center, Tucson, Arizona, U.S.A.

INTRODUCTION

Noncardiac chest pain (NCCP) is defined as recurring angina-like retrosternal chest pain of noncardiac origin. Patient's history does not reliably distinguish between cardiac and esophageal cause of chest pain (1). This is compounded by the fact that patients with a history of coronary artery disease may also experience chest pain of noncardiac origin. Consequently, an initial evaluation by a cardiologist is needed in all patients with NCCP (2).

NCCP is common in the general population. However, epidemiological studies describing the demographics, such as ethnic, gender, or age distribution as well as potential risk factors for NCCP are still scarce. Furthermore, there are very limited data about referral patterns of patients with NCCP.

An important step forward in understanding the underlying mechanisms of NCCP was the recognition that gastroesophageal reflux disease (GERD) is the most common contributing factor for chest pain. While chest pain has been considered as an atypical manifestation of GERD, it is an integral part of the limited repertoire of symptoms of the esophagus.

HISTORY AND CLINICAL PRESENTATION

Patients with NCCP may report recurring, squeezing, or burning substernal chest pain, which may radiate to the back, neck, arms, and jaws (2). History of retrosternal chest discomfort, pressure or heaviness that lasts several minutes, pain induced by exertion, emotion, exposure to cold, or a large meal, and pain that is relieved by rest or nitroglycerin usually signify typical cardiac angina. Any two of these clinical characteristics are suggestive of atypical cardiac angina and only one or none of these characteristics is indicative of NCCP.

Chest pain is one of the most common reasons for patient visits to emergency room and admissions into coronary care units. However, only 15% to 34% of ambulatory care patients who present with chest pain are ultimately diagnosed with coronary artery disease (3). Importantly, coronary artery disease is found in up to 25% of the patients defined as having atypical chest pain (4). Therefore, all patients who present with chest pain, regardless of its character, should undergo a proper cardiac evaluation before being referred to a gastroenterologist for further work-up.

The clinical attitudes of primary care physicians (PCPs) toward NCCP patients were recently evaluated (5,6). Wong et al. (6), found that most NCCP patients were diagnosed and treated by PCPs (79.5%), without referring them to a gastroenterologist. The most preferred subspecialty for the diagnostic evaluation of a patient presenting with chest pain was cardiology (62%), followed by gastroenterology (17%). However, the mean percentage of such referrals was only 22%. The most preferred subspecialty for further management of a patient with NCCP was gastroenterology (76%), followed by cardiology (8%). However, the mean percentage of actual referral rate was 29.8% for gastroenterologists and 14% for cardiologists (6). Eslick et al. (5) assessed the types of health-care professionals consulted for chest pain. In this study, the main health-care professionals seen were PCPs (85%), cardiologists (74%), and gastroenterologists (30%).

The presence of heartburn and/or acid regurgitation appears to be predictive of GERD-related NCCP, reported in 10% to 70% of the patients with GERD-related NCCP (7). This wide range in the prevalence of associated GERD-related symptoms is probably secondary to an assessment of different patient populations. Patients with GERD-related NCCP often report chest pain provoked by meals or recumbency and relieved by antireflux medications (8). However, many studies reported that the majority of patients who present with GERD-related NCCP lack classic symptoms of GERD (heartburn and acid regurgitation). Additionally, studies of endoscopically evaluated patients with NCCP, revealed a very low incidence of esophageal mucosal injury, such as erosive esophagitis, peptic stricture, ulceration, Barrett's esophagus, or adenocarcinoma of the esophagus (9–11). Consequently, endoscopic screening of NCCP patients, who lack alarm symptoms, is a low-yield procedure.

The impact of NCCP on patients' quality of life is likely to match other functional gastrointestinal (GI) disorders, such as irritable bowel syndrome (IBS). As with other functional bowel disorders, the prognosis of patients with NCCP is favorable. Nevertheless, the natural history of NCCP in most patients is characterized by the persistence of symptoms, repeated clinic visits or hospital admissions, chronic use of medications, repeated cardiac catheterizations, interruptions of daily activities, and impaired quality of life.

EPIDEMIOLOGY

Unfortunately, there are only a few studies that have evaluated the prevalence of NCCP in the general population. The mean annual prevalence of NCCP in six population-based studies was approximately 25%. However, these studies differ in many aspects, such as NCCP definition, geography, sample size, sampling order, and ethnic disparities (3). Some of the important findings of these different population-based studies include: high prevalence rate of NCCP in the general population and decreased prevalence of NCCP with increasing age (12–14). Females under 25 years of age and those between 45 and 55 years of age were found to have the highest prevalence rates of NCCP (15). Kennedy et al. (16) reported that females are more likely to present to hospital emergency rooms with NCCP than males. NCCP patients in Asia are more likely than NCCP patients in Europe to seek medical attention for chest pain (17). In the United States, African-Americans are less likely to report chest pain symptoms than Caucasians (5). To illustrate further how common NCCP is, it is estimated that approximately 65 million subjects in the United States are currently or had been diagnosed with NCCP (mean prevalence of 24%); making NCCP the most common atypical/extraesophageal manifestation of GERD.

While NCCP is very common in the general population, it is still unclear what percentage of patients seek medical attention, and whether the health-care–seeking behavior of these patients differs from those with cardiac-related chest pain. Tew et al. (18) reported that patients with NCCP were younger, consumed greater amounts of alcohol, smoked more, and were more likely to suffer from psychiatric disorder (anxiety) than their counterparts with ischemic heart disease. These patients continued to seek treatment on a regular basis after diagnosis for both chest pain and other unrelated symptoms.

Many patients with NCCP report poor quality of life and admit taking cardiac medications despite lack of evidence for a cardiac cause. Only a small fraction of patients feel reassured. Consequently, NCCP has become a costly disorder, resulting in significant economic burden on the health-care system (5). In one study, the health-care cost for NCCP was estimated at over $315 million annually, primarily because of multiple clinic and emergency room visits, hospitalizations, and prescription medications (19). This cost estimate does not include indirect cost such as lost days of work or intangible cost, such as the impact of symptoms on patients' quality of life, which have been demonstrated to have a significantly greater financial impact than direct cost when evaluating the economic burden of a functional bowel disorder.

DIAGNOSIS
Overview

Currently, the burden of making the diagnosis of NCCP is placed on the cardiologist because symptoms of NCCP are indistinguishable clinically from those of patients with cardiac angina. Once a cardiac cause has been properly excluded, patients may be referred to a gastroenterologist for further evaluation because the esophagus is one of the most common causes of symptoms in patients with NCCP. Other nonesophageal-related abnormalities that make part of the differential diagnosis of chest pain should be ruled out. These include musculoskeletal disorders of the chest, pulmonary/pleuritic abnormalities, panic disorder, and gastric or biliary diseases. Different tests are currently available to assess patients with NCCP (Table 1). The tests are designed primarily to evaluate for gastroesophageal reflux, esophageal dysmotility, and visceral hypersensitivity as the possible underlying mechanism for patient's symptoms.

Although GERD is by far the most common underlying esophageal cause for NCCP, there is currently no gold standard for diagnosing this disorder. The diagnostic tests available for GERD in patients with NCCP include: barium esophagram, upper endoscopy, the acid perfusion test, ambulatory 24-hour esophageal pH monitoring, and the proton pump inhibitor (PPI) test. Most of the tests are not readily available for many physicians and are invasive, costly, and inconvenient to patients. This is compounded by lack of consistent data about the value of these tests in NCCP. Furthermore, the recent introduction of the PPI test has changed the diagnostic and therapeutic approach to NCCP because of its simplicity, reduced cost, and availability at the primary care level. Additionally, the PPI test is highly sensitive and specific and unlike the other tests for NCCP, noninvasive. In patients who failed the PPI test or an empirical therapy with a PPI, pH testing on therapy has been suggested. However, recent studies have demonstrated that most of the patients with NCCP, who failed PPI twice daily, have no evidence of abnormal esophageal acid exposure while on therapy (20).

The role of esophageal manometry in NCCP has been limited in recent years to solely diagnosing achalasia or the related disorder, diffuse esophageal spasm (DES). This is primarily due to lack of association between patients' documented spastic motility disorders and chest pain symptoms. Furthermore, studies have consistently demonstrated that in patients with esophageal motility disorders (except achalasia), pain modulators are more effective in controlling symptoms than smooth muscle relaxants.

Table 1 Diagnostic Tests for Noncardiac Chest Pain

Gastroesophageal reflux
  Barium swallow
  Upper endoscopy
  Acid perfusion test (Bernstein test)
  Ambulatory 24-hour esophageal pH monitoring
  Proton pump inhibitor test
Esophageal dysmotility
  Esophageal manometry
  Edrophonium (Tensilon) test
  Ergonovine test
Visceral hypersensitivity
  Acid perfusion test (Bernstein test)
  Balloon distension test

Diagnostic Tools for Gastroesophageal Reflux Disease-Related Noncardiac Chest Pain

Barium Esophagram

Barium esophagram has a very low sensitivity (20%) in diagnosing GERD-related NCCP, because it is normal in most of the patients (21). Furthermore, the significance of barium reflux during the procedure as diagnostic of GERD is questionable. Johnston et al. (22) found that the proportion of patients with spontaneous barium reflux and abnormal pH test is similar to controls with normal 24-hour esophageal pH monitoring. Furthermore, spontaneous barium reflux has also been demonstrated in up to 20% of healthy subjects (23).

The role of barium esophagram in patients with GERD-related NCCP is likely limited to those who also report dysphagia. In these patients, barium esophagram may be ordered as the first diagnostic test in order to serve as a "road map" for future upper endoscopy.

Upper Endoscopy

Upper endoscopy is the gold standard for diagnosing esophageal mucosal involvement in NCCP. Upper endoscopy can diagnose erosive esophagitis, peptic stricture, esophageal ulcer, and Barrett's esophagus. Additionally, in the presence of alarm symptoms (weight loss, dysphagia, vomiting, and anemia) upper endoscopy should be considered as the initial evaluative test to exclude malignancy as well as other mucosal disorders of the upper gut. However, most patients with GERD-related NCCP do not demonstrate esophageal mucosal injury. Thus, endoscopy has been considered noncontributory as the initial diagnostic test in NCCP (22,23). Interestingly, despite the limited clinical value, community-based gastroenterologists still commonly use endoscopy as the initial diagnostic test in NCCP, regardless of whether alarm symptoms are reported (24).

Ambulatory 24-Hour Esophageal pH Monitoring

Ambulatory 24-hour esophageal pH monitoring with symptom correlation [symptom index (SI)] is commonly used to diagnose GERD-related NCCP. SI is the percentage of symptoms that correlate with acid reflux events. Reported sensitivity and specificity of the test in GERD patients has ranged from 60% to 96% and 85% to 100%, respectively (23). However, there are currently no studies that assess the sensitivity of the test in NCCP patients. Additionally, the test is invasive, costly, inconvenient to most patients, and unavailable for many physicians.

It has been estimated that up to 60% of NCCP patients have pathological esophageal acid exposure or a positive SI alone. Hewson et al. (25) examined 100 consecutive patients with NCCP and detected abnormal esophageal acid exposure in 48 patients (48%). Of the 83 patients with spontaneous chest pain during the pH test, 37 patients (46%) had abnormal pH test parameters, and 50 patients (60%) had a positive SI. In contrast, Dekel et al. (26) found that only a minority of NCCP patients have a positive SI (19% in GERD-related NCCP and 10.6% in non–GERD-related NCCP), primarily because most subjects did not experience chest pain during the pH study.

A wireless system for pH monitoring was recently introduced into the market. It involves the per oral or transnasal insertion of a radiotelemetry pH capsule and its attachment onto the esophageal mucosa. The pH capsule measures intraesophageal pH and simultaneously transmits recorded data to a pager-sized receiver clipped onto the patient's belt, thereby circumventing the need for a nasally placed catheter, which is uncomfortable for many patients. In comparison with the conventional pH test, the wireless pH monitoring is better tolerated (6). The wireless pH system may prove to be helpful in further clarifying the extent of GERD in NCCP and in better determining the relationship between chest pain symptoms and acid reflux events. A recent study demonstrated that the 48 hours recording provided by the wireless pH capsule improves the assessment of sensed acid reflux events (27).

Since the introduction of the PPI test, the role of pH testing in NCCP has significantly diminished. Additionally, studies have suggested that the sensitivity of the PPI test is similar to the sensitivity of the pH test (9).

Acid Perfusion Test (Bernstein Test)

The acid perfusion test was originally devised to distinguish between chest pain of cardiac and esophageal origin. The basic principal of the test is to assess objectively the esophageal chemosensitivity to acid exposure (28). Fass et al. (29) placed a manometry catheter 10 cm above the upper border of the lower esophageal sphincter (LES) to ensure sufficient exposure of the esophageal mucosa to acid. Saline was infused initially for two minutes and then without the patient's knowledge, 0.1 N HCl was infused for 10 minutes at a rate of 10 mL per minute. Patients were instructed to report whenever their typical symptoms were reproduced. Esophageal chemosensitivity to acid was assessed by both the duration until typical symptom perception was induced (expressed in seconds) and the total sensory intensity rating reported by the subject at the end of acid perfusion by using a verbal descriptor scale.

The acid perfusion test is highly specific but the sensitivity ranges from 6% to 60%. A negative test has no clinical relevance and does not exclude esophageal origin for patients' chest pain.

Presently, the acid perfusion test is rarely performed in clinical practice because of its limited diagnostic value in NCCP and other esophageal disorders. Because of the low sensitivity and the emergence of noninvasive modalities, such as the PPI test and empirical therapy with PPI, many authors have considered the acid perfusion test to be obsolete.

The Proton Pump Inhibitor Test

The limitations of the currently available diagnostic modalities for GERD-related NCCP make a therapeutic trial with a PPI an attractive option. The test uses a short course of high-dose PPI in diagnosing GERD-related NCCP. Overall, the PPI test is a simple, readily available and clinically practical diagnostic tool (30). However, no standardized use of the PPI test has been documented in the literature.

The main requirement of a therapeutic trial is to achieve a significant improvement in symptoms of as many patients as possible within a relatively short period of drug administration. Thus far, only PPIs have been used in studies assessing therapeutic trials, because of their profound and consistent effect on acid secretion (24,31–36). Originally, omeprazole was the first PPI used as a test in NCCP patients leading to the term "the omeprazole test."

The sensitivity of the PPI test for GERD-related NCCP ranges from 69% to 95% and the specificity from 67% to 86% (10,31,32,37–40). The dosages of PPIs used ranged from 60 to 80 mg daily for omeprazole; 30 to 90 mg daily for lansoprazole; and 40 mg daily for rabeprazole. The trial duration ranged from 1 to 28 days (Fig. 1).

In a double-blind, placebo-controlled trial, Fass et al. randomized 37 patients with NCCP to either placebo or high-dose omeprazole (40 mg in the morning, and 20 mg in the evening) for seven days (24). After a washout period and repeated baseline symptom assessment, patients crossed over to the opposite arm. The PPI test was considered positive if the chest pain improved by at least 50% after treatment. The combination of upper endoscopy and 24-hour esophageal pH monitoring was used as the gold standard. Sixty-two percent (23/37) of the patients had evidence of GERD. Of the GERD-positive group, 78.3% had a positive PPI test, and 22.7% had a positive placebo response. In contrast, of the GERD-negative group, 14.2% had a positive PPI test, and 7.1% had a positive placebo response. Thus, the calculated sensitivity was 78.3%, specificity 85.7%, and the positive predictive value 90% (24). Using similar design, other investigators confirmed the usefulness of the PPI test for diagnosing GERD-related NCCP (10,38). Furthermore, in subsequent studies, Fass et al. demonstrated that therapeutic trials with lansoprazole and rabeprazole achieve similar efficacy for the diagnosis of GERD-related NCCP (40,41). A recent study in the Chinese population showed that the PPI test, using lansoprazole 30 mg daily for a period of four weeks, was useful in diagnosing endoscopy-negative GERD-related NCCP (10).

When using the PPI test, there was a significant correlation between the extent of esophageal acid exposure in the distal esophagus as determined by ambulatory 24-hour esophageal pH monitoring and the change in symptom intensity score after treatment, suggesting that the higher the esophageal acid exposure, the greater the response to the PPI test in patients with GERD-related NCCP (42).

Economic analysis showed that the PPI test for GERD-related NCCP is a cost-saving approach primarily due to a significant reduction in the usage of various costly and invasive diagnostic tests (24).

Multichannel Intraluminal Impedance

Impedance probes with integrated pH sensor allowed further assessment of esophageal function as well as refluxate composition and its relationship to symptoms (43,44). Because the

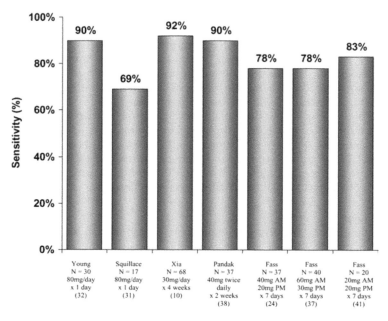

Figure 1 Reported sensitivity of the proton pump inhibitor test in noncardiac chest pain by different investigators.

electrical conductivity of the esophageal muscular wall, air, and any given bolus is different, the presence of different substances in the esophageal lumen provides a different impedance pattern (44). With a highly conductive bolus (e.g., saliva), the impedance decreases; with poorly conductive material (e.g., air) the impedance increases (45,46).

The combination of impedance catheter and a pH probe provides a unique opportunity to study physiological events within the esophagus and their relationship to symptoms. In addition, the recording assembly can disclose the characteristics of the gastric refluxate (acid, nonacid, gas, liquid, and mixed gas and liquid). The value of such a technique has been demonstrated by recent studies that documented that nonacid reflux is not uncommon in GERD patients and may lead to classic heartburn symptoms (43,44). However, thus far, there are no studies that have evaluated the value of multichannel intraluminal impedance in patients with NCCP.

Diagnostic Tools for Esophageal Dysmotility
Esophageal Manometry

Chest pain only, or more commonly in combination with other esophageal-related symptoms, may be caused by various esophageal motility abnormalities. These include DES, nutcracker esophagus, achalasia, long-duration contractions, multipeaked waves, and hypertensive LES (Fig. 2) (49).

However, the reported sensitivity of esophageal manometry appears to be very low in evaluating patients with NCCP. In fact, most patients with NCCP who have been evaluated by esophageal manometry demonstrate normal esophageal motor function. Furthermore, patients rarely experience chest pain during esophageal manometry regardless if esophageal dysmotility is documented (50). To improve the sensitivity of the test in patients with NCCP, some authorities have suggested prolonging the duration of the test to 24 hours. However, the results from this approach vary considerably (51,52). A significant number of patients reported no symptoms at all during the recording period (only 27–43% reported symptoms during the test). Moreover, the investigators were able to relate the pain episodes to a recorded esophageal dysmotility in only 13% to 24% of the patients. These results question the routine usage in clinical practice of ambulatory 24-hour esophageal manometry for the evaluation of patients with NCCP.

Presently, patients who did not respond to antireflux treatment (non–GERD-related NCCP) are likely to undergo manometry. However, it was found that NCCP patients with

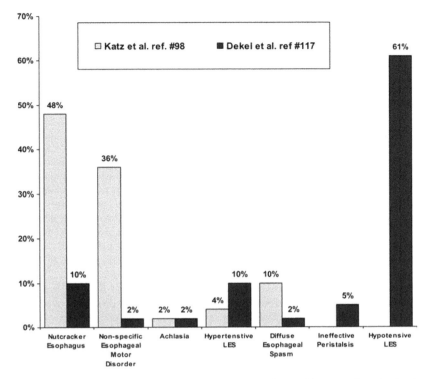

Figure 2 Distribution of esophageal dysmotility in patients with noncardiac chest pain and abnormal esophageal manometry as reported by two studies. *Abbreviation*: LES, lower esophageal sphincter. *Source*: From Refs. 47,48.

esophageal motility abnormalities (primarily spastic motor disorders), other than achalasia, responded better to pain modulators than to any of the smooth muscle relaxants. As a result, the usefulness of esophageal manometry in NCCP is likely limited to excluding achalasia as the underlying cause of patients' chest pain.

Edrophonium Test (Tensilon Test)
Edrophonium is an anticholinesterase that increases cholinergic activity at muscarinic receptors (53). Its effect occurs within 30 to 60 seconds after injection and lasts for an average period of 10 minutes. The test is used to induce greater esophageal body amplitude contractions in the hope of provoking patient's typical chest pain (54). During the test, either 80 mg/kg or a total of 10 mg edrophonium is injected intravenously, immediately followed by 5 to 10 swallows of 5 to 10 mL of water over a period of 5 to 10 minutes. Commonly, subjects experience pain within five minutes after administration of the edrophonium test. Because of the rapid metabolism of edrophonium, pain usually resolves quickly. Side effects may include increased salivation, nausea, vomiting, and abdominal cramps, which are chiefly due to an excessive cholinergic stimulation. Overall, side effects are minimal and the antidote atropine is rarely needed. The drug seems to have no effect on coronary artery diameter (55).

The reported sensitivity of the edrophonium test in NCCP has varied from 9% to 55% (56,57). The exact sensitivity is unknown because of the lack of a gold standard. Overall, it seems that if the edrophonium test is positive, then the esophagus is the likely origin of chest pain. However, due to lack of differences in esophageal contractile activity after the edrophonium test between NCCP patients and normal healthy subjects, several authorities have suggested to perform the test with concomitant esophageal manometry.

Other Provocative Tests
The intravenous ergonovine stimulation test causes chest pain in NCCP patients by inducing an augmented esophageal motor activity (19). Ergonovine is a sympathomimetic agent that is used by cardiologists to diagnose Prinzmetal angina. The drug has been shown to induce chest

pain in patients with NCCP and demonstrated similar sensitivity as edrophonium. Presently, ergonovine is rarely used for esophageal testing due to potential serious side effects, including severe cardiac effects and even death.

The bethanechol test is presently rarely performed in clinical practice because of its questionable diagnostic value and frequent side effects.

Additionally, unlike GERD, we still lack highly effective drugs that can easily correct motility abnormalities and consequently can be used to demonstrate a causal relationship.

Diagnostic Tools for Visceral Hypersensitivity
Balloon Distension

Balloon studies are primarily designed to assess the presence of visceral hyperalgesia in various functional bowel disorders. Early studies with intraesophageal balloon distension demonstrated that pain develops more frequently in NCCP patients than in normal controls, and that their pain occurs at lower balloon volumes (58,59). Balloon distension has been used primarily in the setting of research protocols in order to determine perception thresholds for pain. This modality has been used extensively in studies assessing various functional bowel disorders, most notably, IBS and functional dyspepsia (58,60,61). Additionally, balloon distension has been commonly used to evaluate the effect of various drugs on esophageal perception thresholds for pain in normal controls or patients with NCCP (62).

Early data indicated that, in patients with documented ischemic heart disease, balloon distension of the esophagus produced pain indistinguishable from anginal pain, but without electrocardiogram changes (63). This may be explained by convergence of sensory pathways at the level of the spinal cord or the midbrain. Despite the similarity in pain, it seems that esophageal distension has no effect on coronary blood flow (64).

The procedure includes the insertion of a manometric catheter that is connected to a latex balloon, into the esophagus. The balloon is positioned 10 cm above the LES and distended in a stepwise fashion using an electronic barostat (65). The basic principle of the barostat is to maintain a constant pressure within the balloon/bag in the lumen despite muscular contractions and relaxations or changes in compliance of the esophageal wall (65,66).

The usage of balloon distension protocols in clinical practice has been hampered by limited expertise, cost, concerns about adverse events (such as perforation), and unclear clinical utility.

Impedance Planimetry

This technique was introduced for the assessment of biomechanical characteristics of the esophagus (67,68). The system includes a thin latex balloon, which is used to assess esophageal sensory thresholds. Balloon pressure was increased stepwise by 5 cm H_2O increments from 0 to determine sensory thresholds for pain in several studies (43,68–70). After each inflation, the balloon is completely deflated for a rest period of three minutes. Balloon distensions are maintained each for three to five minutes. In this protocol, at each level of distension, the cross-sectional area is measured and sensory response is determined using verbal descriptor. Presently, impedance planimetry is used for research purposes only, and it is unlikely to find its way into clinical practice.

Brain Imaging

Brain–gut relationship in patients with esophageal disorders is an area of intense research. The GI tract is intricately connected to the central nervous system by pathways that are continuously sampling and modulating gut function (71). Imaging techniques such as positron emission tomography (PET) and functional magnetic resonance imaging (fMRI) have been increasingly used to evaluate the brain–gut axis.

PET scanning is an established method to study the functional neuroanatomy of the human brain (72,73). Radiolabeled compounds allow the study of biochemical and physiologic processes involved in cerebral metabolism (71). Topographic images represent spatial distribution of radioisotopes in the brain. Regional cerebral blood flow is studied with labeled water ($H_2^{15}O$) and glucose metabolism with ^{18}Fl-labeled fluorodeoxyglucose. Unlike PET, fMRI does not require radioisotopes, and hence is considered a safer imaging technique. fMRI detects increase in oxygen concentration in areas of heightened neuronal activity (73–75).

This imaging technique is best suited for locating the site, but not the sequence or duration of neuronal activity. Overall, fMRI provides both anatomic and functional information.

Further studies are needed to assess cerebral activation in patients with different esophageal disorders. In addition, it would be of great interest to determine whether there are differences in central processing of an intraesophageal stimulus in patients with NCCP. It is also important to begin to examine the role of psychophysiologic states such as stress, anxiety, and depression and their effects on central nuclei involved with perception of esophageal stimuli.

Psychological Evaluation

Some of the patients with NCCP require psychological evaluation by an expert psychologist or psychiatrist, because of the high prevalence rate of psychological abnormalities in this group of patients. Deciding who should be referred is individually determined, but the likely candidates are those who appear to be refractory to therapeutic interventions or those that display clear features of a psychological disorder. Physicians can use a structured psychiatric interview to determine if psychological comorbidity is present (76). There are various diagnostic psychological tools, such as the Symptom Checklist-90R (SCL-90R) and the Beck Depression Inventory questionnaires that can be used at the clinical level, but are unlikely to find a place in a busy GI practice. Regardless, when evaluating a patient with NCCP, the presence of coexisting psychological comorbidity should always be entertained.

TREATMENT
Overview

Treatment in NCCP should be directed to the likely underlying mechanism of patients' symptoms (Table 2). Treatment of gastroesophageal reflux has been repeatedly shown to be effective in relieving symptoms of patients with GERD-related NCCP. For patients with non–GERD-related NCCP, pain modulators are the mainstay of therapy. In contrast, muscle relaxants have shown only a limited efficacy in patients with esophageal dysmotility. Figure 3 provides a suggested treatment algorithm.

Treatment of Gastroesophageal Reflux Disease-Related Noncardiac Chest Pain

The treatment of GERD should involve lifestyle modifications and pharmacological intervention. Lifestyle modifications such as elevating the head of the bed at night, reducing fat intake, smoking cessation, and avoiding foods that exacerbate gastroesophageal reflux may decrease reflux-related symptoms (77). Unlike classical GERD, we are still devoid of studies assessing the specific value of lifestyle modifications in patients with GERD-related NCCP.

Most of the studies that compared histamine-2 receptor antagonists (H$_2$RA) to placebo or omeprazole are small and uncontrolled. The reported efficacy of H$_2$RAs in GERD-related NCCP has ranged from 54% to 83% (78). As compared with PPIs, H$_2$RAs have demonstrated a limited response in patients with NCCP. In one study, 13 patients with GERD-related NCCP were treated with high-dose ranitidine (150 mg qid) for a period of eight weeks (79). Of those,

Table 2 Proposed Underlying Mechanisms of Noncardiac Chest Pain

Gastroesophageal reflux
Esophageal dysmotility
Abnormal mechanophysical properties
   Hyperactive
   Compliance
Sustained longitudinal muscle contractions
Visceral hypersensitivity
Altered central processing of visceral stimuli
Altered autonomic activity
Psychological abnormalities
   Panic attack
   Anxiety
   Depression

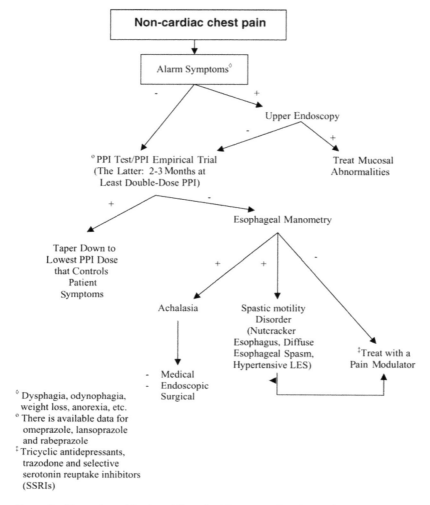

Figure 3 Diagnosis and treatment flow chart for noncardiac chest pain. *Abbreviations*: PPI, proton pump inhibitor; LES, lower esophageal sphincter.

seven patients failed lower doses of ranitidine previously. Whilst all patients improved with high-dose ranitidine, two patients required 300 mg four times daily. DeMeester et al. (80) followed 23 patients with GERD-related NCCP for two to three years. Twelve patients were treated medically with antacids and cimetidine, and 11 were treated with an antireflux surgical procedure. Of the medically treated patients, only five (42%) were chest pain free at follow-up. Overall, H_2RAs provide very limited benefit to patients with GERD-related NCCP primarily due to rapid development of tolerance and a relatively short duration of action. Tolerance to these drugs generally develops within two weeks of repeated administration, resulting in a decline in the acid suppression effect (81).

PPI therapy, on the other hand, results in a more profound and longer duration of acid suppression, and tolerance has not been observed. In one study, omeprazole 20 mg twice daily was administered over a period of eight weeks to GERD-related NCCP patients in a double-blind, placebo-controlled trial. Those who received omeprazole had a significant reduction in the number of days with chest pain when compared with patients who received placebo. Although data regarding the long-term efficacy of PPIs in NCCP are limited to omeprazole, it is highly likely that all other PPIs will demonstrate similar benefits (82). Patients with GERD-related NCCP should be treated initially with at least double-dose PPI until symptoms remit, followed by dose tapering to determine the lowest PPI dose that controls patient's symptoms.

As with other extraesophageal manifestations of GERD, NCCP patients may require more than two months of therapy for optimal symptom control. Long-term treatment with a PPI has been shown to be highly efficacious (83). Borzecki et al. (84) developed a decision analysis that compared empirical treatment for NCCP patients with H_2RAs or standard dose PPI for eight weeks versus initial investigation (upper endoscopy or upper GI series). The cost of empirical therapy was $849 per patient versus $2187 per patient for an initial investigative strategy.

Very few studies have examined the value of laparoscopic Nissen fundoplication in patients with GERD-related NCCP. Patti et al. (85) followed patients with chest pain and other GERD-related symptoms, who underwent antireflux surgery. In patients who did not report episodes of chest pain during the preoperative pH study, surgery resulted in improvement of this symptom in 65% of the patients. However, the response rate was 96% in those patients whose chest pain correlated with gastroesophageal reflux events during preoperative testing. Farrell et al. (86) evaluated the effectiveness of antireflux surgery in patients with atypical manifestations of GERD. Chest pain improved in 90% of the patients with complete symptom resolution reported by 50% of the patients. Although these surgical studies demonstrate a high success rate of antireflux surgery in GERD-related NCCP patients, it should be borne in mind that the patients included were usually carefully selected.

Several endoscopic techniques designed to bolster the antireflux barrier at the gastroesophageal junction are under investigation (87). There are three basic types of endoscopic treatments: suturing, radiofrequency, and injection (88). Sham trials with all endoscopic techniques revealed subjective improvement (heartburn severity, quality of life, etc.), but little or no objective improvement (esophageal acid exposure, PPI consumption, LES basal pressure, etc.). No studies thus far have specifically evaluated patients with GERD-related NCCP. These endoscopic methods are still considered experimental and should not be routinely performed even in patients with confirmed GERD-related NCCP until further data are obtained.

Treatment of Esophageal Dysmotility

The treatment of esophageal dysmotility in patients with NCCP remains an area of intense controversy. This is primarily due to mounting data that patients with NCCP and spastic motility disorders other than achalasia respond better to pain modulators than to muscle relaxants. Furthermore, response to pain modulators in NCCP patients appears to be unrelated to the presence or absence of esophageal dysmotility. This is compounded by lack of an effective treatment for esophageal spastic motility disorders.

Esophageal motor disorders associated with NCCP includes nutcracker esophagus, nonspecific esophageal motility disorders, DES, hypertensive LES, and achalasia (48). Manometrically defined as high amplitude contractions in the distal esophagus (greater than 180 mmHg), nutcracker esophagus remains an area of intense controversy. Investigators have long argued about the clinical relevance of such a manometric phenomenon (39). However, Achem et al. (89) reported that most patients with chest pain associated with nutcracker esophagus responded symptomatically to antireflux treatment. Normalization of the nutcracker motility phenomenon was documented only in the minority of the patients, suggesting that GERD was the likely cause of their symptoms rather than the high amplitude contractions in the distal esophagus. Thus, in patients with nutcracker esophagus, antireflux treatment should be tried first, before smooth muscle relaxants are considered (90). Smooth muscle relaxants have a limited role, if any, in patients with NCCP and esophageal dysmotility.

Data supporting the usage of nitrates are scarce and not uncommonly based on anecdotal experience. Sublingual nitroglycerin and long-acting nitrate preparations appear to have no effect on esophageal amplitude contractions of healthy subjects (91). In a case report, 0.4 mg sublingual nitroglycerin was reported to have a short-lived effect on esophageal dysmotility that was associated with relief of chest pain (92). Reports about the value of long-acting nitrates in patients with NCCP and esophageal dysmotility are conflicting. In an old study, the authors reported complete symptom resolution of chest pain with sublingual nitroglycerin and isosorbide dinitrate during a period of up to seven years (93). However, other investigators were unable to reproduce these findings (94).

Calcium channel blockers (diltiazem, nifedipine, and verapamil) are the most studied smooth muscle relaxants in patients with NCCP and presumed esophageal dysmotility. These drugs, although commonly used in clinical practice, appear to be of limited value in this condition. Furthermore, their usage might be complicated by side effects, such as hypotension, constipation, and pedal edema. In small clinical trials, diltiazem 60 to 90 mg four times daily has been shown significantly to improve chest pain score in patients with NCCP and documented nutcracker esophagus on esophageal manometry (95,96). Nifedipine (10–30 mg trice daily) also demonstrated a limited symptomatic response in patients with NCCP and nutcracker esophagus (97). The drug provided symptom improvement that lasted only two weeks and was noted only after a lag time of three weeks. By the end of the sixth week of therapy, the drug appeared to lose its efficacy completely. The limited effect of calcium channel blockers on symptoms was also demonstrated in NCCP patients with other spastic motility disorders (95,98,99).

Data about the usage of other therapeutic modalities in NCCP patients with esophageal dysmotility are even scarcer. The antispasmodic cimetropium bromide was used in eight patients with NCCP and nutcracker esophagus (100). The drug reduced esophageal amplitude contraction, but it is unclear if chest pain improved as well. Hydralazine, a hypertensive drug that directly dilates peripheral vessels, was shown to improve chest pain and dysphagia as well as decrease the amplitude and duration of esophageal contractions in five patients with NCCP (94).

Botulinum toxin binds irreversibly to acetylcholine-containing neurons, interfering with the release of the neurotransmitter. When injected into the LES in patients with achalasia, the toxin decreases LES basal pressure and consequently improves symptoms. Botulinum toxin injection into the LES was used in a few uncontrolled trials that included patients with NCCP and documented esophageal spastic motility disorder. Injection of botulinum toxin into the LES in one study resulted in 50% reduction of chest pain in 72% of the subjects (101). A total of 100 units of botulinum toxin were injected circumferentially, using five injections at the gastroesophageal junction of 20 units each. In this study, the mean chest pain free duration was seven months. However, 50% of the patients required a second intervention to maintain remission, such as repeat botulinum toxin injection (43%), pneumatic dilation, and bougienage. Overall, it appears that botulinum toxin injection may lead to a short-term symptomatic improvement in NCCP patients with spastic esophageal motility disorders but controlled trials are needed.

Similarly, the role of pneumatic dilation or long esophageal myotomy (Heller myotomy) with or without antireflux surgery in patients with NCCP and nonachalasic dysmotility remains controversial and is best avoided.

Treatment of Visceral Hypersensitivity

Pain modulators or visceral analgesics have been shown to improve symptoms significantly in NCCP patients as compared to placebo. Several classes of drugs have been evaluated and they include the tricyclic antidepressants (TCAs), trazodone, selective serotonin reuptake inhibitors (SSRI), and theophylline. Antidepressants have been used as pain modulators for almost two decades to treat patients with chest pain of a presumed esophageal origin.

The mechanism by which tricyclics reduce visceral pain remains poorly understood. Some authors suggested a central effect, while others a peripheral effect (89). Regardless, TCAs demonstrate a varied receptor affinity to acetylcholine, histamine 1 and α adrenergic receptors (89). Nortriptyline and desipramine are secondary amines (metabolites of tertiary amines) that have less affinity to receptors that result in bothersome side effects (102). The tertiary amines include amitriptyline, imipramine, doxepin, and others. Imipramine has been shown to increase esophageal perception thresholds for pain in normal subjects, without affecting esophageal tone, suggesting a visceral analgesic effect (103). A similar effect that was independent of cardiac, esophageal, or psychiatric testing results at baseline was noted in NCCP patients (62). Additionally, TCAs provide a long-term effect in NCCP patients, although dropout rate due to side effects may reach 30% (104). Treatment with TCAs should start at a low dose (10–25 mg) that is administered at bedtime, and then increased by 10 to 25 mg increments per week to a non–mood-altering goal of 50 to 75 mg per day (102). Because of the varied effect of tricyclics on their respective receptors, failure of one tricyclic to improve symptoms is not indicative of future failure of other tricyclics.

The usage of SSRIs in NCCP has scarcely been studied. As with the TCAs, a neuromodulatory effect has been proposed to mediate their effect on visceral pain. Varia et al. (105)

conducted a randomized, double blind, placebo-controlled trial that assessed the efficacy, tolerability, and safety of the SSRI sertraline in patients with NCCP. Patients were randomly selected to receive sertraline or placebo in doses starting at 50 mg daily and adjusted to a maximum of 200 mg. Dosage was adjusted by the investigator based on patient's clinical response. By using intention-to-treat analysis, investigators have demonstrated that patients receiving sertraline reported a significant reduction in their pain scores as compared with those who received placebo, regardless of concomitant improvement in psychological scores (106). The study confirms the potential role of SSRIs in treatment of patients with non–GERD-related NCCP.

Low-dose trazodone (100-150 mg/day), an antidepressant and anxiolytic, has been shown to improve symptoms of non-GERD-related NCCP patients with esophageal dysmotility, without affecting esophageal amplitude contractions. Clouse et al. (104) in a double blind, placebo-controlled trial (100-150 mg/day) treated 15 patients with NCCP and esophageal dysmotility with trazodone for six weeks and compared their response with that of 14 patients received placebo. The treatment group demonstrated a significantly greater global improvement compared with the placebo group suggesting that trazodone may be of therapeutic value in patients with NCCP and esophageal spastic motility disorders (64-12). Information about other compounds with visceral analgesic effect has been limited to isolated reports in the literature. Infusion of theophylline in an open-labeled trial alleviated chest pain in patients with functional chest pain of presumed esophageal origin (107). It is assumed that theophylline improves esophageal pain by blocking adenosine receptors. Using a balloon distension protocol, octreotide (a somatostatin analog) given subcutaneously (100 mg) has been shown to increase esophageal perception thresholds for pain in normal subjects (108). The effect is unrelated to a change in esophageal compliance.

Table 3 summarizes the medical therapeutic modalities for NCCP.

Treatment of Psychological Comorbidity

A subset of patients with NCCP may report psychological or psychiatric abnormalities, as either the cause or an effect of their chest pain. Reassurance about the benign nature of the disorder has been emphasized as an important mode of early therapeutic intervention in patients with NCCP. However, patients' symptoms are seldom relieved by reassurance only, resulting in the need for additional therapeutic modalities (109). In patients who suffer from panic disorder, treatment with alprazolam and clonazepam has been demonstrated to reduce panic attack frequency, chest pain episodes, and anxiety scores (110,111). However, benzodiazepines should be used cautiously in NCCP patients, primarily due to their addictive effect. Studies with buspirone, an anxiolytic without dependency potential, in patients with NCCP are still unavailable (102).

Table 3 Medical Therapeutic Modalities for Noncardiac Chest Pain

Gastroesophageal reflux	
Proton pump inhibitors	
Omeprazole (Prilosec)	20 mg PO b.i.d.
Rabeprazole (Aciphex)	20 mg PO b.i.d.
Pantoprazole (Protonix)	40 mg PO b.i.d.
Lansoprazole (Prevacid)	30 mg PO b.i.d.
Esomeprazole (Nexium)	40 mg PO b.i.d.
Esophageal dysmotility	
Diltiazem (Cardizem)	60–90 mg PO q.i.d.
Nifedipine (Adalate/Procardia)	10–30 mg PO t.i.d.
Isosorbide dinitrate (Isordil)	10–20 mg PO b.i.d.– t.i.d.
Visceral hypersensitivity	
Tricyclics (commonly used)	50 mg PO q.h.
Nortriptyline (Aventyl/Pamelor)	
Amitriptyline (Elavil/Endep)	
Doxepin (Sinequan)	
Trazodone (Desyrel)	100–150 mg PO q.d.
Sertraline (Zoloft)	50–200 mg PO q.d.

Young patients and males with NCCP appear to be open to medical psychological treatment (112). However, management of psychological comorbidity in these patients should be reserved for experts in the field. That includes prescribing medications for panic attack, depression, and anxiety.

Several studies have suggested that behavioral therapy can be effective in patients with NCCP. Hegel et al. reported about three patients with chest pain and anxiety disorder who were treated with muscle relaxation techniques and controlled diaphragmatic breathing exercise (the techniques were practiced during increasingly complex activities) (113). Two of the patients had substantial reduction in the frequency and intensity of their chest pain that was maintained for 12 months after treatment. Klimes et al. performed the only controlled study of behavioral therapy in patients with chest pain (114). This treatment consisted of education, controlled breathing, training in relaxation and diversion of attention from pain, and practice of the newly learned skills in their home environment. When compared with controls, who were on a waiting list, the treatment program resulted in a significant improvement in chest pain episodes, functional disability, and psychological distress that was maintained for 46 months past intervention.

Future Therapy

Future research in NCCP will continue to focus on mechanisms for pain and will attempt to identify new therapeutic modalities aimed to reduce visceral pain. Research will likely concentrate primarily on the role of central and peripheral sensitization in enhancing perception of intraesophageal stimuli. Furthermore, currently available treatments for other functional GI disorders, such as IBS and nonulcer dyspepsia, may be tested in NCCP as well (44).

Alosetron, a 5-hydroxytryptamine (5HT) type 3 antagonist, which was previously available for the treatment of female patients with diarrhea-predominant IBS, raised the hope for a therapeutic potential in patients with NCCP (115). This serotonin-related class of drugs appears to have a pain-modulatory effect, probably by altering the initiation, transmission, or processing of extrinsic sensory information from the GI tract. New $5HT_3$ antagonists with improved safety profile are in development and may eventually play a therapeutic role in non–GERD-related NCCP. The role of the new partial 5HT type 4 agonist, tegaserod, in modulating pain that originates form the esophagus remains to be elucidated.

Phosphorylation of N-methyl-d-asparate (NMDA) receptors expressed by dorsal-horn neurons leads to central sensitization via increase in their excitability and receptive field size (116). Potentially, this central sensitization may be prevented or even reversed by antagonism of NMDA receptors within the spinal cord. However, it is important to remember that central nervous system mechanisms that mediate visceral hyperalgesia are sensitive to both NMDA and non-NMDA receptor antagonists (6).

Other neuromodulators such as fedotozine and asimadoline, kappa opioid receptor agonists (produce a peripheral antinociceptive effect in patients with IBS); neurokinin receptor antagonists, NK_1 and NK_2 (reduce gut motility and pain) and cholecystokinin-A receptor antagonist, loxiglumide, may all have a future role in non–GERD-related NCCP.

Lastly, acid pump antagonists (APAs) are likely to be introduced into the market by the end of 2010. This class of drugs, which exhibits a rapid onset of action independent of meal stimulation, predictable dose response effect and profound acid secretion blockage, may play an important role in GERD-related NCCP as a diagnostic tool (the "APA test") or as an improved short- and long-term treatment for GERD-related NCCP.

SUMMARY

NCCP is the most common atypical/extraesophageal manifestation of GERD. Diagnosis in the last decade has shifted primarily to noninvasive modalities—the PPI test or the PPI empirical trial. The new role of pH testing in NCCP patients is under evaluation. The role of esophageal manometry has been limited to diagnosing achalasia.

The availability of highly potent antireflux medications has improved our capability to treat patients with GERD-related NCCP. In those patients with non–GERD-related NCCP, regardless if esophageal dysmotility is present or absent, pain modulators remain the cornerstone of therapy.

REFERENCES

1. Nevens F, Janssens J, Piessens J, et al. Prospective study on prevalence of esophageal chest pain in patients referred on an elective basis to a cardiac unit for suspected myocardial ischemia. Dig Dis Sci 1991; 36:229–235.
2. Richter JE. Chest pain and gastroesophageal reflux disease. J Clin Gastroenterol 2000; 30:S39–S41.
3. Katerndahl DA, Trammell C. Prevalence and recognition of panic states in STARNET patients presenting with chest pain. J Fam Pract 1997; 45:54–63.
4. Faybush EM, Fass R. Gastroesophageal reflux disease in noncardiac chest pain. Gastroenterol Clin North Am 2004; 33:41–54.
5. Eslick GD, Talley NJ. Non-cardiac chest pain: predictors of health care seeking, the types of health care professional consultation, work absenteeism and interruption of dial activities. Aliment Pharmacol Ther 2004; 20:909–915.
6. Wong WM, Beeler J, Risner-Adler S, et al. Attitudes and referral patterns of primary care physicians when evaluating subjects with noncardiac chest pain - a national survey. Dig Dis Sci 2005; 50.
7. Richter JE. Extraesophageal presentations of gastroesophageal reflux disease: an overview. Am J Gastroenterol 2000; 95(suppl):S1–S3.
8. Shrestha S, Pasricha PJ. Update on noncardiac chest pain. Dig Dis 2000; 18:138–146.
9. Fass R, Ofman JJ, Sample, et al. The omeprazole test is as sensitive as 24-h oesophageal pH monitoring in diagnosing gastro-oesophageal reflux disease in symptomatic patients with erosive oesophagitis. Aliment Pharmacol Ther 2000; 14:389–396.
10. Xia HH, Lai KC, Lam SK, et al. Symptomatic response to lansoprazole predicts abnormal acid reflux in endoscopy-negative patients with non-cardiac chest pain. Aliment Pharmacol Ther 2003; 17:369–377.
11. Garcia-Compean D, Gonzalez MV, Galindo G, et al. Prevalence of gastroesophageal reflux disease in patients with extraesophageal symptoms referred from otolaryngology, allergy, and cardiology practices: a prospective study. Dig Dis 2000; 18:178–182.
12. Locke G III, Talley NJ, Fett S, et al. Prevalence and clinical spectrum of gastroesophageal reflux: a population-based study in Olmsted County, Minnesota. Gastroenterology 1997; 112:1448–1456.
13. Drossman DA, Li Z, Andruzzi E, et al. U.S. householder survey of Univ gastrointestinal disorders. Prevalence, sociodemography, and health impact. Dig Dis Sci 1993; 38:1569–1580.
14. Eslick GD. Noncardiac chest pain: epidemiology, natural history, health care seeking, and quality of life. Gastroenterol Clin North Am 2004; 33:1–23.
15. Eslick GD, Jones MP, Talley NJ. Non-cardiac chest pain: prevalence, risk factors, impact and consulting–a population-based study. Aliment Pharmacol Ther 2003; 17:1115–1124.
16. Kennedy JW, Killip T, Fisher LD, et al. The clinical spectrum of coronary artery disease and its surgical and medical management, 1974–1979. The Coronary Artery Surgery study. Circulation 1982; 66:III 16–23.
17. Wong WM, Lai KC, Lam KF, et al. Prevalence, clinical spectrum and health care utilization of gastro-oesophageal reflux disease in a Chinese population: a population-based study. Aliment Pharmacol Ther 2003; 18:595–604.
18. Tew R, Guthrie EA, Creed FH, et al. A long-term follow-up study of patients with ischaemic heart disease versus patients with nonspecific chest pain. J Psychosom Res 1995; 39:977–985.
19. Richter JE, Bradley LA, Castell DO. Esophageal chest pain: current controversies in pathogenesis, diagnosis, and therapy. Ann Intern Med 1989; 110:66–78.
20. Vaezi MF, Charbel S. On-therapy pH monitoring: usually recommended but should we do it? Gastroenterology 2004; 126:A-82, 640.
21. Prakash C, Clouse RE. Abstract: extended pH monitoring with the Bravo capsule increases diagnostic yield in chest pain patients. Gastroenterology 2004; 126:A-321, M1376.
22. Johnston BT, Troshinsky MB, Castell JA, et al. Comparison of barium radiology with esophageal pH monitoring in the diagnosis of gastroesophageal reflux disease. Am J Gastroenterol 1996; 91: 1181–1185.
23. Eslick GD, Fass R. Noncardiac chest pain: evaluation and treatment. Gastroenterol Clin North Am 2003; 32:531–352.
24. Fass R, Fennerty MB, Ofman JJ, et al. The clinical and economic value of a short course of omeprazole in patients with noncardiac chest pain. Gastroenterology 1998; 115:42–49.
25. Hewson EG, Sinclair JW, Dalton CB, et al. Twenty-four-hour esophageal pH monitoring: the most useful test for evaluating noncardiac chest pain. Am J Med 1991; 90:576–583.
26. Dekel R, SD M-H, Guillen R, et al. Evaluation of symptom index in identifying gastroesophageal reflux disease-related noncardiac chest pain. J Clin Gastroenterol 2004; 38:24–29.
27. Prakash C, Clouse RE. Value of extended recording time with wireless pH monitoring in evaluating gastroesophageal reflux disease. Clin Gastroenterol Hepatol 2005; 3:329–334.
28. Bernstein LM, Baker LA. A clinical test for esophagitis. Gastroenterology 1958; 34:760–781.
29. Fass R, Naliboff B, Higa L, et al. Differential effect of long-term esophageal acid exposure on mechanosensitivity and chemosensitivity in humans. Gastroenterology 1998; 115:1363–1373.
30. Fass R. Empirical trials in treatment of gastroesophageal reflux disease. Dig Dis 2000; 18:20–26.

31. Squillace SJ, Young MF, Sanowski RA. Abstract: single dose omeprazole as a test for noncardiac chest pain. Gastroenterology 1993; 107:A197.
32. Young MF, Sanowski RA, Talbert GA, et al. Abstract: omeprazole administration as a test for gastroesophageal reflux. Gastroenterology 1992; 102:192.
33. Schenk BE, Kuipers EJ, Klinkenberg-Knol EC, et al. Omeprazole as a diagnostic tool in gastroesophageal reflux disease. Am J Gastroenterol 1997; 92:1997–2000.
34. Schindlbeck NC, Klauser AG, Voderholzer WA, et al. Empiric therapy for gastroesophageal reflux disease. Arch Intern Med 1995; 155:1808–1812.
35. Johnsson F, Weywadt L, Solhaug JH, et al. One-week omeprazole treatment in the diagnosis of gastro-oesophageal reflux disease. Scand J Gastroenterol 1998; 33:15–20.
36. Fass R, Ofman JJ, Gralnek IM, et al. Clinical and economic assessment of the omeprazole test in patients with symptoms suggestive of gastroesophageal reflux disease. Arch Intern Med 1999; 159:2161–2168.
37. Fass R, Pulliam G, Hayden CW. (Abstract) Patients with non-cardiac chest pain (NCCP) receiving an empirical trial of high dose lansoprazole, demonstrate early symptom response–a double blind, placebo-controlled trial. Gastroenterology 2001; 122:A580, W1175.
38. Pandak WM, Arezo S, Everett S, et al. Short course of omeprazole: a better first diagnostic approach to noncardiac chest pain than endoscopy, manometry, or 24-hour esophageal pH monitoring. J Clin Gastroenterol 2002; 35:307–314.
39. Kahrilas PJ. Editorial: nutcracker esophagus: an idea whose time has gone?. Am J Gastroenterol 1993; 88:167–169.
40. Bautista J, Fullerton H, Briseno M, et al. The effect of an empirical trial of high-dose lansoprazole on symptom response of patients with non-cardiac chest pain–a randomized, double-blind, placebo-controlled, crossover trial. Aliment Pharmacol Ther 2004; 19:1123–1130.
41. Fass R, Fullerton H, Hayden CW, et al. Abstract: patients with noncardiac chest pain (NCCP) receiving an empirical trial of high dose rabeprazole, demonstrate early symptom response–a double blind, placebo-controlled trial. Gastroenterology 2002; 122:A580, W1175.
42. Fass R, Fennerty MB, Johnson C, et al. Correlation of ambulatory 24-hour esophageal pH monitoring results with symptom improvement in patients with noncardiac chest pain due to gastroesophageal reflux disease. J Clin Gastroenterol 1999; 28:36–39.
43. Sifrim D, Holloway R, Silny J, et al. Acid, nonacid, and gas reflux in patients with gastroesophageal reflux disease during ambulatory 24-hour pH-impedance recordings. Gastroenterology 2001; 120:1588–1598.
44. Vela MF, Camacho-Lobato L, Srinivasan R, et al. Simultaneous intraesophageal impedance and pH measurement of acid and nonacid gastroesophageal reflux: effect of omeprazole. Gastroenterology 2001; 120:1599–1606.
45. Silny J. Intraluminal multiple electric impedance procedure for measurement of gastrointestinal motility. J Gastrointest Motil 1991; 3:151–162.
46. Fass J, Silny J, Braun J, et al. Measuring esophageal motility with a new intraluminal impedance device. First clinical results in reflux patients. Scand J Gastroenterol 1994; 29:693–702.
47. Kahrilas PJ, Clouse RE, Hogan WJ. An American Gastroenterological Association medical position statement on the clinical use of esophageal manometry. Gastroenterology 1994; 107:1865–1884.
48. Katz PO, Dalton CB, Richter JE. Esophageal testing in patients with noncardiac chest pain or dysphagia: results of three years' experience with 1161 patients. Ann Intern Med 1987; 106:593–597.
49. Dekel R, Pearson T, Wendel C, et al. Assessment of oesophageal motor function in patients with dysphagia or chest pain–the Clinical Outcomes Research Initiative experience. Aliment Pharmacol Ther 2003; 18:1083–1089.
50. DiMarino AJJ, Allen ML, Lynn RB, et al. Clinical value of esophageal motility testing. Dig Dis 1998; 16:198–204.
51. Breumelhof R, Nadorp JHSM, Akkemans LMA, et al. Analysis of 24-hour esophageal pressure and pH data in unselected patients with noncardiac chest pain. Gastroenterology 1990; 99:1257–1264.
52. Lam HGT, Dekker W, Kan G, et al. Acute noncardiac chest pain in a coronary care unit: evaluation by 24-hour pressure and pH recording of the esophagus. Gastroenterology 1992; 102:453–460.
53. London RL, Ouyang A, Snape WJJ, et al. Provocation of esophageal pain by ergonovine or edrophonium. Gastroenterology 1981; 81:10–14.
54. Nostrant TT. Provocation testing in noncardiac chest pain. Chest pain of undetermined origin. Am J Gastroenterol 1991; 5A:S56–S64.
55. Richter JE, Hackshaw BT, Wu WC, et al. Edrophonium: a useful provocative test for oesophageal chest pain. Ann Intern Med 1985; 103:14–21.
56. De Caestecker JS, Pryde A, Heading RC. Comparison of intravenous edrophonium and oesophageal acid perfusion during oesophageal manometry in patients with non-cardiac chest pain. Gut 1988; 29:1029–10374.
57. Ghillebert G, Janssens J, Vantrappen G, et al. Ambulatory 24 hour intraesophageal pH and pressure recordings Vs. provocation tests in the diagnosis of chest pain of oesophageal origin. Gut 1990; 31:738–744.
58. Richter JE, Barish CF, Castell DO. Abnormal sensory perception in patients with esophageal chest pain. Gastroenterology 1986; 91:845–852.

59. Barish CF, Castell DO, Richter JE. Graded esophageal balloon distension. A new provocative test for noncardiac chest pain. Dig Dis Sci 1986; 31:1292–1298.
60. Ritchie J. Pain from distension of the pelvic colon by inflating a balloon in the irritable colon syndrome. Gut 1973; 14:125–132.
61. Mertz H, Walsh JH, Sytnik B, et al. The effect of octreotide on human gastric compliance and sensory perception. Neurogastroenterol Motil 1995; 7:175–185.
62. Cannon RO III, Quyyumi AA, Mincemoyer R, et al. Imipramine in patients with chest pain despite normal coronary angiograms. N Engl J Med 1994; 330:1411–1417.
63. Lipkin M, Sleisenger MH. Studies of visceral pain: measurements of stimulus intensity and duration associated with the onset of pain in esophagus, ileum and colon. J Clin Invest 1958; 37.
64. Yakshe PN, et al. Abstract: does provocative esophageal testing influence coronary blood flow or coronary flow reserve? Preliminary results of concurrent esophageal and cardiac testing. Gastroenterology 1993; 104:A227.
65. Whitehead WE, Delvaux M. Standardization of barostat procedures for testing smooth muscle tone and sensory thresholds in the gastrointestinal tract. The Working Team of Glaxo-Wellcome Research, UK. Dig Dis Sci 1997; 42:223–241.
66. Azpiroz F, Malagelada JR. Physiological variations in canine gastric tone measured by an electronic barostat. Am J Physiol 1985; 248:G229–G237.
67. Silny J, Knigge KP, Fass J, et al. Verification of the intraluminal multiple electrical impedance measurement for the recordings of gastrointestinal motility. J Gastrointest Motil 1993; 5:107–122.
68. Rao SSC, Hayek B, Summers RW. Impedance planimetry: an integrated approach for assessing sensory, active, and passive biomechanical properties of the human esophagus. Am J Gastroenterol 1995; 90:431–438.
69. Orvar KB, Gregersen H, Christensen J. Biomechanical characteristics of the human esophagus. Dig Dis Sci 1993; 38:197–205.
70. Rao SS, Hayek B, Summers RW. Functional chest pain of esophageal origin: hyperalgesia or motor dysfunction. Am J Gastroenterol 2001; 96:2584–2589.
71. Aziz Q, Thompson DG. Brain-gut axis in heath and disease. Gastroenterology 1998; 114:559–578.
72. Hartshorne MF. Positron emission tomography. In: Orrison WW, Lewine JD, Sanders JA, Hartshorne MR, eds. Functional Brain Imaging. St. Louis, MO: Mosby-Year Book, 1995:187–212.
73. Aine CJ. A conceptual overview and critique of functional nueroimaging techniques in humans: I. MRI/FMRI and PET. Crit Rev Neurobiol 1995; 9:229–309.
74. Smout AJ, DeVore MS, Castell DO. Cerebral potentials evoked by esophageal distension in human. Am J Physiol 1990; 259:G955–G959.
75. Sanders JA, Orrison WW. Functional magnetic resonance imaging. In: Orrison WW, Lewine JD, Sanders JA, Hartshorne MF, eds. Functional Brain Imaging. St. Louis, MO: Mosby-Year Book, 1995:239–326.
76. Clouse RE. Psychiatric disorders in patients with esophageal disease. Med Clin North Am 1991; 75:1081–1096.
77. Storr M, Meining A, Allescher HD. Pathophysiology and pharmacological treatment of gastroesophageal reflux: effect of omeprazole. Dig Dis 2000; 18:93–102.
78. Fang J, Bjorkman D. A critical approach to noncardiac chest pain: pathophysiology, diagnosis and treatment. Am J Gastroenterol 2001; 96:958–968.
79. Stahl WG, Beton RR, Johnson CS, et al. Diagnosis and treatment of patients with gastroesophageal reflux and noncardiac chest pain. South Med J 1994; 87:739–742.
80. DeMeester TR, O'Sullivan GC, Bermudez G, et al. Esophageal function in patients with angina-type chest pain and normal coronary angiograms. Ann Surg 1982; 196:488–498.
81. Jones R, Bytzer P. Acid suppression in the management of gastro-oesophageal reflux disease: an appraisal of treatment options in primary care. Aliment Pharmacol Ther 2001; 15:765–772.
82. Fass R. Chest pain of esophageal origin. Curr Opin Gastroenterol 2002; 18:464–470.
83. Fass R, Malagon I, Schmulson M. Chest pain of esophageal origin. Curr Opin Gastroenterol 2001; 17:376–380.
84. Borzecki AM, Pedrosa MC, Prashker MJ. Should noncardiac chest pain be treated empirically? A cost-effectiveness analysis. Arch Intern Med 2000; 160:844–852.
85. Patti MG, Molena D, Fisichella PM, et al. Gastroesophageal reflux disease (GERD) and chest pain: results of laparoscopic antireflux surgery. Surg Endosc 2002; 16:563–566.
86. Farrell TM, Richardson WS, Trus TL, et al. Response of atypical symptom as of gastro-oesophageal reflux to antireflux surgery. Bri J Surg 2001; 88:1649–1652.
87. Moss SF, Armstrong D, Arnold R, et al. GERD 2003: a consensus on the way ahead. Digestion 2002; 67:111–117.
88. Waring JP. Surgical and endoscopic treatment of gastroesophageal reflux disease. Gastroenterol Clin North Am 2002; 31:S89–S109.
89. Achem SR, Kolts BE, Wears R, et al. Chest pain associated with nutcracker esophagus: a preliminary study of the role of gastroesophageal reflux. Am J Gastroenterol 1993; 88:187–192.
90. Fass R. Noncardiac chest pain. In: Fass R, ed. GERD/Dyspepsia Fast Facts. Philadelphia, PA: Hanley & Belfus, 2004:183–196.

91. Kikendall JW, Mellow MH. Effect of sublingual nitroglycerin and long-acting nitrate preparations on esophageal motility. Gastroenterology 1980; 79:703–706.

92. Orlando RC, Bozymski EM. Clinical and manometric effects of nitroglycerin in diffuse esophageal spasm. N Engl J Med 1973; 289:23–25.

93. Swamy N. Esophageal spasm: clinical and manometric response to nitroglycerine and long acting nitrates. Gastroenterology 1977; 72:23–27.

94. Mellow MH. Effect of isosorbide and hydralazine in painful primary esophageal motility disorders. Gastroenterology 1982; 83:364–370.

95. Franchtman RL, Botoman VA, Cope CE. A double blind crossover trial of diltiazem shows no benefit in patients with dysphagia and/or chest pain of esophageal origin [abstract]. Gastroenterology 1985; 90.

96. Cattau EL Jr, Castell DO, Johnson DA, et al. Diltiazem therapy for symptoms associated with nutcracker esophagus. Am J Gastroenterol 1991; 86:272–276.

97. Richter JE, Dalton CB, Bradley LA, et al. Oral nifedipine in the treatment of noncardiac chest pain in patients with the nutcracker esophagus. Gastroenterology 1987; 93:21–28.

98. Botoman VA. Noncardiac chest pain. J Clin Gastroenterol 2002; 34:6–14.

99. Drenth JP, Bos LP, Engels LG. Efficacy of diltiazem in the treatment of diffuse oesophageal spasm. Aliment Pharmacol Ther 1990; 4:411–416.

100. Bassotti G, Gaburri M, Imbimbo BP, et al. Manometric evaluation of cimetropium bromide activity in patients with the nutcracker oesophagus. Scand J Gastroenterol 1988; 23:1079–1084.

101. Miller LS, Pullela SV, Parkman HP, et al. Treatment of chest pain in patients with noncardiac, nonreflux, nonachalasia spastic esophageal motor disorders using botulinum toxin injection into the gastroesophageal junction. Am J Gastroenterol 2002; 97:1640–1646.

102. Clouse RE. Psychotropic medications for the treatment of functional gastrointestinal disorders. Clin Perspect Gastroenterol 1999; 2:348–356.

103. Peghini PL, Katz PO, Castell DO. Imipramine decreases oesophageal pain perception in human male volunteers. Gut 1998; 42:807–813.

104. Clouse RE, Lustman PJ, Eckert TC, et al. Low-dose trazodone for symptomatic patients with esophageal contraction abnormalities. A double-blind, placebo-controlled trial. Gastroenterology 1987; 92:1027–1036.

105. Varia I, Logue E, O'connor C, et al. Randomized trial of sertraline in patients with unexplained chest pain of noncardiac origin. Am Heart J 2000; 140:367–372.

106. Krishnan KR. Selected summary: chest pain and serotonin: a possible link. Gastroenterology 2001; 121:495–496.

107. Johnston BT, Shils J, Leite LP, et al. Effects of octreotide on esophageal visceral perception and cerebral evoked potentials induced by balloon distension. Am J Gastroenterol 1999; 94:65–70.

108. Clouse RE, Carney RM. The psychological profile of non-cardiac chest pain patients. Eur J Gastroenterol Hepatol 1995; 7:1160–1165.

109. Beitman BD, Basha IM, Trombka LH, et al. Pharmacotherapeutic treatment of panic disorder in patients presenting with chest pain. J Fam Pract 1989; 28:177–180.

110. Wulsin LR, Maddock R, Beitman B, et al. Clonazepam treatment of panic disorder in patients with recurrent chest pain and normal coronary arteries. Int J Psychiatry Med 1999; 29:97–105.

111. Van Peski-Oosterbaan AS, Spinhoven P, Willem Van Der Does AJ, et al. Noncardiac chest pain: interest in a medical psychological treatment. J Psychosom Res 1998; 45:471–476.

112. Hegel MT, Abel GG, Etscheidt M, et al. Behavioral treatment of angina-like chest pain in patients with hyperventilation syndrome. J Behav Ther Exp Psychiatry 1990; 20:31–39.

113. Klimes I, Mayou RA, Pearce MJ, et al. Psychological treatment for atypical non-cardiac chest pain: a controlled evaluation. Psychol Med 1990; 20:605–611.

114. Burbige EJ. Abstract: use of a 5-HT$_3$ antagonist in a patient with noncardiac chest pain. Gastroenterology 2001; 96:S183, 579.

115. Sarkar S, Aziz Q, Woolf CJ, et al. Contribution of central sensitisation to the development of non-cardiac chest pain. Lancet 2000; 356:1154–1159.

116. Cervero F. Visceral hyperalgesia revised (commentary). Lancet 2000; 356:1127–1128.

26 | Pathophysiology of Functional Dyspepsia

Jan Tack
Department of Internal Medicine, Division of Gastroenterology, University Hospital Gasthuisberg, University of Leuven, Herestraat, Leuven, Belgium

DEFINITIONS

Until recently, *dyspepsia* was defined as the presence of pain or discomfort centered in the upper abdomen (1). The Rome III committee refers to dyspepsia as a symptom or set of symptoms that is considered by most physicians to originate from the gastroduodenal region (2). Specific dyspeptic symptoms include postprandial fullness, early satiation, and epigastric pain or epigastric burning. *Postprandial fullness* is defined as an unpleasant sensation like the prolonged persistence of food in the stomach. *Early satiation* is defined as a feeling that the stomach is overfilled soon after starting to eat, out of proportion to the size of the meal being eaten, so that the meal cannot be finished. Previously, the term "early satiety" was used, but satiation is the correct term for the disappearance of the sensation of appetite during food ingestion. *Epigastric* refers to the region between the umbilicus and lower end of the sternum, and marked by the mid-clavicular lines. *Pain* refers to a subjective, unpleasant sensation, which, in some patients, creates a feeling that tissue damage is occurring. Epigastric pain may or may not have a burning quality. Patients with one or more of these symptoms are referred to as patients with dyspepsia (2).

Dyspeptic symptoms occur very commonly in the general population (3,4). The majority of these patients have no identifiable cause by standard diagnostic tests (5), which is referred to as "*functional dyspepsia (FD).*" According to international consensus, FD is defined as the presence of one or more dyspeptic symptoms (postprandial fullness, early satiation, and epigastric pain or epigastric burning), in the absence of any organic, systemic, or metabolic disease that is likely to explain the symptoms (2).

DYSPEPSIA SYMPTOM PATTERN

Overall, surveys suggest that 15% to 20% of the general population experience dyspepsia over the course a year (3,6–8). Although often chronic, the symptoms in FD are frequently intermittent, even during a period with marked symptoms (9). Both in the general population and in tertiary care, the most prevalent symptoms are postprandial fullness, epigastric pain, and early satiation (10,11). However, there is considerable heterogeneity in the symptom pattern, both in number and in type of symptoms (11).

Most subjects with dyspeptic symptoms indicate that their symptoms are aggravated by food ingestion (12) (Bisschops R, Karamanolis G, Arts J, et al. Relationship between symptoms and ingestion of a meal in functional dyspepsia. Submitted for publication.). Systematic studies have shown that the intensity of dyspeptic symptoms increases immediately after the meal, and that this increase persists for several hours (Bisschops R, Karamanolis G, Arts J, et al. Relationship between symptoms and ingestion of a meal in functional dyspepsia. Submitted for publication.).

SUBGROUPS OF FUNCTIONAL DYSPEPSIA PATIENTS

The variety of symptoms presented by patients with FD is thought to reflect the multifactorial nature of this syndrome. A factor analysis of dyspepsia symptoms in tertiary-care patients did not support the existence of FD as a homogeneous (unidimensional) condition (13). Several pathophysiological studies confirmed the heterogeneity of FD, and some associations between specific pathophysiological disturbances and dyspeptic symptoms have been reported (11).

A pathophysiology-based subdivision of dyspeptic patients would be difficult to implement in clinical practice, and there is no evidence of clinical usefulness. Attempts have been made to simplify the intricate heterogeneity of the dyspepsia symptom complex by subdividing patients according to symptom-based criteria. The Rome II committee proposed a subdivision according to the predominant symptom being pain or discomfort (1). However, this subdivision has been criticised because of the heterogeneity of the discomfort group of symptoms and because of lack of clinically meaningful association with underlying pathophysiological mechanisms (14). A subset of patients reported an acute onset of their dyspeptic symptoms, and this is associated with different symptomatic and pathophysiological characteristics (15). It is unclear whether the subdivision between acute-onset or unspecified-onset dyspepsia has any clinical usefulness.

Dyspeptic symptoms are often aggravated by food ingestion. Based on questionnaires, up to 75% of dyspeptic patients report a relationship between ingestion of a meal and symptom aggravation (12) (Bisschops R, Karamanolis G, Arts J, et al. Relationship between symptoms and ingestion of a meal in functional dyspepsia. Submitted for publication.), and registration of symptoms before and after ingestion of a standardized meal confirmed meal-induced increases in symptom intensity in a majority of patients with FD (Bisschops R, Karamanolis G, Arts J, et al. Relationship between symptoms and ingestion of a meal in functional dyspepsia. Submitted for publication.) (16). The Rome III committee has suggested to use the definition of FD as an umbrella term, mainly for clinical purposes, and while further research on more specific definitions is ongoing. It has been proposed, particularly for clinical research purposes, to replace the term "functional dyspepsia" by the new more distinctively defined diagnostic categories of (i) meal-induced dyspeptic symptoms [*postprandial distress syndrome* (PDS)] and (ii) epigastric pain [*epigastric pain syndrome* or (EPS)] (2). Thus, PDS has been defined as the presence of bothersome postprandial fullness or early satiation in the absence of any organic, systemic, or metabolic disease that is likely to explain the symptoms; EPS has been defined as the presence of pain or burning sensation in the epigastric region, in the absence of any organic, systemic, or metabolic disease that is likely to explain the symptoms. The pain is intermittent, not generalized, or localized to other abdominal or chest regions, is not relieved by defecation or passage of flatus, and does not have the characteristics of biliary pain. The usefulness of distinguishing PDS and EPS awaits further studies.

PUTATIVE PATHOPHYSIOLOGICAL MECHANISMS

Several pathophysiologic mechanisms have been suggested to play a role in the dyspepsia symptom complex. These include delayed gastric emptying, impaired gastric accommodation to a meal, hypersensitivity to gastric distention, *Helicobacter pylori* infection, altered duodenal sensitivity to lipids or acid, abnormal duodenojejunal motility, or central nervous system dysfunction.

Delayed Gastric Emptying

Several studies have addressed the prevalence and role of gastric emptying in FD. In a meta-analysis of 17 studies involving 868 dyspeptic patients and 397 controls, significant delay of solid gastric emptying was present in almost 40% of patients with FD (17). However, most of the studies were performed on small numbers of patients and controls. Recent large studies report delayed gastric emptying in 20% to 30% of dyspeptic patients (18–23). Most small studies have failed to find a convincing relationship between dyspeptic symptoms and presence or severity of delayed emptying (11). Three large-scale European single-center studies found that patients with delayed gastric emptying for solids are more likely to report postprandial fullness, nausea, and vomiting (18–20). On the other hand, large multicenter studies in the United States found no or only a weak association between delayed emptying and postprandial fullness (22,23). Pharmacological induction of delayed gastric emptying in healthy subjects is not associated with increasing dyspeptic type symptoms (Tack J, Coulie B, Verbeke K, Janssens J. Influence of delaying gastric emptying on meal-related symptoms in healthy subjects. Submitted for publication.), and the relationship between symptom improvement and changes in gastric emptying during prokinetic therapy is weak at best (24). Hence, convincing evidence that delayed emptying per se is a source of dyspeptic symptoms is presently lacking.

Impaired Gastric Accommodation

Accommodation of the stomach to a meal consists of a relaxation of the proximal stomach, providing the meal with a reservoir, and enabling a volume increase without an increase in pressure. Scintigraphic and ultrasonographic studies have demonstrated an abnormal intragastric distribution of food in patients with FD, with preferential accumulation in the distal stomach (25–27), and gastric barostat studies have confirmed reduced proximal gastric relaxation in response to a meal in patients with FD (28,29). As the barostat is invasive, attempts have been made to develop noninvasive methods to estimate gastric accommodation. Studies have shown that measurements of pre- and postprandial gastric volumes can be used to estimate gastric accommodation, either using scintigraphy or single-photon emission computed tomography (30–32). Others have challenged the validity of volumetric approaches to the assessment of gastric accommodation (33). A relationship between impaired gastric accommodation and early satiety and weight loss has been reported by some (28,31,32), but has not been confirmed in other studies (34). The prevalence of impaired accommodation is particularly high in patients with acute-onset dyspepsia, and this has been attributed to a defect at the level of gastric intrinsic nitrergic neurons (15).

Hypersensitivity to Gastric Distention

Visceral hypersensitivity has been proposed as a key mechanism underlying symptom generation in functional gastrointestinal disorders (35). Several studies have confirmed that, as a group, patients with FD have enhanced sensitivity to balloon distention of the proximal stomach (34,36–40). It is now clear that hypersensitivity to distention is present in only a subset of patients (34,38–40). According to one large study, hypersensitivity of the proximal stomach was associated with symptoms of postprandial pain, belching, and weight loss (40), but so far, other, be it numerically smaller, studies failed to report significant associations of visceral hypersensitivity and the symptom pattern (34,39). Gastric hypersensitivity is certainly not exclusively associated with pain, as nonpainful symptom intensity is also influenced by hypersensitivity status (41).

Recent studies indicate that not only the proximal stomach but also, and perhaps even more intensely, the distal stomach may be involved in symptom generation due to gastric distention (42–45).

Helicobacter pylori Infection

Many studies have attempted to establish a link between *H. pylori* infection and FD, but the role of *H. pylori* in FD remains to be a subject of controversy. Large mechanistic studies found no association between *H. pylori*-positivity and the symptom pattern, gastric emptying rate, gastric accommodation, or sensitivity to distention in FD (46,47). Most carefully designed studies found no convincing evidence that eradication of *H. pylori* consistently relieves the symptoms of FD (48–51). Meta-analyses suggest that a subset of *H. pylori*–positive patients respond favorably to eradication therapy, with an estimated number needed to treat of approximately 15 (52,53).

Other Mechanisms

A number of other pathophysiological mechanisms have been implicated in the pathophysiology of FD, based on limited numbers of studies, generally in small groups of patients. These include duodenal hypersensitivity to lipids (54,55), increased duodenal acid exposure due to impaired duodenal clearance (56,57), lack of postprandial suppression of phasic contractility of the proximal stomach (58), and abnormalities of gastric electrical rhythm (59,60).

PATHOGENESIS OF FUNCTIONAL DYSPEPSIA

The pathogenesis of FD is obscure, but recent studies indicate a postinfectious origin in a subset of patients. Using a questionnaire in 400 consecutive patients with FD, we found that 17% had a history with acute onset, suggestive of a postinfectious origin (15). These patients had a particularly high prevalence of impaired accommodation, which is attributable to a dysfunction at the level of gastric nitrergic neurons (15). Anecdotal evidence suggests a postviral origin (61), but prospective data are only available for FD that arises after *Salmonella* infection (62).

Important comorbidity exists between FD and psychological disorders (13,63–65). There is evidence of heterogeneity within the FD population with regard to psychopathological comorbidity. A recent factor analysis identified four separate symptom factors within FD, each of which was associated with a measurable abnormality of gastric function, and two of which were associated with specific psychosocial characteristics (13). The factor related to nausea, vomiting, early satiety, and weight loss was associated with female sex, physician visits, and sickness leave, and the factor related to consists of epigastric pain was associated with several psychosocial dimensions, including medically unexplained symptoms and conditions, as well as with low health-related quality of life (13). It is presently unclear whether psychological factors play a pathogenetic role in FD, especially in patients with hypersensitivity to gastric distention, or whether they are disease modulators, determining health-care seeking, perception of symptoms and the outcome of the disorder. In a recent study, experimentally induced anxiety in healthy volunteers was shown to decrease gastric compliance, to inhibit meal-induced accommodation and to increase symptoms after a standardized meal (66). These observations suggest that psychological factors have the potential to play a causal role in the pathogenesis of some dyspeptic symptoms and mechanisms.

Finally, an association between dyspeptic symptoms and a functional polymorphism in a G protein subunit was reported (67). It remains to be established whether this genotype is associated with any specific pathophysiological mechanism, with the likelihood of postinfectious FD or with altered psychosocial features.

REFERENCES

1. Talley NJ, Stanghellini V, Heading RC, Koch KL, Malagelada JR, Tytgat GNJ. Functional gastroduodenal disorders. Gut 1999; 45(suppl II):37–42.
2. Tack J, Talley NJ, Camilleri M, et al. The functional gastroduodenal disorders. Gastroenterology 2006. In press.
3. Talley NJ, Zinsmeister AR, Schleck CD, Melton LJ III. Dyspepsia and dyspepsia subgroups: a population-based study. Gastroenterology 1992; 102:1259–1268.
4. Agreus L, Svardsudd K, Nyren O, et al. Irritable bowel syndrome and dyspepsia in the general population: overlap and lack of stability over time. Gastroenterology 1995; 109:671–680.
5. Klauser AG, Voderholzer WA, Knesewitsch PA, Schindlbeck NE, Muller-Lissner SA. What is behind dyspepsia?. Dig Dis Sci 1993; 38:147–154.
6. Drossman DA, Li Z, Andruzzi E, et al. US householder survey of functional gastrointestinal disorders. Dig Dis Sci 1993; 38:1569–1580.
7. Agreus L, Svardsudd K, Nyren O, Tibblin G. The epidemiology of abdominal symptoms: prevalence and demographic characteristics in a Swedish adult population. Scand J Gastroenterol 1994; 29:102–109.
8. Kay L, Jorgerosen T. Epidemiology of upper dyspepsia in a random population. Scand J Gastroenterol 1994; 29:1–6.
9. Agreus L. Natural history of dyspepsia. Gut 2002; 50(suppl 4):iv2–iv9.
10. Tougas G, Chen Y, Hwang P, Liu MM, Eggleston A. Prevalence and impact of upper gastrointestinal symptoms in the Canadian population: findings from the DIGEST study. Am J Gastroenterol 1999; 94:2845–2854.
11. Tack J, Bisschops R, Sarnelli G. Pathophysiology and treatment of functional dyspepsia. Gastroenterology 2004; 127:1239–1255.
12. Castillo EJ, Camilleri M, Locke GR, et al. A community-based, controlled study of the epidemiology and pathophysiology of dyspepsia. Clin Gastroenterol Hepatol 2004; 2:985–996.
13. Fischler B, Tack J, De Gucht V, et al. Heterogeneity of symptom pattern, psychosocial factors, and pathophysiological mechanisms in severe functional dyspepsia. Gastroenterology 2003; 124:903–910.
14. Karamanolis G, Caenepeel P, Arts J, Tack J. Association of the predominant symptom with clinical characteristics and pathophysiological mechanisms in functional dyspepsia. Gastroenterology 2006. In press.
15. Tack J, Demedts I, Dehondt G, et al. Clinical and pathophysiological characteristics of acute-onset functional dyspepsia. Gastroenterology 2002; 122:1738–1747.
16. Arts J, Caenepeel P, Demedts I, Verbeke K, Tack J. Influence of erythromycin on gastric emptying and meal-related symptoms in functional dyspepsia with delayed gastric emptying. Gut 2005; 54:455–460.
17. Quartero AO, de Wit NJ, Lodder AC, Numans ME, Smout AJ, Hoes AW. Disturbed solid-phase gastric emptying in functional dyspepsia: a meta-analysis. Dig Dis Sci 1998; 43:2028–2033.

18. Stanghellini V, Tosetti C, Paternico A, et al. Risk indicators of delayed gastric emptying of solids in patients with functional dyspepsia. Gastroenterology 1996; 110:1036–1042.
19. Sarnelli G, Caenepeel P, Geypens B, Janssens J, TackJ. Symptoms associated with impaired gastric emptying of solids and liquids in functional dyspepsia. Am J Gastroenterol 2003; 98:783–788.
20. Perri F, Clemente R, Festa V, et al. Patterns of symptoms in functional dyspepsia: Role of *Helicobacter pylori* infection and delayed gastric emptying. Am J Gastroenterol 1998; 93:2082–2088.
21. Maes BD, Ghoos YF, Hiele MI, Rutgeerts PJ. Gastric emptying rate of solids in patients with nonulcer dyspepsia. Dig Dis Sci 1997; 42:1158–1162.
22. Talley NJ, Verlinden M, Jones M. Can symptoms discriminate among those with delayed or normal gastric emptying in dysmostility-like dyspepsia? Am J Gastroenterol 2001; 96:1422–1428.
23. Talley NJ, Locke Iii GR, Lahr B, et al. Functional dyspepsia, delayed gastric emptying and impaired quality of life. Gut 2005. In press.
24. Sturm A, Holtmann G, Goebell H, Gerken G. Prokinetics in patients with gastroparesis: a systematic analysis. Digestion 1999; 60:422–427.
25. Scott AM, Kellow JE, Shuter B, et al. Intragastric distribution and gastric emptying of solids and liquids in functional dyspepsia. Dig Dis Sci 1993; 38:2247–2254.
26. Troncon LEA, Bennett RJM, Ahluwalia NK, Thompson DG. Abnormal distribution of food during gastric emptying in functional dyspepsia patients. Gut 1994; 35:327–332.
27. Gilja OH, Hausken T, Wilhelmsen I, Berstad A. Impaired accommodation of proximal stomach to a meal in functional dyspepsia. Dig Dis Sci 1996; 41:689–696.
28. Tack J, Piessevaux H, Coulie B, Caenepeel P, Janssens J. Role of impaired gastric accommodation to a meal in functional dyspepsia. Gastroenterology 1998; 115:1346–1352.
29. Salet GAM, Samsom M, Roelofs JMM, van Berge Henegouwen GP, Smout AJPM, Akkermans LMA. Responses to gastric distention in functional dyspepsia. Gut 1998; 42:823–829.
30. Kuiken SD, Samsom M, Camilleri M, et al. Development of a test to measure gastric accommodation in humans. Am J Physiol 1999; 277(6 Pt 1):G1217–G1221.
31. Kim DY, Delgado-Aros S, Camilleri M, et al. Noninvasive measurement of gastric accommodation in patients with idiopathic nonulcer dyspepsia. Am J Gastroenterol 2001; 96:3099–3105.
32. Piessevaux H, Tack J, Walrand S, Pauwels S, Geubel A. Intragastric distribution of a standardized meal in health and functional dyspepsia: correlation with specific symptoms. Neurogastroenterol Motil 2003; 15:447–455.
33. van den Elzen BD, Bennink RJ, Wieringa RE, Tytgat GN, Boeckxstaens GE. Fundic accommodation assessed by SPECT scanning: comparison with the gastric barostat. Gut 2003; 52(11):1548–1554.
34. Boeckxstaens GE, Hirsch DP, Kuiken SD, Heisterkamp SH, Tytgat GN. The proximal stomach and postprandial symptoms in functional dyspeptics. Am J Gastroenterol 2002; 97:40–48.
35. Camilleri M, Coulie B, Tack J. Visceral hypersensitivity: facts, speculations and challenges. Gut 2001; 48:125–131.
36. Lemann M, Dederding JP, Flourie B, Franchisseur C, Rambaud JC, Jian R. Abnormal perception of visceral pain in response to gastric distension in chronic idiopathic dyspepsia. The irritable stomach syndrome. Dig Dis Sci 1991; 36:1249–1254.
37. Mearin F, Cucala M, Azpiroz F, Malagelada JR. The origin of symptoms on the brain-gut axis in functional dyspepsia. Gastroenterology 1991; 101:999–1006.
38. Mertz H, Fullerton S, Naliboff B, Mayer EA. Symptoms and visceral perception in severe functional and organic dyspepsia. Gut 1998; 42:814–822.
39. Rhee PL, Kim YH, Son HJ, et al. Evaluation of individual symptoms cannot predict presence of gastric hypersensitivity in functional dyspepsia. Dig Dis Sci 2000; 45:1680–1684.
40. Tack J, Caenepeel P, Fischler B, Piessevaux H, Janssens J. Symptoms associated with hypersensitivity to gastric distention in functional dyspepsia. Gastroenterology 2001; 121:526–535.
41. Vandenberghe J, Vos R, Persoons P, Demyttenaere K, Janssens J, Tack J. Dyspeptic patients with visceral hypersensitivity: sensitisation of pain specific or multimodal pathways?. Gut 2005; 54(7): 914–919.
42. Ladabaum URI, Koshy SS, Woods ML, et al. Differential symptomatic and electrogastrographic effects of distal and proximal human gastric distension. Am J Physiol 1998; 275:G418–G424.
43. Marzio L, Falcucci M, Grossi L, et al. Proximal and distal gastric distension in normal subjects and *H. pylori*-positive and -negative dyspeptic patients and correlation with symptoms. Dig Dis Sci 1998; 43:2757–2763.
44. Caldarella MP, Azpiroz F, Malagelada JR. Antro-fundic dysfunctions in functional dyspepsia. Gastroenterology 2003; 124:1220–1229.
45. Lee KJ, Vos R, Janssens J, Tack J. Differences in the sensorimotor response to distension between the proximal and distal stomach in humans. Gut 2004.
46. Rhee PL, Kim YH, Son HJ, et al. Lack of association of *Helicobacter pylori* infection with gastric hypersensitivity or delayed gastric emptying in functional dyspepsia. Am J Gastroenterol 1999; 94:3165–3169.
47. Sarnelli G, Janssens J, Tack J. *Helicobacter pylori* is not associated with symptoms and pathophysiological mechanisms of functional dyspepsia. Dig Dis Sci 2003; 48:2229–2236.
48. McColl K, Murray L, El-Omar E, et al. Symptomatic benefit from eradicating *Helicobacter pylori* infection in patients with nonulcer dyspepsia. N Engl J Med 1998; 339:1869–1874.

49. Blum AL, Talley NJ, O'Morain C, et al. Lack of effect of treating *Helicobacter pylori* infection in patients with nonulcer dyspepsia. Omeprazole plus Clarithromycin and Amoxicillin Effect One Year after Treatment (OCAY) Study Group. N Engl J Med 1998; 339:1875–1881.
50. Talley NJ, Janssens J, Lauritsen K, Racz I, Bolling-Sternevald E. Eradication of *Helicobacter pylori* in functional dyspepsia: randomized double blind placebo controlled trial with 12 months' follow up. The optimal Regimen Cures Helicobacter Induced Dyspepsia (ORCHID) Study Group. BMJ 1999; 318:833–837.
51. Talley NJ, Vakil N, Ballard ED 2nd, Fennerty MB. Absence of benefit of eradicating *Helicobacter pylori* in patients with nonulcer dyspepsia. N Engl J Med 1999; 341:1106–1111.
52. Moayyedi P, Soo S, Deeks J, et al. Eradication of *Helicobacter pylori* for non-ulcer dyspepsia. Cochrane Database Sys Rev 2003; (1): CD002096.
53. Laheij RJ, van Rossum LG, Verbeek AL, Jansen JB. *Helicobacter pylori* infection treatment of nonulcer dyspepsia: an analysis of meta-analyses. J Clin Gastroenterol 2003; 34(4):315–320.
54. Barbera R, Feinle C, Read NW. Abnormal sensitivity to duodenal lipid infusion in patients with functional dyspepsia. Eur J Gastroenterol Hepatol 1995; 7:1051–1057.
55. Feinle C, Meier O, Otto B, D'Amato M, Fried M. Role of duodenal lipid and cholecystokinin. A receptors in the pathophysiology of functional dyspepsia. Gut 2001; 48:347–355.
56. Samsom M, Verhagen MA, van Berge Henegouwen GP, Smout AJPM. Abnormal clearance of exogenous acid and increased acid sensitivity of the proximal duodenum in dyspeptic patients. Gastroenterology 1999; 116:515–520.
57. Lee K, Demarchi B, Demedts I, et al. A pilot study on duodenal acid exposure and its relationship to symptoms in functional dyspepsia with prominent nausea. Am J Gastroenterol 2004; 99:1765–1773.
58. Simren M, Vos R, Janssens J, Tack J. Unsuppressed postprandial phasic contractility in the proximal stomach in functional dyspepsia: relevance to symptoms. Am J Gastroenterol 2003; 98:2169–2175.
59. Lin W, Eaker EY, Sarosiek I, McCallum RW. Gastric myoelectrical activity and gastric emptying in patients with functional dyspepsia. Am J Gastroenterol 1999; 94:2384–2389.
60. Parkman HP, Miller MA, Trate D, et al. Electrogastrography and gastric emptying scintigraphy are complementary for assessment of dyspepsia. J Clin Gastroenterol 1997; 24:214–219.
61. Bityutskiy LP, Soykan I, McCallum RW. Viral gastroparesis: a subgroup of idiopathic gastroparesis. Clinical characteristics and long-term outcomes. Am J Gastroenterol 1997; 92:1501–1504.
62. Mearin F, Perez-Oliveras M, Perello A, et al. Dyspepsia and irritable bowel syndrome after a Salmonella gastroenteritis outbreak: one-year follow-up cohort study. Gastroenterology 2005; 129(1):98–104.
63. Wilhelmsen I, Haug TT, Ursin H, Berstad A. Discriminant analysis of factors distinguishing patients with functional dyspepsia from patients with duodenal ulcer. Significance of somatization. Dig Dis Sci 1995; 40:1105–1111.
64. Cheng C. Seeking medical consultation: perceptual and behavioral characteristics distinguishing consulters and nonconsulters with functional dyspepsia. Psychosom Med 2000; 62:844–852.
65. Van Oudenhove L, Demyttenaere K, Tack J, Aziz Q. Central nervous system involvement in functional gastrointestinal disorders. Baillieres Best Pract Res Clin Gastroenterol 2004; 18:663–680.
66. Geeraerts B, Vandenberghe J, Van Oudenhove L, et al. Influence of experimentally induced anxiety on gastric sensorimotor function in humans. Gastroenterology 2005; 129(5):1437–1444.
67. Holtmann G, Siffert W, Haag S, et al. G-protein beta 3 subunit 825 CC genotype is associated with unexplained (functional) dyspepsia. Gastroenterology 2004; 126(4):971–979.

Dyspepsia: Clinical Features and Management

Nimish Vakil

University of Wisconsin School of Medicine and Public Health, Madison, Marquette University College of Health Sciences, Milwaukee, Wisconsin, U.S.A.

DEFINITIONS

Dyspepsia is defined as pain or discomfort centered in the upper abdomen by an expert consensus group (Rome definition of dyspepsia) (1). Discomfort is a subjective negative feeling that may not be interpreted by the patient as pain and may include a variety of symptoms including fullness in the upper abdomen, early satiety, bloating, or nausea. Dyspeptic symptoms may be continuous or intermittent and may be of short of long duration. Dyspeptic patients who undergo investigation and have no detectable cause for their symptoms are considered to have *nonulcer dyspepsia or functional dyspepsia*. These patients should be distinguished from those who have symptoms of dyspepsia but have not undergone investigation (*uninvestigated dyspepsia*). To meet the criteria for the definition of this condition, patients must have a chronic course and have no abnormalities at endoscopy that could explain the symptoms. Nonulcer dyspepsia is therefore defined as: at least 12 weeks, which need not be consecutive, within the preceding 12 months of:

1. Persistent or recurrent dyspepsia (as defined above)
2. No evidence of organic disease (including upper endoscopy) that is likely to explain the symptoms
3. No evidence that the dyspepsia is exclusively relieved by defecation or associated with the onset of a change in stool frequency or stool form [i.e., not irritable bowel syndrome (IBS)] (1).

The minimum work-up for a clinical diagnosis of functional dyspepsia is a careful history, physical examination, and upper endoscopy during a symptomatic period of antisecretory therapy. These definitions for dyspepsia are by no means uniformly accepted, and in some countries, dyspepsia is a broad term used to refer to all symptoms from the upper gastrointestinal (GI) tract (2). The Rome II definition excludes patients with predominant reflux symptoms (2). The rationale is that when classic heartburn or regurgitation is the predominant symptom, the underlying cause is gastroesophageal reflux disease (GERD) and the patient should be managed as such.

PREVALENCE

The prevalence of dyspeptic symptoms in a year is in approximately 25% of all adults (3). Of these, one-quarter seek treatment, making dyspepsia the presenting complaint of 4% of patients visiting primary care physicians and one of the commonest conditions encountered by primary care physicians (4,5). The true incidence of dyspepsia has not been well studied, but in the Scandinavian population less than 1% developed symptoms of dyspepsia over a three-month period (6). The number of people who develop dyspeptic symptoms is matched by those who lose their symptoms and the prevalence is therefore stable (7). In the US Householder study, the prevalence of dyspepsia was 13%, but one-third of this population had heartburn and would probably be excluded from the diagnosis by the Rome criteria (8).

DIFFERENTIAL DIAGNOSIS

Several studies have estimated the prevalence of endoscopic abnormalities in unselected dyspeptic patients in primary care. These studies were performed before the widespread eradication of *Helicobacter pylori* and the adoption of test-and-treat strategies in primary care. They probably overestimate the prevalence of ulcer disease in this population. These studies have found that 10% to 20% of dyspeptic patients in primary care have peptic ulcer disease, 5% to 15% have esophagitis, 10% to 12% have abnormalities that are less specific (gastritis and duodenitis), and approximately 50% have no visible abnormalities at endoscopy. Kagevi et al. (9) studied 172 patients with dyspepsia who were evaluated in a primary care center. After history taking, physical examination, laboratory tests, upper endoscopy, and flexible sigmoidoscopy, a final diagnosis was established. Six percent of patients had esophagitis, 13% had peptic ulcer disease, and 64% had nonulcer dyspepsia. In another study, Gear et al. (10) studied 346 patients and found that a gastric ulcer was present in 6% of cases and a duodenal ulcer in 12% of cases presenting with dyspepsia in primary care. Sixty percent of patients in that study did not have specific findings at endoscopy. More recent studies have found a much higher prevalence of esophagitis and a lower prevalence of peptic ulcer disease than in earlier studies. A recent Canadian study evaluated 1040 dyspeptic patients in 49 primary care physician practices (11). The prevalence of *H. pylori* infection was 30%, and aspirin/nonsteroidal anti-inflammatory drug (NSAID) use was reported by 20% to 28% of patients. Clinically significant findings were reported in 58% of the population. Peptic ulcer disease was observed in 5% of cases. Esophagitis was found in 43% with the largest proportion of cases having mild esophagitis (Los Angeles grade A = 51%, grade B = 37.5%, grade C = 10%, and grade D = 3%). Gastric or esophageal cancer is found infrequently (< 2%) in dyspeptic patients in Western countries, but in countries where gastric cancer remains common, dyspeptic symptoms may be a symptom of malignancy. In the Canadian study, two patients were found to have a malignancy based on biopsy of nonspecific findings. Chronic pancreatitis, sprue, and biliary disorders can occasionally be confused with dyspepsia but they are rare causes of dyspepsia. Drugs can cause dyspepsia. NSAIDs are the best-studied drugs in this regard but other drugs may also cause dyspepsia.

CLINICAL DIAGNOSIS

Several studies have evaluated the ability of general practitioners and specialists to diagnose the cause of dyspepsia (12–14). In one study, with endoscopy as the gold standard, the sensitivity and specificity of the clinical evaluation was 61% and 84% for primary care doctors and 73% and 37% for gastroenterologists, respectively (12). Another study of 400 patients in primary care used a one-year follow up as the diagnostic method to determine the correct diagnosis (13). The sensitivity and specificity for a diagnosis of functional dyspepsia were 43% and 69%, respectively. These data suggest that the clinical evaluation of patients has limited utility in determining the underlying cause of dyspepsia.

ALARM FEATURES

Alarm features are symptoms and signs that suggest a more sinister underlying cause for the patients dyspeptic symptoms, e.g., an ulcer or a malignancy. These alarm features are listed in Table 1 and suggest the need for early evaluation of the patients generally with endoscopy or abdominal imaging studies. Despite the importance given to alarm features, it should be recognized that their sensitivity and specificity is low. Two U.K. studies found that cancer was rarely detected in patients under the age of 55 years without alarm symptoms, and when found, the cancer was usually inoperable (15,16). The rate of presentation of malignancy in patients less than 55 years without alarm symptoms was at 1 per million population per year. Data from the United States and Canada have shown similar findings (17,18). In a Danish study of 2479 patients with 13 upper GI cancers, only 1.5% of patients with dysphagia and 1.5% with weight loss had upper GI malignancy (19). The rate of finding colorectal cancer was similar to the rate of finding upper GI cancer in patients with dyspepsia and weight loss.

MANAGEMENT STRATEGIES

The management of dyspepsia is determined by several factors that are unique to this disorder: (i) the disease is very common in primary care settings, (ii) the clinical evaluation of these patients is of limited utility, and (iii) endoscopic evaluation is expensive and changes the management in only a small number of patients.

Table 1 Alarm Features that Suggest a Need for Early Investigation in Dyspepsia

Age > 55 with new-onset dyspepsia
Family history of upper gastrointestinal cancer
Unintended weight loss
Gastrointestinal bleeding or unexplained anemia
Progressive dysphagia
Persistent vomiting
Palpable abdominal mass or lymphadenopathy
Jaundice

Strategies That Have Been Described for the Management of Dyspepsia

Early Endoscopy

Early endoscopy is an expensive strategy that has limited utility because of its high cost in most countries. Endoscopy has been shown to have some benefit in reassuring anxious patients (20). Early endoscopy may also have value in countries where gastric cancer is prevalent in young individuals.

Initial Therapy with H_2 Receptor Antagonists

To simplify management in primary care settings, the American College of Physicians published a guideline on the management of dyspepsia in 1985 (21). This guideline recommended that dyspeptic patients should receive an empirical trial of H_2 receptor antagonists for six to eight weeks. Patients having symptomatic relief would undergo no further diagnostic or therapeutic intervention. Patients who failed to respond in 7 to 10 days or those who relapsed after therapy would undergo endoscopy. This guideline was evaluated by Bytzer et al. when they randomized patients to early endoscopy and empirical H_2 receptor antagonist therapy (22). One year later, most patients in the empirical therapy group had undergone endoscopy for recurrent or persistent symptoms. Costs were higher and patient's satisfaction was poorer in the empirical treatment group. This study showed that many dyspeptic patients have recurrent symptoms despite short courses of treatment with H_2 receptor antagonists and that an empirical treatment strategy may not be associated with reduced costs or improved outcomes.

Helicobacter pylori Testing Strategies

The rationale for the "test-and-treat strategies" is that if a substantial portion of the dyspeptic population is cured by a low-cost, noninvasive test for *H. pylori* followed by antimicrobial therapy, then cost-savings would result (23). The "test-and-scope strategy" is also designed to reduce costs. In this case, endoscopy is limited to patients who test positive with a noninvasive test for *H. pylori*. Both these strategies are limited to patients under the age of 55 years, because the risk of a gastric malignancy presenting with new-onset dyspepsia rises after the age of 55. Noninvasive testing and treatment will resolve symptoms related to peptic ulcer disease (24). There is also a small benefit of eradication over placebo in nonulcer dyspepsia [number needed to treat (NNT)= 15] (25). A Cochrane review concluded that test-and-treat was equivalent to an initial endoscopic management strategy with regard to symptom improvement, and, by reducing the need for endoscopy, was a less expensive strategy (26).

Hybrid Treatment Strategies

Hybrid strategies account for the declining prevalence of *H. pylori* infection in some populations by combining eradication and acid suppression. This allows eradication therapy and the possibility of a "cure" to be offered to the patients who are infected and an alternate approach for those who test negative. The potential, clinical, and economic impact of implementing the four alternative strategies was estimated in separate cost-effectiveness and cost-utility analyses in a recent study (27). The four strategies evaluated were as follows.

1. An empirical trial of proton-pump inhibitor (PPI) with endoscopy reserved for failures of acid suppression,
2. test-and-treat for *H. pylori* with endoscopy for the nonresponders,
3. initial test-and-treat for *H. pylori* with an empirical course of PPI for nonresponders and those who test negative and endoscopy reserved for failures of both strategies, and
4. initial PPI therapy followed by test-and-treat for nonresponders and endoscopy reserved for failures.

Strategies 3 and 4 were most effective, with 83% of patients rendered symptom-free in both analyses and 0.98 quality-adjusted life-years gained, compared with 75% of patients and 0.93 quality-adjusted life-years gained by Strategy 2. Strategy 3 was the optimal approach overall. Recent guidelines from the American College of Gastroenterology and the American Gastroenterological Association have embraced hybrid strategies for the management of dyspepsia (28,29).

Treatment Strategies for Nonulcer Dyspepsia

When *H. pylori*–related diseases and acid-related disorders are removed from the population of patients with dyspepsia, we are left with a group of patients that have no obvious findings at endoscopy. A number of treatment strategies have been evaluated in this population. Treatment studies in nonulcer dyspepsia have had many weaknesses. There is a high placebo response rate and therefore adequate controls are essential to allow appropriate comparisons. As there are no objective findings to evaluate at endoscopy, symptom scales are used to assess response. Scales require validation to ensure their responsiveness and test–retest reliability. Blinding of patients and controls is essential to prevent bias. Prolonged follow up (generally 12 months) is necessary to determine if the effects are truly sustained. Many trials have lacked critical elements in the design that make the results difficult to interpret.

Randomized, Controlled Trials of Helicobacter pylori Eradication in Nonulcer Dyspepsia

There are now several large double-blind, randomized, placebo-controlled trials that evaluate the efficacy of *H. pylori* eradication in nonulcer dyspepsia. Although the overall design of the studies is excellent, the results are not uniform and have resulted in a debate on the usefulness of eradicating *H. pylori* in nonulcer dyspepsia. Blum et al. (30) randomly assigned 438 patients to PPI triple therapy or omeprazole alone for one week and followed patients for one year. The study was carefully designed with appropriate controls and blinding. Treatment success was reported in 27% of patients in the triple therapy group and 21% of patients in the placebo group (not significant). Talley et al. (31) randomly treated 278 patients with triple therapy and placebo for one week. Relief of dyspepsia at one year was similar in the two groups (24% in active treatment and 22% in placebo). Data from another large, U.S. multicenter trial also show no benefit for eradication therapy in nonulcer dyspepsia (32). Of 337 patients randomized to either *H. pylori* eradication therapy or placebo and followed for one year, 46% of patients in the active treatment group and 50% in the placebo group had a successful response to therapy ($p = 0.55$). No significant association was found between the symptom type (ulcer like, reflux like, or dysmotility like) and the outcome, and there was no correlation with improvement in chronic gastritis at 12 months. In contrast, in a single-center study from Scotland, a significant benefit was reported with eradication therapy. McColl et al. (33) reported that symptoms resolved in a significantly greater proportion of patients (21%) with *H. pylori* triple therapy compared to 7% in the placebo group.

Another small recent study from the United States reported no benefit for eradication therapy in nonulcer dyspepsia. One hundred patients were randomized to therapy with omeprazole and clarithromycin or placebo. At one year, reduction in dyspepsia scores was similar in both groups (34). The study however had significant limitations: it did not use a validated symptom scale, was not powered to detect small differences, and used a two-drug treatment regimen (omeprazole and clarithromycin) that is obsolete. The final results from the ELAN study, a large European study of 860 patients randomized to lansoprazole or lansoprazole triple therapy, are not completely published (35). Preliminary data suggest that if patients were classified as responders (dyspepsia score less than or equal to 1) or nonresponders, there was a higher proportion of responders (44%) in patients with successful eradication compared to patients without eradication (36%). These data can only be considered preliminary at this time.

Meta-analyses of Helicobacter pylori Eradication in Nonulcer Dyspepsia

A recent Cochrane review of H. pylori eradication in nonulcer dyspepsia identified 13 trials with 3180 patients with nonulcer dyspepsia (28). Patients were evaluated after 12 months in seven of the trials and after shorter periods in the other trials. Eradication therapy was statistically significantly superior to placebo (RR = 0.91, 0.87–0.96) with an NNT of 17 (95% CI = 11–33).

Acid Suppressive Therapy

PPIs and H₂ Receptor Antagonists

There have been mixed results with the use of H_2 receptor antagonists in nonulcer dyspepsia. A recent meta-analysis concluded that there was some benefit, but a large number of the studies had to be excluded from the analysis (only 18 of 150 studies met the inclusion criteria (36). This suggests that many studies have been poorly conducted. The overall results suggest that H_2 receptor antagonists have a modest effect. With cimetidine, the therapeutic benefit above placebo was 14% (95% CI 3–24%), and with ranitidine, the therapeutic benefit was 33% (95% CI 23–43). A Cochrane review suggested that H_2 receptor antagonists were effective [eight trials generating 1125 patients; relative risk reduction 30% (95% CI 4–48%)] (37). An updated review found 11 trials and the proportion of patients that continued to have dyspeptic symptoms was significantly reduced in patients allocated to H_2RA therapy (RR = 0.78, 95% CI = 0.65–0.93) (28).

Several recent studies evaluated the effectiveness of PPIs in functional dyspepsia. A total of 1262 patients with functional dyspepsia were enrolled in two studies (BOND and OPERA studies) to omeprazole 20 or 10 mg/day or identical placebo for four weeks (38). Complete symptom relief was seen on the last three days of therapy in 38% of patients receiving omeprazole 20 mg, 36% of patients receiving omeprazole 10 mg, and 28% on placebo ($p = 0.002$). Symptom relief was similar in patients who were *H. pylori*–positive or –negative. Similar data have been reported in preliminary form with lansoprazole in a U.S. population. Peura et al.(39) reported complete symptom relief in 44% of patients given lansoprazole 30 mg for eight weeks compared to 29% of controls given placebo in a trial lasting eight weeks. A Cochrane review found four trials with 1248 patients and a relative risk reduction of 12% (95% CI = 1–24%) (11). The Cochrane review has recently been updated. PPI therapy was given for two to eight weeks and was statistically significantly superior to placebo (RR = 0.86, 95% CI 0.78–0.95) with an NNT of 9 (95% CI = 6–25) (28).

Prokinetic Agents
One meta-analysis showed that when cisapride was used, improvement over placebo occurred in 36% (95% CI 28–44%) (40). Cisapride is no longer available in the United States and many other countries because of cardiac toxicity. Metoclopramide has a modest effect but the relatively high incidence of side effects is a significant disadvantage. A Cochrane review found 12 trials with 829 patients with a relative risk reduction of 50% (95% CI 30–65%), but a funnel plot suggested that these results could be due to publication bias alone (11). An update of the Cochrane review found 14 studies with a significant reduction in dyspepsia in the prokinetic group compared to placebo (RR = 0.52; 95% CI = 0.37–0.73) (28).

Antidepressants
A meta-analysis of antidepressant therapy in functional GI disorders has suggested that antidepressant therapy is more effective than placebo in functional GI disorders, with an NNT of 3 (95% CI = 2–7) (40). There are limited data on the efficacy of antidepressants in nonulcer dyspepsia without overlapping IBS, and these agents cannot be considered of proven efficacy at this time (28).

Psychological Therapies
Individual studies have reported benefit with psychological interventions, cognitive behavioral therapy, and hypnotherapy (41–45). There are several problems with the design of the studies including small sample sizes and improvements in symptoms that are small and of questionable value. A systematic review concluded that these therapies are not of proven value at the present time (46).

Simethicone
Simethicone has been shown in one study to be superior to cisapride in resolving the symptoms of dyspepsia in the first two weeks (47).

Herbal Therapies
Limited data suggest that herbal therapies may have efficacy in functional dyspepsia, but these studies need confirmation in other populations (48,49).

Future Directions in Therapy for Nonulcer Dyspepsia
Drugs That Improve Gastric Accommodation
Patients with disordered gastric accommodation may have dyspepsia, early satiety, and weight loss. The exact prevalence of this subgroup of patients is uncertain, but the development of drugs that relax the fundus is an area of considerable interest. 5-hydroxytryptamine (5-HT)

is a neurotransmitter in the enteric nervous system and has been shown to be involved in vagally mediated gastric relaxation. Although a number of 5-HT agonists have been shown to affect gastric accommodation in animals and humans, conclusive evidence for the role of 5-HT in gastric accommodation under physiologic conditions in man is lacking, and the precise receptor involved remains elusive. Receptors that may be relevant to gastric physiology include 5-HT1A, 5-HT1B, 5-HT4, and 5-HT7 receptors. Tegaserod is a 5-HT4 partial agonist and enhances gastric emptying and improves the abnormalities in fundic accommodation that are seen in some dyspeptic individuals (50). Preliminary data suggest that tegaserod may improve symptoms of nonulcer dyspepsia in patients with normal gastric emptying. The overall response rate (relief of symptoms for at least 50% of the time) was 55% in females who received 12 mg tegaserod/day and 42% in placebo-treated patients. Beneficial effects were seen in symptoms of postprandial fullness and early satiety, but these data need to be confirmed in larger trials (51). Another recent study showed that tegaserod had no effect on the balloon pressures or volumes inducing first perception of discomfort, but enhanced fasting gastric compliance compared with placebo (52). Alosetron, a 5-HT3 antagonist, reduces postprandial symptoms such as nausea and bloating in functional dyspepsia without altering gastric accommodation or maximal tolerable volume, suggesting that 5-HT3 antagonism may have a role in upper GI sensation (53). The drug has been withdrawn from the U.S. market because of concerns about ischemic colitis. One study reported enhanced gastric emptying after administration of the 5-HT3 receptor antagonist tropisetron, but another reported no effect on gastric emptying. Ondansetron has no effect on fundic tone, suggesting that the effect seen with alosertron may therefore be due to an effect on sensation rather than due to an increase in motility or accommodation. Drugs that prolong the effect of 5-HT by decreasing its reuptake have also been studied. Paroxetine had a limited effect on gastric accommodation in one study and no effect in another (54,55). Sumatriptan, a 5-HT1 receptor agonist, used in the treatment of migraine, relaxes the proximal stomach in humans and in short-term studies improves gastric accommodation (56). As injectable sumatriptan is inconvenient and expensive for use in dyspepsia, intranasal sumatriptan has been studied but was not effective (57). Second-generation triptans such as naratriptan and rizatriptan have higher bioavailability and may also be effective suggesting a class effect with these agents (58).

New Prokinetics Agents

Itopride is a new prokinetic agent that stimulates gastric emptying and is currently under investigation in the United States. It is marketed in some countries (Japan and Eastern Europe), and its mechanism of action is related to inhibition of dopamine action on D-2 receptors on postsynaptic cholinergic nerves and stimulation of the release of acetylcholine in the myenteric plexus (59). Preliminary data suggest that the drug is well tolerated and improves dyspeptic symptoms, but the results of two large phase III trials in the United States are awaited (60).

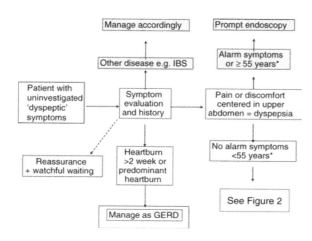

Figure 1 Initial approach to the patient with dyspepsia.

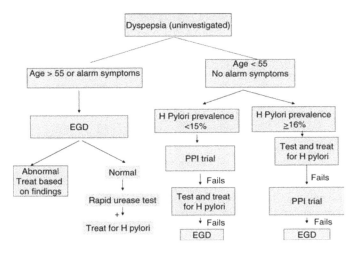

Figure 2 Management of young patients with dyspepsia and no alarm symptoms.

Clinical Management of Dyspepsia

Figure 1 illustrates the initial management strategy for symptoms of dyspepsia in primary care. The initial focus is to identify patients with GERD and alarm features and to manage them appropriately. Due to the increasing risk of a serious underlying condition after the age of 55, early endoscopy is recommended in patients with new symptoms of dyspepsia who are older than 55. The age threshold for this decision must be determined based on local conditions (the incidence of upper GI cancer and the average age at which it is detected). Figure 2 illustrates the recommended management of dyspepsia and is based on the prevalence of *H. pylori* in the community. In communities with a low prevalence of *H. pylori* infection, an empirical treatment strategy with acid suppression is recommended. In areas with a moderate-high prevalence of *H. pylori* infection, an initial test-and-treat strategy is the recommended strategy. Serologic testing for *H. pylori* may be inaccurate in low prevalence areas and active tests such as the urea breath test or the stool antigen test are recommended (61). Hypnotherapy, herbal remedies, and antidepressants are best reserved for refractory patients who fail conventional methods of therapy.

REFERENCES

1. Talley NJ, Stanghellini V, Heading RC, Koch KL, Malagelada J, Tytgat GN. Functional gastroduodenal disorders. In: Drossman DA, ed. Rome II: The Functional Gastrointestinal Disorders. McLean, VA: Degnon, 2000:299–350.
2. Veldhuyzen van Zanten S, Flook N, Chiba N, et al. An evidence-based approach to the management of uninvestigated dyspepsia in the era of *Helicobacter pylori*. CMAJ 2000; 162(12 suppl):S3–S23.
3. Talley NJ, Zinsmeister AR, Schleck CD, Melton LJ. Dyspepsia and dyspepsia subgroups: a population-based study. Gastroenterology 1992; 102:1259–1268.
4. Jones R, Lydeard S. Prevalence of symptoms of dyspepsia in the community. Br Med J 1989; 298:30–32.
5. Marsland DW, Wood M, Mayo F. Content of family practice. Part I. Rank order of diagnoses by frequency. Part II. Diagnosis by disease category and age/sex distribution. J Fam Pract 1976; 3:37–68.
6. Agreus L, Svardsudd K, Nyren O, Tibblin G. Irritable bowel syndrome and dyspepsia in the general population: overlap and lack of stability over time. Gastroenterology 1995; 109:671–680.
7. Talley N, Weaver A, Zinsmeister A, Melton LJ III. Onset and disappearance of gastrointestinal symptoms and functional gastrointestinal disorders. Am J Epidemiol 1992; 136:165–177.
8. Drossman D, Li Z, Andruzzi E, et al. U.S. householder survey of functional gastrointestinal disorders. Prevalence sociodemography, and health impact. Dig Dis Sci 1993; 38:1569–1580.
9. Kagevi I, Lofstedt S, Persson L-G. Endoscopic findings and diagnoses in unselected dyspeptic patients at a primary health care center. Scand J Gastroenterol 1989; 24:145–150.
10. Gear MWL, Barnes RJ. Endoscopic studies of dyspepsia in general practice. BMJ 1980; 1:1136–1137.
11. Thomson A, Barkun A, Armstrong D, et al. The prevalence of clinically significant endoscopic findings in primary care patients with uninvestigated dyspepsia: the Canadian Adult Dyspepsia Empiric treatment-prompt endoscopy (CADET-PE) study. Aliment Pharmacol Ther 2003; 17:1481–1491.

12. The Danish Dyspepsia Group. Value of the unaided clinical diagnosis in dyspeptic patients in primary care. Am J Gastroenterol 2001; 96:1417–1421.
13. Heikkinen M, Pikkarainen P, Takala J, Rasanen H, Julkunen R. Etiology of dyspepsia: four unselected consecutive patients in general practice. Scand J Gastroenterol 1995; 30:519–523.
14. Hansen J, Bytzer P, Schaffalitzky de Muckadell OB. Management of dyspeptic patients in primary care. Scand J Gastroenterol 1998; 33:799–805.
15. Christie J, Shepherd NA, Codling BW, et al. Gastric cancer below the age of 55: implications for screening patients with uncomplicated dyspepsia. Gut 1997; 41:513–517.
16. Gillen D, McColl KE. Does concern about missing malignancy justify endoscopy in uncomplicated dyspepsia in patients aged less than 55?. Am J Gastroenterol 1999; 94:2329–2330.
17. Canga C 3rd, Vakil N. Upper GI malignancy, uncomplicated dyspepsia, and the age threshold for early endoscopy. Am J Gastroenterol 2002; 97:600–603.
18. Breslin NP, Thomson AB, Bailey RJ, et al. Gastric cancer and other endoscopic diagnoses in patients with benign dyspepsia. Gut 2000; 46:93–97.
19. Meineche-Schmidt V, Jorgensen T. 'Alarm symptoms' in patients with dyspepsia: a three-year prospective study from general practice. Scand J Gastroenterol 2002; 37:999–1007.
20. Quadri A, Vakil N. Health-related anxiety and the effect of open-access endoscopy in US patients with dyspepsia. Aliment Pharmacol Ther 2003; 17:835–840.
21. Health and Policy Committee. American College of Physicians. Endoscopy in the evaluation of dyspepsia. Ann Intern Med 1985; 102:266–269.
22. Bytzer P, Hansen J, de Muckadell O. Empirical H2 blocker therapy or prompt endoscopy in management of dyspepsia. Lancet 1994; 343:811–815.
23. Silverstein M, Petterson T, Talley N. Initial endoscopy or empirical therapy with or without testing for. Hpylori for dyspepsia: a decision analysis. Gastroenterology 1996; 110:72–83.
24. McColl KE, el-Nujumi A, Murray L, et al. The *Helicobacter pylori* breath test: a surrogate marker for peptic ulcer disease in dyspeptic patients. Gut 1997; 40:302–306.
25. Moayyedi P, Soo S, Deeks J, et al. Eradication of *Helicobacter pylori* for non-ulcer dyspepsia. Cochrane Database Syst Rev 2003; (1):CD002096.
26. Delaney BC, Moayyedi P, Forman D. Initial management strategies for dyspepsia. Cochrane Database Syst Rev 2003(2):CD001961.
27. Spiegel BM, Vakil NB, Ofman JJ. Dyspepsia management in primary care: a decision analysis of competing strategies. Gastroenterology 2002; 122(5):1270–1285.
28. Talley N, Vakil N, Moayyedi P. AGA technical review: evaluation of dyspepsia 2005. Gastroenterology 2005; 129:1756–1780.
29. Talley NJ, Vakil N. Practice Parameters Committee of the American College of Gastroenterology. Guidelines for the management of dyspepsia. Am J Gastroenterol 2005; 100(10):2324–2337.
30. Blum AL et al. Lack of effect of treating *Helicobacter pylori* infection in patients with nonulcer dyspepsia. N Engl J Med 1998; 339:1869–1874.
31. Talley NJ, Jenssens J, Lauritsen K, et al. Eradication of *Helicobacter pylori* in functional dyspepsia-randomized double blind placebo controlled trial with 12 months follow up. BMJ 1999; 318:833–837.
32. Talley NJ, Vakil N, Ballard ED, Fennerty B. Absence of benefit of eradicating *Helicobacter pylori* in patients with nonulcer dyspepsia. N Engl J Med 1999; 341:1106–1111.
33. McColl K, Murray L, El-Omar E, et al. Symptomatic benefit from eradicating *H. pylori* in patients with nonulcer dyspepsia. N Engl J Med 1998; 339:1869–1874.
34. Greenberg P, Cello J. Lack of effect of treatment for *Helicobacter pylori* on symptoms of non-ulcer dyspepsia. Arch Int Med 1999; 159:2283–2288.
35. Malfertheiner P. *Helicobacter pylori* eradication in functional dyspepsia: new evidence for symptomatic benefit. Eur J Gastroenterol Hepatol 2001; 13(suppl 2):S9-S11.
36. Finney JS, Kinnersley N, Hughes M, Bryan-Tear C, Lothian J. Meta-analysis of anti-secretory and gastrokinetic compounds in functional dyspepsia. J Clin Gastroenterol 1998; 26:312–320.
37. Soo S. Pharmacological interventions for non-ulcer dyspepsia. Cochrane Database Syst Rev 2000(2):CD001960.
38. Talley N, Meineche-Schmidt V, Pare P, et al. Effect of omeprazole in functional dyspepsia: double-blind, randomized, placebo-controlled trials (the Bond and Opera studies). Aliment Pharmacol Ther 1998; 12:1055–1065.
39. Peura DA, Kovacs TO, Metz DC, Siepman N, Pilmer BL, Talley NJ. Lansoprazole in the treatment of functional dyspepsia: two double-blind, randomized, placebo-controlled trials. Am J Med 2004; 116(11):740–748.
40. Jackson JL, O'Malley PG, Tomkins G, Balden E, Santoro J, Kroenke K. Treatment of functional gastrointestinal disorders with antidepressant medications: a meta-analysis. Am J Med 2000; 108:65–72.
41. Bates S, Sjoden PO, Nyren O. Behavioral treatment of non-ulcer dyspepsia. Scand J Behav Ther 1988; 17:155–165.
42. Haug TT, Wilhelmsen I, Svebak S, Berstad A, Ursin H. Psychotherapy in functional dyspepsia. J Psychosom Res 1994; 38:735–744.
43. Hamilton J, Guthrie E, Creed F, et al. A randomized controlled trial of psychotherapy in patients with chronic functional dyspepsia. Gastroenterology 2000; 119:661–669.

44. Calvert EL, Houghton LA, Cooper P, Morris J, Whorwell P. Long-term improvement in functional dyspepsia using hypnotherapy. Gastroenterology 2002; 123:1778–1785.
45. Chiarioni G, Benini L, Bonfante F, Menegotti M, Salandini L, Vantini I. Prokinetic effect of a single session of gut oriented hypnotherapy on gastric emptying in normal subjects and dyspeptic patients. Gastroenterology 2001; 120:A133.
46. Soo S, Forman D, Delaney B, Moayyedi P. A systematic review of psychological therapies for nonulcer dyspepsia. Am J Gastroenterol 2004; 99:1817–1822.
47. Holtmann G. Randomized double-blind comparison of simethicone with cisapride in functional dyspepsia. Aliment Pharmacol Ther 1999; 13:1459–1465.
48. Melzer J, Rosch W, Reichling J, Brignoli R, Saller R. Meta-analysis: phytotherapy of functional dyspepsia with the herbal drug preparation STW 5 (Iberogast). Aliment Pharmacol Ther 2004; 20:1279–1287.
49. Madisch A, Holtmann G, Plein K, Hotz J. Treatment of irritable bowel syndrome with herbal preparations: results of a double-blind, randomized, placebo-controlled, multi-centre trial. Aliment Pharmcol Ther 2004; 19:271–279.
50. Tack J, Vos R, Janssens J, Salter J, Jauffret S, Vanddeplassche G. Influence of tegaserod on proximal gastric sensory and motor function in man. Gastroenterology 2002; 122:A20.
51. Tack J, Delia T, Ligozio G, Sue V, Lefkowitz M, Vandeplassche L. A Phase II placebo controlled randomized trial with Tegaserod in functional dyspepsia patients with normal gastric emptying. Gastroenterology 2002; 122:A453.
52. Tack J, Vos R, Janssens J, Salter J, Jauffret S, Vandeplassche G. Influence of tegaserod on proximal gastric tone and on the perception of gastric distension. Aliment Pharmacol Ther 2003; 18(10):1031–1037.
53. Kuo B, Camilleri M, Burton D, et al. 5-HT3 antagonism of upper gastrointestinal symptoms after a dyspepsia inducing meal. Gastroenterology 2001; 120:A134.
54. Tack J, Broekaert D, Coulie B, Fischler B, Janssens J. Influence of the selective serotonin re-uptake inhibitor, paroxetine, on gastric sensorimotor function in humans. Aliment Pharmacol Ther 2003; 17(4):603–608.
55. Chial HJ, Camilleri M, Burton D, Thomforde G, Olden KW, Stephens D. Selective effects of serotonergic psychoactive agents on gastrointestinal functions in health. Am J Physiol Gastrointest Liver Physiol 2003; 284(1):G130–G137.
56. Tack J, Coulie B, Wilmer A, Andrioli A, Janssens J. Influence of sumatriptan on gastric fundus tone and on the perception of gastric distension in man. Gut 2000; 46(4):468–473.
57. Sarnelli G, Janssens J, Tack J. Effect of intranasal sumatriptan on gastric tone and sensitivity to distension. Dig Dis Sci 2001; 46(8):1591–1595.
58. Moro E, Crema F, De Ponti F, Frigo G. Triptans and gastric accommodation: pharmacological and therapeutic aspects. Dig Liver Dis 2004; 36:85–92.
59. Iwanaga Y, Miyashita N, Saito T, Morikawa K, Itoh Z. Gastroprokinetic effect of a new benzamide derivative itopride and its action mechanisms in conscious dogs. Jpn J Pharmacol 1996; 71(2):129–137.
60. Amarapurkar DN, Rane P. Randomised, double-blind, comparative study to evaluate the efficacy and safety of ganaton (itopride hydrochloride) and mosapride citrate in the management of functional dyspepsia. J Indian Med Assoc 2004; 102(12):735–737, 760.
61. Vaira D, Vakil N, Menagatti M, et al. The stool antigen test for the detection of *Helicobacter pylori* after eradication therapy. Ann Intern Med 2002; 136(4):280–287.

27 | Pathophysiology and Management of Pain in Chronic Pancreatitis

John H. Winston and Pankaj Jay Pasricha

Department of Internal Medicine, Division of Gastroenterology and Hepatology, and Enteric Neuromuscular Disorders and Pain Center, University of Texas Medical Branch, Galveston, Texas, U.S.A.

BACKGROUND AND NATURE OF THE PROBLEM
Introduction

Pancreatitis, acute or chronic, is a significant contributor to the "burden of gastrointestinal disease" in this country, according to a recent survey conducted by the American Gastroenterological Association (1). In 1998, there were about 1.2 million cases, with 327,000 inpatients and 530,000 physician office visits. The estimated total direct cost for this group of diseases was $2.1 billion in 1998. Unfortunately, progress in our understanding of the biology of these diseases has been slow, particularly with respect to the pathogenesis of the cardinal symptom of pancreatitis i.e., pain. Any physician who has dealt with these patients is aware of the fact that pain is not only the most important symptom of chronic pancreatitis but also the most difficult to treat: "Painful chronic pancreatitis is poorly understood and its management is controversial" (2). Our lack of knowledge about what causes pain in pancreatitis has been a serious obstacle to improvement of the care of these patients, leading to various empirical approaches that are often based on purely anatomical grounds, are generally highly invasive and at best of marginal value (3). Despite a wide variety of approaches covering innocuous (enzyme therapy), minimally invasive (endoscopic decompression and nerve blocks), and highly aggressive (surgical decompression, pancreatectomy), no consensus has emerged and no form of treatment can be considered satisfactory at the present time.

PATHOGENESIS OF PAIN IN CHRONIC PANCREATITIS
Current and Evolving Theories

A relatively small proportion of patients with chronic pancreatitis and pain have readily identifiable lesions such as pseudocysts that are amenable to surgical or endoscopic treatment. In the others, traditional theories focus on increased pancreatic tissue pressure and possible ischemia either from ductal obstruction ("ductal hypertension") or fibrosing encasement of the pancreas ("compartment syndrome") (4–13). Although these theories still have their adherents, subsequent studies have not confirmed a correlation between ductal pressure and either the severity of pain or its relief after ductal decompression (14,15).

It is likely that these phenomena, while clearly associated with the disease, are not the root cause of the pain. Instead, they probably are inciting factors on a background of neuronal sensitization induced by damage to the perineurium and subsequent exposure of the nerves to mediators and products of inflammation. Many of the elements of the "inflammatory soup" described in somatic pain models [including ions (K^+ and H^+), amines [serotonin (5-HT) and histamine], kinins (bradykinin), prostanoids (PGE_2), purines (adenosine triphosphate), cytokines [tumor necrosis factor, interleukin (IL)-1, and IL-6], nitric oxide, and caloric activity (heat) are likely to result in early sensitization of pancreatic nociceptors in patients with pancreatitis as well.

In keeping with this, attention has shifted more recently to changes in pancreatic nerves that may by themselves perpetuate the pain state. Pancreatic tissue from patients with chronic pancreatitis reveals ultrastructural evidence of damage and edema, along with disruptive changes of the perineurial sheath, potentially exposing the nerve bundles directly to their surroundings (16). In addition, expression of a well-established neurotrophic factor for nociceptive neurons, nerve growth factor (NGF), is increased in chronic pancreatitis and appears to correlate with pain (17). The same group has also found a marked intensification of the immunostaining for substance P and calcitonin gene-related peptide (CGRP) (18), both of which are expressed by NGF-responsive nociceptors and play an important role in pain signaling in several models. The evidence for neuroimmune interactions in the pathogenesis of pain in humans with chronic pancreatitis has recently been reviewed (19) and is summarized in Table 1.

These theories are not mutually exclusive: A useful conceptual framework is to view increases in pressure or minor exacerbations in inflammation as pain "triggers" against a background of a sensitized pain-signaling system. Under normal conditions, such minor degrees of activation may not lead to major episodes of pain. However, nerves which have been structurally and/or functionally altered by previous or ongoing episodes of inflammation may respond to these stimuli in a greatly exaggerated fashion, a phenomenon known as sensitization. Peripheral tissue injury or inflammation results in long-term changes in nociceptive processing that can involve both primary sensory neurons (peripheral sensitization), as well as neurons in the spinal cord and higher structures (central sensitization). The net result of sensitization is that noxious stimuli now elicit a pain response that is much greater when compared with the normal state, a phenomenon termed "hyperalgesia." A further characteristic of the sensitized state is called "allodynia," a phenomenon in which innocuous or physiological stimuli are perceived as painful. As an example, one can postulate that in the setting of pancreatic neuronal sensitization patients will experience mechanical allodynia: pain in response to physiological changes in intraductal pressure, which would otherwise have not been perceived. Similarly, subsequent minor flare-ups of inflammation in such patients could also cause the associated pain to be felt as severe, rather than mild (hyperalgesia). As discussed above, increased intraductal pressure and increased interstitial pressure (leading to pancreatic ischemia) are not uniformly observed in patients with chronic pancreatitis and even when they are, the response to decompression is inconsistent. These discrepancies can be explained by the phenomenon of neural sensitization, where pain signaling may be triggered by pressures and other stimuli in the normal range.

An understanding of the biology of neuronal sensitization in pancreatitis is, therefore, critical. While some lessons can be extrapolated from the somatic literature, given the difficulty in treating the pain medically, the neurochemical changes induced in the afferent nervous system may be different from that of somatic or visceral inflammation in hollow organs and require specific models for analysis.

Experimental Models of Painful Pancreatitis

A significant barrier to understanding the biological basis of pain in pancreatitis has been the lack of suitable animal models and assays. This is due, in part, to the relative inaccessibility of the pancreas and in part, to the lack of validated behavioral or other surrogate markers for pancreatic pain in animals. One approach to studying pancreatic pain is to take advantage of the phenomenon of referred hypersensitivity, which is characteristic of visceral pain. Humans with both acute and chronic pancreatitis can develop severe pain, often associated with areas of referred cutaneous hyperalgesia extending across the upper abdomen and around the back. These findings were exploited to develop two recently described rat models of pancreatitic pain. Vera-Portocarrero et al. induced "persistent" pancreatitis by systemic

Table 1 Pathological Correlates of Pain in Patients with Chronic Pancreatitis

Pain correlated with perineural eosinophils in chronic pancreatitis
Inflammatory foci; damage to perineurium; more enlarged nerves
Increased neuropeptide expression in chronic pancreatitis
Growth-associated protein 43 (GAP-43) expression and neuronal sprouting
Correlate among GAP-43 expression, immune cell infiltration, and pain
Nerve growth factor and its high-affinity receptor, the tyrosine kinase A receptor, in chronic pancreatitis correlates with pain
  intensity
Increased interleukin-8 gene expression
Relation between substance P receptor and pain
Brain derived neurotrophic factor increased expression in chronic pancreatitis correlates with pain score

Source: Adapted From Ref. 19.

dibutylin dichloride in rats and showed an increase in withdrawal events after von Frey filament (VFF) stimulation of the abdomen and decreased withdrawal latency after thermal stimulation during a period of seven days, indicating a "sensitized nociceptive" state accompanied by increased levels of substance P, but not CGRP levels in spinal cords (20). The efficacy of VFF testing as a means to measure nociceptive behavior was also shown by Winston et al. from our group, who induced acute pancreatitis by systemic L-arginine. In this model, referred tactile sensitization occurred during the period of maximum tissue damage and inflammation in the pancreas, developing on day 1 after L-arginine administration and persisting at least through day 7 (21). Lu et al. have also described direct behavioral assays for pancreatic pain using acute noxious stimulation of the pancreas via an indwelling ductal cannula in awake and freely moving rats (22). These assays included cage crossing, rearing, and hind limb extension in response to intrapancreatic bradykinin infusion. Intrathecal administration of either 2-amino-5-phosphonovalerate (D-APV) [N-methyl-D-aspartate (NMDA) receptor antagonist] or morphine alone partially reduced visceral pain behaviors in this model. Combinations of both reduced pain behaviors to baseline. These findings demonstrate the feasibility of making quantitative measures of nociceptive behavior in rats with pancreatitis.

We have also recently assessed a rat model of chronic pancreatitis induced by pancreatic infusion of trinitrobenzene sulfonic acid (TNBS). Rats with pancreatitis exhibited marked increase in sensitivity to mechanical probing of the abdomen and increased sensitivity to noxious electrical stimulation of the pancreas (23).

Mechanisms of Neuronal Sensitization in Experimental Pancreatitis
Potential Role for the Vanilloid Receptor, TRPV1
We have shown that both acute and chronic pancreatitis result in an increase in capsaicin-evoked release of CGRP from thoracic sensory neurons, suggesting involvement of the vanilloid receptor, TRPV1 (21,23). Subsequently, we have confirmed functional sensitization of this receptor in both models, using patch-clamp techniques on pancreas-specific sensory neurons (unpublished). This receptor is expressed by nociceptive primary afferents, responds to and appears to integrate several noxious stimuli produced during tissue injury, including heat, local tissue acidosis, and several proalgesic metabolites. Activation of the receptor results in a cationic, calcium-preferring current, which leads to depolarization of the membrane. Acid and heat are both thought to function as endogenous ligands of this receptor and recent evidence also points to a potential role for other biologically active compounds such as anandamide and related lipid metabolites.

Potential Role for Neurotrophins and Protein Kinases
We had previously described an increased expression of NGF as well as other neurotrophic factors in the pancreas of animals with acute L-arginine-induced inflammation (24,25). Subsequently, we also observed increases in mRNA levels of preprotachykinin (PPT) and CGRP in thoracic dorsal root ganglia (DRG) (T9–T11). No changes were found in cervical or lumbar DRG (data not shown) suggesting that this effect was secondary to the induction of pancreatitis and not a nonspecific response to systemic or peritoneal L-arginine by itself (21). Initial studies with this model, therefore, have produced findings similar to those found in some human studies: increased neuropeptide content of nerve fibers and increased NGF in the pancreas. We have also shown similar results in a more chronic model of pancreatitis induced by TNBS (see above)—significant increases in NGF protein in the pancreas and in expression of neuropeptides CGRP and SP in the sensory neurons from dorsal root ganglia receiving input from the pancreas (21).

NGF may be responsible for the sensitization of TRPV1 in acute pancreatitis (26). In addition, nociceptive sensitization in several somatic pain models has been associated with activation of protein kinases including trypomyosin-related kinase A (trkA)(the high-affinity receptor for NGF), protein kinase C (PKC), and protein kinase A (PKA). In the L-arginine model, increased sensitivity to abdominal stimulation with VFF observed in rats with pancreatitis was associated with an eight-fold increase in levels of phosphorylated trkA in the pancreas. We, therefore, tested the hypothesis that systemic treatment with a kinase inhibitor, k252a, known to inhibit all of these kinases, would alleviate pain in an animal model of pancreatitis. Treatment with the kinase inhibitor k252a suppressed the phosphorylation of trkA in the pancreas as well as reversed both the abdominal sensitivity and the increase in neuropeptide expression associated with pancreatitis (21).

Potential Role for Trypsin

In addition to the somewhat ubiquitous inflammatory elements described above, pancreatitis is also uniquely associated with a significant release and activation of endogenous proteases such as trypsin that may contribute to pain by causing damage to afferent nerves. In addition, these activated proteases exert direct effects on sensory neurons, mediated by specific receptors such as protease-activated receptor-2 (PAR-2), a member of a unique family of G-protein-coupled receptors (27–33). We demonstrated the presence of PAR-2 mRNA and protein expression in adult rat thoracic DRG, as well as an increase in intracellular calcium in response to treatment of cultured DRG neurons with either trypsin or the PAR-2 agonist activating peptide (AcPep) (34). We then showed that activation of PAR-2 in vitro resulted in sensitization of the TRPV1 receptor in the form of enhanced capsaicin-evoked release of CGRP, a marker for nociceptive signaling. Further, when injected directly into the pancreatic duct, AcPep was able to activate directly pancreas-specific afferent neurons in vivo, as well as sensitize them to subsequent applications of capsaicin, as measured by FOS expression in the dorsal horn of the spinal cord. These observations suggest that PAR-2 contributes to nociceptive signaling and may provide a novel link between inflammation and pain in pancreatitis.

The natural agonists for PAR-2 include trypsin and mast cell tryptase, with the former the obvious candidate in the setting of pancreatitis. We therefore, tested the effect of different doses of intraductal pancreatic trypsin injections on FOS expression in vivo and showed that it significantly increased FOS expression over boiled trypsin in a dose-dependent manner in spinal segments receiving signals from the pancreas (35). We also examined whether infusion of trypsin into the pancreatic duct could provoke a behavioral pain response in awake rats. To test this we used a surrogate assay for visceral pain, the visceromotor reflex. Acute visceral pain can cause reflex contractions of somatotopically innervated skeletal muscle, which can be measured by electromyography (EMG). Infusion of trypsin as well as AcPep into the pancreatic duct significantly increased EMG activity of the acromiotrapezius muscle suggesting that trypsin can induce a behavioral nocisponsive effect in conscious rats. To determine whether direct activation of PAR-2 produces a similar nocisponsive effect as trypsin, the PAR-2 agonist, AcPep (1 mM), was injected into the pancreas. We examined cross desensitization of the nocisponsive effect to provide evidence that trypsin and PAR-2 AcPep activate the same receptor. Infusion of the pancreatic duct with AcPep significantly decreased subsequent responses to trypsin.

Potential Role for Mast Cells

Mast cells have been implicated in the pathogenesis of several painful visceral syndromes such as interstitial cystitis and IBS (see respective chapters), where they have been found in close proximity to nerve endings. They are increased in both acute and chronic pancreatitis in humans (36,37). Activated mast cells can release several mediators that increase excitability of neurons such as NGF and tryptase, whose potential role in pancreatitic pain has been alluded to above. In turn, neurotransmitters such as substance P can trigger mast cell degranulation. We hypothesized that mast cells are involved in the pathogenesis of pain in chronic pancreatitis and examined the association of pain with mast cells in autopsy specimens of patients with painful chronic pancreatitis (38). Archival tissues with histological diagnoses of chronic pancreatitis were identified and clinical records reviewed for presence or absence of reported pain in humans. Humans with painful chronic pancreatitis demonstrated a 3.5-fold increase in pancreatic mast cells as compared with those with painless chronic pancreatitis. We also studied this hypothesis using an experimental model of TNBS-induced chronic pancreatitis in both wild type and mast cell deficient mice (MCDM). The presence of pain was assessed using VFFs to measure abdominal withdrawal responses in both wild type and MCDM mice with and without chronic pancreatitis. Wild type mice with chronic pancreatitis were significantly more sensitive as assessed by VFF pain testing of the abdomen, when compared with MCDM.

Summary

Our understanding of the pathogenesis of pain in pancreatitis is still evolving. Recent insights from both human as well as experimental animal studies are beginning to shed light on potential mechanisms of pain. There is growing evidence for a role of neurotrophins and possibly,

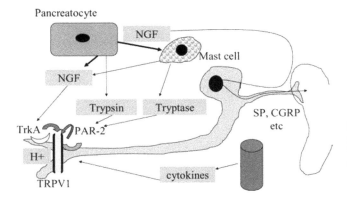

Figure 1 A conceptual paradigm for the pathogenesis of pain in pancreatitis (see text for details). *Abbreviations*: NGF, nerve growth factor; trkA trypomyosin-related kinase A receptor; TRPV1, vanilloid receptor.

trypsin in neuronal sensitization mediated in part at least via the TRPV1 receptor, as illustrated by the conceptual paradigm in Figure 1. If validated, these findings have major implications for the pathogenesis of pain in chronic pancreatitis and will provide novel targets for analgesic therapy.

Clinical Patterns of Pain in Chronic Pancreatitis

The pain in chronic pancreatitis can vary highly from patient to patient as well as over time in the same patient; this fact has made it difficult to reliably interpret the published literature, much of which is in the form of uncontrolled clinical trials of various treatments. Several factors may contribute to this variability, including etiology, natural history of the pancreatitis, and the presence or absence of associated complications (e.g., pseudocysts, biliary obstruction, etc.). In addition, psychosocial factors such as secondary gain and an addiction-prone personality significantly add to the complexity of management of these patients. Pain is present in approximately 75% of patients with alcoholic-chronic pancreatitis, 50% of patients with late-onset idiopathic chronic pancreatitis, and 100% of patients with early-onset idiopathic chronic pancreatitis (2). Most of the published literature deals with pain in patients with alcoholic pancreatitis, because it is the most common form of the disease. Even in these patients, pain is not a uniform symptom, and its pattern may have implications for therapy and prognosis. Thus, in a prospective longitudinal study of 207 patients, Ammann and Muellhaupt (39,40) identified two categories of patients in approximately equal numbers. The first group reported an intermittent, but recurrent pattern of short episodes of pain; none of these patients required surgery. The second group complained of constant pain occurring two or more days per week for at least two months at a time and all of them underwent surgery; the majority of these patients had a pseudocyst and some of the others had biliary obstruction (this was particularly common later in the course of the disease). Most patients (80%) in either group had pain relief after 10 years.

Although it appears that pain will subside spontaneously over time in at least half of patients with alcoholic chronic pancreatitis, in practice such an outcome remains difficult to predict in an individual patient and several studies suggest that most patients will continue to experience pain despite glandular failure, withdrawal of alcohol (41–43). Thus, a decision to withhold surgical or other invasive therapies in the hope of eventual "burn-out" is probably not warranted. This is particularly true of patients with idiopathic forms of chronic pancreatitis, with one series reporting spontaneous cessation of pain in only about 25% (44).

Management of Pancreatic Pain
General Measures and Analgesic Use

As can be appreciated, the treatment of pain in patients with chronic pancreatitis remains unsatisfactory. Even if complicated procedures are attempted, pain relief may not be complete and patients will continue to require medical attention and more often than not, narcotic

Table 2 Current Approaches to Management of Pain in Chronic Pancreatitis

General measures
  Cessation of alcohol intake
  Analgesics
Reduction of intrapancreatic pressure
    Suppression of secretion
      Enzymes
      Octreotide
    Decompression techniques
      Endoscopic dilation and stenting
      Stone removal (endoscopic or ESWL)
    Surgical drainage (Peustow)
Organ resection
Neural interruption
  Percutaneous or endoscopic (EUS) nerve blocks
  Surgical (thorascopic) splanchnic nerve resection

analgesics. The management of these patients requires skills and patience, as well as a clear and realistic understanding of the goals of the treatment (Table 2) and a firm "patient-physician" contract. It is best done in a multidisciplinary pain-management environment, requiring input from mental health professionals, anesthesiologists, social, and rehabilitation workers. However, the gastroenterologist remains central in this process and familiarity with the principles and practice of chronic narcotic prescriptions is essential (Table 2).

Measures Aimed at Reduction of Intrapancreatic Pressure

Suppression of Secretions

The rationale behind enzyme treatment is that activated proteinases in the duodenal lumen cleave the peptide that causes release of CCK and hence, suppress further pancreatic secretion, diminishing intraductal pressures. Although enzymatic therapy has become firmly entrenched for the treatment of painful pancreatitis, the evidence supporting this practice is equivocal at best; only one of six randomized controlled trials showed a statistically significant benefit and only 52% of the pooled patient population expressed a preference for enzyme over placebo (45). Although it has been argued otherwise, it is unlikely that the lack of response in these studies is simply due to the use of delayed release preparations with inadequate concentrations of proteases in the duodenal lumen (3). The response to octreotide in this setting has similarly been disappointing (46).

Decompression Techniques

Endoscopic approaches are increasingly being attempted in many patients as an alternative to surgery for the treatment of pseudocysts (47), stone removal (48), stricture dilation/ stenting, (49) or pancreatic sphincter hypertension (50). Stricture dilation and stenting have been reported to vary widely in efficacy, with persistent pain relief ranging from as low as 11% to nearly 90% (51–53); this variation in part is explained by the divergent nature of the trials and methodology as well as the underlying pathology and techniques used. Endoscopic stone removal is often combined with extracorporeal shock wave lithotripsy, a combination that is clearly of considerable promise at least in a subset of patients with chronic–calcific pancreatitis with successful stone clearance and pain relief varying from approximately 50% to 80% of patients (54). While a strong case can be made for the use of endoscopic drainage of pseudocysts, endoscopy approaches for the other indications, particularly stricture dilation, remains to be validated. This is in large part because to the lack of controlled trials, the limited duration of follow up, questions about the robustness of pain relief (many patients remain on narcotic analgesics despite "relief"), and the dominance of single-center experiences only. Further, the results of more "robust" decompression techniques such as surgical pancreatojejunostomy (see below) are also disappointing in the long term, raising questions about the underlying rationale for these procedures in all these patients.

    If attempted, these procedures are probably best done by experts in major referral centers. This is because they are relatively high risk; pancreatic sphincterotomy is often required, ductal and parenchymal trauma can occur, and indwelling stents themselves can induce chronic changes.

Surgical Decompression for Chronic Pancreatitis

The first widely used surgical approach for painful pancreatitis was the lateral pancreatojejunostomy, first described by Puestow and Gillesby and modified by Partington and Rochelle. This is essentially a decompression procedure, based on relieving putative high intrapancreatic pressures as implied by the presence of a significantly dilated main pancreatic duct (>6–7 mm). Short-term results with this procedure are impressive. Pain relief is achieved in 80% of cases with very low morbidity and mortality (0–5%). However, these results are not sustained over time: As early as two years after surgery, pain relief persists in only 60% of patients (3,55) with perhaps a further decline in the long term. Possible reasons for incomplete or transient relief from this procedure include progression of underlying disease, and failure of the procedure actually to decrease intraparenchymal pressure, as suggested by at least one study (10). Further, a significant proportion (25–66%) of these patients may require concomitant or additional surgery for duodenal and or biliary strictures.

Pancreatic Resection Procedures for Chronic Pancreatitis

Patients without dilated ducts (small-duct disease) do not have the same decompressive options, either endoscopically or surgically. The early surgical approaches in these patients were based on the axiom that the degree of pain was proportional to the amount of (diseased) gland. This led to the evolution of strategies that attempted to maximize the amount of tissue that could be removed, while avoiding the risks of pancreatoduodenectomy and the need for intestinal and biliary anastomoses. Distal subtotal resections were performed from the tail toward the head of the gland resulting in 60% to nearly 95% resections. However, long-term results remained disappointing and were further complicated by the almost inevitable development of exocrine and endocrine insufficiency by extensive resection. Subsequently, interest shifted away from the "left-to-right" approach to the proximal part of the pancreas, based on the concept that the head of the pancreas may function as the "pain pacemaker" of this organ. This coincided with significant improvements in the operative mortality (<5%) after pancreatoduodenectomy. In patients with small duct disease, resection of the pancreatic head by either a conventional or pylorus-preserving pancreaticoduodenectomy will provide pain relief in up to 85% of patients, even if the disease extends into the distal pancreas (46). Again, however, long-term results may not be sustained and fall from 70% to 50% (55). While theoretically able to provide complete relief, total pancreatectomy is not recommended because not only do a significant number of patients continue to have pain, but also the metabolic consequences can be very severe. Although autotransplantation of islet or pancreatic tissue is being performed in combination with this procedure in some centers, low success rates and technical challenges remain formidable obstacles (56–58). Recent data on this procedure from a particular center in the United States suggests a more optimistic picture with 58% of patients becoming narcotic independent and 40% being insulin-free after a mean follow up of 18 months (59). Finally, some centers in Europe advocate duodenum-preserving resection of the pancreatic head in patients with inflammatory masses in the head of the pancreas with short-term pain relief reported in 70% to 90% of cases (60). Although the success rates are similar to pancreaticoduodenectomy, these operations may not have significant nutritional advantages (46) and are not widely practiced in this country.

Comparative Studies

The debate on surgical versus endoscopic approaches has until now been largely conducted along partisan lines. Recently, however, the first prospective, randomized study comparing surgery with endoscopy in patients with painful obstructive chronic pancreatitis was published (61). Surgery was tailored to patient anatomy and consisted of resection (80%) and drainage (20%) procedures, while endotherapy included sphincterotomy and stenting (52%) and/or stone removal (23%), but not extra corporeal shock wave lithotripsy (ESWL). Of 140 eligible patients, only about half agreed to be randomized with the rest opting for one treatment or the other. However, the results were similar regardless of whether the analysis included all 140 patients or only those randomized. when the analysis included all patients, the initial success rates were around 50% for both groups, but at the five-year follow up, complete absence of pain was seen in about 35% of the surgical group but in only about 15% of the endotherapy group; increase in body weight was also greater by 20% to 25% in the surgical group, while new-onset diabetes developed with similar frequency in both groups (34–43%). The authors concluded that surgery is superior to endotherapy for long-term pain reduction in patients with painful obstructive chronic pancreatitis.

Neural Interruption

As discussed earlier, pancreatic nerves traverse the celiac ganglion and splanchnic nerves and most neurolytic techniques target these areas. These techniques vary widely, ranging from radiological or endoscopic injection of "neurolytic" chemicals such as alcohol or phenol to surgical interruption such as thoracoscopic splanchnicectomy. Celiac plexus "block" typically consists of the use of a local anesthetic such as bupivacaine, usually along with a steroid. These agents are short acting with effects that range from a few days to months at most. True "neurolytic" injections use toxic chemicals such as absolute alcohol or phenol that cause permanent damage to the nerves. However, "permanence" is seldom if ever achieved in practice and most investigators avoid the use of alcohol for fear of potential neurological consequences such as paraplegia.

The cumulative experience with 90 patients undergoing EUS-guided celiac plexus block at a single center is illustrated in Figure 2 (62). As can be seen, most patients had relapsed within a month of treatment. In general, the response rate was poorer in younger patients (<45 years) and those with a history of prior pancreatic surgery for chronic pancreatitis were least likely to benefit. There are many potential explanations for the short duration of response including the choice of drugs (see above), anatomical variability in the celiac plexus itself, and the fact that nerves proximal to the block remain intact and can set up independent foci of excitability. The same group of investigators has also reported a prospective randomized comparison of EUS and CT (transposterior) approaches (63). EUS-guided celiac plexus block was more effective, as attested by the proportion of patients reporting short-term relief (50% vs. 25%), the absolute posttreatment mean pain scores (1 vs. 9, on a scale of 1–10), and duration of treatment (15 weeks vs. four weeks). Further, EUS-guided celiac block was also less expensive ($1100 vs. $1400). Thus, on the basis of very limited data, it appears that the EUS-guided approach is more cost effective than that using CT. However, the percutaneous method may be the preferred method for the occasional patient who is at high risk for conscious sedation or general anesthesia.

Thoracoscopic "splanchnicectomy" is a recent surgical approach to neural interruption (64–66). As with other procedures, early enthusiasm for this treatment has been tempered by experience with recent studies suggesting that initial short-term reductions in pain, degree of disability, and narcotics are not sustained in the long term (67–69). The risks of this procedure include atelactasis, intercostal neuralgia, pneumothorax, chlyothorax, bleeding,

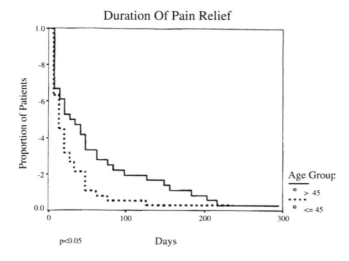

Figure 2 Kaplan-Meier plot comparing subjects less than 45 years if age to patients greater than 45 years of age. A positive response was identified a priori, as a decrease in the pain score greater than or equal to three points. The older patients had a more significant response to the EUS-guided celiac block ($p = 0.04$). *Source*: From Ref. 62.

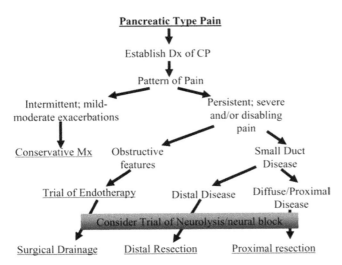

Figure 3 Suggested approach to the management of pain in chronic pancreatitis. See text for details.

postural hypotension, and pneumonia. Although the overall rate of complications is low, it remains to be seen whether this remains true as the procedure begins to be practiced outside of major medical centers.

Conclusions

Painful chronic pancreatitis remains a major clinical challenge. A suggested clinical algorithm to the approach of these patients is provided in Figure 3. As discussed in this chapter, management of these patients is difficult and all currently available measures have significant shortcomings. However, recent insights from both human as well as experimental animal studies are beginning to shed light on potential mechanisms of pain and it is hoped that they will provide novel targets for analgesic therapy in the near future. Such targets will likely include TRPV1, NGF-trkA signaling, and perhaps PAR-2.

- Setting realistic expectations (e.g., reduction not elimination of pain)
  - ✓ Improvement in physical functioning
  - ✓ Improvement in mood and associated symptoms such as sleep
  - ✓ Development of active coping skills
  - ✓ Return to work
- Opioid management
  - ✓ Only one practitioner takes responsibility for opioid prescription
  - ✓ Opioid prescription is contingent upon certain agreed obligations or goals being met by the patient e.g., return to work or alteration of inappropriate behaviors, etc. This could take then form of a written contractual arrangement
  - ✓ Unauthorized demands for emergency injectable opioids will not be tolerated although some provision can be made for "rescue analgesia" for brief exacerbations of pain

REFERENCES

1. The Burden of Gastrointestinal Diseases. AGA Publications, 2001.
2. DiMagno EP. Toward understanding (and management) of painful chronic pancreatitis. Gastroenterology 1999; 116:1252–1257.
3. American Gastroenterological Association Medical Position Statement: treatment of pain in chronic pancreatitis. Gastroenterology 1998; 115:763–764.
4. Ebbehoj N, Borly L, Madsen P, Svendsen LB. Pancreatic tissue pressure and pain in chronic pancreatitis. Pancreas 1986; 1:556–558.
5. Ebbehoj N, Christensen E, Madsen P. Prediction of outcome of pancreaticogastrostomy for pain in chronic pancreatitis. Scand J Gastroenterol 1987; 22:337–342.
6. Ebbehoj N, Klaaborg KE, Kronborg O, Madsen P. Pancreaticogastrostomy for chronic pancreatitis. Am J Surg 1989; 157:315–317.

7. Ebbehoj N, Borly L, Bulow J, Henriksen JH, Heyeraas KJ, Rasmussen SG. Evaluation of pancreatic tissue fluid pressure measurements intraoperatively and by sonographically guided fine-needle puncture. Scand J Gastroenterol 1990; 25:1097–1102.

8. Ebbehoj N, Borly L, Bulow J, et al. Pancreatic tissue fluid pressure in chronic pancreatitis. Relation to pain, morphology, and function. Scand J Gastroenterol 1990; 25:1046–1051.

9. Ebbehoj N, Borly L, Madsen P, Matzen P. Pancreatic tissue fluid pressure during drainage operations for chronic pancreatitis. Scand J Gastroenterol 1990; 25:1041–1045.

10. Ebbehoj N, Borly L, Bulow J, Rasmussen SG, Madsen P. Evaluation of pancreatic tissue fluid pressure and pain in chronic pancreatitis. A longitudinal study. Scand J Gastroenterol 1990; 25:462–466.

11. Ebbehoj N. Pancreatic tissue fluid pressure and pain in chronic pancreatitis. Dan Med Bull 1992; 39:128–133.

12. Karanjia ND, Reber HA. The cause and management of the pain of chronic pancreatitis. Gastroenterol Clin North Am 1990; 19:895–904.

13. Karanjia ND, Widdison AL, Leung F, Alvarez C, Lutrin FJ, Reber HA. Compartment syndrome in experimental chronic obstructive pancreatitis: effect of decompressing the main pancreatic duct. Br J Surg 1994; 81:259–264.

14. Manes G, Buchler M, Pieramico O, Di Sebastiano P, Malfertheiner P. Is increased pancreatic pressure related to pain in chronic pancreatitis. Int J Pancreatol 1994; 15:113–117.

15. Renou C, Grandval P, Ville E, Laugier R. Endoscopic treatment of the main pancreatic duct: correlations among morphology, manometry, and clinical follow-up. Int J Pancreatol 2000; 27:143–149.

16. Bockman DE, Buchler M, Malfertheiner P, Beger HG. Analysis of nerves in chronic pancreatitis. Gastroenterology 1988; 94:1459–1469.

17. Friess H, Zhu ZW, di Mola FF, et al. Nerve growth factor and its high-affinity receptor in chronic pancreatitis. Ann Surg 1999; 230:615–624.

18. Buchler M, Weihe E, Friess H, et al. Changes in peptidergic innervation in chronic pancreatitis. Pancreas 1992; 7:183–192.

19. Di Sebastiano P, di Mola FF, Bockman DE, Friess H, Buchler MW. Chronic pancreatitis: the perspective of pain generation by neuroimmune interaction. Gut 2003; 52:907–911.

20. Vera-Portocarrero LP, Lu Y, Westlund KN. Nociception in persistent pancreatitis in rats: effects of morphine and neuropeptide alterations. Anesthesiology 2003; 98:474–484.

21. Winston JH, Toma H, Shenoy M, et al. Acute pancreatitis results in referred mechanical hypersensitivity and neuropeptide up-regulation that can be suppressed by the protein kinase inhibitor k252a. J Pain 2003; 4:329–337.

22. Lu Y, Vera-Portocarrero LP, Westlund KN. Intrathecal coadministration of D-APV and morphine is maximally effective in a rat experimental pancreatitis model. Anesthesiology 2003; 98:734–740.

23. Winston JH, He ZJ, Shenoy M, Xiao SY, Pasricha PJ. Molecular and behavioral changes in nociception in a novel rat model of chronic pancreatitis for the study of pain. Pain 2005; 117:214–222.

24. Toma H, Winston J, Micci MA, Shenoy M, Pasricha PJ. Nerve growth factor expression is up-regulated in the rat model of L-arginine-induced acute pancreatitis. Gastroenterology 2000; 119:1373–1381.

25. Toma H, Winston JH, Micci MA, Li H, Hellmich HL, Pasricha PJ. Characterization of the neurotrophic response to acute pancreatitis. Pancreas 2002; 25:31–38.

26. Winston J, Wang W, Palade P, et al. NGF induces sensitization of the vanilloid receptor (TRPV1) response in sensory neurons in acute pancreatitis by recruiting silent nociceptors. Gastroenterology 2005; 128:A86.

27. Dery O, Bunnett NW. Proteinase-activated receptors: a growing family of heptahelical receptors for thrombin, trypsin, and tryptase. Biochem Soc Trans 1999; 27:246–254.

28. Saito T, Bunnett NW. Protease-activated receptors: regulation of neuronal function. Neuromolecular Med 2005; 7:79–99.

29. Jacob C, Yang PC, Darmoul D, et al. Mast cell tryptase controls paracellular permeability of the intestine. Role of protease-activated receptor 2 and beta-arrestins. J Biol Chem 2005; 280:31936–31948.

30. Amadesi S, Bunnett N. Protease-activated receptors: protease signaling in the gastrointestinal tract. Curr Opin Pharmacol 2004; 4:551–556.

31. Coelho AM, Ossovskaya V, Bunnett NW. Proteinase-activated receptor-2: physiological and pathophysiological roles. Curr Med Chem Cardiovasc Hematol Agents 2003; 1:61–72.

32. Ossovskaya VS, Bunnett NW. Protease-activated receptors: contribution to physiology and disease. Physiol Rev 2004; 84:579–621.

33. Cottrell GS, Amadesi S, Schmidlin F, Bunnett N. Protease-activated receptor 2: activation, signalling and function. Biochem Soc Trans 2003; 31:1191–1197.

34. Hoogerwerf WA, Zou L, Shenoy M, et al. The proteinase-activated receptor 2 is involved in nociception. J Neuroscience 2001; 21:9036–9042.

35. Hoogerwerf WA, Shenoy M, Winston JH, Xiao SY, He Z, Pasricha PJ. Trypsin mediates nociception via the proteinase-activated receptor 2: a potentially novel role in pancreatic pain. Gastroenterology 2004; 127:883–891.

36. Braganza JM. Mast cell: pivotal player in lethal acute pancreatitis. QJM 2000; 93:469–476.

37. Esposito I, Friess H, Kappeler A, et al. Mast cell distribution and activation in chronic pancreatitis. Hum Pathol 2001; 32:1174–1183.

38. Hoogerwerf WA, Gondesen K, Xiao SY, Winston JH, Willis WD, Pasricha PJ. The role of mast cells in the pathogenesis of pain in chronic pancreatitis. BMC Gastroenterol 2005; 5:8.
39. Ammann RW. The natural history of alcoholic chronic pancreatitis. Intern Med 2001; 40: 368–375.
40. Ammann RW, Muellhaupt B. The natural history of pain in alcoholic chronic pancreatitis. Gastroenterology 1999; 116:1132–1140.
41. Di Sebastiano P, Friess H, Di Mola FF, Innocenti P, Buchler MW. Mechanisms of pain in chronic pancreatitis. Ann Ital Chir 2000; 71:11–16.
42. Malfertheiner P, Buchler M, Stanescu A, Ditschuneit H. Pancreatic morphology and function in relationship to pain in chronic pancreatitis. Int J Pancreatol 1987; 2:59–66.
43. Malfertheiner P, Pieramico O, Buchler M, Ditschuneit H. Relationship between pancreatic function and pain in chronic pancreatitis. Acta Chir Scand 1990; 156:267–270; discussion 270–271.
44. Lankisch PG, Seidensticker F, Lohr-Happe A, Otto J, Creutzfeldt W. The course of pain is the same in alcohol- and nonalcohol-induced chronic pancreatitis. Pancreas 1995; 10:338–341.
45. Brown A, Hughes M, Tenner S, Banks PA. Does pancreatic enzyme supplementation reduce pain in patients with chronic pancreatitis: a meta-analysis [see comments]. Am J Gastroenterol 1997; 92:2032–2035.
46. Apfel SC, Kessler JA, Adornato BT, Litchy WJ, Sanders C, Rask CA. Recombinant human nerve growth factor in the treatment of diabetic polyneuropathy. NGF Study Group [see comments]. Neurology 1998; 51:695–702.
47. Mark DH, Lefevre F, Flamm CR, Aronson N. Evidence-based assessment of ERCP in the treatment of pancreatitis. Gastrointest Endosc 2002; 56:S249–S254.
48. Kozarek RA, Brandabur JJ, Ball TJ, et al. Clinical outcomes in patients who undergo extracorporeal shock wave lithotripsy for chronic calcific pancreatitis. Gastrointest Endosc 2002; 56:496–500.
49. Boerma D, Huibregtse K, Gulik TM, Rauws EA, Obertop H, Gouma DJ. Long-term outcome of endoscopic stent placement for chronic pancreatitis associated with pancreas divisum. Endoscopy 2000; 32:452–456.
50. Okolo PI 3rd, Pasricha PJ, Kalloo AN. What are the long-term results of endoscopic pancreatic sphincterotomy. Gastrointest Endosc 2000; 52:15–19.
51. Lehman GA. Role of ERCP and other endoscopic modalities in chronic pancreatitis. Gastrointest Endosc 2002; 56:S237–S240.
52. Hammarstrom LE. Endoscopic management of chronic and non-biliary recurrent pancreatitis. Scand J Gastroenterol 2004; 39:5–13.
53. Rosch T, Daniel S, Scholz M, et al. Endoscopic treatment of chronic pancreatitis: a multicenter study of 1000 patients with long-term follow-up. Endoscopy 2002; 34:765–771.
54. Brand B, Kahl M, Sidhu S, et al. Prospective evaluation of morphology, function, and quality of life after extracorporeal shockwave lithotripsy and endoscopic treatment of chronic calcific pancreatitis. Am J Gastroenterol 2000; 95:3428–3438.
55. Sarr MG, Sakorafas GH. Incapacitating pain of chronic pancreatitis: a surgical perspective of what is known and what needs to be known. Gastrointest Endosc 1999; 49:S85–S89.
56. White SA, Davies JE, Pollard C, et al. Pancreas resection and islet autotransplantation for end-stage chronic pancreatitis. Ann Surg 2001; 233:423–431.
57. Bell RH Jr. Surgical options in the patient with chronic pancreatitis. Curr Gastroenterol Rep 2000; 2:146–151.
58. Johnson PR, White SA, Robertson GS, et al. Pancreatic islet autotransplantation combined with total pancreatectomy for the treatment of chronic pancreatitis–the Leicester experience. J Mol Med 1999; 77:130–132.
59. Ahmad SA, Lowy AM, Wray CJ, et al. Factors associated with insulin and narcotic independence after islet autotransplantation in patients with severe chronic pancreatitis. J Am Coll Surg 2005; 201:680–687.
60. Cunha JE, Penteado S, Jukemura J, Machado MC, Bacchella T. Surgical and interventional treatment of chronic pancreatitis. Pancreatology 2004; 4:540–550.
61. Dite P, Ruzicka M, Zboril V, Novotny I. A prospective, randomized trial comparing endoscopic and surgical therapy for chronic pancreatitis. Endoscopy 2003; 35:553–558.
62. Gress F, Schmitt C, Sherman S, Ciaccia D, Ikenberry S, Lehman G. Endoscopic ultrasound-guided celiac plexus block for managing abdominal pain associated with chronic pancreatitis: a prospective single center experience. Am J Gastroenterol 2001; 96:409–416.
63. Gress F, Schmitt C, Sherman S, Ikenberry S, Lehman G. A prospective randomized comparison of endoscopic ultrasound- and computed tomography-guided celiac plexus block for managing chronic pancreatitis pain. Am J Gastroenterol 1999; 94:900–905.
64. Leksowski K. Thoracoscopic splanchnicectomy for the relief of pain due to chronic pancreatitis. Surg Endosc 2001; 15:592–596.
65. Bradley EL 3rd, Reynhout JA, Peer GL. Thoracoscopic splanchnicectomy for "small duct" chronic pancreatitis: case selection by differential epidural analgesia. J Gastrointest Surg 1998; 2:88–94.
66. Bradley EL 3rd, Bem J. Nerve blocks and neuroablative surgery for chronic pancreatitis. World J Surg 2003; 27:1241–1248.

67. Buscher HC, Jansen JB, van Dongen R, Bleichrodt RP, van Goor H. Long-term results of bilateral thoracoscopic splanchnicectomy in patients with chronic pancreatitis. Br J Surg 2002; 89:158–162.
68. Howard TJ, Swofford JB, Wagner DL, Sherman S, Lehman GA. Quality of life after bilateral thoracoscopic splanchnicectomy: long-term evaluation in patients with chronic pancreatitis. J Gastrointest Surg 2002; 6:845–852; discussion 853–854.
69. Maher JW, Johlin FC, Pearson D. Thoracoscopic splanchnicectomy for chronic pancreatitis pain. Surgery 1996; 120:603–609; discussion 609–610.

28 | Abdominal Wall Pain[a]

David S. Greenbaum
College of Human Medicine, Michigan State University, Michigan, U.S.A.

"...following up a positive Carnett's sign with a successful injection of local anesthetic must be one of the most cost effective procedures in gastroenterology" (1).

■ Case

You see a 46-year-old woman in the Emergency Department for the third time in the past month because of severe right upper quadrant pain. For two months, she has needed hydrocodone with acetaminophen every four to six hours to "take the edge off" the pain that interfered with sleep and her work as a high school teacher. Nonsteroidal anti-inflammatory drugs (NSAIDs) had been unhelpful. A selective serotonin reuptake inhibitor was started two weeks ago. Beginning two years ago, the pain varied from dull to sharp and from moderate to "excruciating...11/10." Initially, it was intermittent but has been constant for the last six months. She has not identified accentuating or alleviating factors. Except for a 15-lb weight gain over the past three years, she had been without complaints.

Five months ago a laparoscopic cholecystectomy was performed. An acalculous gall bladder with "minimal mucosal inflammatory reaction" was removed. Earlier ultrasonic examination had suggested a "slightly thickened gall bladder wall" and "possible sludge." Upper gastrointestinal series, hepatobiliary scan, esophagogastroduodenoscopy and, endoscopic retrograde cholangiopancreatography were normal. No cholesterol crystals were found in the duodenal aspirate after cholecystokinin stimulation. Abdominal computerized tomography showed mild hepatic steatosis and absence of the gall bladder. Numerous laboratory tests were normal.

The obviously uncomfortable patient is sitting with her left hand pressed to her right upper quadrant. Her vital signs are normal. On examination you find tenderness localized to a 2-cm area in the right upper quadrant at the lateral border of the rectus abdominis, 5 cm from the nearest laparoscopy scar. With the examining finger fixed on the tender point, the pain becomes unbearable as she tenses the recti abdominis by lifting her head off the pillow—a positive Carnett sign. After two years, chronic abdominal wall pain (CAWP) has been diagnosed!

ECONOMIC COSTS

The charges for the patient's imaging and endoscopic procedures and cholecystectomy were approximately $11,000. Laboratory tests, postoperative care, physician office and Emergency Department visits, and drugs were additional costs. Although it can be debated which tests were unnecessary, even with concerns about potential litigation, it is difficult to justify multiple procedures to exclude rather than support suspected diagnoses.

The problem of economic costs in relation to abdominal wall pain was raised in 1991 by an editorial in The Lancet titled in part "Could Carnett cut costs?" that suggested economic savings if more physicians were aware of this source of pain (2). In 1994, we reported the estimated average charge for tests to exclude visceral lesions as $880 (2004 dollars) in 56 patients ultimately diagnosed with abdominal wall pain. For the 30 patients in the group who had procedures, the average charge was $2070 (2004 dollars) (3). Thompson et al. in 2001 reported the mean charge to be $6727 before the diagnosis was made (4). A retrospective Kaiser-Permanente study of 133 patients seen in consultation over a five-year period compared a number of outcomes during the year before and the year after CAWP was diagnosed. Health-care usage decreased by almost fourfold, and costs for abdominal pain–related charges dropped a mean of 48%. The decrease would have been even greater if upper gastrointestinal endoscopy had not been carried out in about 20% of the patients after CAWP was identified (5). The senior author acknowledged that although he was confident of the CAWP diagnosis, he felt

---

[a] Dedicated to Radhika Srinivasan, M.D.

it necessary to exclude peptic ulcer in order to satisfy patients and referring doctors (Longstreth GF, Personal communication, 2004). The cost data from this prepaid plan with salaried physicians is not be directly applicable to other systems where the costs may well be greater.

PREVALENCE

If CAWP was rare, there would be less concern about missing the diagnosis. However, it appears to be relatively frequent in certain groups of patients, being highest in those individuals referred to specialty practices for their pain. Aware physicians have reported seeing one to two such patients in a week and even three in one day (6,7). Thomson et al. estimated that about 1% of all general surgical referrals were eventually considered to be CAWP (8). Applegate speculated that for every 150 patients seen in a primary care practice one to two had abdominal wall pain (9). Over 14 years of obstetrical-gynecological practice, Shute reported seeing 269 such patients (10). CAWP was diagnosed in 100 patients during 15 years and 74 patients over five years in separate university gastroenterology practices (3,11). During a seven-month period, 38% (68 of 226) of patients referred for abdominal pain to a university gastroenterology clinic were identified as having a "myofascial" origin of the complaint. Forty-two had been referred for biliary manometry, and of these, 38 (91%) had postcholecystectomy right upper quadrant pain that was the same as the preoperative pain (12). Thirty-two of 43 (74%) patients referred to a pain clinic by gastroenterologists for persistent abdominal pain of obscure origin were diagnosed with abdominal wall pain (13). In a gynecological clinic specializing in abdominal-pelvic pain, 131 of 177 (74%) women had localized superficial tender areas, mainly abdominal (14). The abdominal wall was the source of pain in 19 of 67 (28%) patients admitted to a surgical service over a six-month period with "nonspecific" abdominal pain and in 24 of 120 (20%) emergency surgical admissions in another study (15,16). Hall and Lee reported that about 15% of patients referred to a pain clinic for abdominal pain suffered from parietal pain (17). In an unpublished prospective survey of 162 patients seen in two private gastroenterology practices with chronic abdominal pain, 22 (13.6%) fulfilled the CAWP diagnostic criteria (Greenbaum DS, Greenbaum RB, unpublished data, 1995). Seventeen patients of 156 (11%) with pain of obscure etiology in an academic gastroenterology practice were considered to have wall pain (18). The previously-noted 133 Kaiser-Permanente patients diagnosed as CAWP comprised 7.8% of 1705 patients referred with abdominal symptoms (5).

NONRECOGNITION OF CAWP

When presented with a classic case history of abdominal wall pain, only 6 of 23 (26%) medical residents correctly identified the source of symptoms (4). Just 34% of gastroenterologists referring patients to a pain clinic for undiagnosed abdominal pain later found to arise from the wall had made the correct diagnosis (13). Merely 3% of all physicians referring patients to a gastroenterology clinic for the same complaint suspected CAWP (5). Although chest wall pain is readily recognized, pain arising from the abdominal wall is not. Why is an entity that is usually easily diagnosed so often undetected? The problem appears to be lack of awareness of diagnostic findings rather than ignorance of CAWP. Is this because most physicians are trained to think in terms of abdominal visceral disease and its potential life-threatening implications? Could this be because there are potentially more intra-abdominal than intrathoracic causes of pain? Since the diagnosis of CAWP is entirely dependent on history and physical examination, it may be often overlooked in an environment of great dependence on endoscopy, imaging, and biochemical testing. Ironically, even in 1926, Carnett commented on the frequency of the missed diagnosis (6).

ETIOLOGIES

Probably the most common putative cause of CAWP is entrapment of the anterior cutaneous branch of one of the T7–T12 intercostal nerves in its tortuous course through the rectus abdominis. After negotiating a 90° angle, the nerve passes from the posterior rectus sheath through a fibrous foramen in the muscle and then again branches at right angles following passage

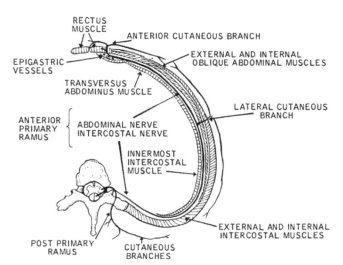

Figure 1 Intercostal nerve course. *Source*: From Ref. 19.

through the anterior rectus sheath just below the overlying aponeurosis (Figs. 1 and 2). Applegate, who has championed this etiology of abdominal wall pain, termed it "anterior cutaneous nerve syndrome" (19). He postulated that when there is increased intra-abdominal pressure, the fatty "plug" that accompanies the neurovascular bundle may herniate into the unyielding fibrous ring causing neural ischemia. He has also posited that stretching the nerve, a thoracic nerve's most distal branch from the spinal cord against the fibrous ring may cause inflammation and edema (20). These hypotheses would fit well with the observations that obesity and edema accompanying pregnancy and use of oral contraceptives have been associated with CAWP in some studies (21,22). Entrapment may involve the lateral cutaneous branch of the thoracic nerves or the ilioinguinal and iliohypogastric nerves, although the pain is not primarily located in the anterior abdominal wall. Other neuropathies that may cause abdominal wall pain are due to diabetes, herpes zoster, trauma, and malignant neoplasia. Myofascial trigger points are implicated, but seem to be less common than neural involvement. Incisional, epigastric and Spigelian (linea semilunaris) hernias, rectus sheath hematomas, endometrial implants are sometimes sources of wall pain and should be

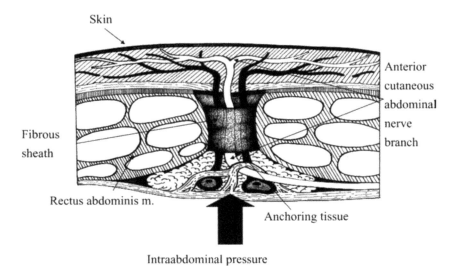

Figure 2 Course of anterior cutaneous nerve in abdominal wall.

identifiable as tender protrusions or nodules. "Slipped rib syndrome" may occasionally account for lateral upper quadrant pain (23,24).

CLINICAL HISTORY

Most studies have reported that CAWP is more often on the right side. The pain is frequently at the linea semilunaris, the lateral edge of the rectus abdominis, or in proximity to surgical scars. However, it may be in any location and is frequently at multiple sites. The diagnosis of somatic pain may be suspected when the patient indicates that pain is very narrowly localized. Visceral sensation cannot be so precisely confined because of its widely overlapping spinal cord representation. However, when wall pain is particularly severe, it is usually diffuse and difficult to localize. It varies from mild to excruciating and constant to intermittent. Although the quality and intensity of abdominal wall pain has no unique features, there often are neuropathic qualities often described as burning, sharp, stabbing, or tingling. Nevertheless, there are some historical cues that may be helpful. Relief afforded by external support of the painful area, particularly if there is a sagging panniculus, is a cue that the pain is likely from the abdominal wall. Twenty-two patients with abdominal pain fulfilling the CAWP diagnostic criteria were compared with 140 whose pain did not meet the criteria. The likelihood ratios in favor of CAWP were 4.7 ($p = 0.016$) if the pain was adjacent to a surgical scar, 3.7 ($p = 0.028$) if accentuated by walking), 2.5 ($p = 0.06$) when relieved by lying down, and against CAWP if heartburn was also present 0.2, ($p = 0.007$) or when abdominal pain was associated with three or more gastrointestinal symptoms 0.14, ($p = 0.005$) (Greenbaum DS, Greenbaum RB, unpublished data, 1995).

Most patients with CAWP are in their late 40s or early 50s, and 60% to more than 80% are women, a proportion that does not appear to be significantly different from patients with abdominal visceral pain. The Kaiser-Permanente study reported that almost 84% of CAWP patients were overweight or obese by body mass index (BMI) criteria (5). We, too, found a high BMI (mean 28.7) in CAWP patients, but it was not significantly different from the patients with non-CAWP pain (Greenbaum DS, Greenbaum RB, unpublished data, 1995).

PHYSICAL EXAMINATION

CAWP can only be diagnosed by the physical findings. Often there is exquisite tenderness and allodynia, with gentle stroking or pinching the skin. This may extend over the course of the corresponding dermatome that contrasts dramatically with the comparable area on the opposite side. If radiculopathy is responsible for the pain, there may be tenderness over the vertebral body and transverse process. The Carnett sign has been considered an essential diagnostic feature. As originally defined, a positive "Test A" is localized abdominal tenderness in the supine relaxed patient while "Test B" is positive when the tenderness is "almost or quite as much" during abdominal wall muscle tensing (6). We have been impressed that pain is usually markedly increased when the supine patient raises the head and shoulders and/or lifts both heels while the palpating finger remains on the area of tenderness (3). Carnett explained that in the case of visceral pain, tightening the abdominal wall protects the underlying tender structure from pressure of the finger, whereas if pain arises from the abdominal wall, contracting its muscles increases pressure and accentuates tenderness. The diagnostic maneuvers are impossible to carry out with young children and uncomprehending or uncooperative adults. Obviously they are inappropriate when there is diffuse abdominal tenderness.

Gallegos and Hobsley devised an algorithm for a diagnostic approach to chronic abdominal pain based with the Carnett test as the first nodal point (25). In essence, if the tenderness is in proximity of a surgical scar and there is no evidence of a hernia, local anesthetic is injected and if the pain is substantially relieved, nerve entrapment is implicated as its cause. Radicular pain is suspected if the symptom is unrelated to a scar and is accentuated by spinal movement. When there is no relationship to a scar, hernia, back motion, or painful rib syndrome, CAWP is implicated. Because we found that the Carnett test alone was insufficiently sensitive, we devised a set of five criteria. At least two must be fulfilled to suggest CAWP (Fig. 3). The diagnosis was considered "confirmed" if the pain was relieved by 50% or more within three days of a local anesthetic corticosteroid injection for three or more months, and no alternative diagnosis was made. If it recurred, there had to be a similar level

Diagnostic Criteria for Abdominal Wall Pain

Patient indicates narrowly localized pain
(most severe component can be covered by fingertip)

OR

Unchanging location of tenderness

AND

Superficial tenderness
(at level of or anterior to abdominal wall muscles)

OR

Point tenderness diameter no greater than 2.5 cm.

OR

Increased point tenderness with abdominal wall
muscle contraction (positive Carnett test)   **Figure 3** Diagnostic criteria for abdominal wall pain.

of alleviation by an anesthetic/steroid reinjection. When 33 patients with confirmed CAWP were compared with 62 patients with abdominal pain but not meeting the criteria, the criteria's sensitivity was 85% and specificity 97% (3). The Carnett test component's sensitivity was 81% with a specificity of 88%. The criteria's inter-rater reliability was 93% ($\kappa = 0.83$), whereas that of the Carnett test alone was 76% ($\kappa = 0.52$) (24). Our recommended approach to the patient with chronic abdominal pain of uncertain etiology is shown as an algorithm in Figure 4, a modification of Gallegos and Hoblsey's.

Although anesthetic injections and nerve blocks have been used to differentiate visceral from somatic pain, this approach is not infallible because a placebo effect may make interpretation difficult or there may be more than one causal element (26–28). However, various reports indicate that when patients are diagnosed with CAWP correctly placed anesthetic injection provides unequivocal pain relief in 70% to more than 90%, whereas, in general, placebo response rates are about 30% (24).

Electromyography has been reported to be abnormal in some patients with abdominal wall pain due to diabetic neuropathy (29,30). A nerve stimulator has been used to locate the injured nerve in obese persons where localization was difficult (31).

RELIABILITY OF DIAGNOSIS

In view of the heavy dependence on technological procedures for the evaluation of abdominal pain, relying on criteria based only on historical and physical findings may cause some physicians considerable anxiety. In a litigious society, the concern that potentially serious visceral diseases must be excluded may be overwhelming, even when the physician believes that it to be very unlikely. Although it is well known that visceral pain can be referred to somatic structures and has been reported to cause a false-positive Carnett sign, the tenderness is usually diffuse and not sharply localized. The accuracy of the CAWP diagnosis is high when the history and physical findings are highly suggestive, especially when there is sustained relief after anesthetic, with or without corticosteroid, injection. Even in patients who were not injected, Longstreth and coworkers found that the diagnosis was unchanged in 97% of 133 on following patients a mean of 47 months (5). After an average follow-up period of 13.8 months, we reported that 4 of 56 (7%) patients with "confirmed" CAWP had visceral disease to explain the pain (3). However, one of the patients had common bile duct stenosis and had been misclassified as CAWP since she had only transient relief after the first of six anesthetic injections by the primary care physician. Over a period of 10 years, Thomson et al. noted that 4 of 62 (6%) patients diagnosed with CAWP were later

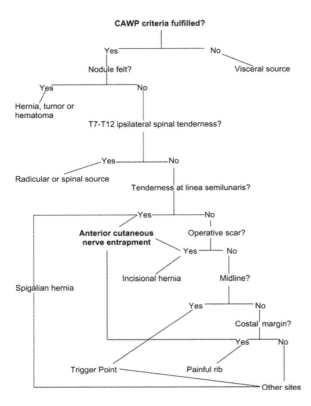

Figure 4 Suggested initial diagnostic approach to patient with chronic abdominal pain to exclude somatic origin. *Abbreviation*: CAWP, chronic abdominal wall pain. *Source*: Modified From Ref. 25.

found to have visceral disease explaining the pain; two were known to have had cancer at the time of consultation (8). Gray et al. reported that 5 of 53 (9.4%) patients with a positive Carnett test had appendicitis, whereas 1 of 24 (4%) patients considered to have pain from the wall was found to have that diagnosis in Thomson and Francis' series (15,16). These older reports predate the use of ultrasonography and helical computerized tomography for finding or excluding acute appendicitis (31–33). Because of their high sensitivity and specificity, these techniques should minimize the probability of misdiagnosing appendicitis. Fulfillment of CAWP criteria could be very helpful in instances where acute appendicitis has been suspected but is excluded by imaging studies. CAWP, by definition, is chronic, making the distinction between it and appendicitis somewhat moot since appendicitis is acute, although it may present recurrently before being recognized.

It is important to emphasize that the presence of CAWP does not exclude coexisting visceral pain; comorbidity with irritable bowel syndrome (IBS) is common (5). Indeed, the recognition of CAWP serves to differentiate the two types of pain by separating somatic from visceral symptoms.

MANAGEMENT

For a number of patients with CAWP, especially for those carrying an invidious "psychosomatic" implication, the accurate identification of prolonged undiagnosed pain is in itself a positive intervention. If the quality of life is not significantly impaired, the recognition and modification or avoidance of precipitants may be sufficient to moderate the symptom. When hand pressure alleviates the pain, an abdominal binder may be helpful. In the corpulent patient, weight loss eventually may be symptomatically effective. Local heat or cold often affords temporary relief during acute exacerbations, but avoidance of skin burns should be stressed. Analgesics, anti-inflammatories, and acetaminophen are commonly used, sometimes with antidepressants, although we have not been impressed with their effectiveness. Concerns about cyclooxygenase (COX2) inhibitors as well as some nonselective non-steroidal anti-inflammatory drugs (NSAIDs) should discourage their profligate use. Narcotic analgesics may be indicated for short term, but if pain intensity necessitates their chronic use, local anesthetic/corticosteroid injection is probably indicated. We have found the technique detailed below to be simple and effective; other variations have been described and apparently give equally successful results (9,14,34).

The patient is instructed in detail as to what to expect, emphasizing that precise localization of the point of maximum tenderness is essential for the injection to achieve optimal results. Indicating that aggravation of the pain will occur when the needle tip reaches the pain source is framed positively since it demonstrates that the needle is accurately placed. After localizing the spot by measuring the distances from the midline and from the level of the umbilicus, costal margin or inguinal ligament, the site is marked. Skin sterilization is accomplished, the area is gently pinched, and a 26-gauge 1½-inch needle is passed perpendicularly through the mark. When the panniculus is especially thick, a lumbar puncture needle may be needed to reach a sufficient depth. Preliminary anesthesia is unnecessary, because the narrow needle is virtually painless until the entrapped nerve is reached. We have had satisfactory results after injection of 2 mL of 0.25% bupivacaine and 20 to 40 mg of triamcinolone or a comparable corticosteroid. If multiple sites are to be injected, we limit the total dose of anesthetic to 10 mL to minimize possible systemic effects. Complications from the injection include small hematomata and localized inflammation and are usually inconsequential. Pain alleviation frequently occurs within a few minutes, and, in most instances, substantial relief occurs by 72 hours following transient accentuation after the anesthetic effect dissipates. Failure to obtain benefit from the injection may be due to (i) depth and/or lateral–medial misplacement of the bolus, (ii) radicular pain arising from a more proximal site, or (iii) an incorrect diagnosis.

For reasons that are not entirely clear, a single anesthetic/corticosteroid injection may provide long-term relief in the majority of patients. This has been observed in a number of studies during follow-up periods from over six months to greater than six years (10,24,34). Anesthetics have been hypothesized to "break" a chronic pain cycle and concomitant corticosteroids to enhance the anesthetic effect by "membrane stabilization." Experimentally they have been found to reduce ectopic neural discharges from neuromas (35). In our experience, fewer than one-third of patients injected with anesthetic/corticosteroid require reinjection. We reassess the situation if within one year the patient obtains satisfactory (> 50%) but only transient pain relief after three injections at the same site. If the CAWP diagnosis still is robust, we consider neurolysis with 5% to 6% phenol, absolute alcohol, or other means. Although some have used phenol as the primary agent, we have rarely found the need for an ablative drug (36,37). On rare occasions surgical freeing the nerve entrapment or neurectomy is needed to provide permanent relief (19,38). If radiculopathy, hernia, or a tumor are found, we refer the patient to an appropriate specialist.

CONCLUSIONS

When chronic abdominal pain is narrowly confined to a small area, the abdominal wall is almost always its source. It appears to be most often from entrapment of the anterior cutaneous branch of a thoracic nerve but may also result from surgical scars, myofascial trigger points, or less common lesions, such as herniations, tumors, or a variety of intercostal neuropathies. The diagnosis is uncommonly made in spite of its relative frequency, often resulting in unnecessary suffering, frustration and considerable expense. The frequency in the general population is unknown. It may account for about 8% to 10% of patients with undiagnosed abdominal pain seen in gastroenterology practice. CAWP afflicts a much larger proportion of patients with persistent pain after surgical procedures, such as cholecystectomy or hysterectomy, specifically undertaken to relieve the symptom.

Although it can be suspected by history, CAWP can only by diagnosed by a physical examination that consistently discloses localized tenderness and finds increased tenderness with the Carnett test or other appropriate criteria. It frequently coexists with visceral abdominal pain; the separate sources can be distinguished when the wall site is identified. A precisely placed local anesthetic/corticosteroid injection affords substantial relief, often for prolonged periods, in more than 75% of those injected and provides confirmation of the diagnosis. When the diagnostic criteria are adhered to and patients are followed for at least three months, there appears to be greater than 93% probability that CAWP is the correct diagnosis and that further investigation is not required. If more physicians become competent in the diagnosis of CAWP and, better still, facile with the simple technique of local anesthetic/corticosteroid injection, these patients would infrequently need to undergo extensive testing or be referred to gastroenterologists or pain clinics.

REFERENCES

1. Sharpston D, Colin-Jones DG. Chronic, non-visceral abdominal pain. Gut 1994; 35:833.
2. Editorial. Abdominal wall tenderness test: could Carnett cut costs? The Lancet 1991; 337:1134.
3. Greenbaum DS, Greenbaum RB, Joseph JG, et al. Chronic abdominal wall pain, diagnostic validity and costs. Dig Dis Sci 1994; 39:1935.
4. Thompson C, Goodman R, Rowe WA. Abdominal wall syndrome: a costly diagnosis of exclusion. Gastroenterol 2001; 120:A637.
5. Costanza CD, Longstreth GF, Liu AL. Chronic abdominal wall pain: clinical features, health care costs, and long-term outcome. Clin Gastroenterol Hepatol 2004; 2:385.
6. Carnett JB. Intercostal neuralgia as a cause of abdominal pain and tenderness. Surg Gynecol Obstet 1926; 42:625.
7. Langdon DE. Letter to the editor. Abdominal wall pain will be missed until examinations change! Am J Gastroenterol 2002; 1998:3207.
8. Thomson WHF, Dawes RFH, Carter S St C. Abdominal wall tenderness test a useful sign in chronic abdominal pain. Br J Surg 1991; 78:223.
9. Applegate WV. Abdominal cutaneous nerve entrapment syndrome (ACNES): a commonly overlooked cause of abdominal pain. Permanente J 2002; 6:20.
10. Shute WB. Abdominal pain—the primary diagnosis. Zentralbl Gynakol 1984; 106:309.
11. Hershfield NB. The abdominal wall, a frequently overlooked source of abdominal pain. J Clin Gastroenterol 1992; 14:199.
12. Johlin FC, Buhac J. Myofascial pain syndromes: an important source of abdominal pain for refractory abdominal pain. Gastroenterol 1996; 110:A6.
13. McGarrity TJ, Peters DJ, Thompson C, et al. Outcome of patients with chronic abdominal pain referred to chronic pain clinic. Am J Gastroenterol 2000; 95:1812.
14. Slocumb JC. Neurological factors in chronic pelvic pain: trigger points and the abdominal pelvic pain syndrome. Am J Obset Gynecol 1984; 149:536.
15. Gray DWR, Seabrook G, Dixon JM, et al. Is abdominal tenderness a useful sign in the diagnosis of non-specific abdominal pain? Ann R Coll Surg Engl 1988; 70:233.
16. Thomson H, Francis DMA. Abdominal-wall tenderness: a useful sign in the acute abdomen. Lancet 1977; 2:1053.
17. Hall PN, Lee APB. Rectus nerve entrapment causing abdominal pain. Br J Surg 1988; 75:917.
18. Rubio M, Gitlin MC, Lambiase LR. Abdominal wall pain as cause of abdominal pain of obscure etiology [abstr]. Am J Gastrenterol 1998; 93:1740.
19. Applegate WV. Abdominal cutaneous nerve entrapment syndrome. Surgery 1972; 71:118.
20. Applegate WV, Buckwalter NR. Microanatomy of the structures contributing to abdominal cutaneus nerve entrapment syndrome. J Am Board Fam Pract 1997; 10:329.
21. Peleg R, Gohar J, Koretz M, et al. Abdominal wall pain in pregnant caused by cutaneous nerve entrapment. Eur J Obstet Gynecol Reprod Biol 1997; 74:1269.
22. Peleg R. Abdominal wall pain caused by cutaneous nerve entrapment in adolescent girl taking oral contraceptive pills. J Adolesc Health 1999; 24:45.
23. Suleiman S, Johnston DE. The abdominal wall: an overlooked source of pain. Am Fam Physician 2001; 64:431.
24. Srinivasan R, Greenbaum DS. Chronic abdominal wall pain: a frequently overlooked problem. Am J Gastroenterol 2002; 97:824.
25. Gallegos NC, Hobsley M. Abdominal wall pain: an alternative diagnosis. Br J Surg 1990; 77:1167.
26. Ashby EC. Abdominal pain of spinal origin, value of intercostal block. Ann R Coll Surg Engl 1977; 59:242.
27. Soffer EE, Kunze GY, Conwell D, et al. Chronic abdominal pain: the diagnostic value of a combined clinical and pain management approach. Gastroenterol 1998; 114:AO40.
28. Hogan QH, Abram SE. Neural blockade for diagnosis and prognosis. Anesthesiol 1997; 86:216.
29. Streib EW, Sun SF, Paustian FF, et al. Diabetic thoracic radiculopathy: electrodiagnostic study. Muscle Nerve 1986; 9:548.
30. Sun SF, Streib EW. Diabetic thoracoabdominal neuropathy: clinical and electrodiagnostic features. Ann Neurol 1981; 9:799.
31. Terasawa T, Blackmore CC, Bent S, et al. Systemic review: computed tomography and ultrasonography to detect acute appendicitis in adults and adolescents. Ann Intern Med 2004; 141:537.
32. Tepel J, Sommerfeld A, Klomp H. J. et al. Perspective evaluation of diagnostic modalities in suspected acute appendicitis. Langenbacks Arch Surg 2004; 389:219.
33. Torbati SS, Guss DA. Impact of helical computed tomography on the outcomes of emergency department patients with suspected appendicitis. Acad Emerg Med 2003; 10:823.
34. Bourne IHJ. Treatment of painful conditions of the abdominal wall with local injections. Practitioner 1980; 24:912.
35. Devor M, Govrin-Lipmann R, Raber R. Corticosteroids supress ectopic neural discharge originating in experimental neuromas. Pain 1985; 22:127.

36. McGrady EM, Marks RL. Treatment of abdominal nerve entrapment syndrome using a nerve stimulator. Ann R Coll Engl 1988; 70:120.
37. Mehta M, Ranger I. Persistent abdominal pain: treatment by nerve block. Anesthesia 1971; 26:330.
38. Hahn L. Clinical findings and results of operative treatment in ilioinguinal nerve entrapment syndrome. Br J Obstet Gynecol 1989; 96:1080.

29 | Unexplained Visceral Pain in Children: Pathophysiology, Clinical Features, and Management

Robert J. Shulman

Department of Pediatrics and Children's Nutrition Research Center, Texas Children's Hospital, Baylor College of Medicine, Houston, Texas, U.S.A.

Danita Czyzewski

Departments of Psychiatry and Behavioral Sciences and Pediatrics, Texas Children's Hospital, Baylor College of Medicine, Houston, Texas, U.S.A.

Margaret Heitkemper

Department of Biobehavioral Nursing, University of Washington, Seattle, Washington, U.S.A.

INTRODUCTION

Although abdominal pain is a common complaint in childhood accounting for a large percentage of health-care visits (10–30%) for children aged 4 to 16 years, there is confusion surrounding definitions related to chronic so-called "nonorganic" abdominal pain in childhood (1–4). An early definition was developed from the seminal work of Apley who defined recurrent abdominal pain (RAP) as intermittent abdominal pain in children between the ages of 4 and 16 years that persists more than three months and affects normal activity (1). This definition has withstood the test of time to denote a population of children that often are brought to medical attention. Recent as well as older data demonstrate that 10% to 25% of children 4 to 16 years of age meet the criteria for RAP, with younger children (4–6 years of age) accounting for the greater percentages (1–6). Recently, these criteria have been defined further by von Baeyer and Walker: (i) the pain occurs at least once each month, in at least three consecutive months, and within the last year and (ii) episodes have been severe enough to cause the child to stay at home, terminate or avoid play, take medication for pain, or rate the pain as moderate or severe ($\geq 3/10$ on a scale of pain intensity) (7). Although this definition appears to work well to define a particular population of children with chronic nonorganic abdominal pain, clinically it has been recognized that as in adults, there probably exist identifiable clinical subtypes of children with chronic nonorganic abdominal pain.

A pediatric working team met in 1997 in an attempt to define these subtypes. From this meeting were developed the Pediatric Rome Criteria for Functional Gastrointestinal Disorders which recently have been updated (8). The majority of the subtypes of chronic nonorganic pain were adapted from adult criteria since little data exist in the pediatric literature to describe epidemiology, etiology, course, or treatment of most of these subtypes. While the Rome criteria declined to use the term RAP, the majority of the information in the literature relates to RAP. Consequently, we will use RAP as described above to denote all children with chronic nonorganic abdominal pain (including its subtypes) recognizing that it may include disorders with disparate symptoms and courses (7).

The Rome III Criteria subtypes of chronic nonorganic abdominal pain include: functional abdominal pain (FAP), functional abdominal pain syndrome (FAPS), irritable bowel syndrome (IBS), functional dyspepsia (FD), abdominal migraine, and aerophagia (8). We will not discuss aerophagia further because the etiology of pain in this disorder is clear (abdominal distention from air swallowing). We also will not discuss abdominal migraine because this condition remains poorly defined in the literature.

Table 1 specifies the Pediatric Rome III Criteria for these disorders. Most published studies of RAP included children with FAP, FAPS, and/or IBS. We will begin with a discussion of FAP and IBS, and then discuss dyspepsia separately.

Table 1   Pediatric Rome III Criteria for Functional Disorders in Which Abdominal Pain Is a Major Characteristic

Disorder	Diagnostic Criteria

Functional dyspepsia	Must include all of the following:
	  Persistent or recurrent pain or discomfort centered in the upper abdomen (above the umbilicus)
	  Not relieved by defecation or associated with the onset of a change in stool frequency or stool form (i.e., not irritable bowel syndrome)
	  No evidence of an inflammatory, anatomic, metabolic, or neoplastic process that explains the subject's symptoms
	  Criteria fulfilled at least once per week for at least 2 mo before diagnosis

Functional abdominal pain	Must include all of the following:
	  Episodic or continuous abdominal pain
	  Insufficient criteria for other functional gastrointestinal disorders
	  No evidence of an inflammatory, anatomic, metabolic, or neoplastic process that explains the subject's symptoms
	  Criteria fulfilled at least once per week for at least 2 mo before diagnosis

Functional abdominal pain syndrome	Must include childhood functional abdominal pain at least 25% of the time and one or more of the following:
	  Some loss of daily functioning
	  Additional somatic symptoms such as headache, limb pain, or difficulty sleeping
	  Criteria fulfilled at least once per week for at least 2 mo before diagnosis

Irritable bowel syndrome	Must include all of the following:
	  Abdominal discomfort (an uncomfortable sensation not described as pain) or pain associated with 2 or more of the following at least 25% of the time
	    Improved with defecation
	    Onset associated with a change in frequency of stool
	    Onset associated with a change in form (appearance) of stool
	  No evidence of an inflammatory, anatomic, metabolic, or neoplastic process that explains the subject's symptoms
	  Criteria fulfilled at least once per week for at least 2 mo before diagnosis

Abdominal migraine	Must include all of the following:
	  Paroxysmal episodes of intense, acute periumbilical pain that lasts for 1 hour or more
	  Intervening periods of usual health lasting weeks or months
	  The pain interferes with normal activities
	  The pain is associated with 2 or more of the following:
	    Anorexia
	    Nausea
	    Vomiting
	    Headache
	    Photophobia
	    Pallor
	  No evidence of an inflammatory, anatomic, metabolic, or neoplastic process considered that explains the subject's symptoms
	  Criteria fulfilled at least once per week for at least 2 mo before diagnosis

Aerophagia	Must include all of the following:
	  Air swallowing
	  Abdominal distention because of intraluminal air
	  Repetitive belching and/or increased flatus

RAP - FUNCTIONAL ABDOMINAL PAIN AND IRRITABLE BOWEL SYNDROME
Epidemiology

As noted above, RAP is a ubiquitous problem. In addition to accounting for a large percentage of visits to the pediatrician or primary care physician, RAP accounts for approximately 50% of office visits for abdominal pain seen by a pediatric gastroenterologist (Shulman RJ, unpublished 2005). The sexes are affected equally in children between five and six years of age (6). After this age, the incidence appears to be greater in girls (1,9). In some studies, the peak incidence is between 11 and 12 years of age after which there is a sharp decline in the incidence in boys but no change in that in girls (10).

In a recent community-based survey of 507 middle and high school students, 75% of the respondents reported abdominal pain with girls and boys affected equally (5). Eleven percent of the boys versus 16% of the girls reported IBS symptoms. The pain occurred weekly in about

15% of the subjects and was severe enough to affect activities in approximately 21%. Eight percent of children had consulted a physician regarding the pain (5). Thus, even in this population-based study, RAP appeared to be common.

Similar findings have been reported recently from Australia (11). Parents of consecutive patients in a two-physician rural general practice completed a questionnaire inquiring, among other things, as to diet history, pain of any kind, and school absences (11). Of the parents of 164 children, 44% reported the child having abdominal pain in the past 12 months, with 18% reporting pain at least four times and 12% at least once a month (11). In a sample of 1549 Malaysian schoolchildren between 11 and 16 years of age, 10% met Apley's criteria for RAP (12). In a group of 439 British five to six year olds, the incidence of children meeting Apley's criteria was 34% (6). A Finnish study of 2246 14- to 16-year-olds demonstrated an incidence of "quite often, often, or continuous(ly)" abdominal pain of approximately 15% in girls and 7% in boys (13). Thus, RAP may be a common condition throughout the world.

There is less clarity regarding the incidence of RAP subtypes. In the community study of American high school and middle school children reported by Hyams et al., 17% and 8% of students, respectively, reported symptoms compatible with IBS (5). The same group reported that, of patients consulting a pediatric gastroenterologist for abdominal pain, 117 of 171 patients with diagnosed RAP also had IBS symptoms (14). Epigastric discomfort, pain radiating to the chest, and regurgitation were more common in the non-IBS RAP group; these symptoms being compatible with the Rome I subtype dyspepsia (14).

A prospective Italian study of 9660 children from 13 pediatricians using a questionnaire reported a 14% incidence of IBS and a 13% incidence of dyspepsia (15). The lower incidence of IBS in this study compared with the American study of Hyams et al. may relate to the fact that no adolescents were included in the Italian study (aged up to 12 years) (5,15).

In a British study, 51% of 52 children over three years of age referred to a pediatric gastroenterologist for evaluation of abdominal pain met the criteria for IBS after an extensive evaluation (16). Another study that consisted of referral for tertiary care noted that 45% of 107 children had met criteria for IBS, 16% functional dyspepsia, 8% FAP, and 5% met criteria for abdominal migraine (17). In a Finnish study of 135 children aged 10 to 11 years referred for extensive evaluation of abdominal pain, somewhere between 30% and 50% of the children had IBS-like symptoms (18). These data in toto suggest that a substantial proportion of children with RAP may meet criteria for IBS. However, more data are needed, particularly from community-based studies.

Long Term Outcome

With regard to long-term follow-up of children with RAP, two main issues need consideration. First, how many children with RAP go on to develop abdominal complaints as adults (e.g., IBS, FAP, etc.). Second, of children initially diagnosed with RAP, how many are identified later with organic disease.

Overall, there are notable similarities between RAP in children and IBS in adults. These include the report of abdominal pain, lack of organic disease findings, prevalence, course, medical and psychiatric comorbidity, family medical and psychiatric history, and association with life events (19). Such findings have led others and us to suggest that RAP and IBS may be the same syndrome at different developmental stages (20,21). It has been observed that RAP and IBS often "run in the family" (22). However, it remains to be determined from prospective studies how many children with RAP actually have FAP or IBS as adults. Further, we do not know what happens to the subtypes of RAP; do children track their same symptoms into adulthood and if so with what frequency (e.g., children with IBS grow up to be adults with IBS vs. FAP). The few available studies have had relatively short follow-up.

Of the 27 children with IBS followed by Miele et al., at three-month follow-up most had improved with education and reassurance alone. One child was eventually diagnosed with *Giardia lamblia*, and of the 21 who were available at one-year follow-up, none had evidence of organic disease (15).

Walker et al. studied 76 children diagnosed with RAP (they excluded those with constipation or IBS) compared with 49 control subjects who had been seen for a minor illness (23). Five years after the initial evaluation, the children and their parents participated in a phone interview. There were no differences between RAP and control males in the number who now met IBS criteria (8%). In contrast, 18% of RAP girls, but no controls, met IBS criteria. In the RAP group, life stress was associated with IBS symptoms (23).

A 10-year follow-up study of 16 children with RAP demonstrated that in 50% the symptoms disappeared, in 25% they persisted, and in the remaining children other painful symptoms developed (24). Six cases of the original 22 had been lost to follow-up. The average age at follow-up was 23 years. Poor outcome was associated with belonging to a "painful family," many surgical procedures, low educational level and social class, and a personality attribute described as poor capacity to control emotions (24).

In, perhaps, the longest follow-up study available, 34 children hospitalized with RAP during 1942 to 1943 were contacted approximately 30 years later and compared with similarly aged adults (22). Fifty-three percent of the former RAP children continued to have pain as adults compared to 29% of the adults with no history of RAP as children.

Unfortunately, in the above-mentioned study, the extent of the medical evaluation that was done in each case to reach a diagnosis of RAP was not specified or as in the case of the 30-year follow-up study (22), the diagnostic techniques were old. Consequently, it is possible that true organic disease may have been missed (see below).

Some studies have evaluated adults to determine the relationship of adult psychological symptoms to a history of RAP as a child. Campo et al. interviewed young adults who had been diagnosed with RAP as children and compared them with a control group of adults who as children had been part of an otolaryngological study (25). Adults who had RAP as children were more likely to be anxious and consider themselves as physically disabled on questionnaire measures (25).

Other Diagnoses

Of children who initially receive a diagnosis of RAP, how many children go on to prove to have another diagnosis? Data from older studies are hard to interpret for several reasons including unavailability of newer diagnostic procedures (e.g., endoscopy) and methods (e.g., stool *G. lamblia* antigen testing) as well as recognition of "new" conditions that can imitate RAP (e.g., *Helicobacter pylori*). Older studies suggest that few children diagnosed with RAP ultimately prove to have another diagnosis to explain their symptoms. In contrast, recent data may suggest otherwise.

Stordal et al. investigated 44 children presenting with RAP. Routine investigation included blood count and chemistries, sedimentation rate and C-reactive protein, *H. pylori* and celiac disease serology, and serum IgE. Other tests included urinalysis, stool examination for pathogens and blood, abdominal ultrasound, plain abdominal radiograph, lactose breath test, and 24-hour esophageal pH-probe testing (26). No organic findings were discovered in 55%, 16% had constipation, 22% had gastroesophageal reflux disease (GERD), 2% had nodular gastritis and lactose intolerance, and 5% had both GERD and lactose intolerance. In a follow-up study, they found that the incidence of IBS symptoms was similar in children with RAP (i.e., no organic etiology) compared with children with organic disease (e.g., GERD), underscoring the importance of considering an organic etiology even when children by report meet the criteria for IBS (27).

Ironically, endoscopic findings including biopsies have complicated the diagnostic process in dealing with RAP. Kokkonen et al. performed upper GI endoscopies on 44 children with RAP (28). Abnormal endoscopic findings were noted in 48% (e.g., esophagitis, gastritis, and duodenitis). However, there was no comparison to control children. In our experience, many children who undergo upper GI endoscopy have mild degrees of gastric and/or duodenal inflammation that ultimately do not appear related to their initial complaints. A similar rate of positive endoscopic findings has been noted in studies from other countries. For example, Ashorn et al. from Finland found that 59% of 82 children with RAP had abnormal upper GI endoscopies (including histology) (29). A similar incidence (52%) of abnormal endoscopies was noted in a study from Thailand, although it appears that only biopsies looking for *H. pylori* were taken (30). In a study from Singapore in which all children presenting with RAP underwent upper GI endoscopy, 39% of 38 children had an abnormal upper GI endoscopy (31). However, these findings are difficult to interpret because 24% of the children were denoted as having an abnormal endoscopy but had a "nonorganic" cause of their pain that was not described in the report.

Soeparto in Indonesia endoscoped children with RAP (32). Of the 42 children between the ages of 6 and 13, 22 (52%) had abnormalities. However, it is not clear if biopsies were done (32). Quak et al. from Singapore demonstrated in 36 children with RAP (9 ± 3 years, mean $\pm$ SD) that 8 (22%) had endoscopic abnormalities confirmed histologically (33). Even greater rates of histologic abnormalities have been found in some studies (34,35). Taken together, these recent reports in which upper GI endoscopy was employed suggest a relatively high rate of pathologic findings in children presenting with RAP. Whether these findings account for the pain requires further study.

More recently, laparoscopy has been suggested as another modality that can be used in the evaluation of children with obscure RAP, although its use and the indications are controversial (36–38). Whether it may serve to further increase the number of children with organic etiologies of RAP remains to be determined.

Although children with RAP may have an abnormal upper GI endoscopy, the findings may not necessarily be the cause of the pain. For example, many children with *H. pylori* are asymptomatic. Therefore, the finding of the organism does not equate with it being the etiology of the pain. Similarly, an abnormal pH probe does not necessarily mean that GERD is the etiology of the pain. More powerful evidence would be that the children are treated and the abnormal organic finding and pain resolve. In fact, in 25 children with RAP, of whom 56% had an abnormal pH probe, treatment of the reflux resolved pain in only 71% of children with reflux (39). In another study, children with RAP underwent upper GI endoscopy (40). *H. pylori* were found in 12 children. Non–*H. pylori* antritis was noted in 16 children who then were treated with an H_2 receptor antagonist (ranitidine) for six weeks. At three months after therapy, 4 of 16 (25%) children continued to have symptoms (40).

Pathophysiology

Because no organic abnormality explains all features of the problem, a biopsychosocial model rather than the traditional biomedical model has been suggested to better understand and describe RAP (41). The biopsychosocial model is one that is concerned not only with the disease but also with a patient's subjective sense of suffering, feeling unwell, or disability. An illness may arise from any one of or a combination of organic disease, functional disorder, somatization (converting emotional distress into physical complaints), the individual's interpretation of symptoms, and peer or family reactions.

Although the cause(s) of RAP is/are not known, several factors are thought to contribute to the symptom. Similar to IBS, these include visceral hypersensitivity, dietary factors, motility disturbances, and psychosocial factors. There is growing evidence that functional GI disturbances may be due to a central nervous system dysfunction that produces autonomic nervous system (ANS) and neuroendocrine alterations that become manifest in the clinical phenomenon of GI symptoms (see discussions below). The importance of psychosocial factors (e.g., child's and parent's pain-coping abilities, parent modeling, and reinforcement of illness behavior) influencing the experience of symptoms and the resultant health-care seeking behavior and disability have been explored in both RAP and other pain syndromes in children and adults (42).

There is some evidence to suggest that certain psychological and social factors relate to greater pain experience and disability in children with RAP, but no studies of RAP in children have examined all aspects of the biopsychosocial model simultaneously.

Motility

A few studies in children with RAP have focused on motility as being an element in the pathogenesis of the disorder. Kopel et al. investigated rectosigmoid activity in children with RAP compared with normal controls and children with inflammatory bowel disease (43). They observed that children with RAP had greater rectosigmoid activity both at baseline and after cholinergic stimulation compared with that in the other two groups (43). However, Dimson measured transit time in children with RAP compared with a group of children with headaches and found delayed transit in the RAP group (44). In a related observation, Feldman et al. carried out a double-blind short-term study in which children with RAP were randomized to either supplementation with corn fiber or placebo in cookies (45). Significantly, more children receiving fiber had a 50% decrease in the frequency of abdominal pain (45).

The authors postulated that the efficacy of the fiber was due to its effect on shortening transit time although this was not measured. Differences in findings among these studies may relate to the fact that subtypes of RAP were not investigated.

Only one study has examined gastroduodenal motility directly in children with RAP. Piñeiro-Carrero et al. carried out motility studies in eight children (ages 9–17 years) with RAP and compared the findings with seven normal adolescents (ages 17–19 years) (46). Compared with the normal adolescents, the children with RAP had more frequent migrating motor complexes that propagated more slowly down the intestine. Interpretation of these results is limited by the disparity in ages between the patients and controls and the small number of subjects. Further, although the differences were statistically significant, the differences between most of the values were small (approximately 10%) and therefore, of questionable clinical significance (46). Indeed, Christensen measured serum motilin (the hormone stimulating motility and the migrating motor complex) in 20 children with RAP (ages 6–15 years) and could not detect differences compared with values in age-matched controls (47).

Olafsdottir et al. measured gastric movement with ultrasound (48). Ten to 20 minutes after a meat-soup meal, children with RAP had a significantly smaller sagittal area of the proximal stomach than did healthy control subjects. They also had significantly higher emptying fractions of the proximal stomach than healthy control subjects at 10 minutes after ingestion of the meal. Unfortunately, again the ages of the children with RAP were different compared with controls (range 3–7 vs. 7–10, respectively), limiting interpretation of the results (48).

Dietary Factors

Lactose intolerance is part of the differential diagnosis of abdominal pain. Although lactose may not be completely absorbed, it is an infrequent cause of abdominal pain, diarrhea, and bloating in children with or without RAP. Studies by Webster et al. in 137 children with RAP demonstrated that symptoms of gas, bloating, diarrhea, and constipation were similar in children with and without lactose malabsorption (49). Lebenthal et al. noted a similar finding, specifically, that children with RAP with or without lactose malabsorption responded similarly in reduction of pain frequency to a trial of a lactose-free diet (50). The response rate in the study by Lebenthal et al. is comparable to children with RAP given no treatment (50). At best, lactose elimination can reduce but not eliminate pain frequency and other abdominal symptoms in some children with RAP as would be expected in any person with lactose malabsorption (51).

As noted above, dietary fiber supplementation has been used in the treatment of children with RAP. However, only one well-controlled study supports its use (45). Although it reduced the frequency of pain in some children with RAP, the severity of pain was not significantly different between groups (45). In contrast, a recent randomized trial demonstrated no benefit with fiber supplementation in children with RAP (52). Based on studies in adults, supplementation with fiber may be most helpful for patients with constipation-predominant IBS (45). Notably, in some patients fiber supplementation can worsen symptoms of gas and bloating, actually provoking pain (53).

Visceral Hyperalgesia

Visceral hyperalgesia is a consistent physiologic finding in one-half to two-thirds of adult patients with IBS. However, little information is available in children. This is particularly unfortunate, given the experimental animal data suggesting that early-life experiences (e.g., stress) can induce visceral hypersensitivity later in life (54).

Two recent studies suggest the presence of visceral hyperalgesia in children with RAP. More striking, there appear to be differences in children with FAP compared with those with IBS.

van Ginkel et al. studied eight children with FAP and eight with IBS and compared them with nine controls matched for age (55). All children underwent rectal barostat testing at baseline and in response to a meal. The children with IBS had a lower threshold for pain following rectal distention compared with children with FAP or controls. Compliance was similar between FAP and IBS children (the former lower than in controls). In contrast, rectal contractile response to a meal was diminished in children with IBS compared with children with FAP and controls, and this decreased response was not different between children with diarrhea or constipation-predominant IBS (55).

Another study reported the same year by Di Lorenzo et al. also pointed to physiologic differences between children with FAP and those with IBS. They reported a study in which children with FAP, IBS, and controls were studied using a gastric and rectal barostat (56). The children were fairly well matched for age but not for gender (mean age 11, 13, 10, and 13 years and 8/10, 8/10, 0/8, and 4/7 females, respectively). Similar to the findings of van Ginkel et al., rectal pain threshold was significantly different among the groups (IBS < FAP < control). In contrast, gastric pain threshold was lower in the FAP group compared with the IBS group and controls (56). In contrast to the findings of van Ginkel et al., there were no differences among groups in rectal (or gastric) compliance. This difference between the two studies may have been due to differences in technique because the actual method for calculating compliance was not spelled out by Di Lorenzo. These two studies suggest that children with FAP and IBS have similar alterations in visceral pain thresholds as do adults with IBS.

Somatic Hyperalgesia

Recent studies by Alfven have demonstrated that children with RAP (3–14 years of age, $n = 27$) have greater skeletal muscle (somatic) tightness and tenderness compared with that in unmatched controls ($n = 16$) (57). Further, Alfven has shown that children (mean age 11 years) with RAP ($n = 49$) have lower muscle pressure pain thresholds compared with that in control children ($n = 50$) (58). Analogous findings were reported by Duarte et al. who compared children with RAP and controls using an algometer to determine pressure pain thresholds in different regions of the body (59). Whether there are differences between children with FAP and IBS remains to be determined.

ANS Dysfunction

One possible interpretation of the motility data in children with RAP is that it reflects, in part, ANS modulation. In the only controlled investigation, Feuerstein et al. studied children with RAP (ages 9–14 years, $n = 10$) and compared them with children hospitalized for other disorders ($n = 9$) and well controls ($n = 9$) (60). They measured autonomic (peripheral vaso-motor and heart rate), somatic (forearm electromyography), subjective (pain intensity and distress), and behavioral (facial expression) reactions during baseline, stressor ($0°C$ water immersion), and recovery periods. No differences were noted among groups (60). However, the small number of subjects studied may have precluded detecting differences. Additionally, only heart rate was measured during the study, whereas 24-hour recordings may have provided different results.

Battistella et al. used electronic pupillometry before and after phenylephrine instillation to determine sympathetic function in children with RAP ($n = 18$) compared with controls ($n = 15$) (61). After treatment, iris dilatation was greater in the children with RAP suggesting that they have sympathetic hypofunction.

Psychosocial Factors

A large literature exists on the psychosocial factors potentially contributing to RAP in children. A detailed review is beyond the scope of this chapter, but we will summarize briefly the main points. The following groups of factors typically differentiate children with RAP from comparison children.

Child Factors

Anxiety: Many research teams including our own using standardized measures (e.g., Child Behavior Checklist, CBCL; Behavioral Assessment System for Children, BASC; and State Trait Anxiety Inventory for Children, STAI-C) have identified elevated levels of anxiety in children with RAP as compared to normal controls (62–65). In a series of studies, Walker et al. compared children with RAP (8–17 years of age) with well controls, children with identifiable organic disease (primarily ulcers), and children with emotional disorders (66,67). Children with RAP had levels of anxiety similar to children with organic disease, higher than well controls, but lower than children with mood and anxiety disorders (67). Our own studies of younger children with RAP (ages 7–10 years) found that only the mother's report of anxiety and not the children's reports differentiated RAP children from well controls (65). Others have found children with RAP similar to children diagnosed with anxiety disorders on many characteristics, including psychological and physiological measures of anxiety (68). Thus, elevated levels of anxiety appear to be a fairly consistent finding, especially in older children with RAP.

Somatization: While typically moderately correlated with measures of anxiety, the concept of somatization or somatic focus has been independently investigated as a factor in RAP. Studies support the idea that children with RAP as compared to normal controls endorse more somatization symptoms (64,65,67,69). Routh and Ernst found that children with RAP (ages 7–17 years) compared with children who had organic GI disease (e.g., ulcer and gastritis) endorsed more somatic complaints on the CBCL (70). Again our data found that only mother's report of child somatization revealed differences between RAP and well controls in a younger age sample (65).

Coping: In a variety of medical conditions, type of coping strategy has been related to level of pain, functionality, and psychological distress (71–73). Specifically, when faced with an uncontrollable stressor such as pain, better outcomes are found for those who attempted to adapt to their situation by regulating their attention and cognitions. While coping is typically studied within groups to predict outcomes, several groups have examined coping between RAP and non-RAP children. Sharrer and Ryan-Wenger found that school-age children with RAP were more likely to endorse passive as opposed to active coping strategies in managing any stressor (74). Further, Davison et al. showed that children with RAP compared with controls were more likely to withdraw from new situations and have more difficulty settling into routines (75). Given the ubiquity of abdominal pain in children, these results suggest that type of coping strategy may be a factor that promotes these children becoming identified as children with RAP.

Parent Factors

Parental somatization: Several research teams have found a higher rate of parental somatization in families of children with RAP than in those without RAP. Studies by Routh et al., Walker et al., and others including our own group have found an increased incidence of somatization in the parents of children with RAP (65–67,70,76,77). On the other hand, McGrath et al. found no differences in the incidence of parental somatization between 30 children with RAP and 30 well children (78). Dispairty between studies may be due to differences in the measure of somatization or to recruitment bias between studies with parents in tertiary care endorsing more somatization than those from primary care. Our research group explored the latter hypothesis, however and did not find evidence to support it (65).

Both biological/hereditary and environmental/learning mechanisms are conceptually related to this positive relationship between incidence of RAP and parental somatization (79). Social learning, typically modeling, has been hypothesized by many to be the environmental mechanism through which parental somatization and child RAP are related (20,67,70). Parents could influence their children's illness experience through modeling of their own illness behaviors, modeling hypervigilance to symptoms, or through their own hypervigilance, and attention to the child's illness behaviors. Levy et al.'s studies of adults with IBS who are known to be high in somatization provide the best empirical exploration of the heredity/environment issue. Their examination of twin data suggests that while there is a genetic contribution to IBS, there is an equally strong or stronger social learning contribution (80). Further, Levy et al. demonstrated that children of parents with IBS ($n = 631$) compared with children of non-IBS parents ($n = 646$) were more likely to have ambulatory visits for non-GI as well as for GI complaints suggesting a more general somatic focus rather than a specific genetic tendency toward abdominal dysfunction (80).

Reinforcement of illness behavior: Walker et al. found that parents of children with RAP were more likely than control parents to reinforce abdominal pain complaints through attention and decreased demands. Our research group did not replicate this finding in younger children with RAP (67,81).

Perception of disability: Parental perception of greater disability differentiated children with RAP seen by their pediatrician from those seen in tertiary care. The children's perception of disability did not differ between these groups or from healthy controls (65).

Interactive Factors

The preceding sections summarized the research on psychological variables that have differentiated children with RAP from well children, or, in fewer cases, from children with emotional or known organic illness. Walker argues that advances in understanding RAP are to be found not in further searching for group differences in psychological factors but by using multivariate individual difference models to examine how children and families experience or manage

RAP (82). In many instances, the relationships between these psychological factors and the course of RAP are not straightforward main effects, but are complex interactions of a number of variables. The following sections summarize the more limited explorations of psychological factors as they impact the course of RAP.

Anxiety: In children with RAP the number of negative life events, which was correlated with anxiety, predicted the chronicity of symptoms (83). Further the relation between daily stressors and somatic complaints was stronger for children with RAP who had higher levels of negative affectivity (84).

Coping: Children with RAP who had the best health, emotional, and functional outcomes are those who actively managed their emotional reactions to pain, rather than withdrawing or catastrophizing (65,72,85,86).

Competence: Low competence moderated the relationship between symptoms and functional disability and moderated the relationship between stressful life events and persistent somatic complaints such those children with RAP and with lower competence had poorer outcomes (87,88).

In summary, although there are factors in the child that affect the experience of RAP, the influence of the parent (mother) needs to be taken into account. The mother's own somatization symptoms, the mother's perception of the child's disability, as well the parent's tendency to reinforce illness behavior are all factors that may affect the adaptation as well as healthcare seeking behavior in children with RAP.

Making the Diagnosis of RAP

Although the differential diagnosis can be extensive, studies have suggested that less than 10% of children have some other diagnosis causing their pain (89). However, these studies have not routinely carried out endoscopic procedures in children presenting with RAP. As noted above, recent studies that have employed upper GI endoscopy have suggested a rate of organic findings greater than previously thought. Unfortunately, the issue remains cloudy, because the criteria (symptoms and/or signs) used to endoscope individual patients are not always clear from the report. It is possible, if not likely, that children (or parents) who complain the most are the ones who are likely to find themselves at the end of an endoscope. Additionally, we would speculate that children with symptoms more suggestive of organic disease (e.g., GERD) or who do not readily respond to reassurance probably are more likely to undergo testing. On the other hand, studies in which upper GI endoscopy is not often employed could easily miss children with mild organic disease who are well at coping and/or derive a greater placebo benefit than other children.

Recent technical and clinical reports from the American Academy of Pediatrics in collaboration with the North American Society for Pediatric Gastroenterology, Hepatology, and Nutrition have been published, which outline recommendations for the evaluation of the child with chronic abdominal pain (90,91). Those are listed in Table 2.

We agree that RAP need not be ruled in or out by a litany of expensive and invasive testing but rather, it should be a positive diagnosis based upon the presence of a compatible patient history, family history, and physical examination in the absence of alarm signs that might suggest another etiology for the pain. Additional alarms signs are listed in Table 3.

Table 2 Recommendations for the Diagnosis of Children with Chronic Abdominal Pain

Functional abdominal pain generally can be diagnosed correctly by the primary care clinician in children 4 to 18 years of age with chronic abdominal pain when there are no alarm symptoms or signs, the physical examination is normal, and the stool sample tests are negative for occult blood, without the requirement of additional diagnostic evaluation

The presence of alarm symptoms or signs, including but not limited to involuntary weight loss, deceleration of linear growth, gastrointestinal blood loss, significant vomiting, chronic severe diarrhea, persistent right upper or right lower quadrant pain, unexplained fever, family history of inflammatory bowel disease, or abnormal or unexplained physical findings, is generally an indication to pursue diagnostic testing for specific anatomic, infectious, inflammatory, or metabolic etiologies on the basis of specific symptoms in an individual case. Significant vomiting includes bilious emesis, protracted vomiting, cyclical vomiting, or a pattern worrisome to the physician. Alarm signs on abdominal examination include localized tenderness in the right upper or right lower quadrants, a localized fullness or mass effect, hepatomegaly, splenomegaly, costovertebral angle tenderness, tenderness over the spine, and perianal abnormalities

Testing may also be performed to reassure the patient, parent, and physician of the absence of organic disease, particularly if the pain significantly diminishes the quality of life of the patient

Source: From Ref. 90, 91.

Table 3 Alarm Signs in the Evaluation of Chronic Abdominal Pain

Well-localized pain away from the umbilicus
Altered bowel pattern (diarrhea and constipation) associated with the abdominal pain
Vomiting
Recurrent isolated episodes of pain which come on suddenly and last several minutes to a few days
Pain awakening patient from sleep
Radiation of pain to back, shoulder, scapula, and lower extremities
Involuntary weight loss or growth deceleration
Rectal bleeding, constitutional symptoms (including temperature above 100°F, arthralgias, and rash)
Intermittent fecal incontinence
Consistent sleepiness following pain attacks
Positive family history of peptic ulcer, inflammatory bowel disease

Source: From Ref. 92.

In the absence of red flags, when should one pursue a more extensive evaluation (i.e., endoscopy)? Partial response or a response to acid suppression that then dissipates could be a marker of organic disease (e.g., GERD and *H. pylori*). Lack of response to the usual treatments (see discussions below) in combination with cognitive behavioral therapy could either mean significant psychopathology or organic disease. Fundamentally, consideration should be given to giving the patient the benefit of the doubt when there is doubt on the part of the physician.

Therapy

In contrast to the exhaustive literature on treatment of IBS in adults, there are few data from trials in children. There are even fewer data from randomized, double-blind trials. Most of the treatments that have been studied have been derived from previous investigations in adults. A recent publication has reviewed available published studies to date (93).

A recent randomized, double-blind, controlled trial in 42 children with IBS demonstrated that pH-dependent, enteric-coated peppermint oil capsules reduced the severity of pain in 75% of those receiving peppermint (94). Unfortunately, the short treatment period of two weeks and lack of follow-up preclude definitive conclusions. The mechanism whereby the peppermint was effective has not been elucidated but may be due to an antispasmodic effect (95,96).

As noted in the previous section on diet, the addition of dietary fiber and the avoidance of lactose in those individuals who are lactose intolerant may be of benefit in the treatment of children with RAP (45,50). Cognitive behavioral therapy also appears to have a role in treatment. In two separate studies, Sanders et al. demonstrated its effectiveness compared with controls who received no therapy (97,98). Humphreys et al. randomized 64 children aged 10 years with RAP to receive one of four treatments (52). Of those who received fiber

Table 4 Recommendations for the Management of Children with Chronic Abdominal Pain

The child with functional abdominal pain is best evaluated and treated in the context of a biopsychosocial model of care. Although psychological factors do not help the clinician distinguish between organic (disease based) and functional pain, it is important to address these factors in the diagnostic evaluation and management of these children
Education of the family is an important part of treatment of the child with functional abdominal pain. It is often helpful to summarize the child's symptoms and explain in simple language that although the pain is real, there is most likely no underlying serious or chronic disease. It may be helpful to explain that chronic abdominal pain is a common symptom in children and adolescents, yet few have a disease. Functional abdominal pain can be likened to a headache, a functional disorder experienced at some time by most adults, which very rarely is associated with serious disease. It is important to provide clear and age-appropriate examples of conditions associated with hyperalgesia, such as a healing scar, and manifestations of the interaction between brain and gut, such as the diarrhea or vomiting children may experience during stressful situations (e.g., before school examinations or important sports competitions)
It is recommended that reasonable treatment goals be established, with the main aim being the return to normal function rather than the complete disappearance of pain. Return to school can be encouraged by identifying and addressing obstacles to school attendance
Medications for functional abdominal pain are best prescribed judiciously as part of a multifaceted, individualized approach to relieve symptoms and disability. It is reasonable to consider the time-limited use of medications that might help to decrease the frequency or severity of symptoms. Treatment might include acid-reduction therapy for pain associated with dyspepsia; antispasmodic agents, smooth muscle relaxants, or low doses of psychotropic agents for pain or nonstimulating laxatives or antidiarrheals for pain associated with altered bowel pattern

Source: From Ref. 90, 91.

supplementation, 79% improved compared with 100% who received fiber and biofeedback, 94% who received fiber, biofeedback, and cognitive behavioral therapy, and 93% who received fiber, biofeedback, cognitive behavioral therapy, and parental support. These data suggest that active support (biofeedback, cognitive behavioral therapy, and parental support) are likely to improve outcome (52). A general outline for management of children with chronic abdominal pain is outlined in Table 4.

FUNCTIONAL DYSPEPSIA

As noted above, the term RAP when used in the literature is a catchall term that includes a number of functional disorders, one of which is likely FD. Unlike the adult literature, there are few studies that clearly define the population being investigated as having FD based on either the adult definition or that contained in the pediatric Rome III criteria (Table 1). Thus, there is limited information that deals specifically with this condition in children.

Epidemiology

Little is known regarding the epidemiology of FD. Hyams et al. investigated children with FD seen in a pediatric gastroenterology practice (99). They administered a questionnaire to all children five years of age or older, who had at least a month of abdominal pain or discomfort, nausea, or vomiting, and their parents, . During a one-year period, 257 patients were screened with 127 subjects fulfilling criteria for dyspepsia (59% girls, 85% white; median age, 12 years; and median duration of symptoms, 8 months). Symptoms were ulcer-like in 26% and dysmotility-like (nausea predominance) in 15% of subjects. As anticipated from the above issues related to terminology, in those with dyspepsia, IBS and gastroesophageal reflux were noted in 24% and 43%, respectively (99). Nausea and abdominal pain are the primary symptoms in FD in children followed in decreasing order by vomiting, bloating, and early satiety (100).

Long Term Outcome

There are few data on the long-term outcome of children with FD. In the study by Hyams et al. in which 127 children were followed, 35 children had a normal upper GI endoscopy, 70% were asymptomatic or much improved six months to two years after diagnosis and 3% were worse (99). Girls appeared to have a somewhat better prognosis but the numbers were small. Of those with the clinical diagnosis who did not undergo upper GI endoscopy, 82% were asymptomatic or much improved six months to two years after diagnosis and none were worse (99).

Miele et al. reevaluated 24 children with FD and 27 children with IBS as defined by the Pediatric Rome Criteria at 1, 3, and 12 months to study the natural history of the illnesses (15). Of the 13 children with FD who were available at one-year follow-up, 10 were pain free and three continued to have symptoms.

Other Diagnoses

As would be anticipated, there is overlap between FAP and FD in terms of the organic conditions that may mimic these conditions. They include gastroesophageal reflux, esophagitis, gastritis, duodenitis, and *H. pylori*. In the study by Hyams et al., mucosal inflammation was found in 21 of 56 children who had an upper GI endoscopy (99). However, similar to the argument above for RAP, it is unclear if these histologic findings equate with symptoms.

Pathophysiology

Few data are available regarding the pathophysiology of FD in children. Riezzo et al. compared 52 children with FD with 112 control children (101). They performed electrogastrography and gastric ultrasound as a proxy of gastric emptying after a meal. Approximately, 20% of the children with FD had pre- and postprandial tachygastria compared with approximately 10% of controls (102). Ultrasound demonstrated that the fasting antral area and half-emptying time were similar in dyspeptic children and controls. However, 32% of dyspeptic children compared with 66% of healthy children had a normal gastric emptying time (cross-sectional antral area vs. time). However, the large number of healthy children with "abnormal gastric emptying" must call into question the validity of the measure. Similar findings were seen in a smaller study (12 FD and 10 controls) carried out by Cucchiara et al. (102).

In a cross-sectional chart review of children who had FD and scintigraphic studies, Chitkara et al. noted that around 20% of 57 children had either slow or rapid gastric emptying (60% were normal) (100). Small bowel transit was slow in around 40% and fast in 15% (100). There was no association between symptoms and the scintigraphic results. Interpretation of the study is limited by the fact that no scintigraphic data for age and sex-matched controls exist (100). In a later study, Chitikara et al. compared 15 children with FD according to Rome II criteria (ages 13–17 years) to 15 healthy controls (103). There was no difference between the two groups in the maximal tolerated volume on drinking a nutrient meal (Ensure®, Ross Laboratories, Columbus, Ohio, U.S.A.), however, the FD subjects had greater aggregate postprandial symptoms (e.g., nausea). They measured gastric emptying with a ^{13}C-Spirulina breath test after a meal of eggs, bread, and milk and with ^{99m}Tc single-photon emission computed tomography after 300 mL of Ensure (103). Compared with controls, FD subjects had higher fasting gastric volume and a lower gastric volume change after a meal. FD subjects with daily symptoms had more delayed gastric emptying compared with those having monthly or weekly complaints. The severity of symptoms and the delay in gastric emptying were related. Given the variability among FD subjects in their responses, it suggests that there is a significant degree of heterogeneity in the pathophysiology of these individuals (103).

Making the Diagnosis of Functional Dyspepsia

The guidelines that apply to making the diagnosis of RAP also are applicable to FD. Given the negligible risk of cancer in children compared with adults, the primary impetus for upper GI endoscopy is to evaluate children who do not respond to empiric therapy with acid blockade and/or a prokinetic agent or who have hematemesis, persistent vomiting, weight loss, and/or intractable pain. Thought also should be given to performing an upper GI radiographic contrast study to assess anatomy (e.g., malrotation, duplication cysts, etc.).

Therapy

Few data are available regarding therapy for children with FD and to our knowledge there are no randomized, controlled trials. The management schema outlined in Table 4 also can be applied to children with FD. Miele et al. treated 12 children with FD using a H_2 receptor antagonist (ranitidine 5–7 mg/kg three times a day for four weeks) and 4 children with a prokinetic agent (cisapride 0.2 mg/g four times a day for four weeks), and all reportedly had improvement in pain symptoms (15). Similarly, Cucchiara et al. showed in three children that an eight-week course of cisapride could improve symptoms and normalize the electrogastrographic recording (104). Unfortunately, because of concerns about its safety, cisapride is available only on a compassionate-use basis.

Di Lorenzo et al. carried out antroduodenal motility studies in six children with FD one of whom had a normal study (105). Treatment with octreotide induced longer and faster phase III motor activity, but no information was provided regarding response to symptoms (105).

SUMMARY

RAP (FAP and IRB) and FD cause similar symptoms of pain in children as they do in adults. They are responsible for a large proportion of health-care visits, yet there are few data regarding their pathophysiology, treatment based on randomized, controlled trials, and long-term prognosis. The data available suggest that they may be forerunners of the same or similar entities that appear in adults.

REFERENCES

1. Apley J. The Child with Abdominal Pains. London: Blackwell Scientific, 1975.
2. Zuckerman B, Stevenson J, Bailey V. Stomachaches and headaches in a community sample of preschool children. Pediatrics 1987; 79:677–682.
3. Arnhold RG, Calllos ER. Composition of a suburban pediatric office practice: an analysis of patient visits during one year. Clin Pediatr 1966; 5:722–727.

4. Levine M. Recurrent abdominal pain in school children: the loneliness of the long-distance physician. Pediatr Clin North Am 1978; 31:969–991.

5. Hyams JS, Burke G, Davis PM, Rzepski B, Andrulonis PA. Abdominal pain and irritable bowel syndrome in adolescents: a community-based study. J Pediatr 1996; 129:220–226.

6. Faull C, Nicol AR. Abdominal pain in six-year-olds: an epidemiological study in a new town. J Child Pyschol Psychiatry 1986; 27:251–260.

7. Von Baeyer CL, Walker LS. Children with recurrent abdominal pain: issues in the selection and description of research participants. Develop Behav Pediatr 1999; 20:307–313.

8. Rasquin A, Dilc, Forbes D, et al. Childhood functional gastrointestinal disorders: Child/adolescent. Gastroenterology 2006; 130:1527–1537.

9. Oster J. Recurrent abdominal pain, headache and limb pains in children and adolescents. Pediatrics 1972; 50:429–436.

10. Stickler GB, Murphy DB. Recurrent abdominal pain. Am J Dis Child 1979; 133:486–489.

11. Huang RC, Palmer LJ, Forbes DA. Prevalence and pattern of childhood abdominal pain in an Australian general practice. J Paediatr Child Health 2000; 36(4):349–353.

12. Boey C, Yap S, Goh KL. The prevalence of recurrent abdominal pain in 11- to 16-year-old Malaysian schoolchildren. J Paediatr Child Health 2000; 36(2):114–116.

13. Aro H, Paronen O, Aro S. Psychosomatic symptoms among 14–16 year old Finnish adolescents. Soc Psychiatry 1987; 22(3):171–176.

14. Hyams JS, Treem WR, Justinich CJ, Davis P, Shoup M, Burke G. Characterization of symptoms in children with recurrent abdominal pain: resemblance to irritable bowel syndrome. J Pediatr Gastroenterol Nutr 1995; 20(2):209–214.

15. Miele E, Simeone D, Marino A, et al. Functional gastrointestinal disorders in children: an Italian prospective survey. Pediatrics 2004; 114(1):73–78.

16. El-Matary W, Spray C, Sandhu B. Irritable bowel syndrome: the commonest cause of recurrent abdominal pain in children. Eur J Pediatr 2004; 163(10):584–588.

17. Walker LS, Lipani TA, Greene JW, et al. Recurrent abdominal pain: symptom subtypes based on the Rome II Criteria for pediatric functional gastrointestinal disorders. J Pediatr Gastroenterol Nutr 2004; 38(2):187–191.

18. Kokkonen J, Haapalahti M, Tikkanen S, Karttunen R, Savilahti E. Gastrointestinal complaints and diagnosis in children: a population-based study. Acta Paediatr 2004; 93(7):880–886.

19. Burke P, Elliott M, Fleissner R. Irritable bowel syndrome and recurrent abdominal pain. A comparative review. Psychosomatics 1999; 40:277–285.

20. Scarff L. Recurrent abdominal pain in children: a review of psychological factors and treatment. Clin Psychol Rev 1997; 17:145–166.

21. Jarrett M, Heitkemper M, Czyzewski DI, Shulman RJ. Recurrent abdominal pain in children: forerunner to adult irritable bowel syndrome. J Soc Pediatr Nurs 2003; 8(3):81–89.

22. Christensen MF, Mortensen O. Long term prognosis in children with recurrent abdominal pain. Arch Dis Child 1975; 50(2):110–114.

23. Walker LS, Guite JW, Duke M, Barnard JA, Greene JW. Recurrent abdominal pain: a potential precursor of irritable bowel syndrome in adolescents and young adults. J Pediatr 1998; 132:1010–1015.

24. Magni G, Pierri M, Donzelli F. Recurrent abdominal pain in children: a long term follow-up. Eur J Pediatr 1987; 146(1):72–74.

25. Campo JV, Di Lorenzo C, Chiappetta L, et al. Adult outcomes of pediatric recurrent abdominal pain: do they just grow out of it. Pediatrics 2001; 108(1):E1.

26. Stordal K, Nygaard EA, Bentsen B. Organic abnormalities in recurrent abdominal pain in children. Acta Paediatr 2001; 90:638–642.

27. Nygaard EA, Stordal K, Bentsen BS. Recurrent abdominal pain in children revisited: irritable bowel syndrome and psychosomatic aspects. A prospective study. Scand J Gastroenterol 2004; 39(10): 938–940.

28. Kokkonen J, Tikkanen S, Karttunen TJ, Savilahti E. A similar high level of immunoglobulin A and immunoglobulin G class milk antibodies and increment of local lymphoid tissue on the duodenal mucosa in subjects with cow's milk allergy and recurrent abdominal pains. Pediatr Allergy Immunol 2002; 13(2):129–136.

29. Ashorn M, Maki M, Ruuska T, et al. Upper gastrointestinal endoscopy in recurrent abdominal pain of childhood. J Pediatr Gastroenterol Nutr 1993; 16(3):273–277.

30. Aanpreung P, Atisook K, Suwanagool P, Vajaradul C. Upper gastrointestinal endoscopy in children with recurrent abdominal pain. J Med Assoc Thai 1997; 80(1):22–25.

31. Ukarapol N, Lertprasertsuk N, Wongsawasdi L. Recurrent abdominal pain in children: the utility of upper endoscopy and histopathology. Singapore Med J 2004; 45(3):121–124.

32. Soeparto P. Endoscopic examinations in children with recurrent abdominal pain. Paediatr Indones 1989; 29(11–12):221–227.

33. Quak SH, Low PS, Wong HB. Upper gastrointestinal endoscopy in chidlren with abdominal pain. Ann Acad Med Singapore 1985; 14(4):614–616.

34. Roma E, Panayiotou J, Kafritsa Y, Van-Vliet C, Gianoulia A, Constantopoulos A. Upper gastrointestinal disease, Helicobacter pylori and recurrent abdominal pain. Acta Paediatr 1999; 88(6):598–601.

35. Mavromichalis I, Zaramboukas T, Richman PI, Slavin G. Recurrent abdominal pain of gastrointestinal origin. Eur J Pediatr 1992; 151(8):560–563.
36. Stringel G, Berezin SH, Bostwick HE, Halata MS. Laparoscopy in the management of children with chronic recurrent abdominal pain. JSLS 1999; 3(3):215–219.
37. Stylianos S, Stein JE, Flanigan LM, Hechtman DH. Laparoscopy for diagnosis and treatment of recurrent abdominal pain in children. J Pediatr Surg 1996; 31(8):1158–1160.
38. Hoffenberg EJ, Rothenberg SS, Bensard D, Sondheimer JM, Sokol RJ. Outcome after exploratory laparoscopy for unexplained abdominal pain in childhood. Arch Pediatr Adolsec Med 1997; 151(10):993–998.
39. van der Meer SB, Forget PP, Kuijten RH, Arends JW. Gastroesophageal reflux in children with recurrent abdominal pain. Acta Paediatr 1992; 81(2):137–140.
40. Kumar M, Yachha SK, Khanduri A, Prasad KN, Ayyagari A, Pandey R. Endoscopic, histologic and microbiologic evaluation of upper abdominal pain with special reference to Helicobacter pylori infection. Indian Pediatr 1996; 33(11):905–909.
41. Hyams JS. Recurrent abdominal pain and the biopsychosocial model of medical practice. J Pediatr 1998; 133:473–478.
42. Garralda ME. Somatisation in children. J Child Pyschol Psychiatry 1996; 37:12–33.
43. Kopel FB, Kim IC, Barbero GJ. Comparison of rectosigmoid motility in normal children with recurrent abdominal pain, and children with ulcerative colitis. Pediatrics 1967; 39:539–545.
44. Dimson SB. Transit time related to clinical findings in children with recurrent abdominal pain. Pediatrics 1971; 47(4):666–674.
45. Feldman W, McGrath P, Hodgson C, Ritter H, Shipman RT. The use of dietary fiber in the management of simple, childhood, idiopathic, recurrent abdominal pain. Results in a prospective, double-blind, randomized, controlled trial. Am J Dis Child 1985; 139:1216–1218.
46. Pineiro-Carrero VM, Andres JM, Davis RH, Mathias JR. Abnormal gastroduodenal motility in children and adolescents with recurrent abdominal pain. J Pediatr 1988; 113:820–825.
47. Christensen MF. Motilin in children with recurrent abdominal pain: a controlled study. Acta Paediatr 1994; 83(5):542–544.
48. Olafsdottir E, Gilja OH, Aslaksen A, Berstad A, Fluge G. Impaired accommodation of the proximal stomach in children with recurrent abdominal pain. J Pediatr Gastroenterol Nutr 2000; 30(2):157–163.
49. Webster RB, Dipalma JA, Gremse DA. Lactose maldigestion and recurrent abdominal pain in children. Dig Dis Sci 1995; 40:1506–1510.
50. Lebenthal E, Rossi TM, Nord SK, Branski D. Recurrent abdominal pain and lactose absorption in children. Pediatrics 1981; 67:828–832.
51. Gremse DA, Nguyenduc GH, Sacks AI, Dipalma JA. Irritable bowel syndrome and lactose maldigestion in recurrent abdominal pain in childhood. South Med J 1999; 92:778–781.
52. Humphreys PA, Gevirtz RN. Treatment of recurrent abdominal pain: Components analysis of four treatment protocols. J Pediatr Gastroenterol Nutr 2000; 31:47–51.
53. Francis CY, Whorwell PJ. Bran and irritable bowel syndrome: time for reappraisal. Lancet 1994; 344(8914):39–40.
54. Al-Chaer ED, Kawasaki M, Pasricha PJ. A new model of chronic visceral hypersensitivity in adult rats induced by colon irritation during postnatal development. Gastroenterology 2001; 119:1276–1285.
55. van Ginkel R, Voskuijl WP, Benninga MA, Taminiau JA, Boeckxstaens GE. Alterations in rectal sensitivity and motility in childhood irritable bowel syndrome. Gastroenterology 2001; 120:31–38.
56. Di Lorenzo C, Youssef NN, Sigurdsson L, Scharff L, Griffiths J, Wald A. Visceral hyperalgesia in children with functional abdominal pain. J Pediatr 2001; 139(6):838–843.
57. Alfven G. Preliminary findings on increased muscle tension and tenderness, and recurrent abdominal pain in children. Acta Paediatr 1993; 82:400–403.
58. Alfven G. The pressure pain threshold (PPT) of certain muscles in children suffering from recurrent abdominal pain of nonorganic origin: an algometric study. Acta Paediatr 1993; 82(481):483.
59. Duarte MA, Goulart EM, Penna FJ. Pressure pain threshold in children with recurrent abdominal pain. J Pediatr Gastroenterol Nutr 2000; 31(3):280–285.
60. Feuerstein M, Barr RG, Francoeur TE, Houle M, Rafman S. Potential biobehavioral mechanisms of recurrent abdominal pain in children. Pain 1982; 13:287–298.
61. Battistella PA, Carra S, Zaninotto M, Ruffilli R, Da Dalt L. Pupillary reactivity in children with recurrent abdominal pain. Headache 1992; 32(2):105–107.
62. Hodges K, Klines JJ, Barbero G, Woodruff C. Anxiety in children with recurrent abdominal pain. Psychosomatics 1985; 26:859–866.
63. Wasserman AI, Whittington PF, Rivara FP. Psychogenic basis for abdominal pain in children and adolescents. Adolesc Psychiatry 1988; 27:179–184.
64. Robins PM, Schoff KM, Glutting JJ, Abelkop AS. Discriminative validity of the Behavioral Assessment System for Children-parent rating scales in children with recurrent abdominal pain and matched controls. Psychology in the Schools 2003:145–154.
65. Czyzewski DI, Eakin MN, Lane MM, Jarrett M, Shulman RJ. Recurrent Abdominal Pain in Primary and Tertiary Care: Differences and Similarities. Child Health Care [in press].

66. Walker LS, Greene JW. Children with recurrent abdominal pain and their parents: more somatic complaints, anxiety, and depression than other patient families. J Pediatr Psychol 1989; 14:231–243.
67. Walker LS, Garber J, Greene JW. Psychosocial correlates of recurrent childhood pain: a comparison of pediatric patients with recurrent abdominal pain, organic illness, and psychiatric disorders. J Abnorm Psychol 1993; 102:248–258.
68. Dorn LD, Campo JC, Thato S, et al. Psychological comorbidity and stress reactivity in children and adolescents with recurrent abdominal pain and anxiety disorders. J Am Acad Child Adolesc Psychiatry 2003; 42(1):66–75.
69. Robinson JO, Averez JH, Dodge JA. Life events and family history in children with recurrent abdominal pain. J Psychsom Res 1990; 34:171–181.
70. Routh DK, Ernst AR. Somatization disorder in relatives of children and adolescents with recurrent abdominal pain. J Pediatr Psychol 1984; 9:427–437.
71. Gil KM, Williams DA, Thompson RJ Jr, Kinney TR. Sickle cell disease in children and adolescents: the relation of child and parent pain coping strategies to adjustment. J Pediatr Psychol 1991; 16:643–663.
72. Compas BE, Thomsen AH. Coping and responses to stress among children with recurrent abdominal pain. J Dev Behav Pediatr 1999; 20:323–324.
73. Cheng C, Hui W, Lam S. Perceptual style and behavioral pattern of individuals with functional gastrointestinal disorders. Health Psychol 2000; 19(2):146–154.
74. Sharrer VW, Ryan-Wenger NM. Measurements of stress and coping among school-aged children with and without recurrent abdominal pain. J Sch Health 1991; 61(2):86–91.
75. Davison IS, Faull C, Nicol AR. Research note: temperament and behaviour in six-year-olds with recurrent abdominal pain: a follow up. J Child Pyschol Psychiatry 1986; 27(4):539–544.
76. Garber J, Zeman J, Walker LS. Recurrent abdominal pain in children: psychiatric diagnoses and parental psychopathology. J Am Acad Child Adolesc Psychiatry 1990; 29:648–656.
77. Walker LS, Garber J, Van Slyke DA, Greene JW. Long-term health outcomes in patients with recurrent abdominal pain. J Pediatr Psychol 1995; 20:233–245.
78. McGrath PJ, Goodman JT, Firestone P, Shipman R, Peters S. Recurrent abdominal pain: a psychogenic disorder. Arch Dis Child 1983; 58:888–890.
79. Levy RL, Whitehead WE, Von Korff MR, Feld AD. Intergenerational transmission of gastrointestinal illness behavior. Am J Gastroenterol 2000; 95:451–456.
80. Levy RL, Jones KR, Whitehead WE, Feld SI, Talley NJ, Corey LA. Irritable bowel syhdrome in twins: heredity and social learning both contribute to etiology. Gastroenterology 2001; 121:799–804.
81. Walker LS, Zeman JL. Parental response to child illness behavior. J Pediatr Psychol 1992; 17:49–71.
82. Walker LS. The evolution of research on recurrent abdominal pain: History, assumptions and new directions. Seattle: International Association for the Study of Pain, 1999:141–172.
83. Walker LS, Greene JW. Negative life events and symptom resolution in pediatric abdominal pain patients. J Pediatr Psychol 1991;16: 341–360.
84. Walker L S, Garber J, Smith CA, Van Slyke DA, Claar RL. The relation of daily stressors to somatic and emotional symptoms in children with and without recurrent abdominal pain. J Consul Clin Psychol 2001;69: 85–91.
85. Greene JW, Walker LS. Psychosomatic problems and stress in adolescence. Pediatr Clin North Am. 1997;44:1557–1572.
86. Thomsen AH, Compas BE, Colletti RB, Stanger C, Boyer MC, Konik BS. Parental reports of coping and stress responses in children with recurrent abdominal pain. J Pediatr Psychol 2002;27:215–226.
87. Claar RL, Walker LS, Smith CA. Functional disability in adolescents and young adults with symptoms of irritable bowel disease: The role of academic, social, and athletic competence. J Pediatr Psychol 1999;24:271–280.
88. Walker LS, Garber J, Greene JW. Somatic complaints in pediatric patients: a prospective study of the role of negative life events, child social and academic competence, and parental somatic symptoms. J Consul Clin Psychol. 1994;62:1213–1221.
89. Bury RG. A study of 111 children with recurrent abdominal pain. Aust Paediatr J 1987; 23:117–119.
90. American Academy of Pediatrics Subcommittee on Chronic Abdominal Pain, NASPGHN. Chronic abdominal pain in children. Pediatrics 2005; 115(3):e370–e381.
91. American Academy of Pediatrics Subcommittee on Chronic Abdominal Pain, NASPGHN. Chronic abdominal pain in children. Pediatrics 2005; 115(3):e812–e815.
92. Weydert JA, Ball TM, Davis MF. Systematic review of treatments for recurrent abdominal pain. Pediatrics 2003; 111(1):e1–e11.
93. Kline RM, Kline JJ, Di Palma J, Barbero GJ. Enteric-coated, pH-dependent peppermint oil capsules for the treatment of irritable bowel syndrome in children. J Pediatr 2001; 138:125–128.
94. Goerg JK, Spilker T. Effect of peppermint oil and caraway oil on gastrointestinal motility in healthy volunteers: a pharmacodynamic study using simultaneous determination of gastric and gall-bladder emptying and orocaecal transit time. Aliment Pharmacol Ther 2003; 17(3):445–451.
95. Hiki N, Kurosaka H, Tatsutomi Y, et al. Pepperint oil reduces gastric spasm during upper endoscopy: a randomized, double-blind, double-dummy controlled trial. Gastrointest Endosc 2003; 57:475–482.

96. Sanders MR, Rebgetz M, Morrison M, et al. Cognitive-behavioral treatment of recurrent nonspecific abdominal pain in children: an analysis of generalization, maintenance, and side effects. J Consul Clin Psychol 1989; 57:294–300.
97. Sanders MR, Shepherd RW, Cleghorn G, Woolford H. The treatment of recurrent abdominal pain in children; a controlled comparison of cognitive-behavioral family intervention and standard pediatric care. J Consul Clin Psychol 1994; 62:306–314.
98. Hyams JS, Davis P, Sylvester FA, Zeiter DK, Justinich CJ, Lerer T. Dyspepsia in children and adolescents: a prospective study. J Pediatr Gastroenterol Nutr 2000; 30(4):413–418.
99. Chitkara DK, gado-Aros S, Bredenoord AJ, et al. Functional dyspepsia, upper gastrointestinal symptoms, and transit in children. J Pediatr 2003; 143(5):609–613.
100. Riezzo G, Chiloiro M, Guerra V, Borrelli O, Salvia G, Cucchiara S. Comparison of gastric electrical activity and gastric emptying in healthy and dyspeptic children. Dig Dis Sci 2000; 45(3):517–524.
101. Cucchiara S, Riezzo G, Minella R, Pezzolla F, Giorgio I, Auricchio S. Electrogastrography in non-ulcer dyspepsia. Arch Dis Child 1992; 67(5):613–617.
102. Chitkara DK, Camilleri M, Zinsmeister AR, et al. Gastric sensory and motor dysfunction in adolescents with functional dyspepsia. J Pediatr 2005; 146(4):500–505.
103. Cucchiara S, Minella R, Riezzo G, et al. Reversal of gastric electrical dysarhythmias by cisapride in children with functional dyspepsia. Report of three cases. Dig Dis Sci 1992; 37(7):1136–1140.
104. Di Lorenzo C, Lucanto C, Flores AF, Idries S, Hyman PE. Effect of octreotide on gastrointestinal motility in children with functional gastrointestinal symptoms. J Pediatr Gastroenterol Nutr 1998; 27(5):508–512.
105. Boyle JT. Abdominal Pain. In: Walker WA, Durie PR, Hamilton JR, Walker-Smith JA, Watkins JB, eds. Pediatric Gastrointestinal Disease. Vol. 1. 2nd ed. New York: Mosby, 1996:205–226.

30 | Functional Biliary Type Pain Syndromes

Arnold Wald

Department of Medicine, Section of Gastroenterology and Hepatology, University of Wisconsin School of Medicine and Public Health, Madison, Wisconsin, U.S.A.

INTRODUCTION

Recurrent "biliary" type pain is a perplexing clinical dilemma that occurs in two groups of patients. The first is in patients with an acalculous gallbladder in situ in which symptoms are identical to those in patients with cholelithiasis and biliary colic. The second is in patients who have undergone a previous cholecystectomy but continue to have recurrent episodes of pain that are similar in nature to biliary colic. In the first group of patients, attention is mostly centered on the gallbladder and deciding on the need for a cholecystectomy. In the second group, attention is directed more toward the sphincter of Oddi and deciding on the need for endoscopic sphincterotomy (ES). However, the pathogenesis of biliary type pain in either scenario is often uncertain, and consequently, evaluation and management remain controversial. This chapter addresses the broad topic of biliary type pain in both clinical settings with emphasis on evidence-based diagnostic testing and management strategies.

DEFINITIONS

Many nonspecific gastrointestinal (GI) symptoms have been inappropriately attributed to biliary origins. These include fatty food intolerance, heartburn, belching, flatulence, bloating, and nausea. In an attempt to resolve some of this confusion, functional biliary type pain has been defined by the Rome II Committee on Functional Gastrointestinal Disorders (Table 1) (1). The clinical points to emphasize are that episodes of pain are separated by pain-free intervals of weeks to months, symptoms are stereotypical and last at least 30 minutes but not longer than 24 hours, and there are no structural abnormalities or biochemical clues to explain symptoms. Likewise, other nonbiliary disorders may be excluded on clinical grounds. For example, angina pectoris is usually brought on by exercise and does not last for hours, and pain episodes are not interrupted by pain-free intervals of months or years. Acid-peptic disorders are usually relieved with antacids or acid-inhibiting drugs, renal stones are associated with abnormal urinalysis, and abdominal or chest wall syndromes are usually worsened by movement, cough, or deep breathing. Abdominal discomfort in irritable bowel syndrome (IBS) is associated with altered bowel habits and may be partially relieved with defecation.

Biliary type pain has been presumed to be either due to gallbladder disease or sphincter of Oddi dysfunction. According to the Rome II Committee (1), patients with a gallbladder in situ are defined to have "gallbladder dysfunction" on the basis of an abnormal gallbladder-emptying study. In postcholecystectomy patients, sphincter of Oddi dysfunction is assumed to underlie the pathophysiology of biliary type pain (1). Traditionally, such patients are grouped into three categories on the basis of laboratory and biochemical testing (2), as discussed in later sections.

EPIDEMIOLOGY

Persistent abdominal pain occurs in up to 20% of patients after cholecystectomy (3), and about 15% of all cholecystectomies in the United States are performed in patients without gallstones. Over 80% of patients are young to middle-aged women who exhibit risk factors similar to cholelithiasis such as obesity and multiparity.

Table 1 Rome II Criteria for Biliary Type Pain

Episodes of severe steady pain located in the epigastrium and right upper quadrant, and all of the following
   Symptom episodes last 30 min or more, with pain-free intervals
   Symptoms have occurred on one or more occasions in the previous 12 mo
   The pain is steady and interrupts daily activities or requires consultation with a physician
   There is no evidence of structural abnormalities to explain the symptoms

Source: From Ref. 1.

GALLBLADDER AND BILIARY ANATOMY AND PHYSIOLOGY

It is assumed that acalculous biliary type pain arises from events involving gallbladder contractions and passage of bile through the sphincter of Oddi into the duodenum. During fasting, the gallbladder stores bile and concentrates it to reduce volume. Gallbladder emptying involves the integration of smooth muscle contraction with decreased tone of the sphincter of Oddi to allow the passage of bile into the duodenum (Fig. 1). During periods of fasting, some emptying of the gallbladder occurs in association with late phase II of the migrating motor complex in the upper GI tract. However, maximal emptying occurs during eating which is mediated through both neural and hormonal [predominantly cholecystokinin (CCK)] mechanisms. CCK also inhibits sphincter of Oddi basal tone and phasic motor activity through non-adrenergic, noncholinergic inhibitory nerves, via the release of vasoactive intestinal peptide and nitric acid.

FUNCTIONAL (ACALCULOUS) BILIARY TYPE PAIN
Origins of Pain

The diagnosis of "gallbladder dysfunction" is based upon objective evidence of abnormal gallbladder emptying by cholescintigraphy and is predicated upon the concept that altered gallbladder motility underlies many or most cases of functional biliary pain with an in situ gallbladder. Several mechanisms for abnormal gallbladder emptying have been hypothesized. Amaral et al. showed a good correlation between gallbladder emptying in response to an intravenous infusion of CCK in vivo and gallbladder muscle contraction induced by CCK in vitro (4). The authors demonstrated that patients with acalculous gallbladder disease had impaired gallbladder muscle contraction in response to CCK, when compared with those who had pigment gallstones. The gallbladder muscle cells of patients with acalculous biliary

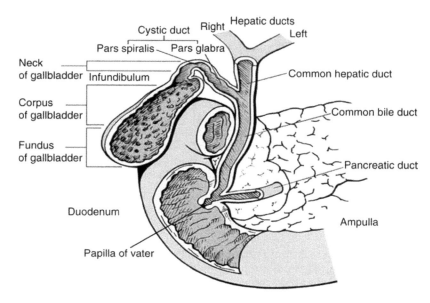

Figure 1 Anatomy of the biliary tract.

pain did not respond normally to receptor-dependent agonists, G-protein activators, and the second messenger diacylglycerol, suggesting that the defect resided in the contractile apparatus. Alternatively, Yap et al. hypothesized that narrowing of the cystic duct may impair emptying of the gallbladder and produce thickening of the gallbladder muscle, fibrosis, and histologic changes consistent with chronic cholecystitis (5). Others also have hypothesized that the mechanism for pain is obstruction leading to distension and inflammation of the gallbladder (1), perhaps resulting from incoordination between gallbladder contraction and relaxation of either the cystic duct or the sphincter of Oddi due to increased resistance or tone. This is analogous to biliary colic caused by intermittent obstruction of the cystic duct by a gallstone.

Some of these patients demonstrate histological evidence of cholesterolosis, which may or may not be of pathophysiologic significance. It has been suggested that an intrinsic defect in gallbladder motility promotes cholesterol monohydrate nucleation and crystal formation within the gallbladder bile before gallstones develop or become demonstrable by imaging studies (6). Crystal growth and entrapment in the mucus layer of the gallbladder wall and associated chronic inflammation together with abnormal motility could then lead to pathologic stretching of the gallbladder and pain.

Finally, central projections from visceral nociceptors to the thalamus and cerebral cortex might lead to visceral hyperalgesia (severe pain evoked by mildly painful stimuli), which in turn might result in allodynia (a state in which innocuous stimuli produce pain) (7). As in other functional disorders of the GI tract, heightened sensitivity in the biliary tree or in adjacent structures may be associated with pain in patients with gallbladder dysfunction. For example, Desautels et al. showed that postcholecystectomy patients with persistent abdominal pain and no evidence of sphincter of oddi dysfunction (SOD) Types I or II exhibited duodenal-specific visceral hyperalgesia and that duodenal distension reproduced symptoms in the vast majority of patients (8). Such mechanisms may be present in patients with acalculous biliary type pain.

Diagnostic Considerations and Testing

It is critically important to exclude gallstone disease and other disorders that can produce biliary type pain. This includes normal laboratory studies including liver and pancreatic biochemical tests and upper endoscopy. Endoscopic ultrasound can detect tiny gallbladder and biliary stones of less than 3 mm, which is superior to transabdominal ultrasound (9). In addition, analysis of duodenal bile after stimulation of gallbladder contraction allows the detection of cholesterol microcrystals or bilirubin granules. Only if all of these tests are normal or negative should a diagnosis of functional biliary pain be made (1).

Efforts to develop a provocative test to elicit gallbladder pain resulted in the advocacy of CCK infusion to reproduce the pain. The CCK-provocation test is neither sensitive nor specific and lacks validity (10). It has no place in the workup of patients with functional biliary pain (11).

Because of the central importance of gallbladder dysfunction in the various theories on pain pathogenesis in this syndrome, much attention has been paid to the assessment of gallbladder emptying. Various techniques have been advocated in the past, including CCK cholecystography and transabdominal ultrasonography employing a meal or CCK to stimulate gallbladder emptying. Cholecystography is now considered obsolete and ultrasound methods are not sufficiently reproducible for clinical use (10).

Currently, the most popular technique to measure gallbladder emptying employs ^{99m}Technetium-labeled hepatobiliary radiopharmaceutical N-alpha(2,6-dimethylacetanilide) iminodiacetic acid (^{99m}Tc HIDA) and CCK octapeptide (12). Gallbladder emptying is expressed in terms of the ejection fraction after stimulation by CCK. In an in vitro model that simulated in vivo gallbladder geometry, gallbladder ejection fraction (GEF) measured by the volume method showed a correlation coefficient of 0.98 compared to that measured by the radioactive counts method (13). Cholescintigraphy can thus accurately measure gallbladder emptying nongeometrically by monitoring changes in ^{99m}Tc HIDA counts as a measure of changes in gallbladder volume.

Unfortunately, the dose and the rate of infusion of CCK to measure the GEF by cholescintigraphy have not been standardized in most published studies. Both dose and rate of infusion of CCK are important, because the GEF varies with different doses and rates of infusion (14). Nevertheless, many studies have used the same definition of abnormal

Table 2   What Is Normal (and Abnormal) GEF?

References	Dose of CCK (ng/kg)	Duration of infusion (min)	GEF (%) (mean± 2SD)	Low GEF (%) (mean - 3SD)
15	20	30	77± 44	< 11
16	10	60	68± 32	< 20
17	20	45	77± 10	< 62
5	20	45	75± 25	< 40

Abbreviations: GEF, gallbladder ejection fraction; CCK, cholecystokinin.

GEF, despite using different doses and rates of CCK infusion. The available evidence suggests that 30- to 60-minute infusions of CCK are more physiologic and therefore clinically more appropriate. However, even employing optimal methods, normative values and definitions of slow GEF vary substantially (Table 2).

It is also important to emphasize that many conditions may be associated with low GEF (Table 3). These include diarrhea-predominant IBS (18,19). Tabet and Anvari observed that patients with gallbladder dysfunction exhibited a higher incidence of symptoms compatible with IBS compared to patients with gallstones (20). This may explain why symptoms may persist after cholecystectomy in patients with "gallbladder dyskinesia" and supports the hypothesis that biliary dyskinesia may be a manifestation of a generalized sensorimotor abnormality of the GI tract. Other conditions in which GEF is decreased include diabetes (21), pregnancy (22), idiopathic slow transit constipation (23), obesity (24,25), cirrhosis (26), impaired gastric emptying, and various drugs (27–30). Failure to recognize these causes may result in unnecessary cholecystectomy if a low GEF is used as an absolute criterion for surgery.

Whether SOD contributes to acalculous biliary type pain in patients with an intact gallbladder is an ongoing controversy, which has not been well investigated. The underlying premise of such studies is that SOD may exist before cholecystectomy and may be the underlying cause of symptoms in some of these patients. Two related issues are whether there is a correlation between SOD and low GEF and whether ES rather than laparoscopic cholecystectomy should be performed as first-line therapy in patients with acalculous biliary type pain.

Although there is some evidence to suggest that SOD is present in some patients with biliary type pain and an intact gallbladder, there is a paucity of cause and effect data linking GEF and sphincter of Oddi basal pressures. Based upon the existing literature, there is insufficient evidence to predict whether or which patients with acalculous biliary pain and low GEF will respond to biliary sphincterotomy (31).

Management

The occurrence of biliary type pain in patients with an acalculous gallbladder continues to remain a difficult and confusing problem for clinicians. There is general agreement that gallstone disease and structural abnormalities must be excluded before a diagnosis of a functional disorder can be considered. A widely accepted approach focuses on the evaluation of gallbladder and sphincter of Oddi function (1) with the premise that CCK-cholescintigraphy (CCK-CS)

Table 3   Causes of Abnormal Gallbladder Ejection Fraction (No Gallbladder Disease or Stones)

Metabolic disorders
  Obesity, diabetes, pregnancy, VIPoma, and sickle hemoglobinopathy
Cirrhosis
Denervation
Irritable bowel syndrome
Functional dyspepsia
Deficiency of CCK
Celiac disease, fasting/total parental nutrition
Drugs
  Anticholinergics, calcium channel blockers, opioids, ursodeoxycholic acid, octreotide,
  CCK-A antagonist, nitric oxide donors, and progestins

Abbreviation: CCK, cholecystokinin.

can identify patients who will respond to cholecystectomy and endoscopic retrograde cholangiography and pancreatography (ERCP) with sphincter of oddi manometry (SOM) can identify which patients may respond biliary sphincterotomy either prior to or after cholecystectomy.

Unfortunately, the validity of CCK-CS has not been established and a low GEF (however defined) might not predict a good outcome after cholecystectomy. Two recent reviews (14,31) acknowledged that it cannot be concluded that CCK-CS is without merit; however, even using an optimal technique does not allow a definition of low GEF to be made with confidence (Table 2). ERCP and SOM are invasive and cause significant morbidity, especially in patients with suspected SOD (32,33).

In the absence of reliable and noninvasive methods, I believe that a conservative approach to treatment should be adopted, to include careful evaluation of psychological issues and the use of agents with putative modulating effects on chronic visceral pain, such as tricyclic antidepressant (TCA) agents (34,35) (see postcholecystectomy pain section). High quality trials of such agents in sufficiently large and well-characterized patient populations carried out for sufficiently long durations are needed. Similarly, higher quality trials are needed to assess the validity of CCK-CS to determine if patients with low GEF do benefit from cholecystectomy. A suggested approach to management (Fig. 2) differs from that advocated by the Rome II Committee (1) in that pharmacologic therapy is advocated when a diagnosis of functional biliary type pain is made (14). CCK-CS should be considered only if symptoms

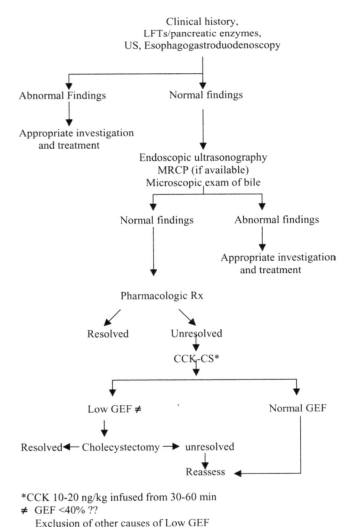

Figure 2 Suggested management of biliary type pain in patients with gallbladder in situ. *Abbreviations*: CCK-CS, cholecystokinin-cholescintigraphy; GEF, gallbladder ejection fraction; CCK, cholecystokinin.

do not resolve. On the basis of current evidence, a precise value for low GEF cannot be given; a value of greater than 40% is probably normal especially in an obese individual and might serve to preclude cholecystectomy.

POSTCHOLECYSTECTOMY FUNCTIONAL BILIARY TYPE PAIN

The acknowledged superiority of laparoscopic versus open cholecystectomy has increased the number of such procedures performed each year and as a result, the number of patients with postcholecystectomy biliary type pain continues to rise. However, the approach to these patients continues to be somewhat controversial.

Diagnostic Considerations and Testing

Patients who complain of intermittent biliary type pain in the absence of structural abnormalities have been considered to have sphincter of Oddi dysfunction. This syndrome has further been classified according to three clinical presentations (Table 4). SOD Type I patients present with typical pain, have elevated liver biochemical tests on at least two occasions, and have a dilated common bile duct of ≥ 12 mm on contrast studies (1). When all are present, a diagnosis of SOD Type I (sphincter of Oddi stenosis) is made with confidence, and sphincterotomy is the accepted treatment without further testing.

SOD Type II patients present with pain and only one of the previously mentioned criteria. In this setting, documentation of SOD is recommended using ERCP manometry to demonstrate resting sphincter of Oddi pressures greater than 40 mmHg (36). Although not proven, it is hypothesized that elevated sphincter of Oddi pressures produce pain by impeding the flow of bile or pancreatic secretions. A high percentage of this subgroup responds to biliary sphincterotomy (36). By contrast, only a small percentage of patients with a type II presentation and normal sphincter of Oddi pressure benefit from sphincterotomy, so that the pathogenesis of pain presumably lies elsewhere.

Most controversial are patients who have biliary type pain with no objective criteria and are labeled as SOD Type III. In this group, sphincterotomy benefits only a minority of patients; furthermore sphincter of Oddi pressures do not reliably predict who will respond. As SOM and ES carry substantial morbidity, the utility of these measures has been challenged. Indeed, the very premise that these patients have a problem localized to the biliary sphincter of Oddi is shaky at best, and alternative explanations concerning the pathophysiology and management of pain should be considered, as discussed next.

Origin of Pain

One possibility is that the origin of pain resides in the duodenum rather than, or in addition to, the biliary tree. For example, Desautels et al. demonstrated that patients diagnosed to have SOD Type III exhibited duodenal-specific visceral hyperalgesia and that duodenal distension reproduced symptoms in all but one of the 11 patients studied (8). This observation is consistent with the concept of visceral hyperalgesia in functional GI disorders, which has emerged as a potentially important factor associated with the development and perpetuation of GI symptoms in affected patients (7,37). Patients with SOD II and III appear to have a higher than expected prevalence of IBS (38), and SOD may occur as part of a more generalized functional disorder of the gut. Indeed, other studies have found that an abnormal sphincter of Oddi

Table 4 Postcholecystectomy "Biliary Type" Pain Classification of Biliary SOD

Type I	Biliary pain
	Abnormal liver enzyme levels
	Fixed stenosis on radiograph
Type II	Biliary pain and
	Transient elevation of enzyme level and/or
	Dilated duct and/or
	Delay in emptying of duct
Type III	Biliary pain only

Source: From Ref. 2.

response to CCK (a so-called paradoxical contraction rather than the expected relaxation) is much more often found in patients with SOD Type II and concomitant IBS (39). Treatment directed against the sphincter of Oddi alone therefore cannot be expected to provide symptom resolution in such patients and may account for the high failure rate of sphincterotomy in many patients with SOD Types II and III.

Duodenal hyperalgesia occurring by itself can produce a similar pain pattern as reported for biliary type pain. Further, biliary hyperalgesia with or without sphincter of Oddi dysfunction could exist concomitantly. The neurobiological basis of this overlap is poorly understood, but could involve both sphincter of Oddi-intestinal neural connections as well as sensory convergence of afferent fibers in the dorsal horn of the spinal cord. With respect to the former, evidence exists for bidirectional neural communications between the duodenum and sphincter of Oddi. In one small study, small bowel dysmotility occurred with greater frequency in patients with SOD Types II and III who did not respond to sphincterotomy than in patients who did respond (40). Similar findings of intestinal dysmotility were found in patients with SOD Types I and II, especially those with abnormal SOM (41). Utsonomiya et al. demonstrated a temporal relationship between phase III of the migrating motor complex and transient elevations of biliary pressure and pain in 89% of patients with SOD compared to only 20% of control subjects (42). Sensory convergence in the dorsal horn of the spinal cord (7) could result in duodenal hyperalgesia in the presence of biliary hyperalgesia after cholecystectomy or even before cholecystectomy, so that both areas would exhibit hypersensitivity to normal stimuli.

A related issue is the influence of psychologic factors on visceral perception and GI functions. Previous studies in IBS have demonstrated that jejunal sensitivity was associated with highly characteristic psychological profiles (39) similar to those of patients with SOD Type III who were studied by Desautels et al. (7). However, they found that jejunal hyperalgesia was not confined only to patients who exhibited psychological distress. More attention must be paid to the psychological and behavioral characteristics in patients with functional biliary type pain, both prior to and after cholecystectomy. As outlined in Chapter 15, failure to incorporate these factors in the management approach often leads to long-term ineffectiveness.

Management

These scenarios suggest that in patients with functional postcholecystectomy pain syndrome, treatment directed toward pharmacologic desensitization prior to invasive therapies with their attendant risks is highly recommended. Controversy exists as to whether only patients with SOD Type II and elevated sphincter of Oddi pressures require SOM or whether sphincterotomy should be performed on all patients (43). It has been argued that 80% of patients with SOD Type II will have sphincter of Oddi pressures greater than 40 mmHg and most of these will respond to ES; at least 20% of the remaining patients with normal sphincter of Oddi pressures will also respond to ES. Therefore, in all patients with SOD II, direct ES will result in an overall response rate of 70% to 80%. The classical approach to SOD Type II utilizing SOM to distinguish patients who should undergo ES is shown in Figure 3.

In contrast, it is difficult to support the use of ERCP with SOM in patients with SOD Type III, nor is there evidence to strongly support the use of ES regardless of sphincter of Oddi pressures. This is an especially critical issue because these patients now make up the majority of referrals to tertiary centers. The relatively low response rates of patients with SOD Type III occur in the context of an increased risk of ERCP, SOM, and sphincterotomy in these patients (32). A pharmacotherapeutic approach using putative visceral pain modulators similar to other functional GI disorders seems appropriate, albeit with little evidence to support their efficacy in functional biliary type pain syndromes. These patients should also be carefully evaluated for psychological dysfunction and the presence of symptoms of IBS.

TCAs have been reported to be of benefit in noncardiac chest pain (44), IBS (44), and other visceral pain syndromes. These agents are given on a continual rather than an as-needed basis and would appear to be more appropriate for patients with chronic or frequently recurring symptoms. This is not characteristic of many patients with biliary type pain in whom there may be long intervals between attacks. In patients with frequent attacks and in those with symptoms of IBS, in addition to biliary type pain, low doses of TCA (10–75 mg/day) should be used. Side effects common to TCAs as a class of drugs include sedation, constipation, mouth dryness, and dizziness, but these symptoms are less likely to occur with

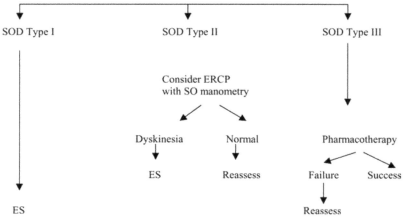

Figure 3 Suggested management of postcholecystectomy biliary type pain. *Abbreviations*: SO, sphincter of Oddi; ES, endoscopic sphincterotomy.

nortriptyline and desipramine than with amitriptyline and imipramine (45). On the other hand, patients with functional GI disorders may be more susceptible to side effects, and it may be necessary to switch to other TCAs if side effects are unacceptable (44). Use of these agents should be monitored by physicians, and increases in dose made no more often than every three to four weeks.

As many patients with functional biliary type pain exhibit mood disorders or evidence of psychosocial distress, antidepressants may offer additional benefits besides pain control. Considerations of selective serotonin reuptake inhibitors or other antidepressants in full doses may be indicated when such conditions are discovered.

This is an area in which sufficiently large studies of high quality are needed to address optimal therapy in an important clinical population. At present, TCAs appear to be an inexpensive form of therapy, which may benefit some patients with little risk or potential for serious harm.

CONCLUSIONS

Recurrent biliary type pain syndromes represent a perplexing clinical dilemma for which there is little evidence-based data to guide diagnostic testing and management strategies. The emphasis on invasive management strategies such as cholecystectomy and biliary sphincterotomy remains controversial. Evaluation of patients should emphasize specific symptoms, consideration of multiple origins of abdominal pain, and expanded use of putative visceral pain modulating drugs prior to more invasive therapies. This is an area of clinical medicine in need of further investigation and high quality studies to determine optimal management strategies.

ACKNOWLEDGMENT

The author thanks Ms Helen Gibson for preparation of the manuscript and Dr. Adam Slivka for his helpful suggestions concerning management issues.

REFERENCES

1. Corazziari E, Shaffer EA, Hogan WJ, et al. Functional disorders of the biliary tract and pancreas. Gut 1999; 45(suppl II):II48–II54.
2. Hogan WJ, Geenen JE. Biliary dyskinesia. Endoscopy 1998; 20:179–183.

3. Black NA, Thompson E, Sanderson CFB. ECHSS Group. Symptoms and health status before and 6 weeks after open cholecystectomy. A European cohort study. Gut 1994; 35:1301–1305.

4. Amaral J, Xiao Z, Chen Q, Yu P, et al. Gallbladder muscle dysfunction in patients with chronic acalculous disease. Gastroenterology 2001; 120:506–511.

5. Yap L, Wycherly AG, Morphett AD, et al. Acalculous biliary pain: cholecystectomy alleviates symptoms in patients with abnormal cholescintigraphy. Gastroenterology 1991; 101:786–793.

6. Velanovich V. Biliary dyskinesia and biliary crystals: a prospective study. Am Surg 1997; 63:69–74.

7. Mayer EA, Gebhart GF. Basic and clinical aspects of visceral hyperalgesia. Gastroenterology 1994; 101:271093.

8. Desautels SG, Slivka A, Hutson WR, et al. Postcholecystectomy pain syndrome: pathophysiology of abdominal pain in sphincter of Oddi type III. Gastroenterology 1999; 116:900–905.

9. Dahan P, Andant C, Levy P, et al. Prospective evaluation of endoscopic ultrasonography and microscopic examination of duodenal bile in the diagnosis of cholecystolithiasis in 45 patients with normal conventional ultrasonography. Gut 1996; 38:277–281.

10. Shaffer E. Acalculous biliary pain: new concepts for an old entity. Dig Liver Dis 2003; 35(suppl 3): S20–S25.

11. Smythe A, Majeed AW, FitzhenRy M, et al. A requiem for the cholecystokinin provocation test? Gut 1998; 43:571–574.

12. Krishnamurthy GT, Bobba VR, Kingston E. Radionuclide ejection fraction: a technique for quantitative analysis of motor function of the human gallbladder. Gastroenterology 1981; 80:482–490.

13. Krishnamurthy GT, Bobba VR, Kingston E, et al. Measurement of gallbladder emptying sequentially using a single dose of ^{99m}Tc-labelled hepatobiliary agent. Gastroenterology 1982; 83:773–776.

14. Rastogi A, Slivka AS, Moser AJ, et al. Controversies concerning pathophysiology and management of acalculous biliary type abdominal pain. Dig Dis Sci 2005; 50:1391–1401.

15. Ziessman HA, Fahey FH, Hixson DJ. Calculation of a gallbladder ejection fraction: advantage of continuous Sincalide infusion over the three-minute infusion method. J Nucl Med 1992; 33:537–541.

16. Ziessman HA, Muenz LR, Agarwal AK, et al. Normal values for Sincalide cholescintigraphy: comparison of two methods. Radiology 2001; 221:404–410.

17. Sarva RP, Shreiner DP, Van Thiel D, et al. Gallbladder function: methods for measuring filling and emptying. J Nucl Med 1985; 26:140–144.

18. Kellow JE, Miller LJ, Phillips SF, et al. Altered sensitivity of the gallbladder to cholecystokinin octapeptide in irritable bowel syndrome. Am J Physiol 1987; G650–G655.

19. Sood GK, Baijal SS, Lahoti D, et al. Abnormal gallbladder function in patients with irritable bowel syndrome. Am J Gastroenterol 1993; 88:1387–1390.

20. Tabet J, Anvari M. Laparoscopic cholecystectomy for gallbladder dyskinesia: clinical outcome and patient satisfaction. Surg Laparosc Endosc 1999:382–387.

21. Schreiber DP, Sarva RP, Van Thiel D, et al. Gallbladder function in diabetic patients. J Nucl Med 1986; 27:357–360.

22. Braverman DJ, Johnson ML, Kern F. Effects of pregnancy and contraceptive steroids on gallbladder function. N Engl J Med 1980; 302:362–364.

23. Hemingway D, Neilly JB, Finlay IG. Biliary dyskinesia in idiopathic slow-transit constipation. Dis Col Rectum 1996; 39:1303–1307.

24. Marzio L, Capone F, Neri M, et al. Gallbladder kinetics in obese patients. Effect of a regular meal and low caloric meal. Dig Dis Sci 1988; 33:4–9.

25. Vezina WC, Paradis RL, Grace DM, et al. Increased volume and decreased emptying of the gallbladder in large (morbidly obese, tall normal, and muscular normal) people. Gastroenterology 1990; 98:1000–1007.

26. Kao CH, Hsieh JF, Tsai SC, et al. Evidence of impaired gallbladder function in patients with liver cirrhosis by quantitative radionuclide scintigraphy. Am J Gastroenterol 2000; 95:1301–1304.

27. Garrigues V, Ponce J, Cano C, et al. Effect of selective and non-selective muscarinic blockade on cholecystokinin-induced gallbladder emptying in man. Dig Dis Sci 1992; 37:101–104.

28. Worobetz LJ, Baker RJ, McCallum JA, et al. The effect of naloxone, morphine and an enkephalin analogue on cholecystokinin octapeptide stimulated gallbladder emptying. Am J Gastroenterol 1982; 77:509–511.

29. Clas D, Hould FS, Rosenthal L, et al. Nifedipine inhibits cholecystokinin-induced gallbladder contraction. J Surg Res 1989; 46:479–483.

30. Shaffer EA, Taylor PJ, Logan K, et al. The effect of progestin on gallbladder function in young women. Am J Obstet Gynecol 1984; 148:504–507.

31. DiBaise JK, Oleynikov D. Does gallbladder ejection fraction predict outcomes after cholecystectomy for suspected chronic acalculous gallbladder dysfunction? A systematic review. Am J Gastro 2003; 98:2605–2611.

32. Freeman ML, Nelson DB, Sherman S, et al. Complications of endoscopic biliary sphincterotomy. N Engl J Med 1996; 335:909–918.

33. Freeman ML, DiSario JA, Neslon DB, et al. Risk factors for post-ERCP pancreatitis: a prospective multicenter study. Gastrointest Endosc 2001; 54:425–434.

34. Cannon RO III, Quyyumi A, Mincemoyer R, et al. Imipramine in patients with chest pain despite normal coronary angiograms. N Engl J Med 1996; 330:1411–1417.

35. Wald A. Psychotropic agents in irritable bowel syndrome. J Clin Gastroenterology 2002; 35(1 suppl): 553–557.
36. Geenen JE, Hogan WJ, Dodds WJ. The efficacy of endoscopic sphincterotomy after cholecystectomy in patients with suspected sphincter of Oddi dysfunction. N Engl J Med 1989; 320:828–837.
37. Kellow JE. Sphincter of Oddi dysfunction Type III: another manifestation of visceral hyperalgesia? Gastroenterology 1999; 116:996–1000.
38. Evans PR, Dowsett JF, Bak Y-T, et al. Abnormal sphincter of Oddi response to cholecystokinin in post-cholecystectomy syndrome patients with irritable bowel syndrome – the "irritable sphincter". Dig Dis Sci 1995; 40:1149–1156.
39. Evans PR, Bennett EJ, Bak Y-T, et al. Jejunal sensorimotor dysfunction in irritable bowel syndrome: psychological influences on pain perception. Gastroenterology 1998; 115:123–171.
40. Soffer EE, Johlin FC. Intestinal dysmotility in patients with Sphincter of Oddi dysfunction: a reason for failed response to sphincterotomy. Dig Dis Sci 1994; 39:1942–1946.
41. Evans PR, Bak Y-T, Dowsett JF, et al. Small bowel dysmotility in patients with postcholecystectomy Sphincter of Oddi dysfunction. Dig Dis Sci 1997; 42:1507–1512.
42. Utsonomiya N, Tanaka M, Ogawa Y. Pain associated with phase III of the duodenal migrating motor complex. Gastrointest Endosc 2000; 51:528–534.
43. Varadarajulu S, Hawes R. Key issues in sphincter of Oddi dysfunction. Gastrointest Endosc Clin N Am 2003; 13:671–694.
44. Clouse RE. Antidepressants for functional gastrointestinal syndromes. Dig Dis Sci 1994; 39: 2352–2363.
45. Richelson E. Pharmacology of antidepressants. Mayo Clinic Proc 2004; 76:511–527.

31 | Pelvic Pain Syndromes: Pathophysiology

Charles H. Hubscher, Harpreet K. Chadha, and Ezidin G. Kaddumi
Department of Anatomical Sciences and Neurobiology, University of Louisville School of Medicine, Louisville, Kentucky, U.S.A.

INTRODUCTION

There are many different types of pelvic pain syndromes, with different etiologies and functional consequences. Many of these syndromes are sex specific, while some are common to both women and men. In the present chapter, some of the more commonly known pelvic pain syndromes are discussed. An overview (male and female) of the anatomy of the pelvis, the peripheral innervation of the reproductive organs, and the central pathways that process and convey nociceptive information originating from the pelvic reproductive organs to higher centers is published elsewhere (1–4).

FEMALES
Dyspareunia

"Dyspareunia" is a term used to describe genital pain experienced during or after sexual intercourse (5–7) and has been reported to be the most common female sexual dysfunction, affecting between 10% and 15% of sexually active women (8). Women with dyspareunia also complain of pain associated with nonsexual activities such as tampon insertion, urination, and gynecological examinations (9). Dyspareunia leads to general disinterest in sexual intercourse and fear of the pain associated with penetration (6,10,11).

Dyspareunia is a symptom that is associated with a number of underlying pathologies (12), including vulvar vestibulitis, vaginismus (involuntary spasms), endometriosis, interstitial cystitis, and pelvic inflammatory disease. Pain originating from the vaginal opening itself (entry dyspareunia), for example, occurs with vulvar vestibulitis. Entry dyspareunia, however, can also be associated with inadequate lubrication (12). Postmenopausal women also experience dyspareunia due to vaginal atrophy, which is the result of hormonal changes (10).

Vulvar vestibulitis syndrome is the predominant cause of dyspareunia in women of reproductive age and prevents patients from having a normal sexual life (13–16). Pain occurs either upon vaginal entry or with touching of the vestibular region (severe "stinging/burning" sensation of the moist pink skin area in front of the hymen) (13,16). Clinical studies demonstrate abnormal thresholds in patients with vulvar vestibulitis syndrome as compared to normal control patients, as tested with von Frey filaments for sensitivity to touch and using the Marstock Method for measuring thermal sensitivity (17,18). Excision of the vestibular tissue (vestibulectomy) or application of 5% lidocaine ointment to the affected region has been shown to be a useful treatment (14,18,19).

In histopathologic comparative studies, it is shown that the peripheral innervation of the vestibular mucosa is significantly increased in women with vulvar vestibulitis syndrome compared to the vestibular area of normal healthy women (15,18,20). Vulvar vestibule tissue samples from pelvic pain patients, when compared with normal specimens, show increased densities and number of nerve fiber bundles and free nerve endings between epithelial cells, as revealed by S-100 neural protein and PGP 9.5 immunohistochemistry, respectively (15,20). These histopathological studies show a linear relation between the extensive increase in the number of nerve fibers and the extent of inflammation (15,20). The underlying mechanisms, however, are not known. The only neuropeptide shown to be contained within the nerve fiber population of the vestibular epithelium was calcitonin gene-related peptide (CGRP), suggesting the involvement of nociceptors in vulvar vestibulitis (21). There was no evidence found suggesting sprouting of sympathetic fibers (21). Lidocaine (5%), which blocks transmission of C-fiber activity, has been shown to provide pain relief when applied to the vestibular region of patients with vulvar vestibulitis (14).

Dysmenorrhea

Dysmenorrhea involves painful menstrual cramps associated with or without heavy menstrual flow (22,23). Pain during menses can occur in the absence of an identifiable pathologic lesion, which is referred to as primary dysmenorrhea, which is highly prevalent in adolescents and found to be associated with spastic hypercontractility of uterine tissue (24–27). Secondary dysmenorrhea, however, refers to painful menses where some form of underlying pelvic pathology has been identified (22,23). Common disorders that are associated with secondary dysmenorrhea include endometriosis, pelvic inflammatory disease, ovarian cysts, adenomyosis (ingrowth of the endometrium into the uterine musculature), and uterine myomas (23). Both primary and secondary dysmenorrhea, however, are associated with abnormal uterine contractions (28).

Elevated levels of vasopressin, which produces uterine ischemia, has been implicated in the pathogenesis of primary dysmenorrhea (22,29–31). At normal physiological levels, vasopressin is involved in the control of blood flow and myometrial activity in the pregnant and nonpregnant uterus (32). In a study using rats, stimulation of the V_{1A} receptor by vasopressin has been shown to be associated with vasoconstriction of the uterine arteries (33).

Prostaglandins, part of a family of bioactive lipids produced from arachidonic acid, are known to cause uterine contractions and pain when released into the menstrual fluid (22,25,34). Prostaglandins are essential for ovulation, luteolysis, gonadotropin secretion, tubal contractility, egg transport, implantation, and uterine contractions in the normal female (25,32). However, higher concentrations of prostaglandin E_2 (PGE_2) and prostaglandin F2 (PGF2) have been observed in women with dysmenorrhea than without (i.e., in those having nonpainful menses) (27). Cyclooxygenase-2 (COX-2) inhibitors, which inhibit the synthesis of prostaglandins, significantly reduce the pain associated with primary dysmenorrhea (35).

Surgical therapies include laparoscopic uterine nerve ablation or presacral neurectomy (bilateral hypogastric neurectomy) (36). The effectiveness of these kinds of therapies is consistent with animal studies. For example, hypogastric neurectomy in rats has been shown to eliminate completely escape responses to uterine distention in animals that show no signs of abnormal pelvic pathology (34). The hypogastric nerve of the rat has been shown to be important for transmitting nociceptive information centrally from the uterus (34,37,38). The peripheral and central pathways conveying this information are reviewed elsewhere (1,4).

Endometriosis

Endometriosis is characterized by the outgrowth of tissue lining the inside of the uterus onto the surfaces of organs in the pelvic and abdominal regions, where such tissue does not normally grow (39,40). The exact cause of the outgrowth is not fully understood, but is believed to involve the reflux of endometrial tissue within the menstrual fluid through the fallopian tubes during menstruation (41–43). Both immunological and genetic factors may contribute to the pathogenesis of endometriosis (41,42). Symptoms of endometriosis include infertility as well as various types of acute and chronic pelvic pains, including dysmenorrhea, dyschezia (pain with defecation), and dyspareunia, although many women are asymptomatic (39,41,42).

Estrogen levels are known to increase in endometriosis, due to the abnormal activity of the enzyme aromatase, which is normally not seen in the endometrium (40). The increase in estradiol levels in endometriosis is also due to the activity of 17β-hydroxysteroid dehydrogenase type 1, an enzyme which converts the estrone (inactive form of estrogen) into estrogen (40). An increase in circulating estrogen levels increases the excitability in gonadotropin–releasing hormone (GnRH) neurons (40) and leads to continuous GnRH secretion (44). The pulsatile activity of the GnRH neurons, however, is essential for the normal secretion of the gonadotropes (44,45).

A rat model of endometriosis involves the autotransplantation of uterine tissue into the peritoneum (46). Endometriotic tissue obtained both from rats induced with endometriosis and humans having endometriosis show similar alterations in gene expression and protein production (47). Also, the pregnancy rate is reduced in rats induced with endometriosis

(65.7% in experimental vs. 100% in controls) (48). The ectopic implants have been shown to regress completely following ovariectomy and during pregnancy in rats (49) and recur following estradiol supplementation in ovariectomized rats as well as one month following parturition. The vascular endothelial growth factor (VEGF) levels are higher in women with endometriosis, which has been shown to enhance the growth of endometrial cells (43).

A recent study conducted using this rat model examined the cysts that were induced. The cyst epithelium was shown to be heavily vascularized and to be innervated by both sensory and autonomic nerve fibers (50). The fibers contained within the cysts were found positive for CGRP, substance P, and vesicular monoamine transporter, which are specific markers for C fibers, Aδ fibers, and sympathetic fibers respectively (50). Similar findings were observed for human ectopic implants (39). The exact mechanism for the innervation of these ectopic endometriotic cysts is not known, but the C-fiber innervation likely contributes to the symptoms of pelvic pain associated with endometriosis. One likely candidate is the splanchnic nerve, which is in proximity to the cysts in the abdominal cavity (50). Once within the central nervous system, the information is likely processed at multiple levels of the neural axis, before reaching higher levels. Regions known to process pelvic visceral information include numerous spinal segmental levels as well as regions within the rostral and caudal medulla, thalamus, and hypothalamus (1,51). For example, afferents of the splanchnic nerve reach neurons both in the spinal dorsal horn at the T7-T11 level as well as the nucleus gracilis within the caudal medulla (52). Nucleus gracilis neurons are known to respond to uterine and vaginal distension (53), as well as neurons at the next level, the ventroposterolateral nucleus of the thalamus (54).

A number of medical and surgical treatments are used to treat patients with endometriosis. Medical therapies include using danazol (a testosterone derivative having androgenic adverse effects, thus, reduced use) and GnRH agonists. GnRH agonists function by ultimately reducing the serum estrogen levels in patients with endometriosis (41,55). The agonists bind to the GnRH receptors in the pituitary and remain for a long time, thus resulting in an initial surge of follicle-stimulating hormone and luteinizing hormone secretion and thereafter, down-regulation of pituitary gonadotropin secretion (41,55). Danazol action results in a chronic anovulatory stage due to its effect on suppression of the luteinizing hormone surge required for ovulation (41,55). These medical therapies induce an anovulatory and hypoestrogenic state and are thus not used when fertility is an issue for the patient with endometriosis (41,56). Surgical therapies that have been shown to reduce pelvic pain include laser vaporization of deposits and more radical surgeries such as hysterectomy (41).

Vulvodynia

Vulvodynia, which often coexists with dyspareunia, is characterized by pain and discomfort due to burning, itching, and rawness of the female genitalia in the absence of either a skin disease or infection. Pain may occur spontaneously or may be induced with direct stimulation (touch, pressure, or friction) of the vulvar area. Early detection and treatment prevents this disorder from becoming chronic (57–60). Vulvodynia has been diagnosed exclusively in Caucasian women (16) and is classified into five subtypes. Classifications include vulvar dermatoses (e.g., chronic dermatitis and eczema), cyclic vulvovaginitis (candida infections of the vulvar region; pain is cyclic—worse in luteal phase), vulvar papillomatosis (may be seen with human papillomavirus infection), dysesthetic (essential) vulvodynia (diffuse hyperesthesia), and vulvar vestibulitis syndrome (characterized by dyspareunia and pain to touch and pressure) (16,57,58,60).

Although the mechanisms underlying vulvodynia are unknown, a number of factors are likely involved, including neuropathic pain associated with multiple nerves (pelvic, levator ani, and pudendal nerves; pudendal neuralgia is discussed later in this chapter) (61). The mammalian vagina has a rich supply of sensory, parasympathetic, and sympathetic nerve fibers (37,62,63). In humans, the nerve supply to the vaginal wall is mainly from the uterovaginal (Frankenhauser's plexus) plexus (63). The vagina receives a rich supply of nerve fibers containing substance P, which is a neuropeptide found in nociceptive afferents (38).

In rats, sensory fibers in the dermis and connective tissue of the vagina and sympathetic and parasympathetic fibers in the vaginal smooth muscle and vasculature contribute to mechanical sensitivity and blood flow (62). In a study done using ovariectomized rats, estradiol was shown to mediate vaginal neuroplasticity. The density of sympathetic (immunostained for tyrosine hydroxylase), parasympathetic (immunostained for vesicular acetylcholine transporter), and sensory (immunostained for CGRP, a specific marker for nociceptive fibers) nerve fibers was shown to increase with ovariectomy. The fiber density was shown, with estradiol supplementation, to return to amounts that are equivalent to those found in cycling animals in estrus (62). Behavioral studies (also on rats), which utilize an operant escape response paradigm support these findings. Increased vaginal hypersensitivity occurred following ovariectomy, which was reversed with estradiol supplementation (64). Thus, the low levels of estradiol that contribute to increases in the number of vaginal nociceptive fibers and increases in behavioral escape responses to vaginal distention may be associated with dysesthetic vulvodynia (59,61). Estrogen administration has been shown to have therapeutic value in reducing pain from vulvodynia (61). In addition, dysesthetic vulvodynia occurs mainly in postmenopausal women, where estrogen levels have declined (57,59).

Uterine Fibroids

Uterine leiomyomas are the most common form of neoplasm seen in women of reproductive age (65,66). They are benign tumors (also called fibroids) derived from smooth muscle (66). The majority of uterine fibroids are asymptomatic. For many women, however, symptoms found to be associated with fibroids include one or more of the following: infertility, abnormal uterine bleeding, chronic pelvic pain, menorrhagia, and complications during pregnancy (65–68). Chronic pelvic pain symptoms associated with fibroids are dysmenorrhea or pressure due to growth of the myomas (66). The location of the myoma can be important regarding the type(s) of symptoms that present. For example, ureteral compression can produce back pain (66).

The leiomyomas express estrogen and progesterone receptors similar to what is seen in the normal myometrium (65). The "Eker" rat is a model developed by mutation of a tumor suppressor gene, Tsc-2 (tuberous sclerosis 2), which spontaneously develops uterine leiomyoma in addition to renal cell carcinoma and splenic tumors (68,69). Studies in an Eker rat model of uterine leiomyoma have shown that the tumor development is hormone dependent and high steroid hormone levels enhance its growth. Pregnancy or reduction in hormone levels due to drug therapy (administration of GNRH agonists to create a hypoestrogenic state) results in reduction of the size of the tumor (65,68,70).

Gynecologic Cancer and Pelvic Pain

Cervical, ovarian, endometrial, vulvar, vaginal, and fallopian tube cancers are types of reproductive cancers seen in either premenopausal or postmenopausal women. Ovarian cancer is the leading cause of death from gynecological cancers (71) due to difficulty in associating it with some of the early nonspecific symptoms that present (72). Vulvar and vaginal cancers are relatively uncommon and comprise about 3% to 4% and 1% to 2% of all gynecologic cancers, respectively (73). Women suffering from these cancers experience severe pelvic pain, which could be visceral, somatic, or neuropathic (74,75). As with males (see below), neuropathic pain is due to the infiltration of the perineal nerves by the malignant tumor (74,75). Somatic pain is due to the metastases of the tumor to the pelvic bones, joints, and the lymphatic supply.

Pelvic pain due to cancer is controlled pharmacologically with the administration of opioids and nonsteroidal anti-inflammatory drugs, although their continuous use can impact quality of life (74,76–79). In order to alleviate pain associated with reproductive organ cancers, the most effective treatment has been surgical blockade of the superior hypogastric or sympathetic plexus, which innervates the pelvic region (74,76–79). Celiac plexus block, in contrast, is carried out for patients with upper abdominal pain, which occurs with pancreatic cancer for example (80). In addition, relief from pelvic pain in a case study of a patient with cancer of the uterine cervix was found by interrupting ascending fibers in the dorsal columns (78). Acute lesion studies in rats have previously shown, with electrophysiological recordings, that the dorsal columns contain a pathway that conveys information originating from the uterine cervix to the caudal medulla (81).

The superior hypogastric (presacral nerve) plexus originates from the aortic plexus and carries nociceptive information from the body of the uterus and cervix (4,75). The afferent fibers from the uterus, cervix and the fallopian tubes ascend from the T10 to L1 level of the spinal cord (75). Afferent fibers from the pelvic visceral organs reach the ventral postero-lateral nucleus of the thalamus via the medial part of the posterior column at the T10 level of the spinal cord (52,82–84). The surgical therapies involved in relieving patients from cancer pain involve interrupting nociceptive information conveyed by this and other pathways. The surgical interruption of the superior hypogastric plexus or the interruption of the dorsal column pathway in the spinal cord provides relief from chronic pelvic pain associated with cancer. In addition, the treatment also results in considerable reduction in the need to take opioids (76,78,80) and thus results in improvements in the quality of life of pelvic cancer patients.

Males Testicular Pain

Testicular pain (orchialgia) is a diffuse type of visceral pain. Because it is referred to the lower back and groin area, it is often misdiagnosed (85). Testicular pain has many underlying causes, but its pathophysiology is not well understood. Examples of precipitating events include infection, tumor, testicular torsion, or trauma, but many of the cases are idiopathic (3,86). The terms "testicular pain"/ "orchialgia," involving the spermatic nerves, which innervate the contents of the scrotum, are often interchanged in the literature with the term "scrotal pain." The scrotum, however, is innervated by the genitofemoral (see section on genitofemoral neuralgia) and pudendal nerves (1). It is important to note, however, that pain originating from other pelvic areas can refer to the testis and/or scrotum and thus are considered second-ary causes of testicular and/or scrotal pain (86,87).

Studies in primates, cats, and rats show that the superior spermatic nerves innervate mainly the testis, but to some extent also the epididymis, whereas the inferior spermatic nerves innervate mainly the epididymis (3,88,89). The axons of these afferents show some branching between the tunica albuginea and the seminiferous tubules; the fine structural features of their nociceptive endings have been described in detail (90). About 93% of the afferent components of the superior spermatic nerve in cats are myelinated fibers (mainly Aδ as determined by nerve latencies) with less than 4% being C fibers (89). In the same study, Peterson and Brown differentiated between afferents that convey normal physiological inputs (those that respond to nonnoxious levels of mechanical stimulation) and those that convey nociceptive inputs centrally (those responding to noxious levels of mechanical stimulation).

As seen in the studies using cats, the afferents in the superior spermatic nerve of dogs are mainly Aδ fibers (91) and are predominantly polymodal (92). These afferents respond not only to graded intensities of mechanical stimulation of the testis and epididymis but also to heat and chemical stimuli. For example, bradykinin, a chemical mediator that is released during inflammation, was investigated using an in vitro preparation of the testis and superior spermatic nerve from dogs. Dose-dependent response discharges were obtained from the tes-ticular afferents of the superior spermatic nerve, which indicates a possible mechanism through which these mediators excite testicular nociceptors in some pathological conditions (91,93). These excitatory responses have been shown to involve the activation of protein kinase C (94). In addition, the effect of bradykinin on activating the afferents in the superior spermatic nerve has been shown to involve the B$_2$ receptor subtype (93,94).

Afferents originating from the testis and epididymis enter the spinal cord at the thora-columber and lumbosacral segments (3,95,96). Substance P and CGRP, two neuropeptides involved in nociception, are found in most of the testicular afferent fibers in the L1 and L2 dor-sal root ganglia (97). Their release in the spinal cord has been shown to increase after noxious stimulation of other visceral organs, including colon and pancreas (98–100). The spinal term-inals of the superior spermatic nerve afferents show an extensive branching caudally and rostrally, relative to their entry into the spinal cord, thereby allowing for extensive connections within the dorsal horn (101). Most of the spinothalamic dorsal horn neurons (as determined by their response to electrical stimulation of the thalamus) in laminae I and III to VII that have testicular inputs respond to one or more types of noxious stimuli applied to the testis (i.e., mechanical and/or thermal and/or chemical). Most of these spinal neurons have cutaneous convergent inputs from the scrotum and perineum (95,96).

Chronic Prostatitis

Prostatitis is a common condition that affects up to 50% of all men at some point during their lifespan (102). According to the National Institute of Diabetes and Digestive and Kidney Diseases, prostatitis is classified into four categories: acute bacterial prostatitis, chronic bacterial prostatitis, chronic nonbacterial prostatitis/chronic pelvic pain syndrome (which is subdivided into inflammatory and noninflammatory chronic pelvic pain syndrome), and asymptomatic inflammatory prostatitis (103). The chronic nonbacterial prostatitis represents most of the prostatitis cases (103–105), and most of these cases are idiopathic (105). The term "prostatodynia" is also used to describe noninflammatory nonbacterial prostatitis (106).

The use of more specific investigation techniques appears to make it possible to better classify chronic prostatitis cases, such as bacterial forms being misclassified as nonbacterial or inflammatory cases being misclassified as noninflammatory prostatitis. For example, DNA fragments (16S ribosomal DNA) of pathogens have been identified in 77% of patients with chronic prostatitis, using broad spectrum polymerase chain reaction (107). Also, just increasing the culture time for the prostate secretions and semen from two to six days revealed more cases of bacterial prostatitis (108). Looking for more specific indicators of inflammatory reaction (other than just counting white blood cells) in the prostate secretions has shown the presence of inflammatory reaction in some of the patients classified with noninflammatory chronic prostatitis (105). Proinflammatory cytokines and tumor necrosis factor-α are examples of these indicators. Some studies show that cytokines (interleukin-1β and interleukin-8) and tumor necrosis factor-α are increased significantly in the prostate of chronic prostatitis patients compared to controls (109,110).

Most of the studies about chronic prostatitis concentrate on the etiology and the underlying pathophysiology of the disease. It has been hypothesized that chronic prostatitis is due to an interplay among neurological, immunological, neuroendocrine, and psychological factors (as depicted in a summary diagram published by others) (105). One animal model of prostatitis, for example, is autoimmune-induced. This model involves the injection of prostatic acid phosphatase, a prostate specific antigen (105,111). This autoimmune-induced prostatitis in rats has been shown to be mainly mediated by CD4 T cells (105,112). In humans, CD4 T cells are found in the seminal fluid in some chronic prostatits patients (113). Another animal model of prostatitis involves injection of a bacterial suspension into the prostatic urethra (114). This model has been used to examine the effects of hormones (androgen deprivation in particular) on bacterial growth and prostatic inflammation, in order to devise an effective treatment for chronic bacterial prostatitis.

In a study of 103 male patients who came to a clinic complaining of pelvic pain in general, more than 45% had pain localized to the prostate and/or the perineal region (115). Patients diagnosed with chronic prostatitis report pain most frequently as being located in the perineum, as well as tenderness in the prostate (102). Pain in the penis, testis, and, lower abdomen are also reported (116). Some chronic prostatitis patients also report some urogenital symptoms, such as increase in urinary frequency and pain during ejaculation (3,102,116).

Experimental studies using cats and rats indicate that the afferent fibers innervating the prostate gland, which would be responsible for conveying nociceptive information centrally, are mainly contained within the pelvic nerve, with the remaining fibers being contained within the pudendal and hypogastric nerves (117,118). Afferents innervating the prostate gland enter the spinal cord at T13-L2 and L5-S2 segments (118,119), which reflects hypogastric and pelvic/pudendal nerve inputs, respectively. Nociceptive afferents to the L6-S2 spinal segments contain substance P, which was shown to increase after chemical irritation of the prostate gland with formalin (120,121). In another study, inflammation of the prostate was shown to induce a similar spinal response pattern (using c-fos and plasma extravasation) as bladder inflammation (120). These findings are consistent with some clinical cases, which present with chronic prostatitis symptoms but turn out to have interstitial cystitis (122). Note that there is a substantial amount of convergence at all levels of the neural axis. For example, electrophysiological studies in rats using electrical stimulation of the pelvic nerve, which conveys information originating from different pelvic organs including the prostate gland, produces responses in many regions of the brain, such as various subregions of the medullary reticular formation (123) and thalamus (124). Both of these supraspinal regions are known to be involved in processing nociceptive information.

Penile Pain

Penile pain is considered a rare form of chronic pelvic pain (3). Most cases of penile pain result from pain being referred from other areas, such as the prostate (prostatitis—see above) and scrotum (genitofemoral neuralgia—see below). The cause of penile pain could result from one of the many conditions that can affect the penis, such as Peyronie's disease (formation of fibrosis in the erectile tissue causing curvature in the penis at erection) (125), paraphimosis (restriction of glans penis with retracted foreskin), and priapism (painful, persistent erection) (126,127). Some reported cases of penile pain are due to penile fracture (128,129), which involves the rupturing of the tunica albuginea of the corpus cavernosa when the penis is erect.

The dorsal nerve of the penis provides most of the sensory innervation of the penis (127,130). Gross dissection of human cadavers showed that the ilioinguinal nerve participates in innervating part of the proximal penile skin in about 30% of the examined specimens (131). The cavernous nerve, which exits from the pelvic plexus, may also contain some afferent fibers originating from the penis, which reach the spinal cord via the pelvic nerve after passing through the pelvic plexus (132,133).

Neuroanatomical studies on rats show that sensory innervation of the penis by the dorsal nerve of the penis (134) contains afferent fibers with cell bodies located mainly in the L6 dorsal root ganglion (135). The dorsal nerve of the penis is the last branch of the pudendal nerve (134), which innervates other regions such as the scrotum and perineum (136,137). The penile afferents terminate in a large area in the spinal cord. Studies in rats show that stimulation of the dorsal nerve of the penis produce c-fos labeling in the dorsal horn and dorsal gray commissure throughout the L5-S1 spinal cord (138). Some studies have revealed some of the supraspinal areas that receive nociceptive inputs from the penis, which could participate in nociceptive processing and ultimately perception of penile pain. For example, electrophysiological studies on rats showed that single neurons in the medullary reticular formation (123) and different thalamic subnuclei (124) respond to electrical stimulation of the dorsal nerve of the penis and mechanical stimulation of penis, including pinch. The location of ascending spinal projections includes pathways located in the dorsal half of the spinal cord (1,139,140).

Prostatic Cancer

Cancer of the prostate is the most common type of cancer affecting males. Pain is one of the symptoms that affects these cancer patients and is often times the reason for seeking medical attention. A study of 540 individuals showed that 75% of patients having urogenital tumors suffer from cancer pain compared, for example, with 5% and 20% in leukemia and lymphoma cases, respectively (141).

Prostate cancer in the early stages is mostly asymptomatic (142). Prostatic cancer pain appears once the tumor has progressed. Prostatic cancer pain is mostly associated with tumor metastasis to bone (141,143), both to the pelvic bones and/or lumber and sacral vertebrae (75,141). This type of pain could be produced due to an increase in osteoclastic activity (bone resorption by osteoclasts). Studies using mice, for example, show that therapies suppressing osteoclastic activity decrease pain associated with bone cancer (144,145). Substances produced with bone cancer, such as prostaglandins and endothelines, also likely contribute to the pain that ensues (146).

Tumor invasion of nervous tissue is another direct cause of cancer pain. More than 90% of patients who have lumbosacral plexus invasion due to pelvic cancer experience pain (147). Prostatic cancer invasion to lumber and sacral plexuses cause pain in the groin and perineum (141). In addition, tumor invasion of the nervous tissue produces neuropathic pain. Blocking the superior hypogastric plexus, which provides innervation to/from the pelvic visceral organs including the prostate gland (75), with alcohol/phenol explains the effective relief of pain in some pelvic cancer patients (74,148).

Cancer pain, in general, can also result as a side effect of cancer therapy, including surgical, chemical, or radiotherapy interventions (141,149). For example, some prostatic cancer patients report pelvic pain after surgical excision of the prostate, but usually this pain subsides with time and is believed to be more related to psychological than pathological conditions (150). Another example is pelvic pain following radiotherapy for prostate cancer.

Radiotherapy can cause pelvic pain due to recurrence of the tumor in the prostate itself (151) or due to development of a sarcoma in the surrounding tissue (152). Pelvic pain after brachytherapy (a type of confined radiotherapy using implanted radioactive material) of the prostate cancer is also reported (153).

Patients with prostate cancer have been shown to have significantly elevated plasma concentrations of certain molecules, such as endothelin-1 (154), which is a substance that is known to stimulate osteoblasts and to be involved in nociception. For example, in mice, intraperitoneal injection of endothelin-1 induces contractions of abdominal and limb muscles, which is relieved by morphine treatment (155). In another study, applying endothelin-1 to the epineurial surface of the sciatic nerve of rats causes retraction of the hindpaw on the same side as shown during subsequent postsurgical behavioral testing (156). Another molecule that may produce pain is polyamines, which are important for cell growth, and so, are believed to be necessary for tumor growth (157,158). Rats that have polyamine deficient food show a decrease in the perception of noxious stimuli, as determined using the Randall-Selitto test (hindpaw) and the tail-flick test (157).

Males and Females

Pudendal neuralgia occurs in both men and women. In males, pudendal nerve injury can produce pain that is felt in the penis and/or scrotum (137,159), which could be mistaken for penile pain and/or orchialgia (testicular pain), respectively. In females, pudendal nerve injury can produce pain that is localized to the external genitalia (labia), which can be mistaken for vulvodynia (137,160). In addition, there will usually be perineal pain with pudendal neuralgia in both males and females (3,137), which is aggravated by sitting and relieved by standing and/or walking (159,161). About 80% of patients having proctalgia fugax (idiopathic, spontaneous pain in the anorectal area, which attacks mostly at night) show signs of pudendal nerve injury (162).

The pudendal nerve in humans innervates the perineal and genital areas, and enters the spinal cord at the S2–S4 segments (136). The pudendal nerve consists of three main branches: the inferior rectal nerve, dorsal nerve of the penis/clitoris, and perineal nerve, which innervates the perineal area and scrotum (136,137). Most cases of pudendal neuralgia result from compression, either of the pudendal nerve itself or one of its branches (163). The compression of the pudendal nerve can be due to nerve entrapment between the sacrospinous and sacrotuberous ligaments while entering the pelvis, or compression of the nerve in the pudendal canal (Alcock syndrome, which can happen, for example, with very frequent use of a bicycle) (137,164). Relief can occur with surgical decompression of the nerve (161) or with cortisone and/or local anesthetic injections at the site of compression (137,162). In a study by Benson and Griffis (163), about 67% of pudendal neuralgia cases were found by neurophysiological tests to have axonal demyelination and/or axonal loss due to nerve compression, the degree of which may contribute to the severity of the symptoms.

Pudendal neuralgia can be due to other pathologies. For example, some cases of diabetes show symptoms of pudendal neuralgia due to diabetic neuropathy (165). In addition, with some types of cancer (e.g., prostate and vulvar cancers), patients suffer from pudendal neuralgia, either due to direct tumor invasion of the pudendal nerve or after radiological treatment of the cancer (153,165). Because herpes simplex infections in the genital area can also cause pudendal neuralgia-like symptoms (166,167), it is recommended that cases of pudendal neuralgia should be examined for the presence of recent herpetic eruptions and other herpes simplex symptoms. Also, neurofibroma (benign tumor derived from the cells surrounding nervous tissue) is another pathology that is reported to produce pudendal neuralgia (168), and so, it too is recommended for consideration in the differential diagnosis of pudendal neuralgia.

Coccygodynia

Coccygodynia is a condition where there is pain in the coccyx and sacrum and the surrounding areas especially upon sitting or palpation (3,169). Coccygodynia is almost five times more prevalent in females than males (170). The coccyx in females is more susceptible to trauma because it is less curved interiorly and less protected by the ischial tuberosities, which have a wider distance between them in females versus males (171). The etiology of this condition is controversial, as is the treatment approach.

It has been estimated (172) that most (70%) of the coccygodynia cases are due to trauma, with an improper sitting position as the main cause (171). Coccygectomy or local injections of corticosteroids and/or anesthetic agents are shown to be an effective treatment for more than 87% of coccygodynia patients (173,174). Pain associated with coccygodynia has also been hypothesized to be related to the surrounding tissues (and thus is "referred" to the coccyx) (169). In Thiele's (169) study, most of the cases were due to anorectal infections, causing muscle spasms in the levator ani and/or coccygeus muscles, which resulted in pain being referred to the coccyx (coccygodynia). The levator ani muscle, innervated by the levator ani nerve, originates from the S3-S5 sacral roots (175). The coccygodynia cases that are caused by muscle spasms were treated by physical therapy (muscle massage) of the levator ani muscle (170,176) without the need for surgical intervention.

Pregnancy is considered one of the main causes of coccygodynia in women, which develops after delivery due to trauma to the coccyx. This type of coccygodynia is considered acute and goes away with time and/or conservative treatment such as massage and avoiding improper sitting (170,177).

Several pathological conditions have been shown to be potential causes that underlie coccygodynia, such as cancer of the coccyx (178), perineural cysts (179), intraosseous lipoma (180), coccygeal fracture due to delivery (181), and congenital abnormalities of the coccyx (182). Some forms of the coccygodynia, however, are considered idiopathic and do not have any apparent related pathology. Most (70%) of the idiopathic coccygodynial pain is believed to emanate from the coccygeal disc (183). Radiological investigations revealed that the coccyx, in patients with idiopathic coccygodynia, is significantly more curved inward compared with the coccyx in patients with traumatic coccygodynia (184). Thus, an abnormal coccyx is a potential underlying cause of coccygodynia in cases classified as being idiopathic.

Genitofemoral Neuralgia

Genitofemoral neuralgia is a rare pathology (originally defined in 1942 as genitofemoral causalgia) (185), where patients suffer from pain and burning sensation in the inguinal region (the area at the inferior, anterior border of the abdominal muscles). Pain may extend to the genital areas (scrotum in males and labia in females) and upper medial thigh. Pain usually is exacerbated by walking, running, or hyperextension of the hip (186–188). Genitofemoral neuralgia symptoms follow the distribution of the genitofemoral nerve.

In humans, the genitofemoral nerve originates from L1-L2 of the lumber plexus. The nerve has two end branches: the genital and femoral branches. The genital branch in males supplies motor fibers to the cremasteric muscle and sensory fibers to the lateral scrotum. In females, sensory fibers supply the labia. The femoral branch sensory innervation is to the skin of the upper anteriomedial part of the thigh (186,189).

In rats, neuroanatomical studies show that afferent fibers in the genitofemoral nerve have their cell bodies in L1–L2 dorsal root ganglia (190,191). These afferents terminate in the dorsal horn of T12-L1 spinal cord (191). Immunohistochemical studies in rats show that the afferent fibers in the genitofemoral nerve contain peptides such as substance P, CGRP, and tachykinin (190,191). Besides the innervation of genital regions, the genitofemoral nerve provides sensory innervation to the lower abdominal area both in sheep (192,193) and rats (191).

The main cause of genitofemoral neuralgia is genitofemoral nerve injury and/or compression/entrapment in fibrous tissue secondary to mechanical trauma. Most of the reported cases of genitofemoral neuralgia have a history of a surgical procedure in the inguinal area. The most common surgeries that cause genitofemoral neuralgia are inguinal herniorrhaphy (surgical repair of hernia) and appendectomy (186,187). Other reported surgical procedures that can cause genitofemoral neuralgia are hysterectomy, vasectomy (188), and ureterectomy (187). Other cases are attributed to blunt trauma (187,188) or wearing restrictive clothing, such as tight jeans (189).

The treatment option for genitofemoral neuralgia is excision of part of the genitofemoral nerve. In some cases, the pain could be due to input via the ilioinguinal nerve (ilioinguinal neuralgia), which has almost the same symptoms as genitofemoral neuralgia (thus, ilioinguinal neuralgia should be excluded before excising the genitofemoral nerve) (186). Selective anesthetic blocks are used to differentiate between these two cases; if the local block of the ilioniguinal nerve does not alleviate the pain, then genitofemoral nerve block (l1 and l2 block) can be used to confirm the diagnosis of genitofemoral neuralgia (186).

REFERENCES

1. Hubscher CH. Ascending spinal pathways from sexual organs: effects of chronic spinal lesions. Prog Brain Res 2005; 152:401–414.
2. Berkley KJ, Hubscher CH. Visceral and somatic sensory tracks through the neuraxis and their relation to pain: lessons from the rat female reproductive system. In: Gebhart GF, ed. Visceral Pain. Vol. 5. Seattle: IASP Press, 1995:195–216.
3. Wesselmann U, Burnett AL, Heinberg LJ. The urogenital and rectal pain syndromes. Pain 1997; 73:269–294.
4. Berkley KJ. A life of pelvic pain. Physiol Behav 2005; 86:272–280.
5. Salonia A, Munarriz RM, Naspro R, et al. Women's sexual dysfunction: a pathophysiological review. BJU Int 2004; 93:1156–1164.
6. Heim LJ. Evaluation and differential diagnosis of dyspareunia. Am Fam Physician 2001; 63: 1535–1544.
7. Binik YM, Reissing E, Pukall C, Flory N, Payne KA, Khalife S. The female sexual pain disorders: genital pain or sexual dysfunction? Arch Sex Behav 2002; 31:425–429.
8. Meana M, Binik YM, Khalife S, Cohen D. Dyspareunia: sexual dysfunction or pain syndrome? J Nerv Ment Dis 1997; 185:561–569.
9. Binik YM, Pukall CF, Reissing ED, Khalife S. The sexual pain disorders: a desexualized approach. J Sex Marital Ther 2001; 27:113–116.
10. Meana M, Binik YM. Painful coitus: a review of female dyspareunia. J Nerv Ment Dis 1994; 182: 264–272.
11. Meana M, Binik YM, Khalife S, Cohen DR. Biopsychosocial profile of women with dyspareunia. Obstet Gynecol 1997; 90:583–589.
12. Iioward F. Dyspareunia. In: Pelvic Pain–Diagnosis and Management. Howard F ed. Lippincott: Williams and Wilkins, 2000:112–121.
13. Bornstein J, Goldschmid N, Sabo E. Hyperinnervation and mast cell activation may be used as histopathologic diagnostic criteria for vulvar vestibulitis. Gynecol Obstet Invest 2004; 58:171–178.
14. Zolnoun DA, Hartmann KE, Steege JF. Overnight 5% lidocaine ointment for treatment of vulvar vestibulitis. Obstet Gynecol 2003; 102:84–87.
15. Bohm–Starke N, Hilliges M, Falconer C, Rylander E. Increased intraepithelial innervation in women with vulvar vestibulitis syndrome. Gynecol Obstet Invest 1998; 46:256–260.
16. Bergeron S, Binik YM, Khalife S, Pagidas K. Vulvar vestibulitis syndrome: a critical review. Clin J Pain 1997; 13:27–42.
17. Bohm-Starke N, Hilliges M, Brodda-Jansen G, Rylander E, Torebjork E. Psychophysical evidence of nociceptor sensitization in vulvar vestibulitis syndrome. Pain 2001; 94:177–183.
18. Granot M, Friedman M, Yarnitsky D, Zimmer EZ. Enhancement of the perception of systemic pain in women with vulvar vestibulitis. Bjog 2002; 109:863–866.
19. Halperin R, Zehavi S, Vaknin Z, Ben-Ami I, Pansky M, Schneider D. The major histopathologic characteristics in the vulvar vestibulitis syndrome. Gynecol Obstet Invest 2005; 59:75–79.
20. Westrom LV, Willen R. Vestibular nerve fiber proliferation in vulvar vestibulitis syndrome. Obstet Gynecol 1998; 91:572–576.
21. Bohm-Starke N, Hilliges M, Falconer C, Rylander E. Neurochemical characterization of the vestibular nerves in women with vulvar vestibulitis syndrome. Gynecol Obstet Invest 1999; 48:270–275.
22. French L. Dysmenorrhea. Am Fam Physician 2005; 71:285–291.
23. Dawood MY. Dysmenorrhea. Clin Obstet Gynecol 1990; 33:168–178.
24. Davis AR, Westhoff CL. Primary dysmenorrhea in adolescent girls and treatment with oral contraceptives. J Pediatr Adolesc Gynecol 2001; 14:3–8.
25. Sales KJ, Jabbour HN. Cyclooxygenase enzymes and prostaglandins in pathology of the endometrium. Reproduction 2003; 126:559–567.
26. Rees MC, Turnbull AC. Menstrual disorders—an overview. Baillieres Clin Obstet Gynaecol 1989; 3:217–226.
27. Rees MC. Heavy, painful periods. Baillieres Clin Obstet Gynaecol 1989; 3:341–356.
28. Bulleti C, D DEZ, Setti PL, Cicinelli E, Polli V, Flamigni C. The patterns of uterine contractility in normal menstruating women: from physiology to pathology. Ann N Y Acad Sci 2004; 1034: 64–83.
29. Akerlund M, Melin P, Maggi M. Potential use of oxytocin and vasopressin V1a antagonists in the treatment of preterm labour and primary dysmenorrhoea. Adv Exp Med Biol 1995; 395:595–600.
30. Akerlund M. Can primary dysmenorrhea be alleviated by a vasopressin antagonist? Results of a pilot study. Acta Obstet Gynecol Scand 1987; 66:459–461.

31. Akerlund M. The role of oxytocin and vasopressin in the initiation of preterm and term labour as well as primary dysmenorrhoea. Regul Pept 1993; 45:187–191.
32. Karim SM, Hillier K. Prostaglandins in the control of animal and human reproduction. Br Med Bull 1979; 35:173–180.
33. Chen YL, Shepherd C, Spinelli W, Lai FM. Oxytocin and vasopressin constrict rat isolated uterine resistance arteries by activating vasopressin V1A receptors. Eur J Pharmacol 1999; 376:45–51.
34. Temple JL, Bradshaw HB, Wood E, Berkley KJ. Effects of hypogastric neurectomy on escape responses to uterine distention in the rat. Pain 1999(suppl 6):S13–S20.
35. Daniels SE, Talwalker S, Torri S, Snabes MC, Recker DP, Verburg KM. Valdecoxib, a cyclooxygenase-2-specific inhibitor, is effective in treating primary dysmenorrhea. Obstet Gynecol 2002; 100:350–358.
36. Wilson ML, Farquhar CM, Sinclair OJ, Johnson NP. Surgical interruption of pelvic nerve pathways for primary and secondary dysmenorrhoea. Cochrane Database Syst Rev 2000; CD001896.
37. McKenna KE. The neural control of female sexual function. NeuroRehabilitation 2000; 15:133–143.
38. Kumazawa T. Sensory innervation of reproductive organs. Prog Brain Res 1986; 67:115–131.
39. Berkley KJ, Rapkin AJ, Papka RE. The pains of endometriosis. Science 2005; 308:1587–1589.
40. Bulun SE, Zeitoun KM, Takayama K, Sasano H. Estrogen biosynthesis in endometriosis: molecular basis and clinical relevance. J Mol Endocrinol 2000; 25:35–42.
41. Child TJ, Tan SL. Endometriosis: aetiology, pathogenesis and treatment. Drugs 2001; 61:1735–1750.
42. Valle RF, Sciarra JJ. Endometriosis: treatment strategies. Ann N Y Acad Sci 2003; 997:229–239.
43. Wu MY, Ho HN. The role of cytokines in endometriosis. Am J Reprod Immunol 2003; 49: 285–296.
44. Silberstein SD, Merriam GR. Physiology of the menstrual cycle. Cephalalgia 2000; 20:148–154.
45. Belchetz PE, Plant TM, Nakai Y, Keogh EJ, Knobil E. Hypophysial responses to continuous and intermittent delivery of hypopthalamic gonadotropin-releasing hormone. Science 1978; 202: 631–633.
46. Vernon MW, Wilson EA. Studies on the surgical induction of endometriosis in the rat. Fertil Steril 1985; 44:684–694.
47. Sharpe-Timms KL. Using rats as a research model for the study of endometriosis. Ann N Y Acad Sci 2002; 955:318–327; discussion 340–342, 396–406.
48. Barragan JC, Brotons J, Ruiz JA, Acien P. Experimentally induced endometriosis in rats: effect on fertility and the effects of pregnancy and lactation on the ectopic endometrial tissue. Fertil Steril 1992; 58:1215–1219.
49. Rajkumar K, Schott PW, Simpson CW. The rat as an animal model for endometriosis to examine recurrence of ectopic endometrial tissue after regression. Fertil Steril 1990; 53:921–925.
50. Berkley KJ, Dmitrieva N, Curtis KS, Papka RE. Innervation of ectopic endometrium in a rat model of endometriosis. Proc Natl Acad Sci U S A 2004; 101:11094–11098.
51. Chadha HK, Hubscher CH. Pelvic and pudendal nerve input to hypothalamic neurons in female rats: response variations with stage of estrus. Abstract Viwer/Itinerary Planner, volume Program No. 52.9. Washington, D.C.: Society for Neuroscience, 2005.
52. Al-Chaer ED, Lawand NB, Westlund KN, Willis WD. Visceral nociceptive input into the ventral posterolateral nucleus of the thalamus: a new function for the dorsal column pathway. J Neurophysiol 1996; 76:2661–2674.
53. Berkley KJ, Wood E, Scofield SL, Little M. Behavioral responses to uterine or vaginal distension in the rat. Pain 1995; 61:121–131.
54. Berkley KJ, Guilbaud G, Benoist JM, Gautron M. Responses of neurons in and near the thalamic ventrobasal complex of the rat to stimulation of uterus, cervix, vagina, colon, and skin. J Neurophysiol 1993; 69:557–568.
55. Olive DL. Medical therapy of endometriosis. Semin Reprod Med 2003; 21:209–222.
56. Buyalos RP, Agarwal SK. Endometriosis-associated infertility. Curr Opin Obstet Gynecol 2000; 12:377–381.
57. Paavonen J. Vulvodynia—a complex syndrome of vulvar pain. Acta Obstet Gynecol Scand 1995; 74:243–247.
58. Masheb RM, Nash JM, Brondolo E, Kerns RD. Vulvodynia: an introduction and critical review of a chronic pain condition. Pain 2000; 86:3–10.
59. Welsh BM, Berzins KN, Cook KA, Fairley CK. Management of common vulval conditions. Med J Aust 2003; 178:391–395.
60. Sand PK. Chronic pain syndromes of gynecologic origin. J Reprod Med 2004; 49:230–234.
61. Edwards L. New concepts in vulvodynia. Am J Obstet Gynecol 2003; 189:S24–S30.
62. Ting AY, Blacklock AD, Smith PG. Estrogen regulates vaginal sensory and autonomic nerve density in the rat. Biol Reprod 2004; 71:1397–1404.
63. Gelbaya TA, El-Halwagy HE. Focus on primary care: chronic pelvic pain in women. Obstet Gynecol Surv 2001; 56:757–764.
64. Bradshaw HB, Berkley KJ. Estrogen replacement reverses ovariectomy–induced vaginal hyperalgesia in the rat. Maturitas 2002; 41:157–165.
65. Walker CL. Role of hormonal and reproductive factors in the etiology and treatment of uterine leiomyoma. Recent Prog Horm Res 2002; 57:277–294.

66. Perry CP. Uterine Leiomyomas. In: Howard FM, ed. Pelvic Pain-Diagnosis and Management. Lippincott: Williams and Wilkins, 2000:151–154.
67. Walker CL, Stewart EA. Uterine fibroids: the elephant in the room. Science 2005; 308:1589–1592.
68. Walker CL, Hunter D, Everitt JI. Uterine leiomyoma in the Eker rat: a unique model for important diseases of women. Genes Chromosomes Cancer 2003; 38:349–356.
69. Everitt JI, Wolf DC, Howe SR, Goldsworthy TL, Walker C. Rodent model of reproductive tract leiomyomata. Clinical and pathological features. Am J Pathol 1995; 146:1556–1567.
70. Hunter DS, Hodges LC, Eagon PK, et al. Influence of exogenous estrogen receptor ligands on uterine leiomyoma: evidence from an in vitro/in vivo animal model for uterine fibroids. Environ Health Perspect 2000; 108(suppl 5):829–834.
71. Nijman HW, Lambeck A, Vander Zee AG, Daemen T. Immunologic aspect of ovarian cancer. Tumor antigen. J Transl Med 2005; 34(3):53.
72. Bankhead CR, Kehoe ST, Austoker J. Symptoms associated with diagnosis of ovarian cancer: a systematic review. Bjog 2005; 112:857–865.
73. Burke TW. Vulvar Cancer. In: RR Barakat MB, Gershenson DM, Hoskins WJ, eds. Handbook of Gynecologic Oncology. Londer: Martin Dunitz; Florence KY; Distributed in the USA by fulfilment Center, Taylor & Francis, 2002, 2002:213–221.
74. de Oliveira R, dos Reis MP, Prado WA. The effects of early or late neurolytic sympathetic plexus block on the management of abdominal or pelvic cancer pain. Pain 2004; 110:400–408.
75. Rigor BM Sr. Pelvic cancer pain. J Surg Oncol 2000; 75:280–300.
76. de Leon-Casasola OA, Kent E, Lema MJ. Neurolytic superior hypogastric plexus block for chronic pelvic pain associated with cancer. Pain 1993; 54:145–151.
77. Mercadante S, Fulfaro F, Casuccio A. Pain mechanisms involved and outcome in advanced cancer patients with possible indications for celiac plexus block and superior hypogastric plexus block. Tumori 2002; 88:243–245.
78. Nauta HJ, Hewitt E, Westlund KN, Willis WD Jr. Surgical interruption of a midline dorsal column visceral pain pathway. Case report and review of the literature. J Neurosurg 1997; 86:538–542.
79. Patt RB, Reddy SK, Black RG. Neural blockade for abdominopelvic pain of oncologic origin. Int Anesthesiol Clin 1998; 36:87–104.
80. Mercadante S, Catala E, Arcuri E, Casuccio A. Celiac plexus block for pancreatic cancer pain: factors influencing pain, symptoms and quality of life. J Pain Symptom Manage 2003; 26:1140–1147.
81. Berkley KJ, Hubscher CH. Are there separate central nervous system pathways for touch and pain? Nat Med 1995; 1:766–773.
82. Hirshberg RM, Al-Chaer ED, Lawand NB, Westlund KN, Willis WD. Is there a pathway in the posterior funiculus that signals visceral pain? Pain 1996; 67:291–305.
83. Al-Chaer ED, Lawand NB, Westlund KN, Willis WD. Pelvic visceral input into the nucleus gracilis is largely mediated by the postsynaptic dorsal column pathway. J Neurophysiol 1996; 76:2675–2690.
84. Hubscher CH, Berkley KJ. Spinal and vagal influences on the responses of rat solitary nucleus neurons to stimulation of uterus, cervix and vagina. Brain Res 1995; 702:251–254.
85. Cervero F, Laird JM. Visceral pain. Lancet 1999; 353:2145–2148.
86. Granitsiotis P, Kirk D. Chronic testicular pain: an overview. Eur Urol 2004; 45:430–436.
87. Holland JM, Feldman JL, Gilbert HC. Phantom orchalgia. J Urol 1994; 152:2291–2293.
88. Kuntz A, Morris RE. Components and distribution of the spermatic nerves and the nerves of the vas deferens. J Comp Neurol 1946; 85:33–44.
89. Peterson DF, Brown AM. Functional afferent innervation of testis. J Neurophysiol 1973; 36:425–433.
90. Kruger L, Kavookjian AM, Kumazawa T, Light AR, Mizumura K. Nociceptor structural specialization in canine and rodent testicular "free" nerve endings. J Comp Neurol 2003; 463:197–211.
91. Kumazawa T, Mizumura K, Sato J. Response properties of polymodal receptors studied using in vitro testis superior spermatic nerve preparations of dogs. J Neurophysiol 1987; 57:702–711.
92. Kumazawa T, Mizumura K. The polymodal receptors in the testis of dog. Brain Res 1977; 136:553–558.
93. Kumazawa T, Mizumura K, Koda H, Tamura R, Sato J. Mechanisms of chemical modulation of testicular afferents. In: Gaafar AA, ed. Visceral Pain, Progress in Pain Research and Management. Vol. 5. Seattle: IASP Press, 1995:133–161.
94. Mizumura K, Koda H, Kumazawa T. Evidence that protein kinase C activation is involved in the excitatory and facilitatory effects of bradykinin on canine visceral nociceptors in vitro. Neurosci Lett 1997; 237:29–32.
95. Milne RJ, Foreman RD, Giesler GJ Jr., Willis WD. Convergence of cutaneous and pelvic visceral nociceptive inputs onto primate spinothalamic neurons. Pain 1981; 11:163–183.
96. Kanui TI. Responses of spinal cord neurones to noxious and non-noxious stimulation of the skin and testicle of the rat. Neurosci Lett 1985; 58:315–319.
97. Tamura R, Mizumura K, Kumazawa T. Coexistence of calcitonin gene–related peptide- and substance P-like immunoreactivity in retrogradely labeled superior spermatic neurons in the dog. Neurosci Res 1996; 25:293–299.
98. Traub RJ, Hutchcroft K, Gebhart GF. The peptide content of colonic afferents decreases following colonic inflammation. Peptides 1999; 20:267–273.

99. Roza C, Reeh PW. Substance P, calcitonin gene related peptide and PGE2 coreleased from the mouse colon: a new model to study nociceptive and inflammatory responses in viscera, in vitro. Pain 2001; 93:213–219.
100. Vera-Portocarrero LP, Lu Y, Westlund KN. Nociception in persistent pancreatitis in rats: effects of morphine and neuropeptide alterations. Anesthesiology 2003; 98:474–484.
101. Mizumura K, Sugiura Y, Kumazawa T. Spinal termination patterns of canine identified A-delta and C spermatic polymodal receptors traced by intracellular labeling with Phaseolus vulgaris-leucoagglutinin. J Comp Neurol 1993; 335:460–468.
102. Schaeffer AJ. Epidemiology and demographics of prostatitis. Andrologia 2003; 35:252–257.
103. Krieger JN, Nyberg L Jr., Nickel JC. NIH consensus definition and classification of prostatitis. Jama 1999; 282:236–237.
104. Krieger JN, Egan KJ. Comprehensive evaluation and treatment of 75 men referred to chronic prostatitis clinic. Urology 1991; 38:11–19.
105. Pontari MA, Ruggieri MR. Mechanisms in prostatitis/chronic pelvic pain syndrome. J Urol 2004; 172:839–845.
106. Drach GW, Fair WR, Meares EM, Stamey TA. Classification of benign diseases associated with prostatic pain: prostatitis or prostatodynia? J Urol 1978; 120:266.
107. Krieger JN, Riley DE. Bacteria in the chronic prostatitis-chronic pelvic pain syndrome: molecular approaches to critical research questions. J Urol 2002; 167:2574–2583.
108. Shoskes DA, Mazurick C, Landis R, et al. bacterial cultures in urine, prostatic flouid and semen of men with chronic pelvic pain syndrome: role of culture for 2 vs 5 days. J Urol 2000; 163:24.
109. Nadler RB, Koch AE, Calhoun EA, et al. IL-1beta and TNF-alpha in prostatic secretions are indicators in the evaluation of men with chronic prostatitis. J Urol 2000; 164:214–218.
110. Hochreiter WW, Nadler RB, Koch AE, et al. Evaluation of the cytokines interleukin 8 and epithelial neutrophil activating peptide 78 as indicators of inflammation in prostatic secretions. Urology 2000; 56:1025–1029.
111. Fong L, Ruegg CL, Brockstedt D, Engleman EG, Laus R. Induction of tissue-specific autoimmune prostatitis with prostatic acid phosphatase immunization: implications for immunotherapy of prostate cancer. J Immunol 1997; 159:3113–3117.
112. Vykhovanets EV, Resnick MI, Marengo SR. The healthy rat prostate contains high levels of natural killer-like cells and unique subsets of CD4+ helper-inducer T cells: implications for prostatitis. J Urol 2005; 173:1004–1010.
113. Alexander RB, Brady F, Ponniah S. Autoimmune prostatitis: evidence of T cell reactivity with normal prostatic proteins. Urology 1997; 50:893–899.
114. Seo SI, Lee SJ, Kim JC, et al. Effects of androgen deprivation on chronic bacterial prostatitis in a rat model. Int J Urol 2003; 10:485–491.
115. Zermann DH, Ishigooka M, Doggweiler R, Schmidt RA. Neurourological insights into the etiology of genitourinary pain in men. J Urol 1999; 161:903–908.
116. Krieger JN, Egan KJ, Ross SO, Jacobs R, Berger RE. Chronic pelvic pains represent the most prominent urogenital symptoms of "chronic prostatitis." Urology 1996; 48:715–721; discussion 721–722.
117. Floyd K, Hick VE, Morrison JF. Mechanosensitive afferent units in the hypogastric nerve of the cat. J Physiol 1976; 259:457–471.
118. Danuser H, Springer JP, Katofiasc MA, Thor KB. Extrinsic innervation of the cat prostate gland: a combined tracing and immunohistochemical study. J Urol 1997; 157:1018–1024.
119. McVary KT, McKenna KE, Lee C. Prostate innervation. Prostate Suppl 1998; 8:2–13.
120. Ishigooka M, Zermann DH, Doggweiler R, Schmidt RA. Similarity of distributions of spinal c-Fos and plasma extravasation after acute chemical irritation of the bladder and the prostate. J Urol 2000; 164:1751–1756.
121. Ishigooka M, Nakada T, Hashimoto T, Iijima Y, Yaguchi H. Spinal substance P immunoreactivity is enhanced by acute chemical stimulation of the rat prostate. Urology 2002; 59:139–144.
122. Miller JL, Rothman I, Bavendam TG, Berger RE. Prostatodynia and interstitial cystitis: one and the same? Urology 1995; 45:587–590.
123. Hubscher CH, Johnson RD. Responses of medullary reticular formation neurons to input from the male genitalia. J Neurophysiol 1996; 76:2474–2482.
124. Hubscher CH, Johnson RD. Responses of thalamic neurons to input from the male genitalia. J Neurophysiol 2003; 89:2–11.
125. Chaudhary M, Sheikh N, Asterling S, Ahmad I, Greene D. Peyronie's disease with erectile dysfunction: penile modeling over inflatable penile prostheses. Urology 2005; 65:760–764.
126. Samm BJ, Dmochowski RR. Urologic emergencies. Trauma injuries and conditions affecting the penis, scrotum, and testicles. Postgrad Med 1996; 100:187–190, 193–194, 199–200.
127. Gee WJ, Ansell JS. Pelvic and perineal pain of urologic origin. In: Bonica JJ, ed. The Management of Pain. Vol. 2. Malvern, Pennsylvania: Lea and Febiger, 1990:1368–1382.
128. Asgari MA, Hosseini SY, Safarinejad MR, Samadzadeh B, Bardideh AR. Penile fractures: evaluation, therapeutic approaches and long-term results. J Urol 1996; 155:148–149.
129. El-Taher AM, Aboul-Ella HA, Sayed MA, Gaafar AA. Management of penile fracture. J Trauma 2004; 56:1138–1140; discussion 1140.

130. Kitchell RL, Gilanpour H, Johnson RD. Electrophysiologic studies of penile mechanoreceptors in the rats. Exp Neurol 1982; 75:229–244.
131. Rab M, Ebmer, Dellon AL. Anatomic variability of the ilioinguinal and genitofemoral nerve: implications for the treatment of groin pain. Plast Reconstr Surg 2001; 108:1618–1623.
132. Steers WD. Neural pathways and central sites involved in penile erection: neuroanatomy and clinical implications. Neurosci Biobehav Rev 2000; 24:507–516.
133. Morgan C, Nadelhaft I, de Groat WC. The distribution of visceral primary afferents from the pelvic nerve to Lissauer's tract and the spinal gray matter and its relationship to the sacral parasympathetic nucleus. J Comp Neurol 1981; 201:415–440.
134. Pacheco P, Camacho MA, Garcia LI, Hernandez ME, Carrillo P, Manzo J. Electrophysiological evidence for the nomenclature of the pudendal nerve and sacral plexus in the male rat. Brain Res 1997; 763:202–208.
135. Nunez R, Gross GH, Sachs BD. Origin and central projections of rat dorsal penile nerve: possible direct projection to autonomic and somatic neurons by primary afferents of nonmuscle origin. J Comp Neurol 1986; 247:417–429.
136. Shafik A, el-Sherif M, Youssef A, Olfat ES. Surgical anatomy of the pudendal nerve and its clinical implications. Clin Anat 1995; 8:110–115.
137. Hough DM, Wittenberg KH, Pawlina W, et al. Chronic perineal pain caused by pudendal nerve entrapment: anatomy and CT–guided perineural injection technique. AJR Am J Roentgenol 2003; 181:561–567.
138. Rampin O, Gougis S, Giuliano F, Rousseau JP. Spinal Fos labeling and penile erection elicited by stimulation of dorsal nerve of the rat penis. Am J Physiol 1997; 272:R1425–R1431.
139. Hubscher CH, Johnson RD. Effects of acute and chronic midthoracic spinal cord injury on neural circuits for male sexual function. I. Ascending pathways. J Neurophysiol 1999; 82:1381–1389.
140. Hubscher CH, Johnson RD. Effects of chronic dorsal column lesions on pelvic viscerosomatic convergent medullary reticular formation neurons. J Neurophysiol 2004; 92:3596–3600.
141. Foley KM. Pain syndromes in patients with cancer. In: Bonica JJ, ed. Advances in Pain Research and Therapy. Vol. 2. New York: Raven Press Ltd, 1979:59–75.
142. Miller DC, Hafez KS, Stewart A, Montie JE, Wei JT. Prostate carcinoma presentation, diagnosis, and staging: an update form the National Cancer Data Base. Cancer 2003; 98:1169–1178.
143. Eaton CL, Coleman RE. Pathophysiology of bone metastases from prostate cancer and the role of bisphosphonates in treatment. Cancer Treat Rev 2003; 29:189–198.
144. Luger NM, Honore P, Sabino MA, et al. Osteoprotegerin diminishes advanced bone cancer pain. Cancer Res 2001; 61:4038–4047.
145. Sevcik MA, Luger NM, Mach DB, et al. Bone cancer pain: the effects of the bisphosphonate alendronate on pain, skeletal remodeling, tumor growth and tumor necrosis. Pain 2004; 111:169–180.
146. Sabino MA, Mantyh PW. Pathophysiology of bone cancer pain. J Support Oncol 2005; 3:15–24.
147. Jaeckle KA, Young DF, Foley KM. The natural history of lumbosacral plexopathy in cancer. Neurology 1985; 35:8–15.
148. Plancarte R, Amescua C, Patt RB, Aldrete JA. Superior hypogastric plexus block for pelvic cancer pain. Anesthesiology 1990; 73:236–239.
149. Warfield CA. Cancer pain. In: Warfield CA, ed. Manual of Pain Manegement. Philadelphia: JB. Lippincott Company, 1991.
150. Sall M, Madsen FA, Rhodes PR, Jonler M, Messing EM, Bruskewitz RC. Pelvic pain following radical retropubic prostatectomy: a prospective study. Urology 1997; 49:575–579.
151. Leibovici D, Lee AK, Cheung RM, et al. Symptomatic local recurrence of prostate carcinoma after radiation therapy. Cancer 2005; 103:2060–2066.
152. McKenzie M, MacLennan I, Kostashuk E, Bainbridge T. Postirradiation sarcoma after external beam radiation therapy for localized adenocarcinoma of the prostate: report of three cases. Urology 1999; 53:1228.
153. Antolak SJ, Hough DM, Pawlina W. The chronic pelvic pain syndrome after brachytherapy for carcinoma of the prostate. J Urol 2002; 167:2525.
154. Nelson JB, Hedican SP, George DJ, et al. Identification of endothelin-1 in the pathophysiology of metastatic adenocarcinoma of the prostate. Nat Med 1995; 1:944–949.
155. Raffa RB, Schupsky JJ, Martinez RP, Jacoby HI. Endothelin-1-induced nociception. Life Sci 1991; 49:PL61–PL65.
156. Davar G, Hans G, Fareed MU, Sinnott C, Strichartz G. Behavioral signs of acute pain produced by application of endothelin-1 to rat sciatic nerve. Neuroreport 1998; 9:2279–2283.
157. Kergozien S, Bansard JY, Delcros JG, Havouis R, Moulinoux JP. Polyamine deprivation provokes an antalgic effect. Life Sci 1996; 58:2209–2215.
158. Pegg AE, McCann PP. Polyamine metabolism and function. Am J Physiol 1982; 243:C212–C221.
159. Pisani R, Stubinski R, Datti R. Entrapment neuropathy of the internal pudendal nerve. Report of two cases. Scand J Urol Nephrol 1997; 31:407–410.
160. Turner ML, Marinoff SC. Pudendal neuralgia. Am J Obstet Gynecol 1991; 165:1233–1236.
161. Robert R, Labat JJ, Bensignor M, et al. Decompression and transposition of the pudendal nerve in pudendal neuralgia: a randomized controlled trial and long-term evaluation. Eur Urol 2005; 47: 403–408.

162. Takano M. Proctalgia fugax: caused by pudendal neuropathy? Dis Colon Rectum 2005; 48:114–120.
163. Benson JT, Griffis K. Pudendal neuralgia, a severe pain syndrome. Am J Obstet Gynecol 2005; 192:1663–1668.
164. Oberpenning F, Roth S, Leusmann DB, van Ahlen H, Hertle L. The Alcock syndrome: temporary penile insensitivity due to compression of the pudendal nerve within the Alcock canal. J Urol 1994; 151:423–425.
165. Hagen NA. Sharp, shooting neuropathic pain in the rectum or genitals: pudendal neuralgia. J Pain Symptom Manage 1993; 8:496–501.
166. Layzer RB, Conant MA. Neuralgia in recurrent herpes simplex. Arch Neurol 1974; 31:233–237.
167. Howard EJ. Postherpetic pudendal neuralgia. Jama 1985; 253:2196.
168. Tognetti F, Poppi M, Gaist G, Servadei F. Pudendal neuralgia due to solitary neurofibroma. Case report. J Neurosurg 1982; 56:732–733.
169. Dittrich RJ. Coccygodynia as referred pain. J Bone Joint Surg Am 1951; 33-A:715–718.
170. Thiele GH. Coccygodynia: cause and treatment. Dis Colon Rectum 1963; 11:422–436.
171. Johnson PH. Coccygodynia. J Ark Med Soc 1981; 77:421–424.
172. Torok G. Coccygodynia. J Bone Joint Surg 1974; 56B:386.
173. Postacchini F, Massobrio M. Idiopathic coccygodynia. Analysis of 51 operative cases and a radiographic study of the normal coccyx. J Bone Joint Surg Am 1983; 65:1116–1124.
174. Ramsey ML, Toohey JS, Neidre A, Stromberg LJ, Roberts DA. Coccygodynia: treatment. Orthopedics 2003; 26:403–405; discussion 405.
175. Barber MD, Bremer RE, Thor KB, Dolber PC, Kuehl TJ, Coates KW. Innervation of the female levator ani muscles. Am J Obstet Gynecol 2002; 187:64–71.
176. Peyton FW. Coccygodynia in women. Indiana Med 1988; 81:697–698.
177. Maguire PJ. Coccygodynia. Am J Obstet Gynecol 1963; 87:134–135.
178. Krasin E, Nirkin A, Issakov J, Rabau M, Meller I. Carcinoid tumor of the coccyx: case report and review of the literature. Spine 2001; 26:2165–2167.
179. Ziegler DK, Batnitzky S. Coccygodynia caused by perineural cyst. Neurology 1984; 34:829–830.
180. Dennell LV, Nathan S. Coccygeal retroversion. Spine 2004; 29:E256–E257.
181. Jones ME, Shoaib A, Bircher MD. A case of coccygodynia due to coccygeal fracture secondary to parturition. Injury 1997; 28:549–550.
182. Bar-Maor JA, Kesner KM, Kaftori JK. Human tails. J Bone Joint Surg Br 1980; 62-B:508–510.
183. Maigne JY, Guedj S, Straus C. Idiopathic coccygodynia. Lateral roentgenograms in the sitting position and coccygeal discography. Spine 1994; 19:930–934.
184. Kim NH, Suk KS. Clinical and radiological differences between traumatic and idiopathic coccygodynia. Yonsei Med J 1999; 40:215–220.
185. Magee RK. Genitofemoral causalgia. Canadian Med Assoc J 1942; 46:326–329.
186. Harms BA, DeHaas DR Jr., Starling JR. Diagnosis and management of genitofemoral neuralgia. Arch Surg 1984; 119:339–341.
187. Starling JR, Harms BA, Schroeder ME, Eichman PL. Diagnosis and treatment of genitofemoral and ilioinguinal entrapment neuralgia. Surgery 1987; 102:581–586.
188. Murovic JA, Kim DH, Tiel RL, Kline DG. Surgical management of 10 genitofemoral neuralgias at the Louisiana State University Health Sciences Center. Neurosurgery 2005; 56:298–303; discussion 298–303.
189. O'Brien MD. Genitofemoral neuropathy. Br Med J 1979; 1:1052.
190. Kar S, Gibson SJ, Polak JM. Origins and projections of peptide-immunoreactive nerves in the male rat genitofemoral nerve. Brain Res 1990; 512:229–237.
191. Nagy JI, Senba E. Neural relations of cremaster motoneurons, spinal cord systems and the genitofemoral nerve in the rat. Brain Res Bull 1985; 15:609–627.
192. Kirk EJ, Kitchell RL, Carr DH. Neurophysiologic maps of cutaneous innervation of the external genitalia of the ram. Am J Vet Res 1987; 48:1162–1166.
193. Kirk EJ, Kitchell RL. Neurophysiologic maps of the cutaneous innervation of the external genitalia of the ewe. Am J Vet Res 1988; 49:522–526.

32 | Pelvic Pain Syndromes: Clinical Features and Management

Jane Moore and Stephen Kennedy

Nuffield Department of Obstetrics and Gynecology, University of Oxford, John Radcliffe Hospital, Oxford, U.K.

INTRODUCTION

Chronic pelvic pain (CPP) is common, affecting approximately one in six of the adult female population (1) and can have devastating social and economic consequences. Pain which is very severe even if infrequent may make it difficult to hold down a job or care for one's children. Extra support becomes essential, leading to a loss of confidence and distortion of social roles and responsibilities. Doctors tend to find CPP a difficult symptom to address and many women feel that the response they have received from their doctor has been less than sympathetic (2). All these factors make for a pressing need to improve our understanding and management of this complex symptom.

In this chapter, the factors currently thought to contribute to CPP will be explored and management strategies discussed. Although pelvic pain can occur in men with an incidence of approximately one-sixth of that in women (3), this chapter deals exclusively with pain in women.

Evidence has been collated using a Medline search 1966–2005 and drawing on recent guidelines published by American College of Obstetrics and Gynecology (4), Royal College of Obstetricians and Gynaecologists (5), and European Society for Human Reproduction (6).

DEFINITIONS AND EPIDEMIOLOGY

Pain is defined by the International Association for the Study of Pain as an unpleasant sensory and emotional experience associated with actual or potential tissue damage or described in those terms (7).

The definition of CPP used in this chapter is entirely symptom based. Pelvic pain is experienced in the lower abdomen or pelvis not associated exclusively with menstruation, pregnancy, or intercourse. It is distinct from dysmenorrhea (pain during menstruation), and dyspareunia (pain during sexual intercourse). Pain in the vulva and perineum is considered to be a different condition, and is discussed in a short section at the end of this chapter.

CPP has been defined in a number of different ways in the literature, and this has led to confusion and difficulty in comparing studies (8,9). Some authors use a time frame of three months, others six. Some authors have used other criteria such as the degree of disability caused by the pain, or the identification of pathology or lack of it. Given the huge variation in individuals' responses to pain and our poor understanding of the relevant pathologies, this seems inappropriate.

CPP is common. In a postal community survey of 3106 women identified through the electoral role in the United Kingdom, the three-month prevalence of CPP was 24%. When pain occurring only at the time of ovulation was excluded, the three-month prevalence of CPP was 16.9% (1). In New Zealand, a similar study was undertaken with remarkably similar prevalence (10). In the United States, a telephone survey of 5263 women revealed a three-month prevalence of 14.7% (11). Of course not all of these women will have disabling pain, but many will be seeking an explanation for their pain and making use of health-care resources.

Aetiology of Chronic Pelvic Pain

The conceptualization of CPP is changing as the complexity of its pathogenesis becomes apparent. The "bio-psycho-social model of disease" describes the concept of a number of

Chronic pelvic pain is defined as
intermittent or continuous pain of at least six months duration
felt in the lower abdomen or pelvis not associated
exclusively with menstruation, intercourse, pregnancy or malignancy.

Figure 1 Working definition of chronic pelvic pain.

different factors feeding in to the overall pain experience: physical diseases such as endometriosis, social factors such as job experiences or relationships, and psychological factors such as coping strategies or health beliefs.

More recently, the central role of the "nervous system" in the perception of pain has been recognized (12). Nerve function is influenced by many factors including the presence of an inflammatory condition, the hormonal milieu, and input from the higher centers. The role of the autonomic nervous system is significant (13). These theoretical concepts are explored in much more detail in the first half of this chapter.

CPP is a symptom that is likely to have a number of contributory factors rather than a single cause. The term simply describes the pain rather than being a diagnosis in itself. Pain may arise from any structure in or related to the pelvis. Investigations should seek to identify the various components of pain each of which may be amenable to treatment. One individual may have several types of pain and, as described in Section 4, it is the variation of the pain with functions such as opening the bowels, menstruation, or movement, which may point toward the origin of the pain. Gynecological and some psychological conditions associated with pelvic pain are discussed in this section. Pain arising from the bowel [e.g., irritable bowel syndrome (IBS)], bladder [e.g., interstitial cystitis (IC)], or musculoskeletal system is described in detail in other chapters.

Pain syndromes such as endometriosis, IBS, or IC are common and may coexist in the same individual, but observational studies suggest that this occurs more frequently than would be expected by chance (14,15). The possibility of an underlying regional neurological dysfunction, affecting several systems in the pelvis has been suggested to explain some patients' symptom complex. The etiology of such regional dysfunction could of course be varied, but it is plausible that perhaps the inflammatory stimulus of endometriosis might affect the regional neural network and consequently disrupt bowel function, generating the symptoms known as IBS. This concept is also discussed in more detail in the first half of this chapter.

Endometriosis
What is Endometriosis?

Endometriosis is a condition in which endometrial-like tissue is found in areas outside the uterus such as behind the cervix, within the ovaries, or scattered across the pelvic peritoneum. Rarely, it may also appear at distant sites such as the lungs.

Endometriosis exists in a number of distinct forms and some consider that these different forms represent different disease types (16). Endometriosis may be scattered as superficial peritoneal lesions across the pelvis and cause no distortion of the underlying tissue. Peritoneal disease may have a variety of appearances (17), or may be microscopic (18). Endometriosis may occur within or beneath the ovaries, forming discrete cysts known as endometriomas. These contain dark tar-like material and are sometimes called chocolate cysts.

Endometriosis may form solid nodules located predominantly below the peritoneal surface, which may only appear as small lesions at laparoscopy—like the tip of an iceberg. The lesion may be palpable on vaginal examination, and is often associated with significant distortion of the surrounding tissues. Nodular endometriosis is commonly found in the recto vaginal septum or densely adherent to bowel.

The severity of endometriosis may be assessed by simply describing the findings or by using a classification system such as the one provided by the American Society of Reproductive Medicine (19). However, such systems were never designed to correlate disease severity with pain symptoms.

The diagnosis of endometriosis has traditionally been made visually at diagnostic laparoscopy. It is now recommended that a biopsy should always be taken to confirm the diagnosis because the appearances are so variable. For endometriomas greater than 3 cm in size and for excised nodules, histology should be performed to rule out malignancy (6).

The etiology of endometriosis remains unclear. The most popular theory at present is that retrograde menstruation, which occurs in all women, allows viable endometrial cells to flow through the Fallopian tubes into the pelvis. These cells "seed" in some women leading to the growth of endometriotic tissue. It is thought that genetically determined defects in the immune surveillance system result in a failure to clear the viable endometrial cells (20). The expression of these genetically determined defects may be affected by environmental elements. Other theories have been proposed including the concept that endometrial tissue is a consequence rather than a cause of abnormal nerve function (21). For a fuller discussion of the etiology of endometriosis please see a review by Donnez et al.(22).

The prevalence of endometriosis is uncertain, but estimates suggest that 10% of the general population may be affected (23). Among women suffering from CPP as many as 45% may have the disease (24).

How is Endometriosis Linked to Chronic Pelvic Pain?

Women with endometriosis are more likely to suffer from pain than women without the disease (25) but women may be asymptomatic (26). Different types of pain are experienced: dysmenorrhea, dyspareunia, nonmenstrual pain, dyschezia (pain on opening bowels), and ovulation pain. The hallmark of pain associated with endometriosis is its cyclical variation with nonmenstrual pain increasing markedly in the week prior to menstruation (27).

There is huge variation in the degree of pain experienced by women with seemingly similar amounts of disease—a phenomenon that is not understood. Possible explanations include variation in the site of the lesions (28), the extent of disease (29), and the depth of invasion (30). Some forms of endometriosis may be more painful than others; e.g., certain lesions may cause pain through the release of inflammatory mediators of pain such as bradykinins, prostaglandins, and tumor necrosis factor (31). More fibrous forms may cause pain by tissue traction or constriction of nerves. Endometriosis is known to infiltrate nerves (32). The resulting nerve damage may itself become a source of pain. Even if nerves are not damaged, their function may change in the presence of endometriosis, for example through the recruitment of silent afferents.

However, in a recent multicenter study involving 469 women with CPP, undergoing their first diagnostic procedure, no clear cut link was found between site, morphological characteristics, or severity of disease and severity or frequency of nonmenstrual pelvic pain (33).

It is important to remember that if pain is viewed as a multifactorial condition, then other factors such as comorbidity (e.g., IBS or depression) or psychosocial factors (e.g., health beliefs or coping strategies) may explain some of this variation.

Adenomyosis

Adenomyosis is usually considered a variant of endometriosis, in which endometrial-like tissue is found within the myometrium. The associated symptoms are similar to those of endometriosis with a striking cyclical variation. Women often experience menstrual chaos, and dyspareunia is a prominent symptom. Adenomyosis is less studied than endometriosis because until recently the diagnosis could only be made histologically, i.e., following removal of the uterus.

Pelvic Inflammatory Disease

Sexually transmitted infection is very common particularly among women aged 16 to 24. It is estimated that the prevalence of chlamydia in this group is 9% (34). Chlamydia and gonorrhea colonize the cervix and may be asymptomatic. Infection can then spread into the upper genital tract to infect the uterus, fallopian tubes, and wider tissues in the pelvis. This is referred to as pelvic inflammatory disease (PID). This can present acutely with pain and irregular or post-coital bleeding, but can also be a grumbling or asymptomatic condition. The diagnosis of chronic PID requires evidence of damage to the pelvis usually from laparoscopy and evidence of current or past infection usually of chlamydia. Given its high prevalence, the identification chlamydia at the cervix is not in itself sufficient to attribute the cause of pain to PID (35).

PID can cause extensive anatomical distortion within the pelvis with adhesion formation and permanent damage to the tubes. Fluid may collect within a dilated tube, which is termed "hydrosalpinx." Such damage may cause infertility and an increased risk of ectopic pregnancy.

The etiology of the pain of chronic PID is unclear, but approximately 30% of women who develop PID will go on to have CPP (36). It may be that the adhesions and distortion of the pelvis cause pain, or it could be that pelvic infection damages the nerves and that the pain of chronic PID is neuropathic in origin.

From a public health perspective it is important that chlamydial infection is detected and treated. Women under 25 or those who have recently changed partners should be screened opportunistically (37). However, it is equally important that a woman's pain is not labeled as PID incorrectly. Not only are there social implications of such a diagnosis that may be extremely disruptive, but also the true cause or causes of her pain will remain undetected and therefore inadequately treated.

Adhesions

An adhesion is scar tissue, which sticks one peritoneal surface to another. The surface may be an organ such as bowel or uterus, or it may be the inner lining of the abdominal wall. Adhesions may be dense and fibrous with little movement between the surfaces or they may be filmy like cobwebs. Adhesions may contain nerves or blood vessels. Formation may be provoked by endometriosis, pelvic infection, or previous surgery.

It has long been debated whether adhesions cause pain, but recent evidence seems to suggest that they do not (38). Certainly, it would seem that treating adhesions does not generally result in a reduction in pain. A randomized controlled trial (RCT) of laparotomy with or without adhesiolysis demonstrated no benefit of adhesiolysis except in a small subgroup of patients with dense vascular adhesions (39). A more recent RCT in which 100 women were randomized to receive laparoscopic adhesiolysis or laparoscopy alone, again failed to demonstrate any benefit (40). However, in a study using conscious pain mapping, it was observed that filmy adhesions, which allowed some movement between structures seemed most likely to cause pain. The location of the adhesions was unimportant. This study was retrospective and unblinded and did not have a treatment phase (41).

Two specific forms of adhesive disease relevant to CPP have been described. The retained ovary syndrome occurs when ovaries, conserved at hysterectomy, subsequently become surrounded by dense adhesions associated with the development of new pelvic pain. Ovarian remnant syndrome is similar but arises when a small part of the ovary is inadvertently retained at oophorectomy. In both situations, ovarian suppression may control the pain and removal of all ovarian tissue is then thought to be curative. However the surgery may be extremely difficult.

Musculo-Skeletal Pain

In other chapters, abnormalities of the abdominal wall are described in which trigger points and abnormal muscle function occur in the abdominal wall musculature and could be a primary or secondary source of pain. Nerve entrapments in scar tissue, fascia, or narrow foramina are also common (42). It is proposed that this could also occur in the pelvic floor (43). In addition to pain, the resulting pelvic floor dysfunction may cause impaired bowel or bladder function thereby adding to the overall pain burden.

The bones and joints of the pelvis may be a primary or secondary source of pain. Symphysis pubis dysfunction may persist following pregnancy. There may be congenital or traumatic distortion of the pelvis. Pain from an inflamed sacroiliac joint may be referred to the iliac fossa. Musculo-skeletal structures can also become a secondary source of pain resulting from a sedentary lifestyle perhaps associated with a reduction in activity due to chronic pain (44).

Pelvic Venous Congestion (PVC)

Another proposed cause of pelvic pain is pelvic venous congestion. In this condition, it is postulated that there is local endocrine dysfunction within the ovaries associated with dilated pelvic veins and venous stasis, resulting in pain. These findings are associated with multicystic ovaries. Symptoms are cyclical and get worse with prolonged standing. Women may have pain and tenderness in one or other iliac fossae, deep dyspareunia and a postcoital ache. However, the evidence that venous stasis causes pain is poor (45).

Psychosocial Factors

Depression and sleep disorders are common in patients with chronic pain. This may be a consequence rather than a cause of their pain, but specific treatment may improve the patient's ability to function (46). It has been suggested that certain personality traits may predispose individuals to the development of a pain syndrome or make it harder to cope with the pain. People who "catastrophize" may be particularly at risk. Cognitive behavioral therapy may be helpful (47).

The sufferer's beliefs about the pain are highly relevant. For example, a belief about the origin of the pain, or past family experiences of illness, may heighten anxiety. Stressful life events or circumstances may affect the individual's ability to function around the pain.

Living with chronic pain may lead to the development of unhelpful behavior patterns in the sufferer or their carers, which may become entrenched and persist even when the pain is treated. These behaviors may need to be addressed directly before resolution can occur.

Abuse

The relationship between CPP and sexual or physical abuse is complex. Studies are difficult to interpret because many have a retrospective design and are performed in secondary care. It appears that women with chronic pain in general, when studied in secondary care, are more likely to report childhood physical or sexual abuse than pain-free women. Those who experience CPP specifically are more likely to report sexual abuse than women with another chronic pain complaint (48–51). In a study of 3539 women attending five gynecology clinics, a history of sexual abuse was noted in 20.7%. This history was associated with a complaint of pelvic pain, self-reported poor health, and multiple clinical visits (52). However, using multiple regression analysis, it appears that childhood sexual abuse may be a marker for continuing abuse and development of depression, anxiety, or somatization, which then predispose the individual to the development or presentation of CPP (53,54).

In a primary care population, 26% of women reported childhood sexual abuse and 28% reported adult sexual abuse, but only those reporting both were more likely to have increased pain symptoms (dysmenorrhea, dyspareunia, or CPP) than women reporting no abuse (55). Interestingly, in a prospective study of young adults who had been abused, there was no increase in medically unexplained symptoms (albeit they were only followed into their 20s) compared to those not known to have been abused, but those who did have unexplained symptoms were more likely to report their history of abuse (56).

Summary

CPP should be seen as a condition with contributory causes rather than a single diagnosis. As described in the first part of this chapter, the neural networks within the pelvis may lead to abnormal function of one organ as a result of pain or inflammation in another part of the pelvis.

For some patients, pain will remain unexplained. Either the symptom complex does not fit any existing model of disease or recognized treatments for the condition the patient is supposed to have not worked. In this context, the doctor can still listen with sympathy and accept the validity of the pain. Empirical pain relief may be appropriate. No doubt new diagnoses will be developed and shown to be related to pain such as endosalpingosis or the importance of hernias (57). Whilst there will probably always be patients whose pain is unexplained, it is hoped that the proportion of women who can understand their pain and learn to function around it may be increased.

"It is the theory that should be discounted when the patient's symptoms refuse to fit, not the patient's account of the reality of their experience (58)."

Investigation

The multifactorial nature of CPP should be discussed and explored from the start. The aim should be to develop a partnership between clinician and patient to plan a management programme.

In the only study of its kind, 106 women with CPP were randomized to an integrated management approach or standard treatment, which involved exclusion of organic causes followed by a laparoscopy. Only if the laparoscopy was negative, was attention given to psychological factors. In the integrated management group, a broad approach was adopted from the outset including physical and psychological assessment and treatment. Laparoscopy was performed only if it was indicated at a later stage. After one year, the integrated approach group reported significantly greater pain relief than the standard treatment group (59).

History

All authorities agree that the initial history and examination is crucial in determining the cause(s) of pain (4,27). Time invested at the start may save hours of time and a great deal of money in fruitless investigations. Not only will the history provide the basis for accurate diagnosis but it may also be therapeutic in itself (60). Telling her story to a respected listener may allow a person to make connections she has not previously seen. It also contributes to a sense of validation that her pain and her thoughts about it are being taken seriously. It is important to understand what a patient wants to achieve in consulting at this time and what the patient believes about the origin of the pain.

One of the most important features of the history is the way in which the pain varies over time, for example across the menstrual cycle or during the course of the day. It is also important to note the way in which the pain varies in association with other physiological activities such as urination, defecation, or movement, because it is these variations that indicate the likely origins of the pain. If the patient is unclear about how the pain varies over time, it may be helpful to ask her to keep a pain diary for two or three months.

The history must include a careful exploration of the way the pain began. The patient may have a very clear idea of when it started such as following an accident, a pregnancy, or a period of stress. It may be that the pain reminds the patient of a past event, like an echo. It may be that the patient knows or believes something about the origin of the pain but is not prepared to share this initially. Careful and sensitive questioning and demonstration of a willingness to listen may yield a fuller picture at a subsequent consultation.

The nature of the pain itself is very telling and, with help, patients can usually give a good description of their pain. It may be cramping or period like, squeezing or bloating. Pain, which is burning, aching, or shooting in nature, may suggest neuropathic pain. It is important to ask carefully about all the functions within the pelvis—bowels, bladder, periods, sexual function, and vaginal discharge, and how they relate to the pain.

Although pelvic pain is not usually caused by progressive or life threatening disease, the physician must be alert to symptoms such as irregular or postcoital bleeding, which may suggest more serious pathology. Some of these so-called red flag symptoms are listed in Figure 2.

Other illnesses such as chronic fatigue syndrome or asthma may be relevant to the origin of the pain or its treatment. Patients should be asked directly for symptoms of depression or sleep disorder. Sensitive past events such as a history of abuse are highly relevant but may

- Bleeding per rectum
- New bowel symptoms over 50
- New pain after the menopause
- Pelvic mass
- Suicidal ideation
- Excessive weight loss
- Irregular vaginal bleeding over 40
- Post coital bleeding

Figure 2   Red flag symptoms.

only be revealed as trust in the doctor–patient relationship grows. Many patients have had extensive investigations and treatments previously and their successes, failures, and side effects are highly relevant.

Examination

In the investigation of CPP, the examination is vital not only because of the physical clues that may be obtained, but also because of the alteration in the doctor–patient relationship as a result of the examination. It is a psychodynamic event and the patient's behavior at this time may show something about the way the patient feels and behaves in other situations.

The abdomen should be carefully inspected for scars. The site of maximum tenderness should be ascertained and then the abdomen carefully palpated usually finishing with the most tender area. The tenderness may be quite diffuse or highly localized. The presence of guarding and rebound tenderness is unusual in the presentation of CPP but may suggest underlying peritonism. Areas of numbness or hyperalgesia in association with the pain or with scars should be noted. If a highly localized spot is found then the patient should be asked to tense the recti by lifting her shoulders off the bed whilst a finger is kept on the tender spot. If the pain is exacerbated by this maneuver, it suggests that it is localized to the abdominal wall rather than within the cavity.

The vaginal examination must be done carefully and sensitively in an unhurried manner. If time or circumstance do not allow, the patient should be asked to return when there is more time available. The skin of the vulva should be inspected and sensation in the area gently tested. If an abnormality is found, a detailed "pain map" should be recorded in the notes. A bimanual examination should be performed exploring systematically all parts of the pelvic cavity. Any tenderness, which may be focal or more diffuse, should be noted along with any masses. Nodularity in the fornices or fixity may suggest endometriosis. This test may be most sensitive at the time of menstruation (61).

A speculum examination may be performed if required to inspect the cervix or to take swabs. It is not required routinely.

Further Investigations

If pelvic infection is suspected then an "infection screen" should be performed. Ideally, cervical samples are taken in a genito-urinary medicine clinic because the rates of detection are higher and contact tracing can be more easily arranged. Women under 25 have a high prevalence of chlamydia and opportunistic screening, even if infection is not thought to be the cause of pain, is well tolerated (37).

"Urinalysis" should be undertaken if urinary symptoms are present. If blood is detected, this should be investigated further even if the bladder is not thought to be the source of pain. A midstream specimen of urine may be appropriate if dipstick suggests nitrites or leucocytes.

"A transvaginal ultrasound scan" should be performed, if the vaginal examination reveals structural abnormalities. It may reveal ovarian cysts or endometriomas, fibroids, hydrosalpinges, or other abnormalities. However, these may not necessarily be the cause of the pain.

"Magnetic resonance imaging" is a good test for adenomyosis. In the best hands, it has a sensitivity of 70% to 78% and a specificity of 86% to 93% (62). For assessing the extent of deep infiltrating endometriosis it has a sensitivity of 90% and specificity of 91% (63). It is no better than ultrasound in differentiating endometriomas from other ovarian cysts (64).

"Diagnostic laparoscopy" has been viewed as the gold standard for the investigation of pelvic pain. It involves general anesthetic and surgical risks, in particular a risk of bowel perforation of 2.4 per 1000. Two-thirds of patients who experience this complication will require a laparotomy to correct the damage (65,66). Diagnostic laparoscopy identifies adhesions and most forms of endometriosis but very few other causes of pain. Figures estimating the detection rate for pathology vary hugely depending on the population studied and the attitudes of the surgeons performing the laparoscopies, but in approximately one-third of patients, no pathology will be identified (67). Finding endometriosis or adhesions should not imply that one or both are necessarily the cause of the pain since both conditions may be asymptomatic. Women find it difficult to understand why no cause can be found and tend to feel that the doctor must think the pain is all in their head if nothing abnormal is found at laparoscopy (68).

Curiously, pain may improve spontaneously following a diagnostic laparoscopy in approximately one-third of patients even when endometriosis is diagnosed and left untreated (69). Some women may be reassured by negative or positive findings. In a study of 71 women undergoing diagnostic laparoscopy for pain, only a change in their beliefs about the origin of the pain predicted an improvement in symptoms (70).

Some authorities have attempted to improve the diagnostic accuracy of diagnostic laparoscopy by using a technique called "conscious pain mapping." This involves giving the patient pain relief and sedation while maintaining sufficient consciousness to ensure that dialogue between the patient and the surgeon is possible. The pelvis is inspected using a narrow laparoscope and abnormal areas touched with laparoscopic instruments under direct vision. It was envisaged that this would improve the accuracy of diagnosis on the grounds that recreating a woman's pain by probing an abnormal tender area would identify the pathology responsible for the pain. In a series of 50 consecutive cases of conscious pain mapping in women whose CPP had previously been treated unsuccessfully, 70% were described as successful procedures. Of the 42 sites identified in 29 women, 45% were associated with endometriosis or adhesions. Interestingly, only about half of the women with endometriosis or adhesions experienced pain from these sites (71).

This technique has not gained widespread acceptance perhaps because of the obvious difficulties of performing surgery on conscious patients. There is a need to demonstrate that outcome is improved as a result of this investigation (72).

Assessment by Other Professionals

The input of gastroenterologists, urologists, physiotherapists, psychologists, and genitourinary medicine physicians may be very helpful in trying to understand the contributory factors in the complex web of pain. Appropriate referral should be made according to the symptoms.

Therapeutic Trials

It may be difficult to decipher the cause of the pain from the history, examination, or further investigations. Reduced pain following treatment for a clinically suspected diagnosis may help to confirm that diagnosis.

In an RCT, 100 women with clinically suspected endometriosis received either a gonadotrophin-releasing hormone (GnRH) analogue or placebo without a pretreatment laparoscopy. After 12 weeks, the treatment group had significantly less pain than women taking placebo (73). This RCT is the only study in which the effectiveness of this treatment approach has been evaluated. However, there is a growing consensus, which supports this strategy (27,74). An economic evaluation of the use of GnRH analogues as empirical treatment for cyclical pain prior to laparoscopy demonstrated improved patient and physician satisfaction at reduced cost (75).

TREATMENT
The Expert Patient

In this chapter a pain management approach will be described as well as the specific management of those components of pelvic pain with a strongly cyclical pattern. The management of IBS, IC, and musculoskeletal disorders is described elsewhere. The origin of the pain is commonly, perhaps always, multifactorial: consequently it may be necessary to address a number of factors simultaneously and often in different ways.

In the management of chronic illness, the patient must become the center of the decision-making process rather than a passive recipient of advice or information. Her own ideas must be taken into account (76). Ideally, the patient takes responsibility for decision making, balancing risks and benefits according to her own priorities. The doctor's role is as information giver and guide.

In a qualitative and quantitative study of 53 women with CPP undergoing weekly psychological and physiotherapy-based treatment in small groups over 10 weeks, significant and sustained improvement was seen in pain scores, analgesia intake, use of health service resources, and ability to work. Over the course of treatment, women seemed to develop self-knowledge and to take greater responsibility for, and control over, their own health (77).

Pain Management Approach

For some patients either accurate diagnosis remains elusive or despite treatment, their pain persists. At this point, the patient and doctor may choose to adopt a purely symptom-based approach rather than continuing to pursue a diagnosis. The emphasis is then on restoring function. This emphasis may be appropriate in parallel with other interventions.

Various programs have been described but in essence the patient can be taught techniques for managing their own pain from relaxation techniques to the appropriate use of pain killers. Mobility and stamina are improved through physical exercise. The patient is introduced to the central importance of the effect of the brain on one's pain experience and encouraged to look at psychosocial factors in her own pain experience. In a meta-analysis of over 3000 patients, this approach has been demonstrated to be effective in restoring function for chronic back pain sufferers (78). When an interdisciplinary approach is adopted to the management of CPP, improvement is only seen when all components of the program are in place (79).

Analgesia

Patients may choose to control their CPP with analgesia alone. Women may choose to avoid hormones for a variety of reasons such as wanting to become pregnant. They may prefer to use analgesia just for the few of days of the month when the pain is disruptive rather than take medication throughout the month.

Nonsteroidal anti-inflammatory drugs (NSAIDs) are particularly useful because they reduce inflammation as well as reducing pain. No particular NSAID is recommended over another (5) but whichever is chosen it should be taken regularly on the painful days, to achieve the anti-inflammatory effect. Paracetamol is an excellent analgesic and again should be taken regularly when pain is severe. If these two compounds are not sufficient, codeine can be added to the cocktail, perhaps splitting up the doses of the different drugs so that some form of analgesia can be taken every few hours.

If simple analgesics are not sufficient, adjuvant analgesics, such as antidepressants and antiepileptics should be considered (4). "Amitriptyline" is very effective but has a difficult side effect profile with anticholinergic side effects such as constipation and blurred vision. It often causes sleepiness but this effect can be harnessed to improve sleep patterns for some individuals. The side effects generally fade with time and should be discussed with the patient before treatment. It may take six to eight weeks for the therapeutic benefit to become apparent particularly because the drug should be increased slowly to reduce the impact of side effects. Other antidepressants such as venlafaxine may have similar benefits and may be considered if amitriptyline is unsuccessful or poorly tolerated.

If depression is a significant feature this should be discussed directly and treated accordingly either by harnessing the effect of amitriptyline or by using a selective serotonin reuptake inhibitor (SSRI). SSRIs seem to be less effective for pain relief than amitriptyline.

The use of antiepileptics such as "gabapentin" has been described in the chronic pain literature, but there is little information about its use in the management of CPP. It is generally well tolerated (80).

If additional medication is required, morphine-based drugs can be explored starting with tramadol and including morphine if appropriate. However, very careful consideration should be given before initiating opiate therapy for benign pain and consideration should be given to seeking a second opinion before this is done. Pethidine (meperidine in the United States) should be avoided because it is highly addictive and a poor pain killer inducing dissociation rather than analgesia (81).

"Complementary medicine" can have an important role in the management of CPP. Many remedies have been suggested, and there is some evidence to suggest that some modalities may be effective at least for dysmenorrhea (82). An important benefit of complementary medicine is that the patient is taking control of her own management. Patients should be aware that with some exceptions there is no evidence that the therapies work and that some may do harm.

Hormonal Treatment

Hormonal treatments aim to suppress ovarian function and to reduce or obliterate menstruation. Their use is indicated where pain is strongly cyclical in nature. In the treatment of endometriosis, hormonal treatment should be viewed as a way to control the pain, not as a cure. After treatment has ended, the endometriotic deposits may reactivate bringing a recurrence of pain: within one year of stopping treatment, 18% of patients who responded have recurrent symptoms as severe as their pretreatment pain (83). After five years, 30% to 40% will have experienced a recurrence of symptoms (84).

The pain of endometriosis can be well controlled using the combined oral contraceptive pill (COCP) (85). It can be used in the conventional fashion or in the "tricycle regimen" where three or four packets are run together so that the patient only experiences three or four withdrawal bleeds a year. Where symptoms are particularly associated with menstruation, the combination of tricycling the pill and simple analgesia may be all that is required.

Gonadotrophin-releasing hormone analogues (GnRH-a) induce a reversible, menopause-like state of hypogonadotropic hypogonadism. They control pain symptoms as effectively as other hormonal treatments in endometriosis-associated pain (86). The principal side effects are essentially the symptoms of hypoestrogenism, including hot flushes, night sweats, dry vagina, loss of libido, and most importantly loss of bone density. These side effects can be almost completely controlled by the concurrent use of hormone replacement therapy (HRT) as "add-back" therapy, although in a small proportion of women, HRT will bring back the pain. A recent study of 133 women with relapsed endometriosis randomized to three groups, suggested that pain control and quality of life was highest in the group treated with GnRH-a and HRT rather than the COCP or GnRH-a alone (87). The safety and efficacy of GnRH-a with add back HRT over two years has been established (88). Bone mass remained stable and symptoms were well controlled but the long-term consequences of this regimen are not known. Patients should be warned about the side effects, and about the so-called flare effect in which symptoms may get worse in the first month of treatment.

"Danazol" is an effective treatment for pain associated with endometriosis, achieving comparable pain reduction to GnRH–a (89). However, its side effect profile is androgenic and may be troublesome: acne, hirsutism, weight gain, malaise, etc. Danazol can cause irreversible deepening of the voice and is avoided by many gynecologists. Long-term use has also been linked to the formation of hepatomas and an adverse lipid profile. Treatment for longer than six months is not recommended.

"Progestogens" (e.g., norethisterone, medroxy progesterone acetate, and dydrogesterone) are also effective in the treatment of endometriosis associated pain (90). Side effects include weight gain or fluid retention, mood disturbance or skin changes. Long term, there is concern about the effect of treatment on lipid profiles and bone density in some women. Treatment is usually limited to six months.

Progestogen can be delivered locally to the uterus using the levonorgestrel-releasing intrauterine system (LNG-IUS). This method has distinct appeal because systemic side effects are largely avoided. Amenorrhea is achieved in the majority of women and this may be a very effective treatment, particularly when symptoms are mainly menstrual. In a RCT of 82 women with endometriosis-associated dysmenorrhea or pelvic pain, GnRH-a and the LNG-IUS were equally effective in relieving pain. At six months, 70% of women using the LNG-IUS were amenorrheic (91). If successful in the first six months, continuation rates at three years were high (92).

None of the hormonal treatments described for pain have any beneficial effect on fertility. It is thought, however, that remaining on the pill or another long-term hormonal medication to suppress menstruation may be the best way to preserve fertility.

Other interventions such as the use of aromatase inhibitors have been suggested (93), but these remain experimental.

Fertility Sparing Surgery

Endometriosis can be treated surgically with good effect. The endometriosis is visualized laparoscopically and then destroyed by excision, cautery, or laser energy. In a blinded study, 39 women with histologically proven endometriosis were randomized to receive either diagnostic laparoscopy alone or laparoscopic surgery to excise the endometriosis. At six months, 80% of the treatment group reported symptomatic improvement versus 32% in the diagnosis only group (69). Results suggest improvement rates similar to medical therapy and importantly similar recurrence rates (94).

Just as with medical therapy, ablative surgery should not be viewed as a cure but rather as a treatment whose effects may persist for months or years. It is a particularly appropriate choice when a patient wishes to become pregnant and is therefore unable to use hormonal treatment. Surgery is also the treatment of choice when extensive adhesive disease is present. Endometriomas and recto-vaginal disease are best treated surgically to excise the abnormal tissue, as hormonal treatment is less effective in these circumstances. A cystectomy should be performed for endometriomas greater than 3 cm in size as fenestration and ablation is associated with higher recurrence of pain and cyst reformation (95). Definitive surgery for recto-vaginal disease is reported to have a low recurrence rate (96,97).

Hysterectomy and Bilateral Salpingo-Oophorectomy

When a patient's family is complete she may be seeking a definitive solution to her pain, and if GnRH analogue with add back therapy has controlled the pain well, then a hysterectomy with bilateral salpingo-oophorectomy and HRT may be an appropriate step. In a small proportion of patients, however, the pain will return with HRT (98). Patients need to be aware of the risks and benefits of long-term HRT.

Modification of Nerve Pathways

Some clinicians have suggested that pain can be relieved by dividing the nerve pathways to diseased areas. The utero-sacral ligaments can be cut laparoscopically to ablate the pain fibers thought to supply the uterus: laparoscopic utero-sacral nerve ablation or "LUNA." However, there is no evidence of benefit for endometriosis-associated pain or endometriosis-associated dysmenorrhea. It may be effective for women with non–endometriosis-associated dysmenorrhea (99).

The fibers can be cut higher up in the presacral plexus: presacral neurectomy (PSN). In a study of 141 women, patients were randomized to undergo laparoscopic ablation of endometriosis with or without PSN. Cure rates and quality of life were higher in the group who underwent PSN in addition to their endometriosis surgery (100). However, surgery in this area is complex and the possibility of complications is high—damage to bladder or bowel function through disruption of the nerve supply to these organs and the risk of serious hemorrhage. Opinion remains divided as to the justification for this procedure.

Techniques such as "peripheral nerve stimulation" or "TENS" have been used to harness the changes that occur within the CNS when peripheral nerves are stimulated repeatedly. In a retrospective study of 50 women with CPP, vaginal stimulation was used to treat levator ani spasm. Fifty-two percent showed an improvement in the level of pain at a mean follow up of only 14 weeks (101). Others have used spinal cord stimulation to reduce pain (102).

VULVAL PAIN

The prevalence of vulval pain is unknown but clinical experience would suggest that it is less common than pelvic pain but by no means rare. Pain may occur secondary to neurological or dermatological disease, or infection such as herpes. The term "vulval dysaesthesia" is used where no pathology to explain the pain can be identified. It is considered to be a pain syndrome and is a diagnosis of exclusion.

Vulval dysaesthesia has been classified in two main forms: generalized and localized. In the generalized form, which tends to occur in older women, pain occurs all the time and is not particularly associated with exacerbations through touch or sexual intercourse. The pain is typically burning or stinging in nature. In the localized form, touch usually at one particular site causes excruciating pain as does intercourse and the insertion of tampons. Pain is not present all the time. Vulval pain typically takes a relapsing course and many women will experience spontaneous resolution of their symptoms.

Many of the management approaches described above for CPP such as the need for an explanation and the role of health beliefs are also relevant to vulval pain. Topical local anesthetic can be helpful, but the main stay of treatment is amitriptyline as described above. Some women and their partners may need psychosexual help to explore their feelings. Biofeedback techniques to improve control over the pelvic floor may be helpful. There is no evidence of benefit from surgery in the management of vulval pain.

CONCLUSION

CPP is a common problem that has often been poorly managed. The reasons for this are no doubt complex but at least one component is that doctors have found it difficult to understand what may be causing the pain. With new understanding of the many possible components which contribute to pelvic pain and particularly neuropathic pain, it is hoped that more women will receive help for this most disabling and disruptive symptom.

Many women consult health-care professionals because they want an explanation for their pain as much as pain relief. They find it soul destroying to be told there is nothing wrong with them. It seems that one role health professionals are asked to play is as validators of the pain. Simply being allowed to tell her story may not only give clues to the etiology of the pain but also contribute to a sense of being valued and respected. Early successful intervention may help women avoid the disastrous social and economic consequences of CPP.

REFERENCES

1. Zondervan KT, Yudkin PL, Vessey MP, et al. The community prevalence of chronic pelvic pain in women and associated illness behaviour. Br J Gen Pract 2001; 51(468):541–547.
2. Grace VM. Problems women patients experience in the medical encounter for chronic pelvic pain: a New Zealand study. Health Care Women Int 1995; 16(6):509–519.
3. Luzzi GA. Chronic prostatitis and chronic pelvic pain in men: aetiology, diagnosis and management. J Eur Acad Dermatol Venereol 2002; 16(3):253–256.
4. ACOG Practice Bulletin No. 51. Chronic pelvic pain. Obstet Gynecol 2004; 103(3):589–605.
5. Royal College of Obstetricians and Gynaecologists. The Investigation and Management of Endometriosis Guideline. London: RCOG, 2005:24.
6. Kennedy SH, Bergqvist A, Chapron C, et al. Guideline for the diagnosis and treatment of endometriosis. Hum Reprod 2005; 20(10):2698–2704.
7. Classification of chronic pain. Descriptions of chronic pain syndromes and definitions of pain terms. Prepared by the International Association for the Study of Pain, Subcommittee on Taxonomy. Pain Suppl 1986; 3:S217.
8. Williams RE, Hartmann KE, Steege JF. Documenting the current definitions of chronic pelvic pain: implications for research. Obstet Gynecol 2004; 103(4):686–691.
9. Howard FM. The role of laparoscopy in the chronic pelvic pain patient. Clin Obstet Gynecol 2003; 46(4):749–766.
10. Grace VM, Zondervan KT. Chronic pelvic pain in New Zealand: prevalence, pain severity, diagnoses and use of the health services. Aust N Z J Public Health 2004; 28(4):369–375.
11. Mathias SD, Kuppermann M, Liberman RF, Lipschutz RC, Steege JF. Chronic pelvic pain: prevalence, health–related quality of life, and economic correlates. Obstet Gynecol 1996; 87(3):321–327.
12. Stones RW. Chronic pelvic pain in women: new perspectives on pathophysiology and management. Reprod Med Rev 2000; 8(3):229–240.
13. Janicki TI. Chronic pelvic pain as a form of complex regional pain syndrome. Clin Obstet Gynecol 2003; 46(4):797–803.
14. Pezzone MA, Liang R, Fraser MO. A model of neural cross–talk and irritation in the pelvis: implications for the overlap of chronic pelvic pain disorders. Gastroenterology 2005; 128(7):1953–1964.
15. Cukier JM, Cortina–Borja M, Brading AF. A case–control study to examine any association between idiopathic detrusor instability and gastrointestinal tract disorder, and between irritable bowel syndrome and urinary tract disorder. Br J Urol 1997; 79(6):865–878.
16. Nisolle M, Donnez J. Peritoneal endometriosis, ovarian endometriosis, and adenomyotic nodules of the rectovaginal septum are three different entities. Fertil Steril 1997; 68(4):585–596.
17. Jansen RP, Russell P. Nonpigmented endometriosis: clinical, laparoscopic, and pathologic definition. Am J Obstet Gynecol 1986; 155(6):1154–1159.
18. Nisolle M, Paindaveine B, Bourdon A, Berliere M, Casanas–Roux F, Donnez J. Histologic study of peritoneal endometriosis in infertile women. Fertil Steril 1990; 53(6):984–988.
19. Revised American Society for Reproductive Medicine classification of endometriosis: 1996. Fertil Steril 1997; 67(5):817–821.
20. Bedaiwy MA, Falcone T. Peritoneal fluid environment in endometriosis. Clinicopathological implications. Minerva Ginecol 2003; 55(4):333–345.
21. Quinn M. Endometriosis: the consequence of neurological dysfunction. Med Hypotheses 2004; 63(4):602–608.
22. Donnez J, Van Langendonckt A, Casanas–Roux F, et al. Current thinking on the pathogenesis of endometriosis. Gynecol Obstet Invest 2002; 54(suppl 1):52–58.
23. Vigano P, Parazzini F, Somigliana E, Vercellini P. Endometriosis: epidemiology and aetiological factors. Best Pract Res Clin Obstet Gynaecol 2004; 18(2):177–200.

24. Prevalence and anatomical distribution of endometriosis in women with selected gynaecological conditions: results from a multicentric Italian study. Gruppo italiano per lo studio dell'endometriosi. Hum Reprod 1994; 9(6):1158–1162.
25. Mahmood TA, Templeton AA, Thomson L, Fraser C. Menstrual symptoms in women with pelvic endometriosis. Br J Obstet Gynaecol 1991; 98(6):558–563.
26. Balasch J, Creus M, Fabregues F, et al. Visible and non-visible endometriosis at laparoscopy in fertile and infertile women and in patients with chronic pelvic pain: a prospective study. Hum Reprod 1996; 11(2):387–391.
27. Scialli AR. Evaluating chronic pelvic pain. A consensus recommendation. Pelvic Pain Expert Working Group. J Reprod Med 1999; 44(11):945–952.
28. Vercellini P, Trespidi L, De Giorgi O, Cortesi I, Parazzini F, Crosignani PG. Endometriosis and pelvic pain: relation to disease stage and localization. Fertil Steril 1996; 65(2):299–304.
29. Fedele L, Bianchi S, Bocciolone L, Di Nola G, Parazzini F. Pain symptoms associated with endometriosis. Obstet Gynecol 1992; 79(5 Pt 1):767–769.
30. Porpora MG, Koninckx PR, Piazze J, Natili M, Colagrande S, Cosmi EV. Correlation between endometriosis and pelvic pain. J Am Assoc Gynecol Laparosc 1999; 6(4):429–434.
31. Gazvani R, Templeton A. Peritoneal environment, cytokines and angiogenesis in the pathophysiology of endometriosis. Reproduction 2002; 123(2):217–226.
32. Anaf V, Simon P, El NI, et al. Relationship between endometriotic foci and nerves in rectovaginal endometriotic nodules. Hum Reprod 2000; 15(8):1744–1750.
33. Relationship between stage, site and morphological characteristics of pelvic endometriosis and pain. Hum Reprod 2001; 16(12):2668–2671.
34. Pimenta JM, Catchpole M, Rogers PA, et al. Opportunistic screening for genital chlamydial infection. II: prevalence among healthcare attenders, outcome, and evaluation of positive cases. Sex Transm Infect 2003; 79(1):22–27.
35. Royal College of Obstetricians and Gynaecologists. Management of Acute Pelvic Inflammatory Disease Guideline. London: RCOG, 2003:32.
36. Ness RB, Soper DE, Holley RL, et al. Effectiveness of inpatient and outpatient treatment strategies for women with pelvic inflammatory disease: results from the Pelvic Inflammatory Disease Evaluation and Clinical Health (PEACH) Randomized Trial. Am J Obstet Gynecol 2002; 186(5):929–937.
37. Pimenta JM, Catchpole M, Rogers PA, et al. Opportunistic screening for genital chlamydial infection. I: acceptability of urine testing in primary and secondary healthcare settings. Sex Transm Infect 2003; 79(1):16–21.
38. Hammoud A, Gago LA, Diamond MP. Adhesions in patients with chronic pelvic pain: a role for adhesiolysis. Fertil Steril 2004; 82(6):1483–1491.
39. Peters AA, Trimbos-Kemper GC, Admiraal C, Trimbos JB, Hermans J. A randomized clinical trial on the benefit of adhesiolysis in patients with intraperitoneal adhesions and chronic pelvic pain. Br J Obstet Gynaecol 1992; 99(1):59–62.
40. Swank, DJ, Swank-Bordewijk SCG, Hop WCJ, van Erp WFM, Bonjer HJ, Jeekel J. Laparoscopic adhesiolysis in patients with chronic abdominal pain: a blinded randomised controlled multicentre trial. Lancet 2003; 361:1247–1251.
41. Demco L. Pain mapping of adhesions. J Am Assoc Gynecol Laparosc 2004; 11(2):181–183.
42. Perry CP. Peripheral neuropathies and pelvic pain: diagnosis and management. Clin Obstet Gynecol 2003; 46(4):789–796.
43. Prendergast SA, Weiss JM. Screening for musculoskeletal causes of pelvic pain. Clin Obstet Gynecol 2003; 46(4):773–782.
44. Baker PK. Musculoskeletal origins of chronic pelvic pain. Diagnosis and treatment. Obstet Gynecol Clin North Am 1993; 20(4):719–742.
45. Beard RW, Reginald PW, Wadsworth J. Clinical features of women with chronic lower abdominal pain and pelvic congestion. Br J Obstet Gynaecol 1988; 95(2):153–161.
46. McGowan LP, Clark-Carter DD, Pitts MK. Chronic pelvic pain. Psychological health 1998; 13:937–951.
47. Walsh TM, LeBlanc L, McGrath PJ. Menstrual pain intensity, coping, and disability: the role of pain catastrophizing. Pain Med 2003; 4(4):352–361.
48. Collett BJ, Cordle CJ, Stewart CR, Jagger C. A comparative study of women with chronic pelvic pain, chronic nonpelvic pain and those with no history of pain attending general practitioners. Br J Obstet Gynaecol 1998; 105(1):87–92.
49. Walling MK, Reiter RC, O'Hara MW, Milburn AK, Lilly G, Vincent SD. Abuse history and chronic pain in women: i. prevalences of sexual abuse and physical abuse. Obstet Gynecol 1994; 84(2):193–199.
50. Lampe A, Solder E, Ennemoser A, Schubert C, Rumpold G, Sollner W. Chronic pelvic pain and previous sexual abuse. Obstet Gynecol 2000; 96(6):929–933.
51. Lampe A, Doering S, Rumpold G, et al. Chronic pain syndromes and their relation to childhood abuse and stressful life events. J Psychosom Res 2003; 54(4):361–367.
52. Hilden M, Schei B, Swahnberg K, et al. A history of sexual abuse and health: a nordic multicentre study. BJOG 2004; 111(10):1121–1127.
53. Walling MK, O'Hara MW, Reiter RC, Milburn AK, Lilly G, Vincent SD. Abuse history and chronic pain in women: ii. A multivariate analysis of abuse and psychological morbidity. Obstet Gynecol 1994; 84(2):200–206.

54. Toomey TC, Seville JL, Mann JD, Abashian SW, Grant JR. Relationship of sexual and physical abuse to pain description, coping, psychological distress, and health–care utilization in a chronic pain sample. Clin J Pain 1995; 11(4):307–315.
55. Jamieson DJ, Steege JF. The association of sexual abuse with pelvic pain complaints in a primary care population. Am J Obstet Gynecol 1997; 177(6):1408–1412.
56. Raphael KG, Widom CS, Lange G. Childhood victimization and pain in adulthood: a prospective investigation. Pain 2001; 92(1–2):283–293.
57. Chowbey PK, Bandyopadhyay SK, Khullar R, et al. Endoscopic totally extraperitoneal repair for occult bilateral obturator hernias and multiple groin hernias. J Laparoendosc Adv Surg Tech A 2004; 14(5):313–316.
58. Heath I. Following the story: continuity of care in general practice. In: Greenhalgh T, Hurwitz B, eds. Narrative Based Medicine. London: BMJ Books, 1998:83–92.
59. Peters AA, van Dorst E, Jellis B, van Zuuren E, Hermans J, Trimbos JB. A randomized clinical trial to compare two different approaches in women with chronic pelvic pain. Obstet Gynecol 1991; 77(5):740–744.
60. Selfe SA, Matthews Z, Stones RW. Factors influencing outcome in consultations for chronic pelvic pain. J Womens Health 1998; 7(8):1041–1048.
61. Koninckx PR, Meuleman C, Oosterlynck D, Cornillie FJ. Diagnosis of deep endometriosis by clinical examination during menstruation and plasma CA–125 concentration. Fertil Steril 1996; 65(2):280–287.
62. Bazot M, Cortez A, Darai E, et al. Ultrasonography compared with magnetic resonance imaging for the diagnosis of adenomyosis: correlation with histopathology. Hum Reprod 2001; 16(11):2427–2433.
63. Bazot M, Darai E, Hourani R, et al. Deep pelvic endometriosis: mr imaging for diagnosis and prediction of extension of disease. Radiology 2004; 232(2):379–389.
64. Ang WC, Alvey CM, Maran S, Golding S, Kennedy SH. A systematic review of the accuracy of magnetic resonance imaging (MRI) in te diagnosis of endometriosis. 2005.
65. Jansen FW, Kapiteyn K, Trimbos-Kemper T, Hermans J, Trimbos JB. Complications of laparoscopy: a prospective multicentre observational study. Br J Obstet Gynaecol 1997; 104(5):595–600.
66. Chapron C, Querleu D, Bruhat MA, et al. Surgical complications of diagnostic and operative gynaecological laparoscopy: a series of 29,966 cases. Hum Reprod 1998; 13(4):867–872.
67. Howard FM. The role of laparoscopy as a diagnostic tool in chronic pelvic pain. Baillieres Best Pract Res Clin Obstet Gynaecol 2000; 14(3):467–494.
68. Moore J, Ziebland S, Kennedy S. "People sometimes react funny if they're not told enough": women's views about the risks of diagnostic laparoscopy. Health Expect 2000; 5(4):302–309.
69. Abbott J, Hawe J, Hunter D, Holmes M, Finn P, Garry R. Laparoscopic excision of endometriosis: a randomized, placebo–controlled trial. Fertil Steril 2004; 82:878–884.
70. Elcombe S, Gath D, Day A. The psychological effects of laparoscopy on women with chronic pelvic pain. Psychol Med 1997; 27(5):1041–1050.
71. Howard FM, El Minawi AM, Sanchez RA. Conscious pain mapping by laparoscopy in women with chronic pelvic pain. Obstet Gynecol 2000; 96(6):934–939.
72. Palter SF. Microlaparoscopy under local anesthesia and conscious pain mapping for the diagnosis and management of pelvic pain. Curr Opin Obstet Gynecol 1999; 11(4):387–393.
73. Ling FW. Randomized controlled trial of depot leuprolide in patients with chronic pelvic pain and clinically suspected endometriosis. Pelvic Pain Study Group Obstet Gynecol 1999; 93(1):51–58.
74. Gambone JC, Mittman BS, Munro MG, Scialli AR, Winkel CA. Consensus statement for the management of chronic pelvic pain and endometriosis: proceedings of an expert–panel consensus process. Fertil Steril 2002; 78(5):961–972.
75. Kephart W. Evaluation of Lovelace Health Systems chronic pelvic pain protocol. Am J Manag Care 1999; 5(5 suppl):S309–S315.
76. Silverman JD, Kurtz SM, Draper J. Skills for communicating with patients. Oxford: Radcliffe Medical Press, 1998.
77. Albert H. Psychosomatic group treatment helps women with chronic pelvic pain. J Psychosom Obstet Gynaecol 1999; 20(4):216–225.
78. Flor H, Fydrich T, Turk DC. Efficacy of multidisciplinary pain treatment centers: a meta–analytic review. Pain 1992; 49(2):221–230.
79. Kames LD, Rapkin AJ, Naliboff BD, Afifi S, Ferrer–Brechner T. Effectiveness of an interdisciplinary pain management program for the treatment of chronic pelvic pain. Pain 1990; 41(1):41–46.
80. Saarto T, Wiffen PJ. Antidepressants for neuropathic pain. Cochrane Database Syst Rev 2005; 20(3):CD005454.
81. The Pain Society. Recommendations for the appropriate use of opioids for persistent non–cancer pain. A Consensus Statement Pain Society, the Royal College of Anaesthetists, the Royal College of General Practitioners and the Royal College of Psychiatrists, 2004.
82. Proctor ML, Smith CA, Farquhar CM, Stones RW. Transcutaneous electrical nerve stimulation and acupuncture for primary dysmenorrhoea. Cochrane Database Syst Rev 2002; (1):CD002123.
83. Mori H, Taketani Y, Uemura T, Miyake A, Tango T. Rates of endometriosis recurrence and pregnancy 1 year after treatment with intranasal buserelin acetate (Suprecur) (a prospective study). J Obstet Gynaecol Res 1999; 25(3):153–164.

84. Nieto A, Tacuri C, Serra M, Keller J, Cortes–Prieto J. Long–term follow–up of endometriosis after two different therapies (Gestrinone and Buserelin). Clin Exp Obstet Gynecol 1996; 23(4):198–204.
85. Vercellini P, Trespidi L, Colombo A, Vendola N, Marchini M, Crosignani PG. A gonadotropin–releasing hormone agonist versus a low–dose oral contraceptive for pelvic pain associated with endometriosis. Fertil Steril 1993; 60(1):75–79.
86. Prentice A, Deary AJ, Goldbeck-Wood S, Farquhar C, Smith SK. Gonadotrophin–releasing hormone analogues for pain associated with endometriosis. Cochrane Database Syst Rev 2000; 2:CD000346.
87. Zupi E, Marconi D, Sbracia M, et al. Add–back therapy in the treatment of endometriosis–associated pain. Fertil Steril 2004; 82(5):1303–1308.
88. Sagsveen M, Farmer JE, Prentice A, Breeze A. Gonadotrophin–releasing hormone analogues for endometriosis: bone mineral density. Cochrane Database Syst Rev 2003; (4):CD001297.
89. Selak V, Farquhar C, Prentice A, Singla A. Danazol for pelvic pain associated with endometriosis. Cochrane Database Syst Rev 2001; (4):CD000068.
90. Prentice A, Deary AJ, Bland E. Progestagens and anti–progestagens for pain associated with endometriosis. Cochrane Database Syst Rev 2000; (2):CD002122.
91. Petta CA, Ferriani RA, Abrao MS, et al. Randomized clinical trial of a levonorgestrel–releasing intrauterine system and a depot GnRH analogue for the treatment of chronic pelvic pain in women with endometriosis. Hum Reprod 2005; 20(7):1993–1998.
92. Lockhat FB, Emembolu JO, Konje JC. The efficacy, side–effects and continuation rates in women with symptomatic endometriosis undergoing treatment with an intra–uterine administered progestogen (levonorgestrel): a 3 year follow–up. Obstet Gynecol Surv 2005; 60(7):443–445.
93. Ailawadi RK, Jobanputra S, Kataria M, Gurates B, Bulun SE. Treatment of endometriosis and chronic pelvic pain with letrozole and norethindrone acetate: a pilot study. Fertil Steril 2004; 81(2):290–296.
94. Busacca M, Bianchi S, Agnoli B, et al. Follow–up of laparoscopic treatment of stage III–IV endometriosis. J Am Assoc Gynecol Laparosc 1999; 6(1):55–58.
95. Alborzi S, Momtahan M, Parsanezhad ME, Dehbashi S, Zolghadri J, Alborzi S. A prospective, randomized study comparing laparoscopic ovarian cystectomy versus fenestration and coagulation in patients with endometriomas. Fertil Steril 2004; 82(6):1633–1637.
96. Redwine DB, Wright JT. Laparoscopic treatment of complete obliteration of the cul–de–sac associated with endometriosis: long–term follow–up of en bloc resection. Fertil Steril 2001; 76(2):358–365.
97. Fedele L, Bianchi S, Zanconato G, Bettoni G, Gotsch F. Long–term follow–up after conservative surgery for rectovaginal endometriosis. Am J Obstet Gynecol 2004; 190(4):1020–1024.
98. Matorras R, Elorriaga MA, Pijoan JI, Ramon O, Rodriguez–Escudero FJ. Recurrence of endometriosis in women with bilateral adnexectomy (with or without total hysterectomy) who received hormone replacement therapy. Fertil Steril 2002; 77(2):303–308.
99. Johnson NP, Farquhar CM, Crossley S, et al. A double–blind randomised controlled trial of laparoscopic uterine nerve ablation for women with chronic pelvic pain. BJOG 2004; 111(9):950–959.
100. Zullo F, Palomba S, Zupi E, et al. Long–term effectiveness of presacral neurectomy for the treatment of severe dysmenorrhea due to endometriosis. J Am Assoc Gynecol Laparosc 2004; 11(1):23–28.
101. Fitzwater JB, Kuehl TJ, Schrier JJ. Electrical stimulation in the treatment of pelvic pain due to levator ani spasm. J Reprod Med 2003; 48(8):573–577.
102. Deer TR. Current and future trends in spinal cord stimulation for chronic pain. Curr Pain Headache Rep 2001; 5(6):503–509.

33 | Interstitial Cystitis and Related Painful Bladder Syndromes: Pathophysiology

Naoki Yoshimura
Departments of Urology and Pharmacology, University of Pittsburgh School of Medicine, Pittsburgh, Pennsylvania, U.S.A.

Lori A. Birder
Departments of Medicine and Pharmacology, University of Pittsburgh School of Medicine, Pittsburgh, Pennsylvania, U.S.A.

INTRODUCTION

Painful bladder syndrome (PBS), or interstitial cystitis (IC), is a debilitating chronic disease characterized by suprapubic pain related to bladder filling, coupled with additional symptoms such as increased day- and night-time urinary frequency, without proven urinary infection or other obvious pathology. Although the symptoms presented may appear similar to those of a urinary tract infection, urine culture reveals no underlying infection, and there is no response to antibiotic treatment (1–3). Between 700,000 and 1 million people in the United States have IC, the preponderance of whom are women (3). Moreover, it has been estimated that a 60% increase in the number of cases would be identified by experienced clinicians who do not strictly apply the strict National Institute of Diabetes, Digestive, and Kidney Diseases definition of IC (2). While IC may be merely annoying for some patients, when severe, it can render those affected homebound due to extreme urinary frequency (3,4). While the etiology is unknown, theories explaining the pathology of IC include altered barrier lining, afferent, and/or central nervous system (CNS) abnormalities, possible contribution of inflammatory or bacterial agents and abnormal urothelial signaling. These and other factors will be explored in greater detail in this review.

DISEASE PROCESS

The etiology of PBS/IC is unknown; however, several causes have been postulated, including epithelial dysfunction (i.e., leaky urothelium), infection, autoimmune response, allergic reaction, neurogenic inflammation, and inherited susceptibility (3,5). Figure 1 presents the proposed pathogenesis of IC in which there is bladder insult and damage to the urothelial layer that, for example, allows substances in urine such as potassium to leak into the suburothelium and to prompt a cascade of events, each contributing to bladder inflammation and pain (4).

Leaky Epithelium

Increased permeability of the urothelial layer of the bladder, thereby permitting irritating substances in the urine, such as allergens, chemicals, drugs, toxins, potassium, and bacteria, to enter the bladder and causing irritative symptoms has been considered as a major pathogenesis of PBS/IC (3,4,6). This irritation may serve as a "windup" injury that sets up other reactions, including an increase in and activation of mast cells (7), a sign of a neurogenic or allergic reaction (5).

Permeability changes of the bladder urothelium were first noted by Lilly and Parsons (8) who instilled a urea solution into the bladders of IC and control patients. The solutions were drained 45 minutes after urea instillation into the bladders. The urea concentration of the drained IC urine was markedly lower compared with the control group, suggesting enhanced urea absorption (8). In another study, blood fluorescein levels were higher in IC patients than controls after fluorescein was administered orally, suggesting increased absorption of the agent from the bladder surface upon excretion (9). In addition, the instillation of KCl into the bladders of IC patients reportedly worsened symptoms, while the control group

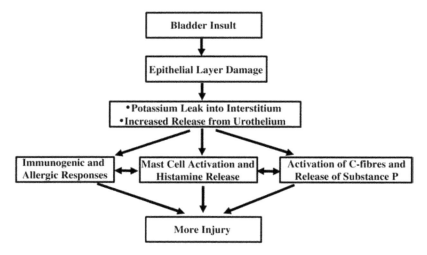

Figure 1   Proposed pathogenesis of painful bladder syndrome/interstitial cystitis.

did not exhibit significant responses to KCl bladder instillation, indicating some alterations in urothelial absorption in PBS/IC (10). Thus, it is likely that increased permeability of the urothelium is an important contributor to pathogenesis of PBS/IC.

Glycosaminoglycans Layers

The urothelial surface is lined by surface mucin, a heterogeneous, gel-like substance composed of numerous sulfonated glycosaminoglycans (GAGs) and glycoproteins. Many clinicians believe that a defect in the protective GAG layer of the bladder that lines the epithelium of the bladder is responsible for the permeability changes of the bladder in PBS/IC. However, the urothelial barrier function of the GAG layer has been a controversial subject. Lilly and Parsons reported that intravesical treatment of the rabbit bladder with protamine sulfate increased urothelial permeability to water, urea, and calcium both in vivo and in vitro (8). This effect was reversed with pentosanpolysulfate (PPS) (8). They concluded that the protamine sulfate affected the GAG layer and that this was repaired by PPS. However, no microscopic evidence of the anatomical changes was presented in this paper. This study was later confirmed by Nickel et al. (11) who compared PPS, heparin, and hyaluronic acid as treatments. The authors concluded that heparin was the best of the three agents in efficacy, but pointed out that this may be due to its anti-inflammatory properties. Indeed the role of the GAG layer may be more in line with an antibacterial adherence function as outlined by Hanno et al. (12). The GAG layer may also be important for the formation and attachment of particulates to the urothelium and stone formation (13,14). However, there are a number of problems with the theory of the GAG layer being the urothelial plasma barrier:

1. The GAG layer does not prevent small molecules such as amiloride reaching and blocking the sodium channels expressed on the surface of the umbrella cells, which form the outer layer of the urothelium (15).
2. The polyene antibiotic nystatin can reach the urothelium as evidenced by increases in the short circuit currents and reduction in transepithelial resistance to insignificant values. This effect is due to generation of nonspecific cation pores in the cholesterol-containing luminal membrane of the umbrella cells.
3. Microelectrode recording has revealed that the first resistive barrier is detected upon penetration of the umbrella cell plasma membrane.
4. Monomeric arginine or polyvalent cations that disrupt the GAG layer do not alter trans-epithelial ion permeability based on electrical measurements.
5. Use of hydrolytic agents such as neuraminidase, hyaluronidase or chondroitonase, or proteolytic agents such as trypsin or kallikrein (to strip the urothelium of the GAG layer) does not alter the ability of protamine to increase the urothelial permeability (16).

Overall, it seems that protamine sulfate does not act at the level of the GAG layer but rather at the surface of the luminal cells, the so-called "umbrella cells" (see also Structure and Function of the Bladder Urothelium), thus enhancing urea absorption by other mechanisms. Protamine sulfate increases the permeability of the apical membrane (luminal surface of umbrella cells) to both monovalent cations and anions. This effect may be reversible depending on the concentration of the protamine, the composition of the bathing solution, and the exposure time of the urothelium to protamine. Prolonged exposure to protamine (>15 minutes) is poorly reversible and is thought to be due to a decrease in paracellular resistance due to cell lysis (17,18).

In summary, the GAG layer may have importance in bacterial antiadherence and prevention of urothelial damage by large macromolecules. However, there is no definite evidence that the GAG layer acts as the primary epithelial barrier between urine and plasma.

Epithelial Mechanisms

Structure and Function of the Bladder Urothelium

The urinary bladder urothelium is a specialized lining of the urinary tract, extending from the renal pelvis to the urethra. The urothelium is composed of at least three layers: a basal cell layer attached to a basement membrane, an intermediate layer, and a superficial apical layer with large hexagonal cells (diameters of 25–250 μm), which are also termed "umbrella cells" (19,20) (Fig. 2). The umbrella cells and perhaps intermediate cells may have projections to the basement membrane (19,21,22). Basal cells, which are thought to be precursors for other cell types, normally exhibit a low (three to six months) turnover rate; however, accelerated proliferation can occur in pathology. For example, using the protamine sulfate injury model that selectively damages the umbrella cell layer, it has been shown that the urothelium rapidly undergoes both functional and structural changes in order to restore the barrier in response to injury (23).

Apical urothelial cells function as a barrier against most substances found in urine, thus protecting the underlying tissues (19,20,24,25). When this function is compromised during injury or inflammation, it can result in the passage of toxic substances into the underlying tissue (neural/muscle layers), resulting in urgency, frequency, and pain during voiding. The superficial umbrella cells play a prominent role in maintaining this barrier, and exhibit a number of properties including specialized membrane lipids, asymmetric unit membrane particles, and a plasmalemma with stiff plaques (19,20,26). These plaques are thought to cover nearly 90% of the urothelial cell surface, and each plaque is composed of nearly 1000 subunits. The proteins uroplakins (UPs) that make up these subunits consist of two tetraspan proteins UPIa and UPIb and two type 1 proteins UPII and UPIII, which are organized into two heterodimer pairs (UPIa/II and UPIb/III) (26,27). These cells are also interconnected with extensive junctional complexes that include cytoskeletal elements and various cytoplasmic as well as transmembrane proteins, which play a role in cell–cell adhesion (19,20,28,29). The "watertight" function of the apical membrane is due in part to these specialized lipid molecules

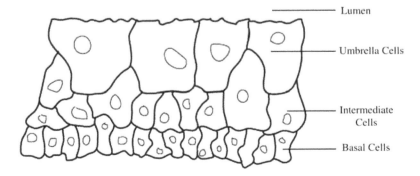

Figure 2 Ultrastructure of the apical surface of the urothelium. Shown is a schematic of unstretched urinary bladder epithelium composed of three layers: basal cells (5–10 μm in diameter), intermediate cells (20 μm in diameter), and superficial umbrella cells (diameter depends upon degree of bladder stretch). *Source*: From Ref. 21.

and UP proteins, which reduce the permeability of the urothelium to small molecules (water, urea, and protons) while the tight junction complexes reduce the movement of ions and solutes between cells (Fig. 2) (19,20,30,31).

"Neuron-Like" Properties of the Urothelium

While the urothelium has been historically viewed as primarily a "barrier," it is becoming increasingly appreciated as a responsive structure capable of detecting physiological and chemical stimuli, and releasing a number of signaling molecules. Data accumulated over the last several years now indicate that urothelial cells display a number of properties similar to sensory neurons (nociceptors/mechanoreceptors), and that both types of cells use diverse signal-transduction mechanisms to detect physiological stimuli. Examples of "sensor molecules" (i.e., receptors/ion channels) associated with neurons that have been identified in urothelium include receptors for bradykinin (32), neurotrophins (trkA and p75) (33,34), purines (P2X and P2Y) (26,35–38), norepinephrine (α and β) (39,40), acetylcholine (nicotinic and muscarinic) (41,42), protease-activated receptors (PARs) (43), amiloride/mechanosensitive Na^+ channels (31,44–47), and a number of transient receptor potential (TRP) channels (TRPV1, TRPV2, TRPV4, TRPM8) (48–51).

TRP Channels: Mediators of Sensory Transduction in Urothelial Cells

The TRP superfamily is a diverse family of proteins that are expressed in many cell types, including neurons, smooth muscle, and nonexcitable cells. These channels, which share sequence homology and structural similarities including six predicted transmembrane segments, can be divided into three main classes (TRPC, TRPV, and TRPM). TRP channels are thought to have an important sensory function in various tissues including the bladder.

One example of a urothelial sensor molecule is the TRP channel, TRPV1, known to play a prominent role in nociception (52). It is well established that painful sensations induced by capsaicin, the pungent substance in hot peppers, are caused by the stimulation of TRPV1, an ion channel protein (53,54), which is activated by capsaicin as well as by moderate heat, protons, and lipid metabolites such as anandamide (endogenous ligand of both cannabinoid and vanilloid receptors). TRPV1 is expressed throughout the afferent limb of the micturition reflex pathway including urinary bladder unmyelinated (C-fiber) nerves that detect bladder distension as well as the presence of irritant chemicals (55). In the urinary bladder, one of the more remarkable findings is that TRPV1 is not only expressed by afferent nerves that form close contact with urothelial cells but also by the urothelial cells themselves (Fig. 3) (49). Urothelial TRPV1 receptor expression correlates with the sensitivity to vanilloid compounds, as exogenous application of capsaicin or resiniferatoxin (RTX) increases intracellular calcium and evokes transmitter (NO) release (49,50) in cultured cells. These responses were eliminated in TRPV1 null mice. In neurons, TRPV1 is thought to integrate/amplify the response to various stimuli and thus play an essential role in the development of inflammation-induced

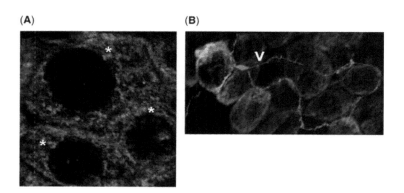

Figure 3 (*See color insert*) TRPV1 is expressed in both urothelial cells as well as in bladder afferents. (**A**) TRPV1-immunoreactivity (cy-3, red, asterisks) in basal epithelial cells (cyt 17, FITC green). (**B**) TRPV1-immunoreactivity in nerve fibers (*arrow*, cy-3, red) located in close proximity to basal cells (FITC, green). Punctate TRPV1 staining in urothelial cells was electronically subtracted to facilitate imaging of the TRPV1-immunoreactive nerve fiber.

hyperalgesia (56,57). Thus, it seems likely that urothelial-TRPV1 might participate in a similar manner, in the detection of irritant stimuli following bladder inflammation or infection.

While anatomically normal, TRPV1 null mice exhibited a number of alterations in bladder function, including a reduction of in vitro, stretch-evoked adenosine 5′-triphosphate (ATP) release and membrane capacitance as well as a decrease in hypotonic-evoked ATP release from cultured TRPV1 null urothelial cells (50). These findings demonstrate that the functional significance of TRPV1 in the bladder extends beyond pain sensation to include participation in the response to normal bladder distension, and is essential for normal mechanically evoked purinergic signaling by the urothelium. Mechanosensitive release of ATP from the urothelium has a number of consequences such as the activation of P2X or P2Y receptors on bladder nerves, or promotion of autocrine activation of P2Y receptors on urothelial cell surface.

In contrast to TRPV1, TRPV2, and TRPV4, which are all detectors of warm temperatures (58–60), another member of the TRP family, TRPM8, has been shown to be activated by cold (25–28°C) temperatures as well as by cooling agents (menthol and icilin) and is expressed in a subset of sensory neurons as well as in non-neural cells. TRPV1, TRPV4, and TRPM8 are localized throughout the urothelium, in contrast to TRPV2, which seems to be expressed primarily in apical cells. This expression suggests that these cells express a range of thermoreceptors responsive to both "cold" and "heat" stimuli (49,51). While the functional role of these thermosensitive channels in urothelium remains to be clarified, it seems likely that a primary role for these proteins may be to recognize noxious stimuli in the bladder. However, the diversity of stimuli, which can activate these proteins, suggests a much broader sensory and/or cellular role. For example, TRPM8 expression has been shown to be increased in some epithelia in malignant disorders (prostate tumors), suggesting a role in proliferating cells (61). Thus, further studies are needed to elucidate fully the role of TRP channels in urothelium and their influence on bladder function.

"Transducer" Function of the Urothelium and Cell–Cell Signaling

Release of chemical mediators [nitric oxide (NO), ATP, acetylcholine, substance P, and prostaglandins (PGs)] (36,39,62–65) from urothelial cells suggests that these cells exhibit specialized sensory and signaling properties that could allow reciprocal communication with neighboring urothelial cells as well as nerves or other cells (i.e., immune, myofibroblasts, and inflammatory) in the bladder wall (Fig. 4). Recent studies have shown that both afferent and autonomic

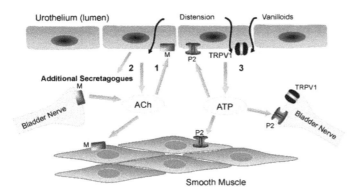

Figure 4   Schematic depicting possible involvement of urothelial "sensor molecules" and/or release mechanisms in bladder function. During bladder storage, increased pressure can lead to release of ACh from both neural and non-neural (urothelial) sources. Released ACh can stimulate muscarinic receptors on smooth muscle cells. Muscarinic receptors present on bladder nerves as well as on urothelium may also be activated by released ACh. Targeting muscarinic receptors activated by urothelial-derived release of ACh (1) and/or other urothelial release mechanisms (2), including additional "secretagogues" may be important in chronic bladder conditions and in the aging bladder. Urothelial cells also express TRPV1 receptors, which can be activated during bladder distension as well as by vanilloid compounds. Stimulation of urothelial TRPV1 can lead to release of transmitters such as ATP, which can activate purinergic (P2X$_3$) receptors on nearby bladder afferents. These afferents also contain TRPV1, which are activated by vanilloid compounds. Other purinergic receptors present on smooth muscle cells as well as on urothelium may also be activated by urothelial-derived ATP. Intravesical vanilloid treatment could lead to activation/desensitization of urothelial TRPV1 or depletion of urothelial-derived mediators (3). *Abbreviations*: ACh, acetylcholine; ATP, adenosine 5′-triphosphate; TRPV1, transient receptor potential channel V1.

axons are located in proximity to the urothelium (49,66). For example, peptide- and TRPV1-immunoreactive nerve fibers have been found localized throughout the urinary bladder musculature and in a plexi beneath and extending into the urothelium (Fig. 3) (49,67). Confocal microscopy revealed that TRPV1-immunoreactive nerve fibers are in close association with basal urothelial cells such that their fluorescent signals overlapped within 0.5-μm optical sections. This type of communication suggests that these urothelial cells may be targets for transmitters released from bladder nerves or other cells, or that chemicals released by urothelial cells may also alter the excitability of bladder nerves. In support of this idea is evidence that ATP (released from urothelial cells during stretch) can activate a population of suburothelial bladder afferents expressing $P2X_3$ receptors, signaling changes in bladder fullness and pain (36,65). Accordingly, $P2X_3$ null mice exhibit a urinary bladder hyporeflexia, suggesting that this receptor as well as neural–epithelial interactions is essential for normal bladder function (68). This type of regulation may be similar to epithelial-dependent secretion of mediators in airway epithelial cells, which are thought to modulate submucosal nerves and bronchial smooth muscle tone and may play an important role in inflammation (69,70). Thus, it is possible that activation of bladder nerves and urothelial cells can modulate bladder function directly or indirectly via the release of chemical factors in the urothelial layer.

ATP released from the urothelium or surrounding tissues may also play a role in the regulation of membrane trafficking. This is supported by recent studies in the urinary bladder where urothelial-derived ATP release purportedly acts as a trigger for exocytosis—in part via autocrine activation of urothelial purinergic (P2X; P2Y) receptors (71). These findings suggest a mechanism whereby urothelial cells sense or respond to $[ATP]_o$ and thereby translate extracellular stimuli into functional processes.

Pathology-Induced Urothelial Plasticity and Effect on Barrier Function

Recent evidence has demonstrated that inflammation or injury can alter the expression and/or sensitivity of a number of urothelial-sensor molecules (32–34,72,73). Sensitization can be triggered by various mediators [ATP, NO, nerve growth factor (NGF), and PGE2, which may be released by both neuronal and non-neuronal cells (urothelial cells, fibroblasts, and mast cells] located near the bladder luminal surface. For example, an important component of the inflammatory response is ATP release from various cell types including urothelium, which can initiate painful sensations by exciting purinergic (P2X) receptors on sensory fibers (36,68). Recently, it has been shown in sensory neurons that ATP can potentiate the response of TRPV1 channels by lowering the threshold for protons, capsaicin, and heat (74). This represents a novel mechanism by which large amounts of ATP released from damaged or sensitized cells in response to injury or inflammation may trigger the sensation of pain. These findings have clinical significance and suggest that alterations in afferents or epithelial cells in pelvic viscera may contribute to the sensory abnormalities in a number of pelvic disorders, such as IC (75–77). A comparable disease in cats is termed "feline interstitial cystitis" (78–81), which is characterized by alterations in stretch-evoked release of urothelially derived ATP (62) consistent with augmented release of ATP from urothelial cells from some patients with IC (82). These cats also exhibit a heightened sensitivity of bladder afferents to bladder distension (83).

Although the urothelium maintains a tight barrier to ion and solute flux, a number of factors such as tissue pH, mechanical or chemical trauma, or bacterial infection can modulate this barrier function of the urothelium (21,84). For example, NO has been demonstrated to be a marker for inflammatory bladder disorders. Endogenous NO levels have been shown to be significantly elevated in patients with classical IC as well as in cats diagnosed with IC. Excess NO levels in the urinary bladder can increase permeability to water/urea in addition to producing ultrastructural changes in the apical cell layer (85–87). Although the pathological mechanism is unknown, these findings appear to be similar to that in other epithelia where excess production of NO has been linked to changes in epithelial integrity (88). Disruption of epithelial integrity may also be due to substances such as antiproliferative factor, which has been recently characterized as a frizzled-8–related sialoglycopeptide. This frizzled-related peptide, which acts via regulation of cell adhesion protein and growth factor production, has been shown to be secreted by bladder epithelial cells from IC patients and can inhibit epithelial proliferation, thereby adversely affecting barrier function (89,90). Taken together, modification of the urothelium and/or loss of epithelial integrity in a number of bladder pathologies could result in passage of toxic/irritating urinary constituents through the epithelium, leading to changes in the properties of sensory pathways.

It is conceivable that the effectiveness of some agents currently used in the treatment of bladder disorders may involve urothelial receptors and/or release mechanisms. For example, antimuscarinic drugs, the standard treatment for detrusor overactivity (91), are generally thought to act by targeting muscarinic receptors on bladder smooth muscle. These agents prevent receptor stimulation by acetylcholine released from bladder efferent nerves and result in increased bladder capacity. Since these drugs are thought to be effective during the storage phase of micturition, when parasympathetic nerves are silent, it has recently been postulated that the release of acetylcholine from the urothelium may contribute to detrusor overactivity (91). In addition, release of acetylcholine from various cell sources could also evoke the release of a number of urothelial-derived mediators such as ATP suggesting a sensory function for urothelial muscarinic receptors. Accordingly, targeting muscarinic receptors activated by acetylcholine released from the urothelium and/or other urothelial-release mechanisms may prove to be an effective therapy. Intravesical instillation of vanilloids (capsaicin or RTX) improves urodynamic parameters in patients with detrusor overactivity and reduces bladder pain in patients with hypersensitivity disorders, presumably by desensitizing bladder nerves (92,93). This treatment could also target TRPV1 on urothelial cells, whereby a persistent activation might lead to receptor desensitization or depletion of urothelial transmitters.

In summary, these findings suggest that urothelial cells exhibit specialized sensory and signaling properties that could allow them to respond to their chemical and physical environments and to engage in reciprocal communication with neighboring urothelial cells as well as nerves within the bladder well. Taken together, pharmacologic interventions aimed at targeting urothelial receptor/ion channel expression or transmitter release mechanisms may provide a new strategy for the clinical management of bladder disorders such as PBS/IC.

Occult Infection

Although infection has been proposed as an etiologic agent of IC, studies have been unable to validate this hypothesis (94). IC has symptoms similar to bacterial cystitis; however, urinalyses and urine cultures have not exhibited any evidence of infection, or no organism has been consistently isolated in the urine or bladder biopsy specimens of IC patients, although it is not known whether an occult infection similar to the *Helicobacter pylori* infection found in chronic gastritis is involved in PBS/IC. Nevertheless, many IC patients have had an episode of urinary tract infection before chronic PBS/IC symptoms began, suggesting that bacterial infection might have triggered bladder injury or insults and subsequently developed irritative voiding symptoms in PBS/IC even after bladder infection subsided (95,96).

Neurogenic Inflammation

Neurogenic inflammation is a process by which sensory nerves secrete inflammatory mediators, resulting in local inflammation and hyperalgesia. Substance P contained predominantly in nociceptive C-fiber neurons including those innervating the bladder (97) is an important mediator of this process, and could be released when the nerve terminal is activated by substances released from the epithelium or when substances in urine penetrate into the bladder wall due to the leaky epithelium (i.e., efferent function of C-fibers) (96). Substance P is a peptide in a family of tachykinins, which share a common C-terminal sequence Phe-Xaa-Gly-Leu-Met-NH$_2$ and also include neurokinin A and B (NKA and NKB). Tachykinins bind to three receptors, termed "tachykinin NK1, NK2, and NK3 receptors," and substance P is the most potent tachykinin for the NK1 receptor (97). An activation of NK1 receptors via locally released substance P is reportedly involved in detrusor muscle contractions (98), as well as an inflammatory cascade including mast cell degranulation, increased capillary permeability, and plasma extravasation and the activation of nearby nerve terminals, thereby resulting in neurogenic inflammation (96). Previous studies in IC patients have shown that the number of substance P–containing nerves in the bladders was increased (99,100) and that urine concentrations of substance P were increased with the concentration of substance P being correlated to the patient's degree of pain (101).

Mast Cell Activation in Neurogenic Inflammation

Mast cell activation has been regarded as an important process in neurogenic inflammation. Mast cells contain many molecules such as histamine and cytokines that contribute to inflammation, bladder mucosal damage, and pain. The release of mast cell contents triggers a loop process, whereby immune cells infiltrate, sensory nerves become sensitized, and cytokines and tachykinins, such as substance P, are released, further activating mast cells to release inflammatory mediators and histamine, which further sensitize the sensory pathway to induce pain (3,6). Histamine and tumor necrosis factor increase vascular permeability, cytokines produce inflammation, kinins and PGs cause pain, and chymase and tryptase generate tissue damage (102).

Sensitization of Bladder Sensory Pathways

Chronic conditions that involve continuous tissue inflammation or irritation can induce changes in sensory pathways that lead to hyperalgesia (heightened response to painful stimuli) and allodynia (pain in response to normally nonpainful stimuli). Thus, continuous tissue inflammation in visceral organs such as the bladder can include sensitization of afferent nerves and increase afferent nerve excitability in response to both noxious and non-noxious stimuli (103,104). Therefore, changes in afferent nerves might contribute to painful symptoms in patients with PBS/IC. While acute sensitization represents early and reversible changes in the excitability of primary afferent pathways mediated by alterations in receptors/ion channels by the activation of intracellular signal transduction cascades, chronic afferent sensitization can induce long-lasting transcriptional changes that can modulate the expression of transmitters/receptors/ion channels in sensory neurons (105,106). In this regard, increased release of substances such as NO or ATP from the urothelium and/or neurogenic inflammation associated with mast cell activation described above can lead to the changes in properties of bladder sensory pathways, resulting in increased pain sensation, the hallmark of in PBS/IC (107).

Anatomy of Bladder Sensory Pathways

Sensory information from the lower urinary tract including the feeling of bladder fullness or bladder pain is conveyed to the spinal cord via afferent axons in the pelvic, pudendal, and hypogastric nerves (103,108). Neuronal somata of these afferent nerves are located in the dorsal root ganglia (DRG) at S2–S4 and T11-L2 spinal segmental levels in humans. The afferent fibers carry impulses from tension receptors and nociceptors in the bladder wall and urethra to second-order neurons in the spinal cord (109–112). (Fig. 5) The primary afferent neurons of the pelvic and pudendal nerves are contained in sacral DRG, whereas afferent innervation in the hypogastric nerves arises in the rostral lumbar DRG (Fig. 4) (108,112,113). Visceral afferent fibers of the pelvic (110) and pudendal (111) nerves enter the cord and travel rostrocaudally within Lissauer's tract. Afferent fibers passing in the pelvic nerve to the sacral cord are responsible for initiating the micturition reflex. These bladder afferents have myelinated (Aδ-fiber) or unmyelinated (C-fibers) axons (Fig. 5) (114,115).

In Vivo Function of Bladder Sensory Pathways

Electrophysiological studies in cats and rats have revealed that the normal micturition reflex is mediated by small myelinated Aδ-fiber afferents that respond to bladder distention (103,114,115). In cats, Aδ-bladder afferents appear to be low-threshold mechanoreceptors (116), whereas C-bladder afferents (103) are generally mechanoinsensitive ("silent C-fibers"). Some of the latter may be nociceptive, and have been found to respond to cold stimuli or chemical/noxious stimuli such as high potassium, low pH, high osmolality, and irritants such as capsaicin and turpentine (103,117–120). Following exposure to these substances, the sensitivity of bladder mechanoreceptors to distension increases and some "silent" afferents become mechanoreceptive.

In rats, Sengupta and Gebhart (104) first reported that mechanosensitive bladder afferents, which responded to bladder distension, were detected in both Aδ- and C-fiber groups. They also found that 30% of bladder afferents were not responsive to any mechanical stimuli, and these unresponsive bladder afferents included both Aδ- and C-fibers. However, Dmietrieva and McMahon (121) have demonstrated, using rats, that most myelinated Aδ-fiber

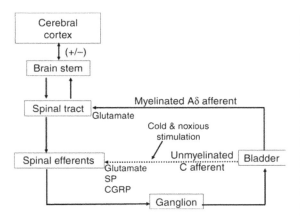

Figure 5 Diagram of reflex pathways that regulate micturition. With intact neuraxis, micturition is initiated by supraspinal reflex pathway passing through the pontine micturition center in the brain stem. The pathway is triggered by myelinated afferents (Aδ-fibers) connected to tension receptors in the bladder wall while the C-fiber reflex pathway is usually weak or undetectable in animals with an intact nervous system. However, cold or noxious stimulation can activate the C-fiber–mediated micturition reflex and induce pain sensation. While glutamate is the main neurotransmitter of afferent fibers to synapse onto spinal cord neurons, C-fiber afferents additionally contain and release neuropeptides such as Substance P or CGRP as neurotransmitters. *Abbreviations*: SP, substance P; CGRP, calcitonin-gene–related peptide.

bladder afferents were mechanosensitive, while about one-half of unmyelinated C-fiber bladder afferents had no clear mechanosensitivity (i.e., silent C-fibers), but responded chemical stimuli. They have also reported that nerve discharges induced by bladder distention were much lower in mechnosensitive C-fiber bladder afferent fibers than myelinated Aδ-fibers, suggesting that C-fiber bladder afferents are less excitable than Aδ-fiber afferents in rats, as shown in cats. Moreover, since capsaicin, a neurotoxin of C-fibers, does not block normal micturition reflexes in both cats and rats, C-fiber afferents are not essential for normal voiding (122–124). In addition, in the rat, there is now evidence that many C-fiber bladder afferents are volume receptors that do not respond to bladder contractions, a property that distinguishes them from "in series tension receptors" (125).

Electrophysiological Properties of Bladder Afferent Neurons
Functional properties of bladder afferent neurons have extensively investigated using patch clamp techniques combined with retrograde axonal transport of fluorescent dyes such as Fast Blue, which can label bladder afferent neurons when injected into the wall of the bladder (Fig. 6) (126–132).

Passive Membrane Properties and Action Potentials of Bladder Afferent Neurons
Based on current clamp recordings, bladder afferent neurons were divided into two populations according to the electrical characteristics of their action potentials (127). The most common population of bladder afferent neurons (greater than 70%) exhibited high-threshold, long-duration action potentials with an inflection on the repolarization phase (Fig. 7). These neurons were small in size, and had action potentials that were resistant to an application of tetrodotoxin (TTX), a Na^+ channel blocker. The other population of bladder afferent neurons, which were larger in size than the neurons with TTX-resistant spikes, exhibited low-threshold, short-duration action potentials that were reversibly blocked by TTX (Fig. 7). In addition, the former population of neurons with TTX-resistant spikes usually exhibits a phasic firing pattern (i.e., one to two spike generation), while the latter with TTX-sensitive spikes have a tonic firing pattern (i.e., multiple spike generation) upon long-duration membrane depolarization. Since the majority of bladder afferent neurons with TTX-resistant spikes are sensitive to capsaicin, TTX-resistant neurons are likely to be the origin of C-fiber afferents (133). The correlation of spike characteristics with other electrical and morphological properties of the neuron, such as somal size, capsaicin sensitivity, action potential thresholds, and duration was also reported by other investigators in unspecified DRG neurons (134–136). Thus, it is assumed that C-fiber bladder afferent neurons with TTX-resistant spikes are less excitable due to higher thresholds for spike activation and phasic firing during prolonged membrane depolarization than the neurons with TTX-sensitive neurons (i.e., Aδ-fiber neurons).

Another distinctive characteristic of bladder afferent neurons with TTX-resistant action potentials was noted in regard to the effect on 4-aminopyridine (4-AP), an A-type K^+ (I_A) channel blocker, on the spike threshold and firing pattern (127,133). When depolarizing currents were injected into the cell, voltage responses in bladder afferent neurons with

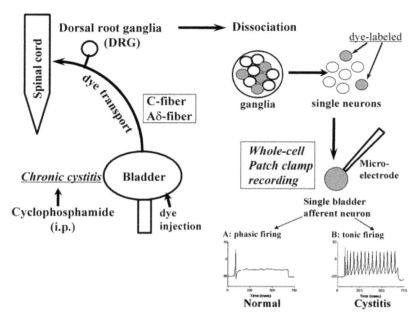

Figure 6 Experimental methods of patch clamp recordings in bladder afferent neurons. Chronic cystitis was induced by IP injection of cyclophosphamide. Fluorescent dye (fast blue) injected into the bladder wall was transported through bladder afferents containing Aδ- and C-fibers to DRG. L6 and S1 DRG were dissected and dissociated into single neurons by enzymatic methods. Whole-cell patch clamp recordings were then performed on fast blue–labeled bladder afferent neurons that were identified by a fluorescent microscope. When long duration (600 msec) depolarizing currents were applied, single action potentials were evoked in neurons from normal rats (**A**), phasic firing while multiple action potential was evoked in neurons from rats with chronic cystitis (**B**), tonic firing. *Abbreviations*: IP, intraperitoneal; DRG, dorsal root ganglia.

TTX-resistant spike, which showed phasic firing during long-duration membrane depolarization, usually exhibited relaxation phenomena at membrane potentials over −45 to −40 mV prior to spike activation. Since an application of 4-AP (1 mM) suppressed this membrane potential relaxation, lowered the threshold for spike activation, and switched the phasic firing pattern to the tonic one (127,133), I_A currents activated from resting membrane potentials are likely to contribute to high thresholds for spike activation and the phasic firing pattern in these TTX-resistant neurons (see details in the following Section).

Ionic Channel Mechanisms in Bladder Afferent Neurons
Na^+ *channels*: Voltage clamp recordings of Na^+ currents in bladder afferent neurons revealed a similar correlation between cell size and sensitivity to TTX (127,137). Both TTX-resistant and TTX-sensitive Na^+ currents could be observed in single neurons, but usually one of the two currents predominated. TTX-resistant currents were prominent (more than 85% of total Na^+ currents) in small-sized bladder neurons, whereas larger bladder afferent neurons had TTX-sensitive currents comprising 60% to 100% of the total Na^+ currents. These two different Na^+ currents exhibited different voltage dependence. The threshold for the activation of TTX-resistant Na^+ currents was shifted by approximately −15 mV in the depolarizing direction when compared with TTX-sensitive Na^+ currents. Steady-state activation and inactivation of TTX-resistant Na^+ currents were also displaced to more depolarized levels by 10 and 30 mV, respectively, in comparison with the TTX-sensitive Na^+ currents. Thus, these different properties in voltage dependence of Na^+ currents likely contribute to the higher spike thresholds in C-fiber bladder afferent neurons with TTX-resistant action potentials than in those with TTX-sensitive action potentials.

It has been documented that two different Na^+ channel subunits ($Na_v1.8$ and $Na_v1.9$) are responsible for TTX-sensitive Na^+ currents in sensory neurons including DRG neurons (138–142). $Na_v1.8$ channels are thought to be more important than $Na_v1.9$ channels in bladder nociceptive mechanisms because of the predominant expression of $Na_v1.8$ channel

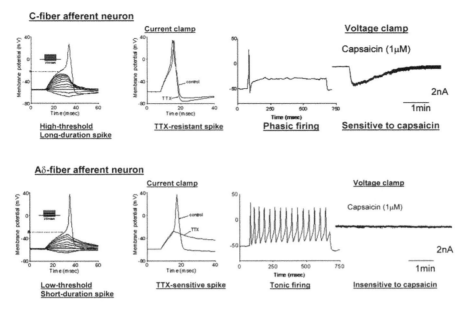

Figure 7 Characteristics of bladder afferent neurons exhibiting TTX-resistant (24 μm diameter) (C-fiber afferent neuron) and TTX-sensitive action potentials (33 μm diameter) (Aδ-fiber afferent neuron). The left panels are voltage responses and action potentials evoked by 30-msec depolarizing current pulses injected through the patch pipette in current-clamp conditions. Asterisks with dashed line indicates the thresholds for spike activation. The second left panels show the effects of TTX application (1 μM) on action potentials. The second right panels show firing patterns during membrane depolarization (700 msec of duration). The right panels show the responses to extracellular application of capsaicin (1 μM) in voltage-clamp conditions. Note that the TTX-resistant bladder afferent neuron (A) exhibited phasic firing (i.e., one to two spikes during prolonged membrane depolarization) and an inward current in response to capsaicin while TTX-sensitive afferent neuron showed tonic firing (i.e., repetitive firing during membrane depolarization) and no response to capsaicin

immunoreactivity in bladder afferent neurons compared with $Na_v1.9$ channels (143) and suppression of bladder nociceptive responses induced by bladder irritation following the treatment with $Na_v1.8$ antisense oligodeoxynucleotides that reduced $Na_v1.8$ expression in lumbosacral DRG neurons as well as the TTX-resistant Na^+ conductance in bladder afferent neurons (137). The relatively greater contribution of the $Na_v1.8$ channel to bladder sensory mechanisms is in line with previous findings that the two types of TTX-resistant channels were expressed in different types of C-fiber afferent neurons: (i) $Na_v1.8$ in peptidergic and isolectin B4 (IB4)-negative neurons and (ii) $Na_v1.9$ in nonpeptidergic, IB4-positive neurons (144,145) and that IB4 staining was present in a smaller number of bladder afferent neurons (10–20%) than in somatic afferent neurons (50%) innervating skin or striated muscles (15,146) (also see Section "Two Different Populations of C-Fiber Bladder Afferents").

K^+ *Channels*: It has been documented that at least two different types of transient A-type K^+ currents (I_A) are expressed in sensory neurons such as nodose ganglia and DRG cells (147–149). One of these I_A currents exhibited slowly inactivating decay kinetics that is quite different from the other typical fast-inactivating I_A currents. This slowly inactivating I_A has an inactivation time constant between 150 and 300 msec and the voltage of half-maximal inactivation is reportedly displaced to a more positive membrane potential when compared with the fast-inactivating I_A. In addition, Gold et al. (149) identified a third transient I_A current, which exhibited activation and inactivation kinetics similar to the fast-inactivating I_A, but had higher thresholds for activation. They have also reported that the slowly inactivating I_A was selectively expressed in DRG neurons that had action potentials with inflections and responded to capsaicin, whereas the fast-inactivating I_A was observed in large diameter DRG neurons without action potential inflections. Bladder afferent neurons exhibited a similar distribution of two types of I_A current; i.e., small-sized neurons with TTX-resistant humped spike expressing slow-inactivating I_A and large-sized neurons with TTX-sensitive spikes exhibiting fast-inactivating I_A currents (Fig. 8) (127,133). It was also observed in bladder afferent

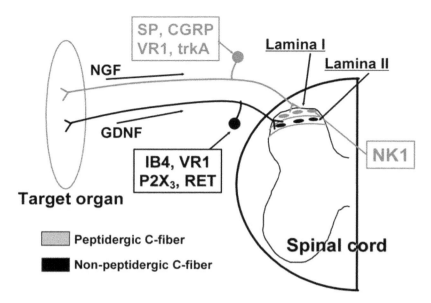

Figure 8 Diagram depicting peripheral and central target fields, trophic factor dependence, and biochemical properties of the two major classes of nociceptive C-fiber afferent pathways. The first subset is a peptidergic population, which expresses the neuropeptides such as SP and CGRP. These peptidergic afferent neurons are regulated by NGF through tyrosine kinase A receptors. The second subset is largely nonpeptidergic and dependent on the glial cell line–derived neurotrophic factor family of growth factors that binds to RET receptors. This subset is also identified by the binding of the Bandaireae simplicifolia isolectin-B4 (IB4) and expresses ATP-binding P2X₃ receptors. There is also a distinguishing characteristic in their central termination patterns. Peptidergic afferent neurons project most heavily to lamina I and the substance P receptor (NK1) is expressed in lamina I where substance P–positive (peptidergic) afferent neurons project, while IB4 binding, nonpeptidergic neurons project most heavily to lamina II of the dorsal horn of the spinal cord. Both populations of afferents express TRPV1 capsaicin receptors *Abbreviations*: CGRP, calcitonin-gene–related peptide; SP, Substance P, NGF, nerve growth factor

neurons that steady-state inactivation of slowly inactivating I_A currents was displaced by approximately 20 mV in a more depolarizing direction than fast-inactivating I_A currents, and that 20% of the slow I_A currents are still available at the resting membrane potential level between −50 and −60 mV, while fast I_A currents were almost completely inactivated at this membrane potential (127,133). This is in accordance with the findings in current clamp recordings that bladder afferent neurons exhibited membrane potential relaxation during depolarization, which was blocked by an application of 4-AP (see Section "Passive Membrane Properties and Action Potentials of Bladder Afferent Neurons"). Thus, in small-sized, C-fiber bladder afferent neurons, TTX-resistant high-threshold Na^+ currents and slow I_A currents contribute to the high thresholds for spike activation.

Ca^{2+} Channels: Voltage-sensitive Ca^{2+} channels are divided into high- and low- voltage–activated types according to their voltage thresholds for activation. High-voltage–activated (HVA) channels, which are known to be involved in neurotransmitter release from nerve terminals, are further classified into L, N, P/Q, and R subtypes based on electrophysiological and pharmacological properties (150,151). N and L channels are major subtypes of HVA Ca^{2+} channels in both types of bladder afferent neurons. However, expression of L-type Ca^{2+} channels is greater in C-fiber bladder afferent neurons than in Aδ-fiber neurons; while the proportion of N-type channels is similar in the two types of neurons (129). Since NO donors inhibited N-type Ca^{2+} currents in bladder afferent neurons (129), it is possible that NO released from the epithelium (see also Section "Transducer Function of the Urothelium and Cell–Cell Signaling") might exert an inhibitory effect on neurotransmitter release from afferent terminals in the bladder. Previous studies have also shown that NK2 tachykinin receptor activation enhanced L- and N-type Ca^{2+} channels via protein kinase C (PKC) phosphorylation in rat DRG neurons (152) as well as bladder afferent nerve firing (153), raising a possibility of autofeedback mechanisms at C-fiber afferent terminals via NK2 receptors. Low-voltage-activated (LVA) T-type Ca^{2+} currents, which are reportedly important in controlling cell

excitability (150,151), were observed in somatic afferent neurons innervating pelvic floor muscles, but not in visceral afferent neurons innervating the bladder or urethra (130).

Histological and Chemical Properties of Bladder Afferent Neurons

Myelinated A-fiber and unmyelinated C-fiber afferent neurons are distinguished by immuno-histochemical staining for neurofilament protein in their somata. Neurofilament is a cytoskeletal protein that is synthesized in cell bodies and delivered to axons by axoplasmic transport. The level of neurofilament expression is known to correlate with axonal caliber and myelination (154,155). It has also been demonstrated that neurofilament, especially the 200 kDa subunit, is exclusively expressed in myelinated A-fiber DRG neurons, but not in unmyelinated C-fiber neurons (156). In bladder afferent neurons from rats, approximately two-thirds of the cells were neurofilament-poor (i.e., C-fiber neurons), while the remaining one-third of cells exhibited intense immunoreactivity for neurofilament (Aδ-fiber neurons) (157). It was also shown that neurofilament immunoreactivity in bladder afferent neurons negatively correlated with the sensitivity to capsaicin. A study using the cobalt uptake assay in DRG cell cultures revealed that approximately 80% of neurofilament-poor C-fiber bladder afferent neurons were sensitive to capsaicin (157), which is similar to the previous findings that the majority of nociceptive C-fiber DRG neurons were sensitive to capsaicin (158). The predominance of neurofilament-poor, C-fiber afferent cells in the bladder afferent population is in line with the finding in other studies such as conduction velocity measurement or histological analysis of the pelvic nerve that unmyelinated C-fiber bladder afferents are more numerous than myelinated Aδ-fiber afferents in bladder afferent pathways (159,160).

Immunohistochemical studies indicate that bladder afferent neurons contain various neuropeptides such as substance P, calcitonin-gene–related peptide (CGRP), pituitary adenylate cyclase–activating polypeptide (PACAP), and vasoactive intestinal pepticle (VIP) (119,161,162). The distribution of these peptidergic C-fiber afferent terminals in the spinal cord is similar to that of central projections of bladder afferent neurons (112,163). The release of these peptides in the bladder wall is known to trigger inflammatory responses, including plasma extravasation or vasodilation (i.e., neurogenic inflammation; also see Section "Neurogenic Inflammation"). The release of neuropeptides in central afferent nerve terminals activates second-order neurons in the spinal cord to transmit nociceptive signals to the brain. Moreover, bladder afferent neurons and fibers, especially C-fiber afferents, express various receptors including TRPV1 capsaicin receptors and $P2X_{2/3}$ ATP receptors that can be activated by low pH or inflammatory mediators (37,40,49,131,164–167). A recent study using patch-clamp recordings from bladder afferent neurons has also demonstrated that a high percentage of bladder neurons not only from lumbosacral DRG (i.e., pelvic nerve afferents) but also thoracolumbar DRG (i.e., hypogastric nerve afferents) responded to ATP, protons, and/or capsaicin (132).

Two Different Populations of C-fiber Bladder Afferents

It has been demonstrated that there are two types of C-fiber afferents distinguished by sensitivity to different growth factors and by the presence of neuropeptides (Fig. 8) (168,169). The first type of afferent is NGF dependent, expresses tyrosine kinase receptors A (trkA), and contains neuropeptides substance P and CGRP (168). The second type is dependent on the glial cell line–derived neurotrophic factor (GDNF) family of growth factors, expresses RET receptor, and is thought to be largely nonpeptidergic (Fig. 8) (169). These two types of C-fibers also have different central terminations. The first type projects primarily to the spinal laminae I and II outer, while the second type projects to the lamina II inner of the spinal dorsal horn (170). The binding of isolectin B4 (IB4) also identifies the latter subtype (171), and IB4-binding neurons reportedly express a specific type of ATP receptor, $P2X_3$ (172,173), TRPV1 (capsaicin) receptor, (183,174). It has been reported that C-fiber afferents innervating the lower urinary tract also seem to be subdivided into two populations based on IB4 binding; i.e., IB4-negative peptidergic and IB4-positive nonpeptidergic subpopulations, and that visceral afferents innervating the bladder or proximal urethra contain a smaller population of IB4-positive, nonpeptidergic C-fiber cells than somatic nerve afferents innervating the distal urethra (20% vs. 49% of C-fiber neurons) (130). Bennett et al. (175) also showed that the percentage of IB4-positive cells was lower in bladder afferent neurons (30%) than in somatic afferent neurons innervating the skin (50%). Thus, there seems to be a considerable heterogeneity in the proportion of IB4-positive and IB4-negative populations in visceral and somatic afferent pathways.

Recent studies have used the neurotoxin, saporin, which is from the seeds of the soapwort plant, from the carnation family, to examine the roles of these two different afferent pathways in the transmission of nociceptive sensory information from the bladder. First, saporin conjugated with IB4 to specifically eliminate the IB4-positive C-fiber population effectively suppressed bladder overactivity induced by bladder irritation in rats (176). Secondly, using saporin conjugated–substance P to eliminate NK1 receptor–expressing pain-related spinal cord neurons, bladder pain responses in the rat model were also effectively suppressed (177). Overall, both IB4-binding, nonpeptidergic and IB4-negative, peptidergic C-fiber afferents seem to play an important role in bladder nociceptive mechanisms, despite the fact that the former is significantly smaller in number than the latter population in bladder afferent pathways.

Plasticity in Bladder Afferent Pathways

Epithelial dysfunction that can increase the amount of urothelially released substances and transurothelial leakage of substances in urine and subsequent neurogenic inflammation associated with mast cell activation can lead to the changes in properties of bladder afferent pathways, resulting in increased pain sensation associated with PBS/IC (Fig. 9). Putative mechanisms involved in the plasticity of bladder afferent pathways in chronic bladder inflammation are reviewed in the following sections.

Hyperexcitability of C-Fiber Afferent Pathways as a Mechanism for Bladder Pain

Pain is a defining characteristic of PBS. One mechanism by which pain is induced is postulated to involve chronic tissue inflammation that can lead to functional changes in C fiber afferents (Fig. 9). These relatively unexcitable fibers appear to have a specific function in signaling noxious events in the bladder as described in the previous sections. Thus, hyperactivity and emergence of mechanosensitivity of C-fiber afferents may, therefore, lead to pain sensation in response to normal non-noxious distension of the bladder.

Indirect evidence for this postulate comes from histologic analysis of bladders from patients with PBS/IC, which revealed marked edema, vasodilation, proliferation of nerve fibers, and infiltration of mast cells (178,179) and from chemically induced cystitis in animals,

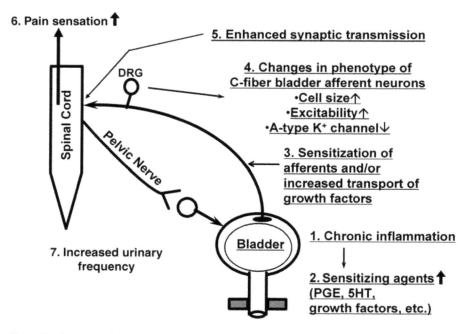

Figure 9 Summary of the events involved in chronic inflammation of the bladder and hyperexcitability of C-fiber bladder afferent neurons. The events that occur following chronic bladder inflammation (1) are indicated in sequential numbers (2–7). *Abbreviations*: DRG, dorsal root ganglia; 5-HT, serotonin; PGE, prostaglandin E..

in which increased urinary frequency is initiated by sensitizing mechanosensitive afferents and/or recruitment of afferents normally unresponsive to mechanical stimulation (103,104, 121,180). Additionally, proinflammatory agents such as PGE2, serotonin (5 HT), histamine, adenosine, and neurotrophic factors such as NGF can induce functional changes in C-fiber afferents that can lead to these relatively unexcitable afferents becoming hyperactive or hyperexcitable (121,136,181,182).

More direct evidence linking chronic inflammation with functional changes in C-fiber afferents has been derived from a rat model of chronic cystitis induced by cyclophosphamide (CYP), which undergoes hepatic metabolism to acrolein, an irritant excreted in the urine (183,184). In this model, the electrical properties of bladder afferent neurons dissociated from L6 and S1 DRG as well as the activity of the inflamed bladder have been measured. DRG neurons that innervate the bladder are identified using fluorescent dye, which undergoes retrograde axonal transport after injection into the bladder wall. The neurons are subsequently dissociated by enzymatic methods, and the membrane properties of single neurons are determined by patch clamp electrophysiologic recording techniques (Fig. 6) (133).

Using such a model, it has been documented that the majority of bladder afferent neurons from both control and CYP-treated rats are capsaicin sensitive and exhibit TTX-resistant action potentials. However, neurons from treated rats exhibit significantly lower thresholds for spike activation (–25.4 mV vs. –21.4 mV) and show tonic rather than phasic firing characteristics (12.3 action potentials vs. 1.2 action potentials per 500-msec depolarization) (Fig. 6) (133). Other significant changes in bladder afferents from CYP-treated rats include increased somal diameter, increased input capacitance, and decreased density of slowly inactivating A-type K^+ currents (I_A) (133). Similar somal hyperexcitability due to reduced I_A current expression after chronic tissue inflammation has also been found in afferent neurons innervating the rat stomach (185) or the guinea pig ileum (186). Thus, the reduction in I_A current size could be a key mechanism inducing afferent hyperexcitability in pain in visceral organs including the bladder.

A recent study using cats with naturally occurring feline-type IC has also demonstrated that capsaicin-sensitive dorsal root ganglion neurons exhibited an increase in cell size and had increased firing rates to depolarizing current pulses due to a reduction in low-threshold K^+ currents elicited by membrane depolarization between –50 and –30 mV (187). Taken together, these data indicated that chronic inflammation in IC/PBS induces both cell hypertrophy and hyperexcitability of C-fiber bladder afferent neurons (Fig. 9) (107). If these changes in neuronal cell bodies similarly occur at C-fiber afferent terminals in the bladder wall, such

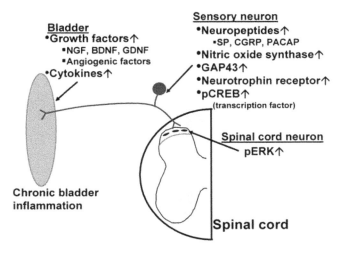

Figure 10 Summary of the neuroplastic changes in the expression of neuronal and chemical markers in the bladder, sensory pathways, and spinal cord following chronic inflammation of the bladder. *Abbreviations*: GAP43, growth-associated protein-43, PACAP: pituitary adenylate cyclase–activating polypeptide; pCREB, phosphorylated CREB; pERK, phosphorylated extracellular signal–regulated kinase; NGF, nerve growth factor; GDNF, glial cell line–derived neurotrophic factor; SP, substance P; CGRP, calcitonin-gene–related peptide.

hyperexcitability may represent an important mechanism for inducing pain in the inflamed bladder (Fig. 10). Therefore, suppression of C-fiber activity represents a mechanism by which to treat bladder pain. This is supported by previous findings that C-fiber desensitization induced by intravesical application of high-dose capsaicin and RTX is effective for treating painful symptoms in patients with IC (188,189), although a recent prospective, randomized clinical trial using intravesical RTX application was not effective in patients with IC (190).

There is also evidence that chronic bladder inflammation can induce changes in functional properties of chemosensitive receptors such as TRPV1 in sensory neurons. Sculptoreanu et al. (191) have recently reported that DRG neurons obtained from cats with feline IC exhibited capsaicin-induced responses that were larger in amplitude and desensitized more slowly compared with those obtained from normal cats, and that altered TRPV1 receptor activity in IC cats was reversed by an application of an inhibitor of PKC, suggesting that PBS/IC could alter TRPV1 activity due to enhanced endogenous PKC activity. Since TRPV1 receptors are reportedly responsible at least in part for bladder overactivity elicited by CYP-induced cystitis due to increased expression of anandamide in the bladder in rats (192), enhanced activity of TRPV1 receptors could contribute to bladder pain in PBS/IC.

Although there is little information available for the neuroplascticity of Aδ-fiber bladder afferents in PBS/IC, a recent study using single nerve fiber recordings has documented that Aδ-fiber bladder afferents are more sensitive to bladder pressure changes in cats with feline type IC compared with normal cats, suggesting that, in addition to neuroplasticity of C-fiber afferents, Aδ-fiber bladder afferents might also undergo functional changes in PBS/IC (83).

Changes in Expression of Neurochemical Markers

It has been shown that tissue inflammation in the bladder can also induce changes in expression of various neurochemical markers in the bladder and bladder afferent pathways (193). Using an animal model of chronic bladder inflammation induced by CYP, it has been reported that expression of NO synthase (194), growth-associated protein (GAP-43) (195), PACAP (162), neuropeptides such as substance P (196), PARs (197), cyclooxygenase-2 (COX-2), and PGs (198) are increased in afferent neurons in lumbosacral DRG innervating the bladder in rats with CYP-induced chronic cystitis (Fig. 10). Thus it is likely that chronic bladder inflammation can induce various changes in expression of inflammation-related proteins/receptors in the bladder and bladder afferent pathways and that these changes can contribute to afferent neuroplasticity, leading to bladder pain symptoms in PBS/IC.

Spinal Mechanisms

Peripheral sensitization of nociceptive afferent pathways due to tissue injury or inflammation is associated with subsequent changes in the excitability of central (spinal) neurons, termed central sensitization to induce secondary hyperalgesia (199). Although this mechanism has been well documented in somatic pain, there are few data available regarding central sensitization in the spinal cord as a mechanism inducing bladder pain. However, it is known that the pain in IC patients can continue after the bladder has been removed, pointing to an important role for a contribution of the CNS to IC symptoms (3). In this regard, a recent study by Cruz et al. (200) has revealed that the expression of phosphorylated extracellular signal–regulated kinases 1 and 2 (phosphoERK), the active form of these kinases, in spinal neurons was increased following CYP-induced cystitis in rats and that increased ERK phosphorylation in spinal neurons was C-fiber dependent because it was blocked by C-fiber desensitization with RTX (Fig. 10). Previous studies have also demonstrated that the number of substance P, CGRP, or GAP-43–positive fibers, as well as Fos protein expression after non-noxious bladder stimulation, were increased in rats with CYP-induced bladder inflammation, suggesting a reorganization of bladder afferent projections and spinal reflex mechanisms controlling bladder function (195,196,201). Further studies are needed in this field to study the mechanisms inducing central sensitization in bladder pain associated with PBS/IC.

Neurotrophic Factors

It has been proposed that elevated expression of neurotrophic factors such as NGF, in the bladder is involved in afferent sensitization inducing bladder pain and overactivity under different pathological conditions including chronic cystitis, spinal cord injury, and bladder outlet obstruction (202–205). NGF is responsible for neuronal growth and function, and is speculated to be a key player in linking inflammation to altered pain signaling (206). NGF is expressed widely in various cells including mast cells, and can activate mast cells to degranulate and proliferate (207). In patients with IC, neurotrophins, including NGF, neurotrophin-3 (NT-3), and GDNF, have been detected in the urine (208). Increased expression of NGF is also present in bladder biopsies from women with IC (209). Thus, target organ–neural interactions mediated by an increase of neurotrophins in the bladder and increased transport of neurotrophins to the neuronal cell bodies in afferent pathways may contribute to the emergence of bladder pain in PBS/IC (Fig. 9) (202).

Using a rat model of chronic cystitis, increased expression of neurotrophic growth factors such as NGF, brain-derived neurotrophic factor (BDNF) and ciliary neurotrophic factor (CNTF) in the bladder, as well as phosphorylation of tyrosine kinase receptors (TrkA and TrkB) in bladder-innervating afferent neurons, has been documented as direct evidence for neurotrophic factor (NT) mediated signal transduction in chronic bladder inflammation (Fig. 10) (210,211). In addition, the enhanced neurotrophic factor mechanisms were also associated with increased phosphorylated CAMP response element-binding protein (CREB) in bladder afferent neurons, and a subpopulation of phosphorylated CREB-positive cells coexpressed phosphorylated Trk in rats with chronic cystitis (Fig. 10) (212). Moreover, RTX, a C-fiber neurotoxin, reduced CYP-induced upregulation of phosphorylated CREB in DRG, suggesting that cystitis can be linked with an altered CREB phosphorylation in capsaicin-sensitive C-fiber bladder afferents (212). These results suggest that upregulation of phosphorylated CREB may be mediated by a NT/Trk signaling pathway, and that CREB phosphorylation may play a role as a transcription factor in lower urinary tract plasticity induced by cystitis (Fig. 10).

Previous studies also demonstrated that exogenous NGF can induce bladder nociceptive responses and bladder overactivity in rats when applied acutely into the bladder lumen (180,213) or chronically to the bladder wall or intrathecal space (214,215). Moreover, it had been shown that an application of NGF-sequestering molecules (trkA-IgG or REN1180) can reduce a referred thermal hyperalgesia elicited by bladder inflammation using turpentine oil (216) or bladder overactivity elicited by CYP-induced cystitis (217), suggesting that increased NGF expression is directly involved in the emergence of bladder-related nociceptive responses in cystitis. Thus, NGF might be a potential target for the treatment of painful symptoms in PBS/IC.

Glomerulation and Angiogenic Growth Factors

It has been reported that not only neurotrophic growth factors but also angiogenic factors such as platelet-derived endothelial cell growth factor/thymidine phosphorylase (PDECGF/TP) and TGF-β were increased in bladder specimens from patients with IC, and that these angiogenic factors were coexpressed with CD44 in the bladder submucosa (Fig. 10) (218). CD44 is one of the heparan sulfate proteoglycans in extracellular matrix (219), and can bind to heparin-binding growth factors and enhance their functions (220). Therefore CD44 is considered to play an important role in inducing prolonged inflammatory changes and overexpression of angiogenic factors in IC bladders. A recent study has also revealed that glomerulations induced by petechial bleeding from distal capillaries following compression by fibrotic bundles during bladder hydrodistension were highly associated with overexpression of angiogenic growth factors such as PDECGF/TP or vascular endothelial growth factor (VEGF) in the bladders from IC patients (221). Thus, it seems likely that neovascularization promoted by angiogenic growth factors plays an important role in the pathogenesis of IC that induces glomerulations during hydrodistension.

Immunogenic Mechanisms (Allergies and Autoimmunity)

It has been is recognized that PBS/IC is often associated with a number of allergic or autoimmune diseases such as allergic rhinitis, asthma, irritable bowel syndrome, fibromyalgia, inflammatory bowel disease (Crohn's disease and ulcerative colitis), systemic lupus erythematosus, and Sjogren's syndrome, suggesting that immunogenic responses might be involved in the pathogenesis of PBS/IC (222). The prevalence of allergies in IC patients is reported to be between 40% and 80% of patients (222). In addition, some clinical studies have reported that treatment of allergy sometimes has a beneficial effect on bladder symptoms of IC (223) and that steroids or other immunosuppressants are occasionally effective in reducing IC symptoms

(224). However, although increased levels of bladder specific autoantigens have been identified in some patients (225), the background of the association is not known, and studies investigating the role of autoimmunity in IC are not conclusive (96,226,227).

Genetic Background of PBS/IC

A recent study by Warren et al. (228) has shown that adult female first-degree relatives of patients with IC may have a prevalence of IC 17 times that found in the general population, suggesting a greater concordance of IC among monozygotic than dizygotic twins and a genetic susceptibility to IC. Another study has also documented some evidence for a possible syndrome in some families with panic disorder, which includes PBS/IC, thyroid disorders, chronic headaches/migraine, and/or mitral valve prolapse (229). However, since these studies are not conclusive, further studies are definitely needed to investigate the genetic background of PBS/IC. It is also reported the a higher incidence of genotype variants are found in α_{1d} and β_2 adrenergic receptor genes as well as interleukin-4 genes in patients with IC, suggesting that variants of these genes might be related to a predisposition to PBS/IC (230).

CONCLUSION

Although various etiologies have been proposed as described in this chapter, no one pathologic process has been identified in every patient with PBS/IC. Thus it is likely that the syndrome of PBS/IC may have multiple etiologies, all of which result in similar clinical manifestations, and that many of the pathologic processes described above may act in concert to produce the clinical features of PBS/IC (Fig. 1).

ACKNOWLEDGMENT

We thank Professor William C. de Groat, Department of Pharmacology, University of Pittsburgh, for his critical review of this article. The authors' research is supported by NIH research grants (DK 54824, DK 57284, DK57267, DK 68557, and P01 HD39768).

REFERENCES

1. Parsons CL, Benson G, Childs SJ, et al. A quantitatively controlled method to study prospectively interstitial cystitis and demonstrate the efficacy of pentosanpolysulfate. J Urol 1993; 150:845–848.
2. Hanno PM, Landis JR, Matthews-Cook Y, et al. The Interstitial Cystitis Database Study Group: The diagnosis of interstitial cystitis revisited: lessons learned from the National Institutes of Health Interstitial Cystitis Database study. J Urol 1999; 161:553–557.
3. Bladder Research Progress Review Group: Overcoming Bladder Disease. A Strategic Plan for Research. Bethesda, Md, National Institute of Diabetes & Digestive & Kidney Diseases (National Institutes of Health), 2002, Chap 8.
4. Chancellor MB, Yoshimura N. Treatment of Interstitial Cystitis. Urology 2004; 63(3 suppl 1):85–92.
5. NIH Publication No. 02–3220; National Kidney and Urologic Diseases Information Clearinghouse. *Interstitial Cystitis*. Bethesda MD, National Institute of Diabetes and Digestive and Kidney Diseases (National Institutes of Health), 2002.
6. Sant GR, Theoharides TC. Interstitial cystitis. Curr Opin Urol 1999; 9:297–302.
7. Theoharides TC, Kempuraj D, Sant GR. Mast cell involvement in interstitial cystitis: a review of human and experimental evidence. Urology 2001; 57(Suppl 6A):47–55.
8. Lilly JD, Parsons CL. Bladder surface glycosaminoglycans is a human epithelial permeability factor. Surg Gynecol Obstet 1990; 171:493–496.
9. Buffington CAT, Woodworth BE. Excretion of fluorescein in the urine of women with interstitial cystitis. J Urol 1997; 158:786–789.
10. Holm-Bentzen M, Sondergaard I, Hald T. Urinary excretion of a metabolite of histamine (1,4-methyl-imidazole-acetic-acid) in painful bladder disease. Br J Urol 1987; 59:230–233.
11. Nickel JC, Downey J, Morales A, Emerson L. Clark J Relative efficacy of various exogenous glycosaminoglycans in providing a bladder surface permeability barrier. J Urol 1998; 160:612–614.
12. Hanno PM, Fritz RW, Mulholland SG, Wein AJ. Heparin – Examination of its antibacterial adsorption properties. Urology 1981; 28(3):273–276.
13. Hurst RE. Structure, function and pathology of proteoglycans and glycosaminoglycans in the urinary tract. World J Urol 1994; 12:3.

14. Grases F, Ferragut LG, Bosta-Bauza A. Study of the early stages of renal stone formation: Experimental model using urothelium of pig urinary bladder. Urol Res 1966; 24:305–311.
15. Niku SD, Stein PC, Scherz HC, Parsons CL. A new method for cytodestrution of bladder epithelium using protamine sulfate and urea. J Urology 1994; 152:1025–1028.
16. Lewis SA, Berg JR, Kleine TJ. Modulation of epithelial permeability by extracellular macromolecules. Physiological reviews 1995; 75(3):561–589.
17. Tzan CJ, Berg JR, Lewis SA. Effect of protamine sulfate on the permeability properties of the mammalian urinary bladder. J membrane Biology 1993; 133:227–242.
18. Tzan CJ, Berg JR, Lewis SA. Mammalian urinary bladder permeability is altered by cationic proteins: modulation by divalent cations. Am J Physiol (Cell Physiol) 1994; 267:C1013–C1026.
19. Apodaca G. The uroepithelium: not just a passive barrier. Traffic 2004; 5:1–12.
20. Lewis SA. Everything you wanted to know about the bladder epithelium but were afraid to ask. Am J Physiol 2000; 278:F867–F874.
21. Hicks M. The mammalian urinary bladder: an accommodating organ. Biol Rev 1975; 50:215–246.
22. Martin BF. Cell replacement and differentiation in transitional epithelium: a histological and autoradiographic study of the guinea-pig bladder and ureter. J Anat 1972; 112:433–455.
23. Lavelle J, Meyers S, Ramage R, et al. Bladder permeability barrier: recovery from selective injury of surface epithelial cells. Am J Physiol 2002; 283:F242–F253.
24. Negrete HO, Lavelle J, Berg J, Lewis SA, Zeidel ML. Permeability properties of the intact mammalian bladder epithelium. Am J Physiol 1996; 271:F886–F894.
25. Zeidel ML. Low permeabilities of apical membranes of barrier epithelia: what makes water-tight membranes water-tight? Am J Physiol 1996; 271:F243–F245.
26. Hu P, Meyers S, Liang FX, et al. Role of membrane proteins in permeability barrier function: uroplakin ablation elevates urothelial permeability. Am J Physiol 2002; 283:F1200–F1207.
27. Wu WR, Lin JH, Walz T, et al. A group of highly conserved urothelial differentiation-related membrane proteins. J Biol Chem 1994; 269:13716–13724.
28. Acharya P, Beckel J, Ruiz WG, et al. Distribution of the tight junction proteins ZO-1, occludin, and claudin-4, -8, and -12 in bladder epithelium. Am J Physiol 2004; 287:F305–F318.
29. Gonzalez-Mariscal L, Betanzos A, Nava P, Jaramillo BE. Tight junction proteins. Progress Biophy Mol Biol 2003; 81:1–44.
30. Tammela T, Wein AJ, Monson FC, Levin RM. Urothelial permeability of the isolated whole bladder. Neurourol Urodyn 1993; 12:39–47.
31. Wang E, Lee JM, Johnson JP, Kleyman T, Bridges R, Apodaca G. Hydrostatic pressure-regulated ion transport in bladder uoepithelium. Am J Physiol 2003; 285:F651–F663.
32. Chopra B, Barrick SR, Meyers S, et al. Expression and function of bradykinin B1/B2 receptors in normal and inflamed rat urinary bladder urothelium. J Physiol 2005; 562:859–871.
33. Murray E, Malley SE, Qiao LY, Hu VY, Vizzard MA. Cyclophosphamide induced cystitis alters neurotrophin and receptor tyrosine kinase expression in pelvic ganglia and bladder. J Urol 2004; 172:2434–2439.
34. Wolf-Johnston AS, Beckel JM, Barrick SR, Kanai AJ, de Groat WC, Birder L. Induction of urinary cystitis results in increased expression of nerve growth factor and its receptors. Soc Neurosci Abstr 2004; 27:742.16.
35. Birder L, Ruan HZ, Chopra B, et al. Alterations in P2X and P2Y purinergic receptor expression in urinary bladder from normal cats and cats with interstitial cystitis. Am J Physiol 2004; 287:F1084–F1091.
36. Burnstock G. Purine-mediated signalling in pain and visceral perception. Trends Pharmacol Sci 2001; 22:182–188.
37. Lee HY, Bardini M, Burnstock G. Distribution of P2X receptors in the urinary bladder and the ureter of the rat. J Urol 2000; 163:2002–2007.
38. Tempest HV, Dixon AK, Turner WH, Elneil S, Sellers LA, Ferguson DR. P2X and P2Y receptor expression in human bladder urothelium and changes in interstitial cystitis. BJU Int 2004; 93:1344–1388.
39. Birder L, Apodaca G, de Groat WC, Kanai AJ. Adrenergic- and capsaicin-evoked nitric oxide release from urothelium and afferent nerves in urinary bladder. Am J Physiol 1998; 275:F226–F229.
40. Birder L, Nealen ML, Kiss S, et al. Beta-adrenoceptor agonists stimulate endothelial nitric oxide synthase in rat urinary bladder urothelial cells. J Neurosci 2002a; 22:8063–8070.
41. Beckel J, Birder L, Kiss S, et al. Expression of nicotinic acetylcholine receptors in rat urothelium. Soc Neurosci Abstr 25: 2002; 538:10.
42. Chess-Williams R. Muscarinic receptors of the urinary bladder: detrusor, urothelial and prejunctional. Auton Autacoid Pharmacol 2002; 22:133–145.
43. D'Andrea MR, Saban MR, Nguyen NB, Andrade-Gordon P, Saban R. Expression of protease-activated receptor-1, -2, -3 and -5 in control and experimentally inflamed mouse bladder. Am J Pathol 2003; 162:907–923.
44. Carattino MD, Sheng S, Kleyman TR. Mutations in the pore region modify epithelial sodium channel gating by shear stress. J Cell Biol 2005; 280:4393–4401.
45. Lewis SA, Clausen C, Wills NK. Transport-related modulation of the membrane properties of urinary bladder epithelium. Biochim Biophys Acta 1991; 1070:99–110.

46. Lewis SA, Hanrahan JW. Apical and basolateral membrane ionic channels in rabbit urinary bladder epithelium. Pflugers Arch 1985; 405:S83–S88.
47. Smith PR, Mackler SA, Weiser PC, et al. Expression and localization of epithelial sodium channel in mammalian urinary bladder. Am J Physiol 1998; 274:F91–F96.
48. Barrick SR, Lee H, Meyers S, et al. Expression and function of TRPV4 in urinary bladder urothelium. Soc Neurosci Abstr 26: 2003; 608:6.
49. Birder L, Kanai AJ, de Groat WC, et al. Vanilloid receptor expression suggests a sensory role for urinary bladder epithelial cells. Proc Natl Acad Sci USA 2001; 98:13396–13401.
50. Birder L, Nakamura Y, Kiss S, et al. Altered urinary bladder function in mice lacking the vanilloid receptor TRPV1. Nat Neurosci 2002b; 5:856–860.
51. Stein RJ, Santos S, Nagatomi J, et al. Cool (TRPM8) and hot (TRPV1) receptors in the bladder and male genital tract. J Urol 2004; 172:1175–1178.
52. Szallasi A. Vanilloid receptor ligands: hopes and realities for the future. Drugs Aging 2001; 18: 561–573.
53. Caterina MJ. The vanilloid receptor: a molecular gateway to the pain pathway. Ann Rev Neurosci 2001; 24:602–607.
54. Caterina MJ, Schumacher MA, Tominaga M, Rosen TA, Levine JD, Julius D. The capsaicin receptor: a heat activated ion channel in the pain pathway. Nature 1997; 389:816–824.
55. Chancellor MB, de Groat WC. Intravesical capsaicin and resiniferatoxin therapy: spicing up the ways to treat the overactive bladder. J Urol 1999; 162:3–11.
56. Ghuang HH, Prescott ED, Kong H, et al. Bradykinin and nerve growth factor release the capsaicin receptor from PtdIns(4,5)P2-mediated inhibition. Nature 2001; 411:957–962.
57. Holzer P. TRPV1 and the gut: from a tasty receptor for a painful vanilloid to a key player in hyperalgesia. Eur J Pharmacol 2004; 500:231–241.
58. Alessandri-Haber N, Yeh JJ, et al. Hypotonicity induces TRPV4-mediated nociception in rat. Neuron 2003; 39:497–511.
59. Liedtke W, Choe Y, Marti-Renom MA, Bell AM, Denis CS, Sali A. Vanilloid receptor-related osmotically activated channel (VR-OAC), a candidate vertebrate osmoreceptor. Cell 2000; 103:525–535.
60. Chung MK, Lee H, Caterina MJ. Warm temperatures activate TRPV4 in mouse 308 Keratinocytes. J Biol Chem 2003; 278:32037–32046.
61. Tsavaler L, Shapero MH, Morkowski S, Laus R. Trp-p8, a novel prostate-specific gene, is up-regulated in prostate cancer and other malignancies and shares high homology with transient receptor potential calcium channel proteins. Cancer Res 2001; 61:3760–3769.
62. Birder L, Barrick SR, Roppolo JR, et al. Feline interstitial cystitis results in mechanical hypersensitivity and altered ATP release from bladder urothelium. Am J Physiol 2003; 285:F423–F429.
63. Chess-Williams R. Potential therapeutic targets for the treatment of detrusor overactivity. Expert Opin Ther Targets 2004; 8:95–106.
64. Chopra B, de Groat WC, Roppolo JR, et al. Alterations in stretch mediated prostacyclin release from bladder urothelium in feline interstitial cystitis. The FASEB Journal 18: 2003; 399:10.
65. Ferguson DR, Kennedy I, Burton TJ. ATP is released from rabbit urinary bladder epithelial cells by hydrostatic pressure changes-a possible sensory mechanism? J Physiol 1997; 505.2:503–511.
66. Beckel J, Barrick SR, Keast JR, et al. Expression and function of urothelial muscarinic receptors and interactions with bladder nerves. Soc Neurosci Abstr 26: 2004; 846:23.
67. Yiangou Y, Facer P, Ford A, Brady C, Wiseman O, Fowler CJ, Anand P. Capsaicin receptor VRI and ATP-gated ion channel P2×3 in human urinary bladder. BJU Int 2001; 87:774–779.
68. Cockayne DA, Hamilton SG, Zhu QM, et al. Urinary bladder hyporeflexia and reduced pain-related behaviour in P2X(3)-deficient mice. Nature 2000; 407:1011–1015.
69. Homolya L, Steinberg TH, Boucher RC. Cell to cell communication in response to mechanical stress via bilateral release of ATP and UTP in polarized epithelia. J Cell Biol 2000; 150:1349–1360.
70. Jallat-Daloz I, Cognard JL, Badet JM, Regnard J. Neural-epithelial cell interplay: in vitro evidence that vagal mediators increase PGE2 production by human nasal epithelial cells. Allergy Asthma Proc 2001; 22:17–23.
71. Wang EC, Lee JM, Ruiz WG, et al. ATP and purinergic receptor-dependent membrane traffic in bladder umbrella cells. J Clin Investigation 2005 115:2412–2422.
72. Sun Y, Chai TC. Up-regulation of P2X3 receptor during stretch of bladder urothelial cells from patients with interstitial cystitis. J Urol 2004; 171:448–452.
73. Wolf-Johnston AS, Buffington CA, Roppolo JR, et al. Increased NGF and TRPV1 expression in urinary bladder and sensory neurons from cats with feline interstitial cystitis. Soc Neurosci Abst 2003; 27:608.4.
74. Tominaga M, Wada M, Masu M. Potentiation of capsaicin receptor activation by metabotropic ATP receptors: a possible mechanism for ATP-evoked pain and hypersensitivity. Proc Natl Acad Sci USA 2001; 29:820–825.
75. Gillenwater JY, Wein AJ. Summary of the national institute of arthritis, diabetes, and kidney diseases workshop on interstitial cystitis. J Urol 1998; 140:205.
76. Nickel JC. Interstitial cystitis–an elusive clinical target? J Urol 2003; 170:816–817.
77. Parsons CL, Greenberger M, Gabal L, Bidair M, Barme G. The role of urinary potassium in the pathogenesis and diagnosis of interstitial cystitis. J Urol 1998; 159:1862–1867.

78. Buffington CA, Chew DJ, Woodworth BE. Feline interstitial cystitis. J Am Vet Med Assoc 1999a; 215:682–687.
79. Buffington CA, Chew DJ, Woodworth BE. Interstitial cystitis in humans, and cats? Urology 1999b; 53:239–240.
80. Buffington CA. Visceral pain in humans: lessons from animals. Curr Pain Headache Rep 2001; 5:44–51.
81. Westropp J, Buffington CA. In vivo models of interstitial cystitis. J Urol 2002; 167:694–702.
82. Sun Y, Keay S, DeDeyne PG, Chai TC. Augmented stretch activated adenosine triphosphate release from bladder uroepithelial cells in patients with interstitial cystitis. J Urol 2001; 166:1951–1956.
83. Roppolo JR, Tai C, Booth AM, Buffington CA, de Groat WC, Birder LA. Bladder Adelta afferent nerve activity in normal cats and cats with feline interstitial cystitis. J Urol 2005; 173:1011–1015.
84. Anderson G, Palermo J, Schilling J, Roth R, Heuser J, Hultgren S. Intracellular bacterial biofilm-like pods in urinary tract infections. Science 2003; 301:105–107.
85. Birder L, Wolf-Johnston AS, Buffington CA, Roppolo JR, de Groat WC, Kanai AJ. Altered Inducible Nitric Oxide Synthase Expression and Nitric Oxide Production in Urinary Bladder from Cats with Feline Interstitial Cystitis. J Urol 2005; 173:625–629.
86. Lavelle J, Meyers SA, Ruiz WG, Buffington CA, Zeidel ML, Apodaca G. Urothelial pathophysiological changes in feline interstitial cystitis: a human model. Am J Physiol 2000; 278:F540–F553.
87. Truschel ST, Ruiz WG, Kanai AJ, et al. Involvement of nitric oxide (NO) in bladder afferent and urothelial abnormalities following chronic spinal cord injury. Soc Neurosci Abstr 2001; 24:842–849.
88. Han X, Fink MP, Uchiyama T, Yang R, Delude RL. Increased iNOS activity is essential for pulmonary epithelial tight junction dysfunction in endotoxemic mice. Am J Physiol 2004; 286:L259–L267.
89. Keay S, Warren JW, Zhang CO, Tu LM, Gordon DA, Whitmore KE. Antiproliferative activity is present in bladder but not renal pelvic urine from interstitial cystitis patients. J Urol 1999; 162:1487–1489.
90. Keay SK, Szekely Z, Conrads TP, et al. An antiproliferative factor from interstitial cystitis patients is a frizzled 8 protein-related sialoglycopeptide. Proc Natl Acad Sci USA 2004; 101:11803–11808.
91. Andersson KE, Yoshida M. Antimuscarinics and the overactive detrusor-which is the main mechanism of action? Eur Urol 2003; 43:1–5.
92. Kim JH, Rivas DA, Shenot PJ, et al. Intravesical resiniferatoxin for refractory detrusor hyperreflexia: a multicenter, blinded, randomized, placebo-controlled trial. J Spinal Cord Med 2003; 26:358–363.
93. Szallasi A, Fowler CJ. After a decade of intravesical vanilloid therapy: still more questions than answers. Lancet Neurol 2002; 1:167–172.
94. Haarala M, Jalava J, Laato M, Kiilholma P, Nurmi M, et al: Absence of bacterial DNA in the bladder of patients with interstitial cystitis. J Urol 1996; 156:1843–1845.
95. Warren JW. Interstitial cystitis as an infectious disease. Urol Clin North Am 1994; 21:31–39.
96. Moldwin RM, Sant GR. Interstitial cystitis: a pathophysiology and treatment update. Clin Obstet Gynecol 2002; 45:259–272.
97. Otsuka M, Yoshioka K. Neurotransmitter functions of mammalian tachykinins. Physiol Rev 1993; 73:229.
98. Lecci A, Maggi CA. Tachykinins as modulators of the micturition reflex in the central and peripheral nervous system. Regul Pept 2001; 101:1.
99. Hohenfellner M, Nunues L, Schmidt RA, et al. Interstitial cystitis: Increased sympathetic innervation and related neuropeptide synthesis. J Urol 1992; 147:587–591.
100. Pang X, Marchand J, Sant GR, et al. Increased number of substance P positive fibers in interstitial cystitis. Br J Urol 1995; 75:744–750.
101. Chen Y, Varghese R, Chiu P, et al. Urinary substance P is elevated in women with interstitial cystitis. J Urol 1999; 161(4):26.
102. Theoharides TC, Sant GR. New agents for the medical treatment of interstitial cystitis. Exp Opin Invest Drugs 2001; 10:521–546.
103. Häbler HJ, Jänig W, Koltzenburg M. Activation of unmyelinated afferent fibres by mechanical stimuli and inflammation of the urinary bladder in the cat. J Physiol (Lond) 1990; 425:545–562.
104. Sengupta JN, Gebhart GF. Mechanosensitive properties of pelvic nerve afferent fibers innervating the urinary bladder of the rat. J Neurophysiol 1994; 72:2420–2430.
105. Woolf CJ, Salter MW. Neuronal plasticity: increasing the gain in pain. Science 2000; 288:1765–1769.
106. Ji RR, Woolf CJ. Neuronal plasticity and signal transduction in nociceptive neurons: implications for the initiation and maintenance of pathological pain. Neurobiol Dis 2001; 8:1–10.
107. Yoshimura N, Seki S, Chancellor MB, de Groat WC, Ueda T. Targeting afferent hyperexcitability for therapy of the painful bladder syndrome. Urology 2002; 59(5 suppl 1):61–67.
108. Janig W. Morrison JFB: Functional properties of spinal visceral afferents supplying abdominal and pelvic organs, with special emphasis on visceral nociception. Prog Brain Res 1986; 67:87–114.
109. de Groat WC. Spinal interneurons and preganglionic neurons in sacral autonomic reflex pathways. In: The Emotional Motor System, Progress in Brain Research edited by Holstege G, Bandler R, Saper C. Amsterdam: Elsevier Science Publishers, 1995.
110. Morgan C, Nadelhaft I, de Groat WC. The distribution of visceral primary afferents from the pelvic nerve to Lissauer's tract and the spinal gray matter and its relationship to the sacral parasympathetic nucleus. J Comp Neurol 1981; 201:415–440.

111. Thor KB, Hisamitsu T, Roppolo JR, Tuttle P, Nagel J, de Groat WC. Selective inhibitory effects of ethylketocyclazocine on reflex pathways to the external urethral sphincter of the cat. J Pharmacol Exp Ther 1989; 248:1018–1025.

112. de Groat WC. Spinal cord projections and neuropeptides in visceral afferent neurons. Prog. Brain Res 1986; 67:165–187.

113. Yoshimura N, de Groat WC. Plasticity of Na^+ channels in afferent neurones innervating rat urinary bladder following spinal cord injury. J Physiol 1997; 503:269–276.

114. de Groat WC, Nadelhaft I, Milne RJ, Booth AM, Morgan C, Thor K. Organization of the sacral parasympathetic reflex pathways to the urinary bladder large intestine. J Auton Nerv Syst 1981; 3:135–160.

115. Mallory B, Steers WD, de Groat WC. Electrophysiological study of micturition reflexes in rats. Am J Physiol 1989; 257:R410–R421.

116. Habler HJ, Janig JW, Koltzenburg M. Myelinated primary afferents of the sacral spinal cord responding to slow filling and distension of the cat urinary bladder. J Physiol 1993; 463:449.

117. McMahon SB, Abel C. A model for the study of visceral pain states: chronic inflammation of the chronic decerebrate rat urinary bladder by irritant chemicals. Pain 1987; 28:109–127.

118. Fall M, Lindstrom S, Mazieres L. A bladder-to-bladder cooling reflex in the cat. J Physiol 1990; 427:281–300.

119. Maggi CA. The dual, sensory and efferent function of the capsaicin-sensitive primary sensory nerves in the bladder and urethra. 1 ed. In: Maggi CA, ed. Vol. 3. The Autonomic Nervous System. Nervous Control of the Urogenital System. London: Harwood Academic Publishers, 1993:383–422.

120. Wen J, Morrison JF. The effects of high urinary potassium concentration on pelvic nerve mechano-receptors and silent afferents from the rat bladder. Adv Exp Med Biol 1995; 385:237–239.

121. Dmietrieva, N, McMahon, SB. Sensitization of visceral afferents by nerve growth factor in the adult rat. Pain 1996; 66:87–97.

122. de Groat WC, Kawatani M., Hisamitsu T, et al. Mechanisms underlying the recovery of urinary bladder function following spinal cord injury. J Auton Nerv Syst 1990; 30:S71–S78.

123. Maggi CA, Conte B. Effect of urethane anesthesia on the micturition reflex in capsaicin–treated rats. J Auton Nerv Syst 1990; 30:247–251.

124. Cheng C.L, Ma C.P, de Groat W.C. The effects of capsaicin on micturition and associated reflexes in the rat. Am J Physiol 1993; 265:R132–R648.

125. Morrison JF. The physiological mechanisms involved in bladder emptying. Scandinavian J Urology & Nephrology 1997; 184:15–18.

126. Yoshimura N, White G, Weight FF, de Groat WC. Patch-clamp recordings from subpopulations of autonomic and afferent neurons identified by axonal tracing techniques. J Auton Nerv Syst 1994; 49:86–92.

127. Yoshimura N, White G, Weight FF, de Groat WC. Different types of Na+ and K+ currents in rat dorsal root ganglion neurons innervating the urinary bladder. J Physiol 1996; 494:1–16.

128. Yoshimura N, de Groat WC. Neural control of lower urinary tract. Int J Urol 1997; 4:101–115.

129. Yoshimura N, Seki S, de Groat WC. Nitric oxide modulates Ca^{2+} channels in dorsal root ganglion neurons innervating rat urinary bladder. J Neurophysiol 2001b; 86:304–311.

130. Yoshimura N, Seki S, Erickson KA, Erickson VL, Chancellor MB, de Groat WC. Histological and electrical properties of rat dorsal root ganglion neurons innervating the lower urinary tract. J Neurosci 2003; 23:4355–4361.

131. Zhong Y, Banning AS, Cockayne DA, Ford AP, Burnstock G, McMahon SB. Bladder and cutaneous sensory neurons of the rat express different functional P2X receptors. Neuroscience 2003; 120: 667–675.

132. Dang K, Bielefeldt K, Gebhart GF. Differential responses of bladder lumbosacral and thoracolumbar dorsal root ganglion neurons to purinergic agonists, protons, and capsaicin. J Neurosci 2005; 25(15):3973–3984.

133. Yoshimura N, de Groat WC. Increased excitability of afferent neurons innervating rat urinary bladder following chronic bladder inflammation. J Neurosci 1999; 19:4644–4653.

134. Waddell PJ, Lawson SN. Electrophysiological properties of subpopulations of rat dorsal root ganglion neurons in vitro. Neuroscience 1990; 36:811–822.

135. Gold MS, Dastmalchi S, Levine JD. Co-expression of nociceptor properties in dorsal root ganglion neurons from the adult rat in vitro. Neuroscience 1996b; 71:265–275.

136. Cardenas CG, Del Mar LP, Cooper BY, Scroggs RS. $5HT_4$ receptors couple positively to tetrodotoxin-insensitive sodium channels in a subpopulation of capsaicin-sensitive rat sensory neurons. J Neurosci 1997; 17:7181–7189.

137. Yoshimura N, Seki S, Novakovic SD, et al. The involvement of the tetradotoxin-resistant sodium channel Nav1.8 (PN3/SNS) in a rat model of visceral pain. J Neurosci 2001a; 21:8690–8696.

138. Akopian AN, Sivilotti L, Wood JN. A tetrodotoxin-resistant voltage-gated sodium channel expressed by sensory neurons. Nature 1996; 379:257–262.

139. Sangameswaran L, Delgado SG, Fish LM, et al. Structure and function of a novel voltage-gated, tetrodotoxin-resistant sodium channel specific to sensory neurons. J Biol Chem 1996; 271:5953–5956.

140. Novakovic SD, Tzoumaka E, McGivern JG, et al. Distribution of the tetrodotoxin-resistant sodium channel PN3 in rat sensory neurons in normal and neuropathic conditions. J Neurosci 1998; 18:2174–2187.

141. Dib-Hajj SD, Tyrrell L, Black JA, Waxman SG. NaN, a novel voltage-gated Na channel, is expressed preferentially in peripheral sensory neurons and down-regulated after axotomy. Proc Natl Acad Sci USA 1998; 95:8963–8968.

142. Tate S, Benn S, Hick C, Trozise D, John V. et al. Two sodium channels contribute to the TTX-R sodium current in primary sensory neurons. Nat Neurosci. 1998 1:653–655.

143. Black JA, Cummins TR, Yoshimura N, de Groat WC, Waxman SG. Tetrodotoxin resistant sodium channels Na(V) 1.8 / SNS and NA(V) 1.9 / NAN in afferent neurons innervating urinary bladder in control and spinal cord injured rats. Brain Res 2003; 963:132–138.

144. Fjell J, Cummins TR, Dib-Hajj SD, Fried K, Black JA, Waxman SG. Differential role of GDNF and NGF in the maintenance of two TTX-resistant sodium channels in adult DRG neurons. Mol Brain Res 1999; 67:267–282.

145. Fjell J, Hjelmstrom P, Hormuzdiar W, et al. Localization of the tetrodotoxin-resistant sodium channel NaN in nociceptors. Neuroreport 2000; 11:199–202.

146. Bennett DL, Dmietrieva N, Priestley JV, Clary D, McMahon SB. trkA, CGRP and IB4 expression in retrogradely labelled cutaneous visceral primary sensory neurones in the rat. Neurosci Lett 1996; 206:33–36.

147. McFarlane S, Cooper E. Kinetics and voltage dependence of A-type currents on neonatal rat sensory neurons. J Neurophysiol 1991; 66:1380–1391.

148. Akins PT, McCleskey EW. Characterization of potassium currents in adult rat sensory neurons and modulation by opioids and cyclic AMP. Neuroscience 1993; 56:759–769.

149. Gold MS, Shuster MJ, Levine JD. Characterization of six voltage-gated K^+ currents in adult rat sensory neurons. J. Neurophysiol 1996a; 75:2629–2646.

150. Catterall WA. Structure and function of neuronal Ca^{2+} channels and their role in neurotransmitter release. Cell Calcium 1998; 24:307–323.

151. Waterman SA. Voltage gated calcium channels in autonomic neuroeffector transmission. Prog Neurobiol 2000; 60:181–210.

152. Sculptoreanu A, de Groat WC. Protein kinase C is involved in neurokinin receptor modulation of N- and L-type Ca^{2+} channels in DRG neurons of the adult rat. J Neurophysiol 2003; 90:21–31.

153. Morrison J, Wen J, Kibble A. Activation of pelvic afferent nerves from the rat bladder during filling. Scand J Urol Nephrol 1999; 201(suppl):73–75.

154. Hoffman PN, Griffin JW, Price DL. Control of axonal caliber by neurofilament transport. J Cell Biol 1984; 99:705–714.

155. Hoffman PN, Cleveland DW, Griffin JW, Landes PW, Cowan, NJ, Price DL. Neurofilament gene expression: a major determinant of axonal caliber. Proc Natl Acad Sci USA 1987; 84:3472–3476.

156. Lawson SN, Perry MJ, Prabhakar E, McCarthy PW. Primary sensory neurones: neurofilament, neuropeptides, and conduction velocity. Brain Res Bull 1993; 30:239–243.

157. Yoshimura N, Erdman SL, Snider MW, de Groat WC. Effects of spinal cord injury on neurofilament immunoreactivity and capsaicin sensitivity in rat dorsal root ganglion neurons innervating the urinary bladder. Neuroscience 1998; 83:633–643.

158. Lundberg JM. Pharmacology of cotransmission in the autonomic nervous system: integrative aspects on amines neuropeptides, adenosine triphosphate, amine acids and nitric oxide. Pharmacol Rev 1996; 48:113–178.

159. Hulsebosch CE, Coggeshall RE. An analysis of the axon populations in the nerves to the viscera in the rat. J Comp Neurol 1982; 211:1–10.

160. Vera PL, Nadelhaft I. Conduction velocity distribution of afferent fibers innervating the rat urinary bladder. Brain Res 1990; 520:83–89.

161. Keast JR, de Groat WC. Segmental distribution and peptide content of primary afferent neurons innervating the urogenital organs and colon of male rats. J Comp Neurol 1992; 319:615–623.

162. Vizzard MA. Up-regulation of pituitary adenylate cyclase-activating polypeptide in urinary bladder pathways after chronic cystitis. J Comp Neurol 2000a; 420:335–348.

163. Steers WD, Mackway AM, Ciambotti J, de Groat WC. Alterations in neural pathways to the urinary bladder of the rat in response to streptozotocin-induced diabetes. J Auton Nerv Syst 1994; 47:83–94.

164. Avelino A, Cruz C, Nagy I, Cruz F. Vanilloid receptor 1 expression in the rat urinary tract. Neuroscience 2002; 109:787–798.

165. Rong W, Spyer KM, Burnstock G. Activation and sensitisation of low and high threshold afferent fibres mediated by P2X receptors in the mouse urinary bladder. J Physiol 2002; 541:591–600.

166. Studeny S, Torabi A, Vizzard MA. P2X2 and P2X3 Receptor expression in postnatal and adult rat urinary bladder and lumbosacral spinal cord. Am J Physiol Regul Integr Comp Physiol 2005 289:R1158–R1160.

167. Nishiguchi J, Hayashi Y, Chancellor MB, et al. Detrusor overactivity induced by intravesical application of adenosine 5'-triphosphate (ATP) under different delivery conditions in rats. Urology 2005 66:1332–1337.

168. Averill, S, McMahon, SB, Clary DO, Reichardt LF, Priestley JV. Immunocytochemical localization of trkA receptors in chemically identified subgroups of adult rat sensory neurons. Eur J Neurosci 1995; 7:1484–1494.
169. Bennett DL, Michael GJ, Ramachandran N, et al. A distinct subgroup of small DRG cells express GDNF receptor components and GDNF is protective for these neurons after nerve injury. J Neurosci 1998; 18:3059–3072.
170. Snider WD, McMahon SB. Tackling pain at the source: new ideas about nociceptors. Neuron 1998; 20:629–632.
171. Kitchener PD, Wilson P, Snow PJ. Selective labelling of primary sensory afferent terminals in lamina II of the dorsal horn by injection of Bandeiraea simplicifolia isolectin B4 into peripheral nerves. Neuroscience 1993; 54:545–551.
172. Vulchanova L, Riedl MS, Shuster SJ, et al. P2X3 is expressed by DRG neurons that terminate in inner lamina II. Eur J Neurosci 1998; 10:3470–3478.
173. Guo A, Vulchanova L, Wang J, Li X, Elde R. Immunocytochemical localization of the vanilloid receptor 1 (VR1): relationship to neuropeptides, the P2X3 purinoceptor and IB4 binding sites. Eur J Neurosci 1999; 11:946–958.
174. Tominaga M, Caterina MJ, Malmberg AB, et al. The cloned capsaicin receptor integrates multiple pain-producing stimuli. Neuron 1998; 21:531–543.
175. Bennett DL, Dmietrieva N, Priestley JV, Clary D, McMahon SB. trkA, CGRP and IB4 expression in retrogradely labelled cutaneous visceral primary sensory neurones in the rat. Neurosci Lett 1996; 206:33–36.
176. Nishiguchi J, Sasaki K, Seki S, et al. Effects of isolectin B4-conjugated saporin, a targeting cytotoxin, on bladder overactivity induced by bladder irritation. Eur J Neurosci 2004; 20:474–482.
177. Seki S, Erickson KA, Seki M, et al. Elimination of rat spinal neurons expressing neurokinin 1 receptors reduces bladder overactivity and spinal c-fos expression induced by bladder irritation. Am J Physiol Renal Physiol 2005; 288:F466–F473.
178. Johansson SL, Ogawa K, Fall M. The pathology of interstitial cystitis. In: Sant GR, ed. Interstitial Cystitis. Philadelphia: Lippincott-Raven, 1997:143–151.
179. Theoharides TC, Kempuraj D, Sant GR. Mast cell involvement in interstitial cystitis: a review of human and experimental evidence. Urology 2001; 57(suppl 6A):47–55.
180. Dmitrieva N, Shelton D, Rice ASC, et al. The role of nerve growth factor in a model of visceral inflammation. Neuroscience 1997; 78:449–459.
181. England S, Bevan S, Docherty RJ. PGE2 modulates the tetrodotoxin-resistant sodium current in neonatal rat dorsal root ganglion neurones via the cyclic AMP–protein kinase A cascade. J Physiol 1996; 495:429–440.
182. Gold MS, Reichling DB, Shuster MJ, et al. Hyperalgesic agents increase a tetrodotoxin-resistant Na^+ current in nociceptors. Proc Natl Acad Sci U S A 1996; 93:1108–1112.
183. Cox PJ. Cyclophosphamide cystitis—identification of acrolein as the causative agent. Biochem Pharmacol 1979; 28:2045–2049.
184. Lantéri-Minet M, Bon K, de Pommery J, et al. Cyclophosphamide cystitis as a model of visceral pain in rats: model elaboration and spinal structures involved as revealed by the expression of c-Fos and Krox-24 proteins. Exp Brain Res 1995; 105:220–232.
185. Dang K, Bielefeldt K, Gebhart GF. Gastric ulcers reduce A-type potassium currents in rat gastric sensory ganglion neurons. Am J Physiol Gastrointest Liver Physiol 2004; 286:G573–G579.
186. Stewart T, Beyak MJ, Vanner S. Ileitis modulates potassium and sodium currents in guinea pig dorsal root ganglia sensory neurons. J Physiol 2003; 552:797–807.
187. Sculptoreanu A, de Groat WC, Buffington CA, Birder LA. Abnormal excitability in capsaicin-responsive DRG neurons from cats with feline interstitial cystitis. Exp Neurol 2005a; 193:437–443.
188. Lazzeri M, Beneforti P, Benaim G, Maggi CA, Lecci A, Turini D. Intravesical capsaicin for treatment of severe bladder pain: a randomized placebo controlled study. J Urol 1996; 156:947–952.
189. Lazzeri M, Beneforti P, Spinelli M, Zanollo A, Barbagli G, Turini D. Intravesical resiniferatoxin for the treatment of hypersensitive disorder: a randomized placebo controlled study. J Urol 2000; 164:676–679.
190. Payne CK, Mosbaugh PG, Forrest JB, et al. ICOS RTX Study Group (Resiniferatoxin Treatment for Interstitial Cystitis). Intravesical resiniferatoxin for the treatment of interstitial cystitis: a randomized, double-blind, placebo controlled trial. J Urol 2005; 173(5):1590–1594.
191. Sculptoreanu A, de Groat WC, Buffington CA, Birder LA. Protein kinase C contributes to abnormal capsaicin responses in DRG neurons from cats with feline interstitial cystitis. Neurosci Lett 2005b; 381:42–46.
192. Dinis P, Charrua A, Avelino A, et al. Anandamide-evoked activation of vanilloid receptor 1 contributes to the development of bladder hyperreflexia and nociceptive transmission to spinal dorsal horn neurons in cystitis. J Neurosci 2004; 24:11253–11263.
193. Sugaya K, Nishijima S, Yamada T, Miyazato M, Hatano T, Ogawa Y. Molecular analysis of adrenergic receptor genes and interleukin-4/interleukin-4 receptor genes in patients with interstitial cystitis. J Urol 2002; 168(6):2668–2671.
194. Vizzard MA, Erdman SL, de Groat WC. Increased expression of neuronal nitric oxide synthase in bladder afferent pathways following chronic bladder irritation. J Comp Neurol 1996; 370:191–202.

195. Vizzard MA, Boyle MM. Increased expression of growth-associated protein (GAP-43) in lower urinary tract pathways following cyclophosphamide (CYP)-induced cystitis. Brain Res 1999; 844:174–187.
196. Vizzard MA. Alterations in neuropeptide expression in lumbosacral bladder pathways following chronic cystitis. J Chem Neuroanat 2001; 21:125–138.
197. Dattilio A, Vizzard MA. Up-regulation of protease activated receptors in bladder after cyclophosphamide induced cystitis and colocalization with capsaicin receptor (VR1) in bladder nerve fibers. J Urol 2005; 173(2):635–639.
198. Hu VY, Malley S, Dattilio A, Folsom JB, Zvara P, Vizzard MA. COX-2 and prostanoid expression in micturition pathways after cyclophosphamide-induced cystitis in the rat. Am J Physiol Regul Integr Comp Physiol 2003; 284:R574–R585.
199. Urban MO, Gebhart GF. Supraspinal contributions to hyperalgesia. Proc Natl Acad Sci U S A 1999; 96:7687–7692.
200. Cruz CD, Avelino A, McMahon SB, Cruz F. Increased spinal cord phosphorylation of extracellular signal-regulated kinases mediates micturition overactivity in rats with chronic bladder inflammation. Eur J Neurosci 2005; 21(3):773–781.
201. Vizzard MA. Alterations in spinal cord Fos protein expression induced by bladder stimulation following cystitis. Am J Physiol Regul Integr Comp Physiol 2000b; 278:R1027–R1039.
202. Yoshimura N. Bladder afferent pathway and spinal cord injury: possible mechanisms inducing hyperreflexia of the urinary bladder. Prog Neurobiol 1999; 57:583–606.
203. Vizzard MA. Changes in urinary bladder neurotrophic factor mRNA and NGF protein following urinary bladder dysfunction. Exp Neurol 2000c; 161:273–284.
204. Steers WD, Kolbeck S, Creedon D, Tuttle JB. Nerve growth factor in the urinary bladder of the adult regulates neuronal form and function. J Clin Invest 1991; 88:1709–1715.
205. Steers WD, Creedon DJ, Tuttle JB. Immunity to nerve growth factor prevents afferent plasticity following urinary bladder hypertrophy. J Urol 1996; 155:379–385.
206. Steers WD, Tuttle JB. Neurogenic inflammation and nerve growth factor: possible roles in interstitial cystitis. In: Sant GR, ed. Interstitial cystitis. Philadelphia: Lippincott-Raven, 1997:67–75.
207. Nilsson G, Forsberg-Nilsson, Xiang Z, et al. Human mast cells express functional TrkA and are a source of nerve growth factor. Eur J Immunol 1997; 27:2295–2930.
208. Okragly AJ, Niles AL, Saban R, et al. Elevated tryptase, nerve growth factor, neurotrophin-3 and glial cell line-derived neurotrophic factor levels in the urine of interstitial cystitis and bladder cancer patients. J Urol 1999; 161:438–441.
209. Lowe EM, Anand P, Terenghi G, Williams-Chestnut RE, Sinicropi DV, Osborne JL. Increased nerve growth factor levels in the urinary bladder of women with idiopathic sensory urgency and interstitial cystitis. Br J Urol 1997; 79:572–577.
210. Qiao LY, Vizzard MA. Cystitis-induced upregulation of tyrosine kinase (TrkA, TrkB) receptor expression and phosphorylation in rat micturition pathways. J Comp Neurol 2002; 454:200–211.
211. Vizzard, 2000.
212. Qiao LY, Vizzard MA. Up-regulation of phosphorylated CREB but not c-Jun in bladder afferent neurons in dorsal root ganglia after cystitis. J Comp Neurol 2004; 469:262–274.
213. Chuang YC, Fraser MO, Yu Y, Chancellor MB, de Groat WC, Yoshimura N. The role of bladder afferent pathways in bladder hyperactivity induced by the intravesical administration of nerve growth factor. J Urol 2001; 165:975–979.
214. Seki S, Sasaki K, Igawa Y, et al. Detrusor overactivity induced by increased levels of nerve growth factor in bladder afferent pathways in rats. Neurourology and Urodynamics 2003; 22:375–377.
215. Lamb K, Gebhart GF, Bielefeldt K. Increased nerve growth factor expression triggers bladder overactivity. J Pain 2004; 5:150–156.
216. Jaggar SI, Scott HC, Rice AS. Inflammation of the rat urinary bladder is associated with a referred thermal hyperalgesia which is nerve growth factor dependent. Br J Anaesth 1999; 83:442–448.
217. Hu VY, Zvara P, Dattilio A, et al. Decrease in bladder overactivity with REN1820 in rats with cyclophosphamide induced cystitis. J Urol 2005; 173:1016–1021.
218. Ueda T, Tamaki M, Ogawa O, Yoshimura N. Over expression of platelet-derived endothelial cell growth factor/thymidine phosphorylase in patients with interstitial cystitis and bladder carcinoma. J Urol 2002; 167:347–351.
219. Jackson RL, Busch SJ, Cardin AD. Glycosaminoglycans: molecular properties protein interactions role in physiological processes. Physiol Rev 1991; 71:481.
220. Bennett KL, Jackson DG, Simon JC, Tanczos E, Peach R, Modrell B, et al. CD44 isoforms containing exon V3 are responsible for the presentation of heparin-binding growth factor. J Cell Biol 1995; 128:687.
221. Tamaki M, Saito R, Ogawa O, Yoshimura N, Ueda T. Possible mechanisms inducing glomerulations in interstitial cystitis: relationship between endoscopic findings and expression of angiogenic growth factors. J Urol 2004; 172:945–948.
222. van de Merwe JP, Yamada T, Sakamoto Y. Systemic aspects of interstitial cystitis, immunology and linkage with autoimmune disorders. Int J Urol 2003; 10(suppl):S35–S38.

223. Ueda T, Tamaki M, Ogawa O, Yamauchi T, Yoshimura N. Improvement of interstitial cystitis symptoms and problems that developed during treatment with oral IPD-1151T. J Urol 2000; 164:1917–1920.

224. Moran PA, Dwyer PL, Carey MP, Maher CF, Radford NJ. Oral methotexate in the management of refractory interstitial cystitis. Aust N Z Obstet 1999; 39:468–471.

225. Silk MR. Bladder antibodies in interstitial cystitis. J Urol 1970; 103:307–309.

226. Jokinen E, Alfthan S, Oravisto K. Antitissue autoantibodies in interstitial cystitis. Clin Exp Immunol 1972; 11:333–339.

227. Anderson JB, Parivar F, Lee G, et al. The enigma of interstitial cystitis- An autoimmune disease? Br J Urol 1989; 63:58–63.

228. Warren JW, Jackson TL, Langenberg P, Meyers DJ, Xu J. Prevalence of interstitial cystitis in first-degree relatives of patients with interstitial cystitis. Urology 12004; 63:17–21.

229. Weissman MM, Gross R, Fyer A, Heiman GA, et al. Interstitial cystitis and panic disorder: a potential genetic syndrome. Arch Gen Psychiatry. 2004; 61(3):273–279.

230. Malley SE, Vizzard MA. Changes in urinary bladder cytokine mRNA and protein after cyclophosphamide-induced cystitis. Physiol Genomics 2002; 9:5–13.

Index

Milton Keynes UK
Ingram Content Group UK Ltd.
UKHW050457071024
449327UK00015B/418

9 780367 389963